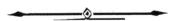

ISBN 978-0-428-99204-0
PIBN 10814157

THE

BOSTON MEDICAL AND SURGICAL JOURNAL.

| Vol. XLVIII. | Wednesday, February 2, 1853. | No. 1. |

DENGUE—YELLOW FEVER, &c.

To the Editor of the Boston Medical and Surgical Journal.

Dear Sir,—We have been visited the past autumn with an ordinary, or rather an extraordinary, endemic fever, somewhat severe withal, but of short duration. It has given rise to considerable speculation among the faculty, as is but too common in such cases, and a great difference of opinion exists as to its nature, and what distinctive appellation is most appropriate to, and characteristic of, the disease. In short, we have had the *dandy yellow fever !*

A similar disease prevailed at Natchez, Miss., in 1848, and in Mobile and other cities in 1850. It has been noticed in different towns and villages of the South, and West Indies, in years past, and described under the fanciful appellations of *dengue, bouquet,* or *dandy fever*, an insignificant and outlandish name of unclassical and uncertain origin.

I witnessed the same at Baton Rouge in 1850, I am sure, and prescribed for a great number of cases, all of which terminated favorably—and, with here and there an exception, without any characteristic symptoms of yellow fever. I described it in my letter to you of Dec., 1850, and gave my mode of treatment, which was simple enough, and the same adopted by myself and others this season as most appropriate to the prevailing disease.

It was to all intents and purposes the dengue, whose name is legion, and, if you please, an illegitimate offspring of yellow fever, partaking now and then of some of its parent features, and, it may be, occasionally terminating in *vomito prieto*, or black vomit.

Season.—Our summer had been unusually dry and pleasant, and though there was more than an ordinary share of disease upon the plantations in the adjoining parishes, in the early part of the season, the city and villages around were particularly healthy. A few cases of ordinary febrile disease were noticed to prevail here and in the neighborhood, in the latter part of the summer, as forerunners of the epidemic, and which seemed to indicate that something severer and more general was to follow. We had no rain of consequence during the summer, and the disease, which commenced about the last of August, continued till the first and only hard rain storm, which fell late in October.

Symptoms.—The invasion, as in the Natchez epidemic—so fully de-

1

scribed by Dr. Stone, in the New Orleans Medical and Surgical Journal, under the caption of Yellow Fever, and to which I would direct the attention of your numerous readers, for some very peculiar features of southern epidemics—was rather sudden, and without much if any previous indisposition. Persons in good health would be abruptly seized, and in the course of a few hours prostrate, and completely delirious with fever, and racked with pain. Sometimes there would precede a slight chill, but pains in the head, eyeballs, back and loins, and always excruciating, were the chief and characteristic symptoms of the disease at the onset, succeeded by cramps in the extremities—calves of the legs especially—with general debility and *malaise*, and sometimes, not always, distress at the epigastrium, together with nausea and vomiting. The bowels were usually constipated. There was a constant disposition, in most cases, to throw the arms above the head, noticed by writers as a common symptom in yellow fever. There was soreness of the throat often, and oppression within the chest, with difficult breathing, and a hawking of mucus from the throat and bronchial tubes, which " was not an unfavorable symptom, though disagreeable to the patient," and continued for some days after recovery—as did the pain in the back and loins, often intermittent, and of long duration in convalescence, and the last to disappear, even when the patient was otherwise well, or apparently free from the disease.

The tongue, pulse, skin, breath, urine, &c., manifested the same indications as mentioned by Dr. Stone, and the consecutive fever, where the disease was prolonged beyond the fifth or sixth day, assumed often a periodical character, intermittent, remittent, &c., requiring full doses of quinine and morphine to complete the cure.

The symptoms continued from 12 to 36 and 48 hours, when an erythematous eruption was sometimes developed, but by no means so general or common as I have witnessed in past epidemics, when all the various forms of *cutanei* were fully and beautifully represented, from the " intense blush of scarlatina to the mottled appearance of roseola, and the actual spots of ephelis itself."

Hemorrhages from the mouth, bowels, &c., were occasionally noticed, while the minor symptoms in the various types of this manifest dengue, as the disease progressed, were as variable and erratic as the disease itself.

Cases.—Two of our physicians in active practice were among the earliest cases, each of them being attacked on the same day, about the last week in September, and considerably in advance of the period when the disease became general. They were comparatively mild, and had no other cases succeeded would have passed off without especial notice.

Case III.—Soon after the above, my attention was particularly directed to the case of a young Parisian, partially acclimated, who was attacked, after much exposure, with violent fever, accompanied with great oppression of breathing, with frequent, deep and prolonged sighing, and partial coma and delirium—without manifest pain or bodily suffering—which continued some 48 hours or longer, when a slight remission occurred, with partial relief to the oppressed organs, but with constant " hawking and spitting," and considerable nausea without vomiting, until towards the close of the fifth day, when the symptoms became aggravated, and he died with unmistakable *black vomit*, but with few if any of the primary and well-marked signs of yellow fever, or the usual phenomena attending the commencement or early periods of this disease.

IV.—Another case, a young creole of the city, who had been exposed to the same general and exciting causes, occurred about the same time in the same family. His attack was light, and the symptoms at first of the mildest character. He was convalescent on the fourth or fifth day, but from fatigue, and anxiety at the sudden death of his associate, relapsed, and was ill with aggravated symptoms for a week or ten days longer. The treatment in this case was entirely *expectant,* and with repose and regimen, chiefly, he recovered, without any of the peculiarities or dangers incident to yellow fever.

V.—A gentleman, who has been a resident here for many years, but had just returned with his family from a visit to Kentucky, was attacked the week following in the most violent maner with high fever and delirium, and all the characteristic pains of the head, back and limbs, followed by vomiting and profuse perspiration, which continued for several hours, to the entire relief of all the morbid symptoms, and restoration to health, with partial medication only, in the course of three or four days.

VI.—A young miss, daughter of the above, who had just recovered from a well-marked intermittent of some days' continuance, and able to attend school, was seized on the first day abroad, and passed through the prevailing epidemic as regularly, and almost as mildly, as she had done in the previous disease.

VII. and VIII.—Dr. R. and his lady were seized about the same period, on the same day, the former, being a creole of the country, very lightly; the latter more violently, and with well-marked symptoms of mild yellow fever. Her case was somewhat critical, but she was restored by the judicious, though simple treatment pursued by her physician, which was uniformly found to be most suited to the disease; yet her convalescence, from personal idiosyncrasy and other circumstances, was tedious and prolonged beyond the usual period of recovery for many days.

IX.—Mrs. F. was another subject, and adds to the number of the acclimated persons who had an attack in a mild form, and who recovered without apprehension of danger, within the usual limits of the disease.

X.—Mrs. D., the wife of the Episcopal clergyman of this town, just returned from a summer trip to New York, was seized soon after her arrival with the prevailing disorder, and died at the end of the sixth day with *vomito prieto,* as reported by her physician.

XI.—I was attacked with the prevailing disease early in October, after considerable fatigue and loss of rest. At first I supposed it to be an attack of the gout, and that an old enemy, whose visits are rarely those of angels' visits, had seized me with unusual violence, and it was hard to persuade myself, even on the second or third day, that I was a subject of dengue, and suffering all the " pains and penalties " of this autumnal disease. I am sure 1 had the same affection, somewhat more lightly it is true, at Baton Rouge in 1850, and what is more singular, after re-covery and being abroad again a full week, attending to my professional duties, I had a relapse, and passed through the same sufferings again, only in a more severe and aggravated form. The fever and pains con-tinued as long and obstinate as before, and called for more active remedies, and more cautious management to prevent its assuming a graver character, and passing into the " sere and yellow " · *leave*—ex-cuse an execrable pun—so often the consequence, not of dengue, but of epidemic yellow fever.

What is still more remarkable in my case, these were the first and only forms of fever ·I have experienced during my residence in the South, a period of more than twenty years.

XII., XIII. and XIV.—Three of my family also passed through the disease, two of them natives of the South, and one acclimated by an attack of dengue two years since. The symptoms in each case were similar, varying but little from those of the epidemic of 1850. The treatment was the same. One of the above cases, however, being con-stitutionally predisposed to erysipelas, exhibited marked signs of this dis-ease, thus favoring the pathology of Dr. Waring, who says that dengue assimilates itself to three different diseases of gastro-enteritic foundation, viz,, gout, erysipelas and yellow fever. In other words, says he, gout may be considered dengue without eruption, erysipelas a dengue without affection of the joints, and yellow fever a dengue concentrated upon the bowels, &c.

There were several other cases, presenting the same general character and symptoms, which came under my notice, but so mild and uniform in their course and treatment that I need not trouble you with details.

Results.—As near as I can learn, there were about forty cases of the disease, and six or eight deaths. I lost but the first case, and this was the only one I saw with *vomito*, though there were several well-authen-ticated cases thus terminating during the prevalence of the disease.

Pathology.—The best descriptions of dengue we have seen are those published by Drs. Waring and Campbell of Georgia, and Drs. Dickson and Wragg of Charleston, S. C., in the southern medical journals; and Dr. Osgood of Havana, and Dr. Dumaresque of New Orleans, in the first volume of this Journal. Besides these there are several valuable papers upon dengue as it appeared in the West Indies in 1827-8, to be found in the London and Edinburgh Medical Journals. Practitioners of the present day will lack no guides to the full comprehension and knowledge of this singular and multiform disease, which has thus far, we believe, been limited chiefly, if not altogether, to the South.

Dr. Dickson, of Charleston, regards dengue as a *contagious eruptive disease* ; while Dr. Waring, of Savannah, considers it a *gastro-enterite*. While one maintains it to be an *eruptive rheumatic fever*, another believes it to be altogether *neuralgic*. One looks upon it as the *offspring of yel-low fever*, and another confidently pronounces it a mild *scarlatina*, modi-fied by tropical climates, &c.

This discrepancy of opinion no doubt results from the fact that den-gue is a disease of tropical climates, being thus far limited to yellow fever districts, and produced by the same causes which give rise to our autumnal fevers, running its course sometimes distinctly, at others being blended with every form and variety of fever, from the mildest remittent to the highest grade of yellow fever.

Dengue can hardly be regarded as a disease *sui generis*, but as a variety of miasmatic fever, whose peculiar characteristics are developed and influenced by climate, locality and other causes—and we can be the more readily reconciled to this opinion, if we keep in view the important fact that every symptom known to attach itself to any fever, may be and often is met with in the several forms of this disease.

I may add, that this disease bears a general resemblance to the epidemic *cerebro-spinal meningitis* observed at Val de Grace, " which was to a certain extent complicated with the influenza of 1847, and the cholera of 1849," reported by Dr. Levy in the Gazette Medicale de Paris. The precursory symptoms and the general character of the disease are similar, and *mutatis mutandis* they might well pass for the same disease. The complications in the epidemic meningitis, it is true, were more numerous and more distinctly marked, and the mortality much greater.

Treatment.—No very active treatment was demanded in this disease. A free use of warm diluents, as lemonade, boneset, &c., pediluvia, laxatives or enemata, morphia and quinine, was nearly all that was required. The disease usually terminated favorably in five or six days.

Conclusions.—1st. This endemic fever is identical with the dengue which has prevailed in the South, at different periods, for years past—in 1848 at Natchez, and in 1850 at Charleston, Mobile, Baton Rouge and New Orleans.

2d. It has been developed under the miasmatic influence which gives rise to periodic fevers.

3d. It has prevailed concurrently with yellow fever, but is distinct in its symptoms, course, lesions and mortality.

4th. It is endemic, and in its uncomplicated form may be classed with the neuralgic affections.

5th. Its true etiology is not well understood, and the contagious character of the disease so confidently insisted upon by some medical writers, is by no means conclusively established.

6th. It is limited, with few exceptions, to a single paroxysm, and may generally be regarded as a self-curing disease.

7th. It is definite in duration, and attacks all indiscriminately, young and old of both sexes, whether acclimated or not. Creoles of the place, and those who had been residents here for forty years, were equally subject to its attack, though in its mildest form. With the unacclimated it sometimes proved fatal.

8th. It has repeated its attack upon the same person, and twice in the same season.

9th. A tedious and protracted convalescence is quite a uniform characteristic of this disease.

10th. Active treatment was seldom required, and in its uncomplicated condition it was rarely fatal.

I find I was mistaken in my late communication to you in saying we seldom have, now-a-days, any of the old-fashioned fevers running their course *according to the books*, for I have since discovered that Rush has described this very form of disease under the head of " bilious remittent," well known to the common people as the *break-bone fever*, which prevailed in Philadelphia in the summer and autumn of 1780 ; and the curious inquirer will there find a full daguerreotype of all the prominent symptoms of this endemic disease ; and, what is more remarkable, we have stumbled upon his very treatment without knowing, or recollecting, that he could do anything in such cases, but bleed and give calomel and jalap. The truth is, after all, that Rush is the magnus Apollo of our profession. He is to medicine what Shakspeare and Milton are to the historic, dramatic and religious world. There is little to be found elsewhere which is not preshadowed in their immortal works ; thus confirming the quaint sentiment of the quaint old Chaucer :—

> " Out of the old fieldes as men saith,
> Cometh al this new corne from yere to yere,
> And out of old bookes, in good faith,
> Cometh al this new science that men lere."

Truly yours, &c.,   Fred. B. Page, M.D.
Ascension, La., December, 1852.

M. RICORD'S LETTERS UPON SYPHILIS.

Addressed to the Editor of L'Union Medicale—Translated from the French by D. D. Slade, M.D., Boston, and communicated for the Boston Medical and Surgical Journal.

SIXTEENTH LETTER.

My Dear Friend,—Most decidedly *we cannot please everybody ;* and this old adage, so ingeniously presented by La Fontaine, is particularly applicable when medical science is concerned. The monkeys have brought me ill luck ; I have not satisfied the experimenters, who have pretended to have inoculated them with syphilis, and I have much less satisfied those who do not believe in this pretended inoculation. However, see how mistaken I am, since I had the naïveté to think that from these two parties I merited some praise. You will see what was my error.

The young Bavarian colleague who has just inoculated his name with syphilis, has reproached us, myself and others, *of having been hasty in our conclusions upon the non-transmissibility of syphilis to animals.* However, if I count correctly, more than *twenty-four hours* have passed by since Hunter, and the time has been sufficiently long for me to reflect, and that, too, without too much precipitation.

On the other hand, the colleagues whom I respect, and who ordinarily entertain the same ideas with me, have reproached me in almost the same way. They have discovered that I have been a little hasty with the monkeys ; they believe—they tell me—that I have yielded to apish tricks. My learned and able colleague of the Hospital du Midi, M. Puche, is yet in a state of perfect incredulity relative to the transmissibility of the syphilis to animals, nor does M. Cullerier, that persevering experimenter, believe the reality of experiments which make so much noise.

What I recounted to you in my last letter, I have seen with my own eyes ; I have also told you the attenuating circumstances, which it is impossible to put to silence, however satisfied of the convictions and good faith of M. Auzias Turenne. But after having told you of this fact of the inoculation of the virulent pus from man to the monkey, all that I know of the matter, *I am astonished at the sudden and premature conclusions which our German colleague draws from the fact ;* and to speak frankly, he who exacts in others so much maturity of reasoning and reflection, has not himself offered the example. After all, the promptitude of his conclusions can be excused on the ground of the very inoculations to which he has courageously submitted himself, and which he would have been very glad not to have made uselessly.

Our German colleague makes much of this proposition : " *One single positive experiment has more value than an innumerable quantity of negative results.*" Without doubt ; but upon one condition, which is that this experiment should be positive, that it should be incontestable, and that it should present all the guarantees of certainty and exactitude, and, more than this, *that it can be repeated ;* without all this, it is worth nothing. The Academy of Science knows the value of this proposition constantly brought forward, and by which, periodically, rash and new experimenters pretend to overthrow the laws of physics. This argument has served for all human deceptions. What says the magnetologist who pretends to transport the sense of sight to the nape of the neck or to the epigastrium ? Precisely what our German colleague says —viz: one single positive experiment, &c. What says the homœopathist, who maintains that an atom of *bryonia* diluted in the immensity of the waters of the ocean can cure pneumonia ? Precisely the same thing as our German colleague.

In the physical and natural sciences, *one isolated fact is worth nothing if it is not susceptible of being repeated.* Here is what all those think who know what the philosophy of science is. Otherwise this would be the most dangerous and the most perfidious stumbling block to progress, if laborious and patient observation did not come in to prove that it was but a sophism, an error, and often only a boast. My honorable colleague and friend, M. Cullerier, ought himself to tell you what he thinks of the experiments of M. Auzias. As to myself, I have established this, that the virulent pus has been transported from man to the monkey, and from the latter it has been inoculated upon man ; nothing more, nothing less. Here is the plain fact ; afterwards comes its interpretation.

I said to you in my last letter, " *Might not the monkey have served herein only as a soil for transplantation ?*" I believe so, for here is what happens—the puncture of the inoculation which has been made upon the monkey, scarcely irritated, scarcely inflamed, and suppurating very little, although soaked in the virulent pus after it has been made, has a constant tendency to heal up, and this happens with astonishing rapidity. We do not see in the inoculation made upon the monkey that ulcerating, continued, increasing progress which is the character of the chancre upon man, especially the chancre which does not become indurated ; we do not find even that period of specific *statu quo*, so tenacious, so long, which nature keeps up in man, and which he has ordinarily so much difficulty to destroy.   There is never in the monkey the least phagedenic tendency ; nothing which resembles the specific induration in its commencement and in its consequences.   A puncture, scarcely any suppuration, a crust, and a cure !   Herein are the effects of inoculation upon the monkey—and all this takes place almost as quick as one of his gestures.   We see that it is for the chancre a refractory and foreign soil ; the virulent seed is there exotic ; in vain we take much precaution to sow it well, water it, to place it in a green-house, or under a bell ; it dies before having thrown out any roots, and consequently without having given forth any fruits.

M. Auzias explains all this by the great vitality of their circulation ; it would be more easy to explain it by their nature so averse to syphilitic virus, upon which I congratulate them.   We can even believe that in the pustule which is produced with so much difficulty, the virulent pus serves there only as an issue-pea which irritates, causes suppuration, but is not combined with the tissues ; it is mixed with the pus which is produced, that is all.   It would be necessary, in fact, to be able to conclude definitely upon any other result, that the pustules produced upon the monkey were broken, that the ulcerated surfaces were frequently cleansed, in order that we should not suppose that there remained some pus of the chancre mixed up, and that we inoculated afterwards the suppuration furnished by these surfaces.   We know what happens in man.   We may in vain cleanse the surface of the chancres, apply to them even medicated substances ; still the virulent secretion continues to be produced.   As long as we shall not have carried out this experimental programme, the sole experiment which has been made will be insufficient to destroy all which has been established by serious men upon numerous and perfectly-established facts.   The sole acquisition made to science, and which I am perfectly ready to recognize, is, that we can place and preserve the virulent pus upon the monkey, and afterwards make use of it to inoculate man, as one transplants a plant from one soil to another.   That is all that I have seen and established, and the only deduction which I can draw from it.

Until a new order of things, then, our German colleague would be in the same condition as regards his inoculation, as if it had been made with virulent pus preserved in tubes or between two layers of glass.

This induces me to tell you what the pus inoculated upon man produces, the course which inoculation follows, and what it teaches as regards the pathology of chancre.   But you inform me that my honorable colleague and friend, M. Cullerier, asks of you permission to speak. I yield to him with pleasure ; we shall all gain from it.

Yours, &c.,

RICORD.

JULY 24, 1850.

To M. Amédée Latour, Editor of l'Union Medicale.

MUCH ESTEEMED COLLEAGUE,—There has been no talk lately, in the special hospitals, but of syphilitic inoculations made from man to the monkey—inoculations which have been pursued with so much ardor by our esteemed colleague, Dr. Auzias Turenne. This question is full of interest to me ; for although certain persons do not appear to hold it of much account, everybody cannot have forgotten the numerous experiments which I made upon this subject a few years since. Satisfied with what those experiments had taught me, I was not a little astonished at the new results announced, when the last letter of M. Ricord came to give them a great value, and to furnish to experimenters a powerful lever to upset all that I have advanced. Permit me, then, to tell you my thoughts upon the facts of M. Auzias. At the time of the first exhibition, which was made in 1845, at the Academies of Science and of Medicine, as also before the Society of Surgery, of a monkey presenting upon the face the results of the inoculation of the chancrous pus taken from man, it was generally granted that these ulcerations presented all the appearance of veritable primitive chancres ; borders cut perpendicularly, greyish bottom, induration at the base ; nothing, in fact, was wanting, and already they ridiculed the experiments of Hunter, of Turnbull, of my father, of M. Ricord, and still of others. I was the only one that was reserved as to the nature of these ulcerations, remembering that I had produced identically similar ones upon certain patients, without an atom of virulence ; and I immediately commenced a series of experiments.

I made them upon different kinds of animals, and especially upon the monkey. I inoculated either by a superficial or profound puncture, by incision, or by a solution of continuity more or less extensive. I constantly failed. M. Auzias attributed my ill success to my manner of manipulating ; he told me that I went the wrong way to work. I begged him to operate himself before my eyes, but established this condition, that he should not continually trouble the wounds he should make. He operated as I did, by puncture, incision, and by excision. Like myself he suffered the virulent pus to macerate for whole days in these solutions of continuity. Two or three times he believed he had obtained a fortunate result, because a little inflammation was manifested ; and in some of the punctures, a raising up of the epidermis, sometimes a purulent secretion ; but soon the negative result was evident to all the world.

How do they now explain the results obtained ? They say that one of the first conditions for success, is to prevent the animal from licking itself, because the action of the tongue might cleanse the wound of the inoculation. But M. Auzias does not remember that in all my experiments this precaution was taken. Let him please to read again my work, which is inserted in the first volume of the *Mémoires de la Societé de Chirurgie,* and he will see that at each instant it is said that the animal was prevented from rubbing itself, and that the wound was made in such a way that the animal could not lick itself. When I gave myself up to experimentation, I did it with as much conscience as any one, and I took all the precautions possible.

At the time when I made my researches, M. Auzias pretended that the skin of animals was endowed with much less irritability than that of man, and that in order to obtain a positive result it was necessary to have a certain amount of irritation in the part where the virus had been deposited ; and heaven knows that there was no lack of irritating the points which had been inoculated both by puncture and by abrasion. This in my eyes explained very well both the delay in the cicatrization, and the appearance of the ulceration kept up by a mechanical cause. There is now no longer a question of the obtuse sensibility of the skin of the monkey ; it is even pretended that it has become much more impressible to the virulence, than the human skin ; but it is said that what caused the experiments to fail is the great plasticity of the blood in animals, which permits it to interpose itself between the bleeding part and the virulent matter ; and in order to succeed, it is advised to constantly soak the puncture of the inoculation with the pus.

Well—what then is done? What has M. Auzias done ? He has caused a solution of continuity which became inflamed, which produced pus perfectly innocent at first, but which afterwards, and that promptly, became virulent by its mixing with the pus with which the wound was constantly covered, or with that which, placed under the epidermis, or in the cellular sub-cutaneous tissue, acted like a thorn and determined in it a phlegmonous inflammation, not as specific pus, but as a foreign body. One can in this way produce successively a certain number of virulent pustules.

What became of the ulcerations upon the monkey ? M. Ricord's letter does not say ; it leaves us to suppose that they dried up and disappeared ; so that there was only, as M. Ricord elsewhere appears disposed to admit, a simple depot of virulent matter upon the animal, which served as a vehicle between the patient of the Hospital du Midi and the courageous German colleague who submitted himself to the experiment. In a word, it is still the history of mediate contagion. The virulent pus, in place of being put upon an inert body, as in the experiments of M. Ricord, and as in some of my own, upon the mediate inoculation, the virulent pus, I say, has been placed and kept warm in the skin, or under the skin, of the monkey.

I have seen only a part of the results obtained by M. Auzias. This was the ulcerated pustules which M. Robert de Welz carried upon his arm, and which he had the goodness to show me one morning at the Hospital de Lourcine. It would have been perhaps in good taste as regards science, if M. Auzias had made me participate in all the stages of the experiment, for he well knew my former labors, in which he took an active part. Does he not know, also, that in all this I am only stimulated by the interests of science, and that I profess the highest esteem for his character and for his talent. If he makes other attempts, I shall be most happy to follow them ; but in spite of what has just passed, I declare in advance, that for me there will be no true inoculation of primitive syphilis from man to the monkey, *until a suppurating ulceration shall be brought about, which can be washed at different times, in order to free it completely of the pus which shall have produced it, and which can be transferred afterwards either to the monkey itself or to man.* Until this, it will not be possible for me to see anything but a depot, with or without production of suppurative inflammation.

This is not an exaggerated scepticism ; it is a strictness of experimentation which appears to me indispensable, and which a *clinicien* of the character of my excellent colleague and friend, M. Ricord, who has accustomed us to so much accuracy in the observation of facts, and to so much logic in their deduction, will not be surprised to see me require.

Yours, &c., CULLERIER.

BIOGRAPHICAL SKETCH OF CALVIN THOMAS, M.D.

BY JOHN O. GREEN, M.D., LOWELL, MASS.

[Communicated for the Boston Medical and Surgical Journal.]

CALVIN THOMAS, M.D., M.M.S.S., Tyngsborough, Mass., was born in Chesterfield, Cheshire County, N. H., Dec. 22, 1765. There were twelve children, of which he was the fifth. His parents dying when he was young, he went to live with an uncle in Rowe, Mass. He subsequently worked on the farm in Chesterfield, until he was 17, then lived two years in Spencer, Mass., and learned the trade of a carpenter. This occupation was relinquished on account of ill health, and he was sent three years to Chesterfield Academy, where he acquired the rudiments of a good English education. At the age of 24 he went to Dr. Josiah Goodhue, of Putney, Vt., to study medicine. After three years of study, he practised one year with Dr. Goodhue, and then came to Massachusetts. His journey on horseback, in November, 1795, was accidentally arrested at Tyngsborough, Mass., where he directly engaged in full practice, and where he died on the 23d day of October, 1851, at the age of 86 years and 10 months, having, for more than fifty-six years, followed his profession with a fidelity and devotion worthy of all praise. In a small country town, on the borders of the Merrimack River, to this day passable in that place only by a ferry, surrounded by a sparse population, such a practice, in a circle of ten or twelve miles, demands an amount of labor, exposure, fatigue, and even of personal peril, which can be only appreciated by those similarly situated. In the midst of incessant occupation he educated fourteen students, several of whom became distinguished in their profession. He joined the Massachusetts Medical Society, under the presidency of Dr. Warren, in 1806, and for more than twenty years was one of its Counsellors. In 1824, he received the honorary degree of M.D. from Harvard University. He was one year a member of the House of Representatives, and Justice of the Peace under commissions from Governors Strong, Gerry, Brooks and Lincoln.

Such is the brief history of a long and laborious life of usefulness and respectability. It resembles most closely that of a class of our aged physicians who are silently dropping away in rapid succession, to be followed by others who, with higher privileges of education, in more refined and cultivated circles of acquaintance, may take a higher rank, but who cannot excel or even equal their predecessors in fidelity and devotion to their profession.

Dr. Thomas wrote but little for the public. He left behind him thirty large day-books or journals, in which are systematically recorded, day by day, the name and residence of every patient, the visit, the medicine prescribed, the disease or accident, and the charge for the service, with frequent notices of the weather, &c. And but very few days are there in fifty years, in which some such service was not rendered and recorded. The day preceding his last sickness, and only a week before his death, being then almost 87 years old, he successfully reduced a dislocated humerus, with only the assistance of a neighbor called in to aid him.

He was naturally zealous and enthusiastic, and followed his business with great industry and earnestness. He had great confidence in remedies—a high estimation of the resources of our art. It is easy to see that such traits would commend him to his patrons. There was no hesitation; no misgivings that the remedy would fail of its expected results : and when the case was unsuccessful, it was attributed to anything rather than the impotency of medicine.

Dr. Thomas made no pretensions to extensive medical learning. Through life he was a reader of the current books of his profession, and he had, what the best-directed education might have failed to supply, an observing mind, a good judgment, and a high sense of responsibility.

He had quick feelings. Amidst the strife of parties and the collision of rival interests, a man, so decided and active, could not be without opponents. His political and religious sympathies were strong and unyielding. Notwithstanding, the conviction that he was a *good physician* was sufficient to overcome the warmth of feeling engendered by such collisions.

In all the interests of the village of his long residence, he was active and public spirited, doing his full share for the advancement of the rising generation, in education, in temperance, in good morals, and all the virtues that adorn the citizen ; and all this, long after every member of his family had been called from earthly scenes.

But to no other claims was Dr. Thomas more alive than to those of the Massachusetts Medical Society. He felt that a great honor was conferred on him in his early election as a Fellow ; and when, subsequently, he became a Counsellor, he made the journey of thirty miles, before railroads were in use, with constancy and alacrity, at no small sacrifice of time and money. His jealousy of all infringement of its rules, his watchfulness of any attempt of unworthy persons to intrude themselves, his scrupulous regard for the rights of others, his delicacy in alluding to their faults and failings, were manifestations of the true spirit of the association.

In his last will he left bequests to the American Unitarian Association, to be expended for the promotion of Unitarian religion in the valley of the Mississippi; to the President of Harvard University, for the benefit of indigent theological students in that institution, to be dispensed at his discretion; to the Unitarian Society in Tyngsborough; and one hundred dollars to the Massachusetts Medical Society, to be expended in the publication of such medical books as said Society shall order.

IMPRACTICABLE THEORIES.

[Communicated for the Boston Medical and Surgical Journal.]

THE age of theorizing and theories, simply, has quite or nearly passed; and a spirit of strict and thorough philosophical investigation has taken its place. The people, and particularly the medical profession, are becoming eminently practical. A utilitarian spirit prevails. No hypotheses or theories can be allowed a place, unless based upon and well built up by facts. No man, from a limited number of experiments, or cases which may have come under his observation, can sit down and draw out a theory—ingenious though it may be, and plausible, but mingled as theories usually are, with conjectures, certainties, and suppositions—without being liable to be called upon to enlighten the public or the profession, relative to what seems to them conflicting principles. There are doubtless things connected with the practice of hydropathy, homœopathy and the botanic systems of medicine, which are good and true; but this by no means proves these several systems to be founded and built upon a true and scientific basis. The true reason why the systems and practices of the humoralist, of the solidist, and of the vitalist, could not exist long, was because they had not sufficient facts to sustain them, and not enough even for any length of time to hide their deformities. The new theory of the motive power of the circulation (the Willardian), though defended with much skill and talent, has, as yet, failed to be established, simply for want of sufficient evidence to prove it, or facts to demonstrate it, and is now either asleep or dead.

The surgical operation which has of late claimed the attention of the medical profession—called " Hullihen's operation," or Miller's operation (as may best please)—has excited considerable interest, and I trust may be productive of much good; but in order to judge correctly of the practicability of any question, or practice, the evils as well as the benefits growing out of it should be considered. The advocates of the new operation claim, I believe, that the surgeon is enabled to plug the carious tooth when the dental pulp is exposed, without pain, and preserve the vitality of the tooth. I do not quite understand how the nerves and bloodvessels can be severed, and, as in some cases stated, the dental pulp removed, without destroying the vitality of the organ. It has always been my impression that when the circulation of the nervous communication is cut off from an organ, it immediately loses its vitality, and nature soon makes effort to remove it. I cannot see why the same rule does not apply to the teeth. So far as my observation goes, it does; for when the vitality of a tooth is destroyed, nature makes effort to rid herself of it, and will do so sooner or later, either by ulceration taking place

around the fang, or by absorption.   Then if the vitality of the tooth
be destroyed by Miller's operation (or Hullihen's), the organ can be in
no better condition than if it had been destroyed through the carious
cavity ; and the only advantage gained, is that it is more convenient,
and an opening is left for the discharge of pus, should any be formed.
It is stated by one of the suggestors of this operation, that when the
dental pulp was removed, the result " in every case, so far as known, has
been as successful as when the pulp was allowed to remain ;" also, that
" when the pulp is removed, the teeth are not sensible to impressions
from heat and cold."   Now if the dental pulp can be removed by ulceration or by mechanical means, and the tooth still retain its vitality,
and not be sensible to impressions from heat and cold, I must confess
that the dental surgeon has made a discovery which must entirely revolutionize all our previous notions of vitality as dependent upon the
nervous system and the circulation.

Dr. Miller, in the second of his reported cases found in the Journal,
Vol. XLVII., No. 12, says, " having amputated the nerve of the cus-
pidatus, a query arose as to what should be done with the bicuspids having *two* nerves.   After a moment's reflection, the drill was carried
deeper, cutting off both branches, and the teeth filled without pain."
If the doctor had reflected two minutes instead of one, he might have
come to the conclusion that the bicuspids are furnished with but *one*
nerve, instead of two, as a general rule—those that have two (as is
sometimes the case) being *exceptions* and not the rule.

The operation requires a careful consideration and examination, before we come to the *grand* conclusion that this is the great ultimatum,
long desired in dental surgery.   There seems to be a tendency with
some minds, in investigating a subject, to first form an opinion, and
then labor to make their experiments prove their opinion correct, which
leads them to receive only such results as may prove their preconceived notions.   This must usually bring a wrong conclusion.

M. M. Frisselle, M.D.
Rockville, Conn., Jan. 20th, 1853.

COMPOUND FRACTURE OF THE SKULL.

To the Editor of the Boston Medical and Surgical Journal.

Sir,—The accompanying very interesting and instructive case of compound fracture of the skull, with depression of bone and wound of the
brain, with perfect recovery, was recently received in a letter from Dr.
Griswold, of West Rutland, Vt., having occurred in the practice of himself and Dr. Sheldon, with whom he is associated.   By giving it a place
in your Journal, you will much oblige   Your obedient Serv't,
Boston, 170 *Tremont st., Jan.* 20.   S. Parkman.

The subject of this fracture was Thomas Carigon, an Irishman, and
laborer in the marble quarries, 26 years of age, who received the injury
Sept. 10th, 1852, by the falling of a derrick guy, which struck him on

the head. I saw the patient 25 minutes after the accident. The hemorrhage, which had been profuse, had nearly subsided; blood, mixed with small portions of brain, was oozing from the wound. The patient was insensible; respiration slow and somewhat stertorous; slow and weak pulse; paralysis of the right side, with loss of speech, but occasional low moaning. The wound presented a contused and lacerated appearance, and upon enlarging it, and laying bare the fractured and depressed portions, the appearance was such as to warrant any one unaccustomed to military surgery, to abandon the case without any farther operation. A large portion of the left parietal bone, with the squamous portion of the temporal bone, and the posterior superior third of the right parietal bone, were fractured into small pieces, except that one large piece, 3 3-4 inches long by 2 1-2 inches wide, on the top of the head, including a portion of both the right and left parietal bones, was depressed and slid under the skull, wounding the dura mater by its being carried under with the bone, and leaving a fissure anterior to the depressed bone where the dura mater could be seen, which aided us materially in removing the depressed and loose pieces, which was done without trephining. The fracture also extended forward, near to the superciliary ridge of the frontal bone. One triangular piece of the internal table penetrated the brain to the depth of 3-4 of an inch, wounding the dura mater to about the same extent. On removing this piece, the patient manifested more sensation, raised his left hand to his head, which he kept in motion by rolling it on the pillow. A small quantity of brain and blood escaped from the wound. The space left uncovered by bone, extended from about the centre of the left parietal bone, obliquely backward, including the posterior superior portion of the right, leaving an oblong, irregular cavity, of 5 1-2 inches in length by 3 1-4 in width. The fracture, extending forward, loosened the main part of the bone forming the left side of the head, but only very slightly, except at the posterior part, including a small part of the temporal bone, where was a piece 2 inches long by 1 1-2 inch in width, completely detached from the surrounding bones but firmly attached to the scalp, which was suffered to remain. The superior edge of this piece was contiguous to the space left uncovered with bone.

The flaps were brought together by suture, leaving sufficient space for the escape of matter, and dressed with water dressing. Four o'clock, 6 hours after, he continued comatose, with less moaning.

11th, 8 A. M.—Reaction coming on; bled to 12 ounces, and gave a purge of calomel. Continues moaning; restless; pulse 100 and firm. 4 P. M.—No operation. Repeated the dose of calomel. Spasms, or partial convulsions of the right, or paralyzed side. Removed the dressings, and applied cold water.

12th.—Had a free evacuation of the bowels.

The convulsions continued at intervals, varying from ten minutes to one hour, till about the fifteenth day, when they gradually subsided in severity and frequency, until the 20th, after which they subsided altogether. During this time the wound discharged healthy matter, but the left side of the head was very much swollen, pressing out the anterior inferior or loosened portion of bone, so that the superior fissure or separation of the bones could be distinctly felt through the scalp.   Profuse hemorrhage from the wound occurred on the 20th, which came near proving fatal.   The blood was venous, and was checked by continued pressure with a pledget of lint.

As the patient recovered from the weakness occasioned by the loss of blood (the swelling of the head being greatly diminished by the hemorrhage), motion of the right side partially returned, he being able to draw up the leg and make slight motion with his toes.   His speech also gradually returned, though but partially, being only able to articulate with difficulty in monosyllables. He continued to improve rapidly both in strength and speech, gradually recovered the use of the paralyzed side, and in five weeks from the time of the accident was able to leave his bed.

Nov. 13*th.*—He is now performing some slight labor, and enjoying a very good degree of health.   His senses seem to be unimpaired.   He frequently hesitates, however, in conversation, forgetting the conclusion of a sentence which he has commenced, and sometimes pronounces several words of a similarity of sound before he gets at the right one.

Jan. 3*d*, 1853.—The wound has completely healed, and the hair grown out, with little or no deformity, there being, however, a space of about four square inches, more or less, where the bone is entirely wanting and the cerebral pulsations seen.   He has now very little inconvenience in consequence of the injury.

THE BOSTON MEDICAL AND SURGICAL JOURNAL.

BOSTON, FEBRUARY 2, 1853.

Drug Inspectors.—The question is not unfrequently asked—Is the country furnished with drugs of a more reliable character, than before the present United States law was enacted ?   And then, again, the question is apt to follow—Do the druggists and apothecaries never dilute or adulterate the articles they purchase ? We cannot undertake to answer interrogatories of this kind.   Those of the trade whom we have the pleasure to know, are honest men ; and, as a body, the druggists and apothecaries of Boston are above any such acts of meanness.   That the inspectors are vigilant officers, is admitted ; and by their close attention to imports, they have been wonderfully successful in designating the good from the bad. Whatever passes the ordeal of their inspection, is unquestionably of the first quality.   After the boxes, bales, bottles and bags leave their custody, their responsibility ceases.   There are ingenious drug brokers in this country, and wholesale merchants, who understand as many mysterious processes for increasing weight and measure, to say nothing of quality, as in Europe, where some of the craft are expert to a proverb.   The post of inspector should in every instance be given to physicians, for they alone are competent to decide grave points in regard to the quality and value of a majority of the imports denominated medicine.   They are more likely to combine the qualifications of chemists and dispensing druggists in addition to their strictly medical attainments, and hence the government and people are both gainers by having such at the post of inspection. It is probable that something like an annual report will emanate from some or all of these gentlemen, before long. Dr. Bailey, of New York, has acquired a prominent reputation for his skill, science, tact and discretion at the Custom House of that port, and it would be gratifying to hear from him in this way.

Broma and Dietetic Cocoa.—Every body in New England, of course, is quite familiar with those two excellent articles of diet for invalids, broma and dietetic cocoa, manufactured by Walter Baker, of Dorchester, Mass. Some years since, the special consideration of medical practitioners was called to these preparations, as appropriate food for the sick, in the various conditions of debility and prostration to which they are at times reduced, leaving the digestive apparatus too feeble to appropriate any but the most delicate nutriment. Medical gentlemen of eminence in this city were delighted with Mr. Baker's broma ; and from that period to this, its good character has been sustained. Another set of physicians have commenced business since that period, who may not have become familiar with the article ; and we therefore refer again to the subject, for the purpose of reminding both our young medical friends at home and those at a distance, that they will derive important advantages from the use of these admirable kinds of food. Druggists in the interior would find their account in always keeping both on hand, with a view to meeting the prescriptions of medical attendants. From our own personal experience of the value of broma particularly, we can speak decidedly in its favor. A dietetic course is not unfrequently quite as necessary as strict medication ; and in recovering from a low state, it is one of the perplexities of a general practitioner's life, to determine what may or may not be safely adopted as regimen.

Uterine Displacements.—Dr. Coale's much valued treatise on the causes, constitutional effects and treatment of uterine displacements, which first appeared in this Journal, has been published in an octavo pamphlet, and is in a convenient form for circulation. The profession will find this an important counsellor in every-day practice, from a source that commands the confidence of judicious physicians. Practical medicine is a common sense business as well as a science, and when men of observation and learning take it in hand, the world is a gainer by their labors. It would be a curious investigation to ascertain how many systems of medical practice have been put forth by persons who never engaged in the duties of a physician. There is an immense difference between curing diseases with pen and ink in an arm chair, and in visiting the victims of disease at the bed side, and studying the symptoms and circumstances of a case. Dr. Coale is a practitioner, whose written opinions and instructions are the result of careful and even laborious research at the only place where facts can be procured — the sick chamber. The originality and importance of his instruction urges us to commend this treatise to the consideration of those who are ambitious to advise judiciously that particular class of patients whose infirmities are the subject of the author's interesting disquisition.

Surgical Apparatus.—Under this term, an endless variety of mechanical contrivances are to be had here at the north, designed to remedy defects, and assist nature in restoring a curved spine, a distorted limb, a weak muscle, or something else equally important to afflicted individuals. Among them may also be found ingeniously devised abdominal supporters, and pessaries without number, which strike the examiner, at first sight, as being eminently appropriate for remedying the misfortunes for which they were constructed. In the midst of these auxiliaries of external surgery, so abundant and skilfully constructed, some distinguished practitioners have dared to call their utility in question. These individuals speak freely against all kinds of apparatus, and even adduce instances in which bad was made worse under the pressure and long-continued action of springs, splints and buckles. This shows, simply, the revolutions to which the opinions even of medical men are subject. At one period, by general consent, the treatment of maladies is after a certain prescribed form, and patients recover all the while. By-and-by, a question is raised in respect to some part or the whole of the treatment, and then new theories and a complete change of medication follow, and the public sentiment goes with the professional current. Something of this kind is now evidently operating in regard to surgical apparatus generally. Even trusses, useful as they are, have their enemies. Correspondents might perhaps profitably discuss the subject; for if the opponents of these artificial aids are in error, and have magnified molehills, or overlooked the good that has been accomplished, it is desirable to have them convinced of the fact. As both medicine and surgery are progressive—the minor details must necessarily be subject to criticism, to alternate objections and praises, according to the ability, enterprise and genius of those who practise them.

Medical Matters at the West.—A correspondent in one of the Western States writes as follows:—

"I have just returned from Cincinnati, where I have been engaged in teaching the present session in the Cincinnati College of Medicine and Surgery. You may not be aware of the existence of this school, as it has gone into operation altogether too quietly for success. The organization of the *Miami College*, with Dr. Mussey at its head, has done something to hinder us. It is intended to give two courses of lectures a year, beginning in November and March.

"I was in the city at the time of the death of Dr. Drake, and attended his funeral. Perhaps no person in that city would have been more missed than the Dr. His advanced age, and his ardent devotion to the profession and to every employment of benevolence, brought him in relation with almost all classes. I am greatly surprised that no one of his cotemporaries has given a more extended obituary notice of him."

Physicians in California.—Among the countless crowd of adventurers who have been wending their way to the regions of gold at the west, physicians have gone in great numbers from the Atlantic States. Some of them, who were early on the ground, have succeeded tolerably well, but not perhaps as well as might have been expected, considering that all charges for personal service have been exorbitantly high there, from the first day the precious metal was discovered. Medicines, of all and every sort, purporting to be of value in the diseases most prevalent among the miners, have been sold at prices beyond precedent in the history of apothecaries. Quack preparations, whether in repute at home or not, have been equally saleable, and sums have been realized by active manufacturers in New

England, whose market has been all over California, that will hereafter constitute memorable anecdotes among the heirs to great estates thus obtained. The high price of drugs and medicines in California may have suggested the idea to some physicians, of becoming homœopathic practitioners. Those who announced themselves as such, have been sought with a confidence that impressed spectators with the idea that economy was thought of by both parties. It has been perhaps the most profitable system of practice there, as many have believed it to be here. Certain it is, that some who were very highly educated, and who went from Boston firm and well schooled in the regular system of practice, on reaching central points in California have raised the flag of Hahnemannism. These are perplexing events, and rather mortifying; but that the dearness of medicine has had some agency in making medical turncoats, seems quite probable.

Napping after Dinner.—"A Constant Reader" in the London Lancet lately requested advice as to the best means of overcoming the disagreeable habit of sleeping after dinner. Among the answers which his request called forth, was the following by a writer with the signature "Wide awake." The remedy is doubtless a good one; but a better one would be some active useful employment during the time mentioned.

"Direct your attendant to procure beforehand a liberal supply of the most pungent nettles, and having arranged them in a suitable form, let him apply them with an energetic hand, following you round and round the apartment until the drowsy god is entirely ousted from the dominion which he had so unwarrantably usurped over you. Allow this process to be repeated daily for some time, and I think you will find the result satisfactory."

Medical Miscellany.—Our importation of wine amounts to six millions of gallons per annum; our consumption to at least twenty millions of gallons.—At Santiago, within the last three months, 3,600 have died of the cholera, says an official report.—Havana is still afflicted with smallpox to a frightful extent.—Cases of scarlet fever are rather on the increase among us.—Cholera seems not to have entirely disappeared from the south.—There are eleven thousand five hundred physicians in France.—Smallpox has extended widely in the eastern world, and the people are dying in vast numbers. — The bills of mortality are unusually favorable for the last month in New England.

ERRATUM —Page 529, line 2 from top, for "ten months since," read *two* months.

MARRIED,—At Philadelphia, 13th ult., Dr. Edward Shippen, U. S. Navy, to Mary Katherine, eldest daughter of Dr. J. Rodman Paul.—James R. Leaming. M.D., of New York, to Jane Helen, eldest daughter of Rev. Lewis Cheeseman.

DIED,—At New Orleans, 31st December (where he had been to seek a climate more congenial to his declining health), Dr. Wallace B. Shelden, formerly of Beverly, Mass.

Deaths in Boston—for the week ending Saturday noon, Jan. 29th, 93 —Males, 44—females, 49. Accidental, 1—inflammation of bowels, 1—inflammation of the brain, 1—consumption, 16—convulsions, 3—croup, 2—dysentery, 1—dropsy, 1—dropsy in head, 5—infantile, 10—puerperal, 2—exhaustion, 1—erysipelas, 1—typhoid fever, 2—scarlet fever, 19—hemorrhage, 1—disease of the heart, 3—intemperance, 1—inflammation of the lungs, 2—congestion of ditto, 1—disease of liver, 2—marasmus, 4—palsy, 1—inflammation of the stomach, 1— teething, 3—thrush, 1—tumor, 1—worms, 1.
Under 5 years, 48—between 5 and 20 years 9—between 20 and 40 years, 13—between 40 and 60 years, 12—over 60 years, 11. Born in the United States, 63—Ireland, 26—England, 3—Br. America, 1. The above includes 8 deaths at the City Institutions.

American Medical Association.—The sixth annual meeting of this Association will be held in the city of New York on Tuesday, May 3, 1853.

The secretaries of all societies and other bodies entitled to representation in the association, are requested to forward to the undersigned correct lists of their respective delegations as soon as they may be appointed ; and it is desired by the committee of arrangements that the appointments be made at as early a period as possible.

The following is an extract from Art. II of the constitution : " Each local society shall have the privilege of sending to the association one delegate for every ten of its regular resident members, and one for every additional fraction of more than half of this number. The faculty of every regularly constituted medical college or chartered school of medicine shall have the privilege of sending two delegates. The professional staff of every chartered or municipal hospital containing a hundred inmates or more, shall have the privilege of sending two delegates ; and every other permanently organized medical institution of good standing shall have the privilege of sending one delegate.' EDW'D L. BEADLE,

One of the Secretaries, No. 42 *Bleecker Street, New York.*

☞ The Medical Press of the United States is respectfully requested to copy the foregoing.

Premium Tract on Tobacco.—The committee of award, Drs. Cox, Lansing and Skinner, have examined sixty to eighty manuscripts, written for the premium of $100, offered through the American missionary association for the best tract against the use of tobacco, and have advised that, if the writers consent to certain conditions, the premium should be divided between three tracts, the writers of which are found to be Elisha Harris, M.D., of New York: William A. Alcott, M.D., of West Newton, Massachusetts ; and A. H. Grimshaw, M.D., of Wilmington, Del.

Changes in the Management of the Paris Hospitals. — L'Union Médicale mentions that the great facility for travelling has so encumbered the hospitals of Paris, that measures will now be taken to make the various departments pay for the people from the provinces who are admitted into the Paris hospitals. The Central Board, which was formerly instituted merely for examining and sending patients to the various hospitals, will now be transformed into a dispensary, without detriment to its former duties ; so that the poor who can be treated at their own residences may be attended to. It should not be forgotten that the municipal body of Paris contributes £350,000 to the expenses of hospitals.—*London Lancet.*

More Poisonous Fungi.—A letter from Montierender (Haute Marne) says :—" The woman who acts as cook to M. de Coucy, a retired officer, brother-in-law to Gen. Oudinot, having last week prepared some mushrooms gathered in a neighboring wood, served up the dish to her master, and partook of it herself, as well as gave a portion to a woman named Voisins, and the son of the latter, a boy of fourteen. In some hours after, symptoms of poisoning appeared, and though every aid was given, the three adult persons expired next day, the boy alone recovering."—*Ib.*

THE

BOSTON MEDICAL AND SURGICAL JOURNAL.

Vol. XLVIII.   Wednesday, February 9, 1853.   No. 2.

CASE OF TÆNIA EXPELLED BY KOUSSO.

[Communicated for the Boston Medical and Surgical Journal.]

November 26th, 1852.—J. H., æt. 14, English, rather tall for his age, slim, of dark complexion. His family are not known to be subject to tænia. Brothers and sisters occasionally pass, and are troubled by, ascarides. First aware of having a tape-worm in 1847, since when discharges of it have, from time to time, occurred, sometimes after taking oil of turpentine, and sometimes without the administration of any medicine. I have had in my possession several yards of the tape-worm evacuated a year or two ago. Subject to occasional attacks of violent abdominal pain, after which he has generally passed a portion of the worm. The discharge, however, is not always preceded by these symptoms, though always by *some* symptoms; as headache and sense of fatigue. His appetite is irregular, and his head frequently affected. Has been prevented by general debility and languor, and occasional distress, attributed to the disturbance caused by the tape-worm, from commencing an apprenticeship, to which his parents have been desirous of binding him.

About three months ago, the patient was attacked with wild delirium, accompanied with loud outcries, the symptoms continuing for a day or two, and being soon followed by the passage of a large portion of the tænia. Since then the patient is reported to have appeared heavy and stupid, pieces of the worm being still occasionally voided.

Now (about 10, A.M., Nov. 26th) the administration of kousso having been resolved upon, the patient is directed to take an ounce of sulphate of magnesia, living on thin porridge, during the day. To take nothing after rising, tomorrow, till my visit.

27th, 9¾, A.M.—Three copious dejections yesterday, in one of which the patient saw a small piece of the worm. Has had no pain, except during the operation of the cathartic. Has, now, just risen, having ingested nothing to-day. To take at once an ounce of lemonade.

10½, A.M—Infusion of kousso administered, preceded and followed by the imbibition of about an ounce of lemonade. The drug was given in a dose of three drachms and fifteen grains, accurate weight, although half an ounce was the quantity written for. The kousso, in powder, was stirred with cold water till a thick paste was formed, when about

2

twelve ounces of hot water were added, the whole being allowed to stand for twenty-five minutes before being administered. A dejection took place in about twenty minutes, containing a few broad joints of the tænia. A second dejection followed in about five minutes after, with a large piece of the broader portion of the worm. A third dejection occurred in five minutes more, with a large portion of the reptile, including the neck. At 2, P.M., there was a fourth dejection, containing a few joints. *No pain* attended the action of the medicine.

At 2, P.M., having carried home the portion of worm discharged, it was found to measure fifty-five inches, without the portion attached to the head, which was not then discovered. It gradually tapered from about the one third of an inch to a line in width. Then its breadth rapidly diminished to half a line, for the space of about four inches of its length, when it was found to have been broken off. Some alcohol being poured upon the reptile, a considerable movement took place.

On a subsequent examination, after the immersion of the worm in alcohol, a slender filament, about a third of a line in width, was found wound around the broad joint, and proved to be a piece of the neck, about an inch and a half in length, with the head attached. The head was hemispherical, or pear-shaped, and, to the naked eye, of the size and appearance depicted in the smaller of the two following figures.

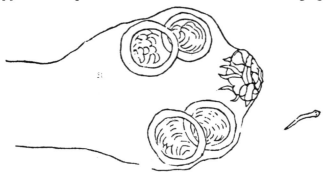

Its appearance is given, as magnified by a low power, and projected in outline by a camera lucida.

The figure below represents the neck, as seen magnified a short distance from the head.

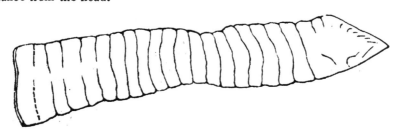

28th.—Slept well; appetite good; more. cheerful. No dejection since 2, P.M. yesterday. Take an ounce of sulphate of magnesia.

30th.—Salts operated well. No pieces of the worm were discharged. Reports himself free from morbid symptoms.

December 23d.—The patient is at school, and is reported to have been well, in all respects, since last visit.

In a paper by Blanchard, in the "Annales des Sciences Naturelles," the circular objects on the head were described as "Ventouses," or "suckers." In Blanchard's plate, on account probably of the original object being less compressed than my specimen, two, only, of the suckers are visible, and those are more prominent than in the representation here given.

These "ventouses" are described, in the monograph referred to, as having behind them cavities communicating with longitudinal canals extending the whole length of the worm, along its borders.

Blanchard describes and illustrates by figures, distinct circulatory, digestive and reproductive systems. But as his views are not generally received, I forbear further quotation from his paper.

In some highly interesting remarks at a late meeting of the Boston Society for Medical Observation, Dr. Dalton spoke of some experiments lately made by Prof. Siebold, in relation to the development of the tapeworm.

Siebold, struck with the resemblance between the head of the cysticercus and that of the tænia, devised and carried out a series of experiments, most ingenious in their conception, and conclusive in their results. This resemblance is so strong, that if the head of the tænia, represented in the above cut, were made to terminate in a sac instead of a succession of joints, it would give a very good idea of the appearance of the cysticercus. The experiments were briefly as follows: A number of dogs were caused to swallow livers (of rats) containing living cysticerci. In the stomachs of the dogs, killed in three or four hours after this scientific repast, the livers were entirely digested, while the heads and necks of the cysticerci were found unharmed, and either retracted within the sacs, or divested of them by the dissolution of the latter. In dogs suffered to live a few hours longer, the cysticerci—minus their sacs —were found in the small intestines. Finally, the remainder of the quadrupeds thus pressed into the service of science, being killed at the end of some fourteen days, contained considerably-developed tapeworms.

Thus is proved the identity between at least one species of cysticerci, and one species of tape-worm, by tracing the development of the former into the latter; and thus are we enabled to understand the mode of introduction of tape-worm into the bodies of animals.

In relation to the drug "kousso," I have only to refer all inquirers to the last edition of "Wood & Bache."

L. PARKS, JR., M.D.

Boston, January 8th, 1853.

SYNCOPE AFTER CHILDBIRTH.

[Communicated for the Boston Medical and Surgical Journal.]

THURSDAY, Nov. 19, 1852.—I was requested to see Mrs. S., in her seventh labor. Nothing unusual occurred, either in its progress or termination. Duration about three hours. After-birth expelled some twenty minutes after the child, with slight assistance. Mrs. S. is corpulent and of lax texture, which, according to the common notion, would predispose to hæmorrhage. About half an hour after the removal of the placenta, the patient appeared to be rapidly sinking, the skin becoming cool, pulse small and weak, countenance pale, &c., asking some one near if it was not night, and saying that the room looked dark—in short, with all the symptoms of syncope. After-pains regular up to the time of fainting, when they became irregular and convulsive. I was very sure, when I saw the woman in such a collapsed state, that hemorrhage must be the cause ; but on examining the uterus through the muscles of the abdomen, it appeared firm and contracted. The vagina at the same time was nearly free from blood. The reverse of this sometimes happens ; although the womb seems to be well contracted, the vagina becomes greatly distended with blood, and alarming syncope follows ; a condition that every physician of ten or fifteen years' practice has witnessed a sufficient number of times to establish a rule, or at least to cause him to be on the look-out. But in the case under consideration we must look for some other cause, and the question may be asked what was it ? Shall we be contented to attribute it to some nervous shock ? This, if possible, involves the subject in still more obscurity. Or is it analogous to what sometimes happens after removing a large quantity of fluid in ascites ? Or shall we say it is on account of a change in the system ? an explanation equal to saying that it is so, because it is. Some of our modern systematic writers, I think Meigs and Ramsbotham, one or both, are among the number who have referred it to the dilatation of the vessels in the vicinity of the uterus, which consequently abstracts an unnatural quantity of blood from distant parts—the brain and other nervous centres in particular; a conclusion which the treatment in the present case corroborates. But if we are not able to describe the correct pathological condition from which the symptoms above referred to result, it is none the less worthy of investigation, considering how suddenly we sometimes lose our patients under similar circumstances—although in the above case recovery took place, and reaction was established in about an hour, the patient several times losing the pulse at the wrist. Stimulants were used, principally brandy and water, alternated with carbonate of ammonia, with camphor friction to the limbs and body, which improved the condition very little. Pressure was immediately made on the lower part of the abdomen, at the same time inclining the bed by elevating the foot, which improved the patient essentially, raising the pulse so as to make it quite perceptible. By changing the position of the bed to its previous state, the circulation at the wrist would be almost imperceptible ; and by again inclining it, the pulse would re-appear. The position was thus changed some three times, while the woman remained in that unnatural condition, which was about one hour. This inclined position of the body, with the head lowest, and pressure as before described, were the only means that seemed effectual in this case. **E. S. Deming.**

Calais, Vt., Nov. 21, 1852.

MELANOSIS IN THE HORSE.

BY CHARLES M. WOOD, VETERINARY SURGEON.

[Communicated for the Boston Medical and Surgical Journal.]

In March last, I was requested to examine a grey horse, with a tumor on the inside of the off, or right thigh, and another within the scrotum on the same side, from which he appeared slightly lame. The tumor on the thigh appeared to partake of the character of a wart; the one in the scrotum, I thought, was probably scirrhus of the spermatic cord. The owner consulted me as to the propriety of having them extirpated. As I considered an operation would be attended with some danger, I advised his continuing his work (which was in a job-wagon), stating that if he was found to be getting worse, I would have no objection to operate on him; but would not be answerable for the consequences that might ensue. I did not see him again for about a month, when he was again brought to me, and in a very emaciated condition, evidently suffering much pain from the rapid growth of the tumors.

The owner now requested me to operate at all hazards. Accordingly the animal was duly prepared, and cast and secured for the operation. On opening the scrotum I found that the tumor was completely enveloped in a sac, composed of cellular membrane, very much thickened, and was firmly attached. I had considerable difficulty in getting to the superior surface; but I excised it, after some trouble, with the loss, to the animal, of about four or five pounds of blood. On introducing my hand into the opening in the scrotum, I could plainly feel another tumor, within the abdomen, and apparently larger than the one I had extracted, which weighed one pound and twelve ounces. As I could, of course, do nothing with this, I allowed the animal to rise. He got up, apparently quite strong, and walked to the stable, a distance of some twenty yards, when he commenced eating. I put up my instruments and casting hobbles, and was about to leave, when the man came from the stable and informed me that the horse had lain down. I went to the stable and found him in that position, and in a few minutes he died, without a struggle. He was immediately removed to the field adjoining; and in making a post-mortem examination, I found within him hundreds of these tumors, of various sizes; some of them as large as a goose egg, and down to the size of a pea. The lungs, liver, spleen, mesentery, kidneys, intestines, and even the peritoneum and pleura, lining the chest and abdomen, were full of them, and there were many dispersed amongst the different muscles. They were of a circular form, of a substance as hard as cartilage, perfectly black, and, by scraping them, you would obtain a black mucus, very much resembling the " nigrum pigmentum " of the eye. Upon further examination of some of the larger ones, I found that they were composed of a number of smaller ones, from the size of a marble down to a very small pea, and apparently united to_ gether by dense cellular membrane. Finding the examination very in_ teresting, I determined on examining the brain, and, strange to say, I found congeries of these tumors, nearly as large as a pin's head, upon the plexus choroides, and in the lateral ventricles.

I could not, however, find anything satisfactory, as to the cause of the sudden death of the animal. It could not have been from loss of blood, as the heart and vessels generally were full. I conclude, there- fore, it must have been from nervous irritation and exhaustion.

Boston, January, 1853.

MEDICAL APPLICATION OF ELECTRICITY.

. *To the Editor of the Boston Medical and Surgical Journal.*

Sir,—I wish to communicate, through your Journal, a few thoughts upon the subject at the head of this article.

Dr. William F. Channing, in a small but very valuable work upon medical electricity, has truly remarked that, " The introduction of elec- tricity into medical practice has been made the subject, within a few years, of many empirical treatises. Original and valuable sources of information have at the same time been multiplied, and the European journals, after a long interval, are again filled with cases of the successful applica- tion of this agent. Professor Wisgrill, in addressing the Medical Asso- ciation of Vienna, remarks, that a revolution has taken place in favor of electricity, which, after its wide celebrity at the commencement of the present century, had fallen into disuse, not from the inefficacy of the means, but from the mode in which they were employed. It will be frequently seen, even in successful cases, quoted hereafter, that the na- ture of the agent and the laws of application have been imperfectly understood ; and many of the failures which have occurred must be as- cribed to this source."

In these quotations from Dr. C. we have a *text* sufficient for a volume. First, " it has been made the subject of many empirical treatises." This fact has prevented its being employed by many scientific physi- cians, who would otherwise have investigated its merits, and thoroughly experimented upon its therapeutical effects. · There is a feeling, perhaps too general, in the profession, to let any medicine or medicinal agent alone, when it has been generally taken up by irregular or empirical practitioners. This should never be the case. The *true eclectic* phy- sician employs, in turn, any and every means of restoring lost health, by whomsoever it might have been discovered, or afterwards used. It is undoubtedly true that multitudes of little or no medical or physiological attainments have taken up this subject, and written upon it, even flood- ing the land with their books. Still, many scientific men have put their pens to it, and sent forth much that is truly valuable ; among whom may be named Drs. Wilson Philip and Golding Bird.

Second. " It failed not for want of efficacy in the means, but from want of knowledge to apply it." While the most ignorant have, doubtless, met with some success, it has more often, when ignorantly applied, utterly failed. This has been the occasion of its failure, in all probability, in nine cases out of ten, where failure has followed its application. I have myself seen an operator apply the magneto-galvanic current, to *stimulate* a nerve, in an opposite direction from that recommended by Matteucci. Of course, he failed to *excite* the nervous energy.

Another cause of its failure has been in the fact, that by this class of operators it has been invariably used *alone ;* not as an *auxiliary* to medicine and therapeutical skill, but as a *sole* recuperative agent. It will be readily seen, by every intelligent physician, that in most cases such an application of electricity would fail. Other treatment was necessary, in conjunction with this. If this " bow is drawn at a venture," and the electric current sent, *pell-mell,* in the right or wrong direction, towards the centres or ramifications of the nerves, or not touching them at all, and irrespective of *quantity* or *intensity,* as the *hobby hydropathist* sends his stream of water, it is to be supposed that the operator would *sometimes* hit right ; but far oftener *wrong,* or *not at all.*

I may add, the whole value of electricity, as a medical agent, depends upon a correct diagnosis of the disease, a proper degree of quantity and intensity of the agent, and its application in the right direction. It should be expected, when applied under these circumstances, to exert a great effect, as a medical agent. How can it be otherwise, when it is acknowledged, by many of the most intelligent physiologists and physicians, to possess a vitalizing and re-active power, an alterative and sedative action, and to promote secretion, absorption, nutrition and capillary circulation. It has been employed successfully in a host of ailments, quite too numerous to be named in this place. The more we study into the philosophy of the electric fluid, and the more we apply it therapeutically to diseases, the more we shall be convinced of the truth of the following declarations of Dr. Philip—" We have seen that galvanism is capable of performing all the functions of the nervous power, properly so called. I have repeatedly seen from it the same effect, when applied to the digestive organs and liver, or biliary system, which arises from calomel ; a copious biliary discharge from the bowels coming on a few hours after its employment."

I have been in the habit of employing this agent, as an auxiliary to other medical treatment, in a large variety of diseases, for several years, and with marked success. In the treatment of many cases 1 would be very unwilling to dispense with its use. I feel well assured that I could not find an equally efficient substitute in the whole range of medical appliances.

Two cases have recently come under my treatment, in which this agent has seemed to be very serviceable. The first, an elderly lady, with a chronic affection of the fingers, but not of very long standing. Upon one hand the fingers were stiff, and considerably swollen. The magneto-galvanic current was applied, for about twenty minutes, each day, for ten days, when the stiffness and swelling were mostly gone. She soon entirely recovered. Other remedies were combined with the use of the machine, but I ascribed the subsidence of the disease chiefly to the electro-galvanic current. The other was that of a young lady with a morbid affection of the eyes. They were very weak, sometimes inflamed and painful. She had been for some time under the care of a very respectable and skilful physician. But still her eyes grew no better. The other treatment which I employed was very ordinary, and I have no reason to suppose it was any better than she had previously received. But I applied the electric current, which remedy she had not previously had. It was administered within the orbit of the eye, and to the ophthalmic branch of the fifth pair of nerves. She expressed herself as relieved at the first sitting, as soon as the sponge was removed (for it was applied through a soft sponge moistened with rose-water). She has wholly recovered under the application, and ascribes her cure entirely to electricity.

While I would be far from making this single branch of medical treatment exclusive, or elevating it above all others, I am constrained to add that its virtues have grown in my estimation, year by year, as it has been medically applied. A sufficient number of well-authenticated cases of recovery under its employment are already before the public, or, rather, the medical profession, to warrant a thorough trial with it in paralysis, partial or total amaurosis, neuralgia, epilepsy, chorea, rheumatism, in the wide range of urinary and uterine diseases, constipation, colica pictonum, general debility, coldness of the extremities, aphonia, and paralysis of the visual and auditory nerves. In narcotism, cases of drowning, and exhaustion from flooding, its use should never be forborne. It no doubt sometimes fails; and what medical treatment does not? Misapplied, like all other active medical appliances, it sometimes does injury; but what medical man would reject a valuable remedy because, when unskilfully used, it did harm? If we were to do this, we must give up every medical agent of the materia medica. Matteucci has shown that the nervous power may be wholly exhausted by an excessive use of electricity. So it may be by an excessive use of the best medicine now known. But " wisdom is profitable to direct," *et verbum sat sapienti.*   W. M. CORNELL, M.D.

Boston, January, 1853.

VACCINATION AT COUNCIL BLUFFS.

[DR. CLARK, of Iowa, furnishes us the following interesting and important facts respecting the practice of vaccination at the West.]

During the spring of 1850, smallpox made its appearance at Kanesville and Council Bluffs, creating much alarm among the thousands of Oregon, California and Utah (Salt Lake) emigrants congregated in this vicinity, preparing for their long journey. There were several cases of confluent smallpox among the emigrants, and one or two of variola among the citizens, before the resident physicians were aware of its existence in the vicinity. At a special meeting of such of the physicians as could be collected together, it was determined to prevent the spreading of the disease by vaccinating all emigrants, citizens, and the Indian tribes belonging to the Council Bluffs Indian sub-agency ; which was no small amount of labor—there being probably five thousand emigrants, as many or more citizens, and some three or four thousand Indians on the Nebraskea side of the river. The physicians went from house to house, from tent to tent, vaccinating all who were unprotected. The missionaries—kind, generous men—at the Omoka and Pawnee Missions, assisted me. We vaccinated some two thousand children and adults, all that we could persuade to submit to the operation. The result crowned our efforts with success. Only two fatal cases of smallpox occurred among the whites, and some half a dozen among the Indians. The progress of the disease was effectually checked, and the alarm and fear of this dread epidemic dispelled.

These cases may be added to those already accumulated, showing the vast amount of good conferred on mankind by the discovery of Jenner, and constitute another conclusive evidence of the fact that if people will adopt the prophylactic course advised by the faculty, this disease will not become epidemic even in localities where every circumstance tends to promote it, as was the case at Council Bluffs and Kanesville at this period.

The red men duly appreciate the benefit of vaccination. Chocopee, the chief of the Ottes, at that time ordered his *braves* to bring to the Mission House all the squaws and children ; and every year since, when the emigrant wagon makes its appearance on the banks of the Missouri River, the chief of the tribe orders the vaccinating process to commence.

ON HOMŒOPATHY.

[Communicated for the Boston Medical and Surgical Journal.]

THE homœopaths, being satisfied of the truth of the doctrine of *similia similibus curantur*, and of the "tremendous potency" of infinitesimal doses, have nothing to do but to experimentalize with various drugs, to ascertain their effect upon the healthy economy. This they have affected to do, and their published results are most entertaining. But for full particulars we refer to Jahr's Manuel of Homœopathic Medicine, and to Dr. Wood's Homœopathy Unmasked. We cannot refrain, however, from narrating a few symptoms, "the undoubted effects of infinitesimal doses."

We have all partaken of salt ; but does our experience of its effects confirm the experiments of homœopathists? According to them it produces, and therefore cures, an immense variety of symptoms ; some of which (for we can't stop to mention all), are "great wasting of the body," "continual shivering," "palsies," "eruption on the skin," "melancholy sadness, with abundant weeping," "hatred of those from whom injuries have long ago been received," "irascibilities and violent rages easily provoked," "desire to laugh," "weakness of memory," and "excessive forgetfulness," "the experimenter blunders in speaking and writing," "falling out of the hair, even of the beard," "ulceration of the chin," "loss of appetite, especially for bread," "repugnance for tobacco-smoke," "warts on the palms of the hands," &c. &c.

Another substance with which most, if not all, of us have experimented upon ourselves, is nutmeg. But according to homœopathy nutmeg produces "bloody perspiration," "a constant flow of facetious ideas," "a strong disposition to make a fool of everybody," "idiocy and madness," shortness of breath," "contraction of the throat," &c.

Lady Bountifuls and "old maids" are fond of giving people camomile tea; but do they know what symptoms camomile produces! "Catalepsy," "epileptic convulsions, with retraction of the thumbs," "a disposition to weep and utter lamentations, with great readiness to take offence," "taciturnity and repugnance for conversation," "music is insupportable," "nostrils ulcerated," lips ditto," "toothache, with pain so insupportable as to drive to despair," "the tongue moves convulsively," and "the head is twisted backwards."

To refute such nonsense as all this, would be an insult to the understanding of all sensible people. Homœopathy is, in fact, only a new name of what has long been known and practised by the regular profession, as the expectant plan of treatment; which consists in standing by and watching the patient, while nature, assisted by an infinitesimal, overcomes the disease; for their minute doses, as they have no visible, or chemical, existence (nothing being detected in a globule save sugar), can have no effect whatever upon the physical system, in a physical or natural way. That their small doses, however, in some cases have a powerful influence upon disease, by influencing the imagination, there can be no doubt.

All physicians and metaphysicians agree on this point, that the imagination has an important agency both in the production and cure of disease. The mind and body are so intimately connected and associated that they mutually affect each other. To give many illustrations of the effect of the imagination, would exceed my space, but one or two we will find room for.

When the powers of nitrous oxide or "laughing gas" were discovered, Dr. Beddoes imagined that it might be useful in chronic paralysis. Accordingly a man affected with this disease was procured, and Sir Humphry Davy was requested to make him inhale the gas. But previous to this, a small thermometer was inserted under his tongue, to ascertain his temperature, with a view to comparing it with that after the inhalation had been begun. The patient was quite ignorant of the process to which he was to be submitted, but was firmly impressed with the idea that it was to cure him. And no sooner was the thermometer placed under his tongue, than he declared that he felt already its benign influence throughout his whole system. This was too tempting an opportunity to lose; so nothing more was done to the man except applying the thermometer, which was repeated every day or every succeeding day for a fortnight, and the man gradually recovered his health.*

Another very striking experiment might be mentioned, which was

* Dr. Paris's Pharmacologia.

tried with some murderers in Russia, since cholera times. They were placed first in beds in which persons had died of the cholera. But they did not take the disease. They were then put in beds that were new, and had not been used at all, but they were told that they were in beds in which persons had died of malignant cholera. Nevertheless, three out of four of them died of the disease in question within four hours.*

The secret, then, of the success of the homœopathic practice, consists, in the first place, in the efforts of nature (which we know are sufficient to the cure in most cases that physicians are called to) ; secondly, in the influence of the imagination ; and thirdly, in the peculiar kind of diseases which they are generally called upon to treat, of which we will presently speak.

The fact that minute portions do great cures, or rather that cures take place under the employment of minute doses, only teaches the regular practitioner the importance of thoroughly understanding his profession —the mental as well as the physical constitution of his patients, so that he may be able to tell, with some degree of certainty, whether it be the mind or the body of his patient that needs his medicine ; or whether both or neither require it.

The most scientific men of the age (physicians) think that too much medicine has generally been given to the sick. And why ? Simply because a large proportion of the diseases for which physicians are called upon to prescribe, have been imaginary, or merely functional, and not organic in their nature ; diseases which belong rather to the movements of the vital machinery, than to its separate organs. For instance, a clock or a watch may be perfect in all its wheels, and yet fail to mark the time accurately, because it is not well regulated. So the human system may be sound and entire in all its parts, and yet its healthy functions may be so deranged as to render the patient really ill. Now what does such a man need ? Does he need active medicine ? Certainly not. But simply the advice of some competent physician, who, if competent, and an honest man, will prescribe, perhaps, a change of diet, a change of place, new objects of attention, increased exercise of both body and mind ; after which, if the above does not succeed in perfecting the cure, or in conjunction with the above, he will prescribe a placebo, which after all may do the patient as much good as the strictest observance of the whole catalogue of hygienic rules. I think no one will doubt that such cases as these do frequently occur.

The existence of this great class of merely functional diseases, gives the homœopathist his wonderful success. But the homœopaths contend that all cures result from the use of their infinitesimals, or at any rate their patients are left to that inference. One event follows the other in the order of time, and the inference is that the consequent was the effect of the antecedent; and this kind of reasoning is the great stumbling block of all ignorant men.

" By education most have been misled,
So they believe because they were so bred."

So it is with at least the majority of the people of these United States.

* We state this on the authority of the London Medical Times.

Their education on such matters has been in perfect keeping with this kind of reasoning, an example of which is to be seen in the case of the Irishman who applied to his physician for a prescription for his wife. He was ordered to apply a blister to the chest. Pat having no chest in the house, applied it to the lid of an old trunk, and the wife happening to recover, was of course ready to certify to the efficacy of the application. The history of charlatanry is full of just such facts. Did any sane man ever persuade himself that the efficacy of a medicine is increased precisely as its quantity is diminished? that the smaller the dose, the more potent in its influence? If the doctrines of the founder of homœopathy be true, an ounce of opium would convert all the water in the Atlantic into an excellent soporific mixture. We will close by saying that we believe as much in the efficacy of a blister when applied to the lid of an old trunk, as in the administration of truly infinitesimal doses.   H. M. ADAMS, M.D.
Hallowell, Maine.

LONDON MEDICAL CELEBRITIES.

[IN the following extract of a letter from London, the individual peculiarities of some of the leading medical and surgical men in that city are humorously illustrated. It will be read with interest by many on this side the Atlantic, who are familiar with the characters of the men alluded to.]

SIR BENJAMIN BRODIE is the most learned man in the profession in London, but the man who has most enemies; Mr. Lawrence, perhaps, the most friends, without any boasted learning. Mr. Guthrie has done more for military surgery than any man who ever lived, and should now be at the head of the medical department of the army; but like Rory O'-More's dreams, all our medical appointments here " go by contraries." The square pegs are ever getting into the round holes, and the round pegs into the square holes. Dr. Marshall Hall has been laughed at and ridiculed till it no longer " pays ;" but his name is now known through the world, and his reputation, if he will only guard it safely, quite equal to Sir Charles Bell's. Men of a certain class deny any force to the excito-motor system of nerves, as Marshall Hall has not given a map and an anatomical description of them. The spiral cord is, no doubt, the centre of these actions. These man wilfully overlook the fact, but were poor Hall to have written from the swamps of the Lower Rhine, or from Vienna, and have a name no one could pronounce, the booksellers' shelves would groan with his discoveries. Mr. Skey is another of the hard grains of our Christmas fruit ; few men of the present day, however, can boast of such a strong masculine intellect. Sitting at the feet of his Gamaliel, whom he half worships (Sir Benjamin Brodie), the combined wisdom of these two great men is something indeed to think of. Mr. Skey laughs at all authorities of the olden time. Mr. South, on the other hand, with his placid mien and hair parted like a woman's, would frame and glaze the washing bills of the ancient surgeons ; would revive *queues,* perpetual pills, red-hot amputating knives, and Ambrose Parè.

Some of the men here (the discordant elements of London medical practice) are perhaps not less singular in their characteristics. As we may not have another opportunity of serving up our currants and raisins again, we may speak of them. A dash of sugar is required, but then there is Mr. Lawrence; a little suet shredded fine, Dr. Ramsbotham; Alfred Smee, and a few fat general practitioners, cut up small; a piece of mistletoe is wanted of course, to stick a-top of our pudding, under the beamy smiles of which we may all love and greet each other, Professor Owen; some thorns to put under the pot, when we have procured a pudding-bag—thorns crackling as is the manner of fools according to high authority, the homœopaths. With a little unanimity and honesty, this desirable consummation might be achieved. A little spirit to burn under the dumpling from the bitter beer testimonials and some of our useless museum preparations. We would wish a place for our prescribing chemists, but it would be very near the thorns under the pot. Then there are others which in time will also prove useful, one way or another. Mr. Coulson, if he would only not aspirate his vowels, invulnerable on the subject of lithotomy and lithotrity; Bence Jones, at St. George's, who would turn everybody's brain he talks to into sulphurets and phosphates; Dr. Robert Lee, from the wintry side of the Tweed, old fashioned, but marvellous in industry, with one arch enemy, Dr. Snow Beck, and one abiding fancy, uterine diseases; Locock, stern and unbending in practice; Bennett, fanciful, ever dreaming of the speculum; Golding Bird, insinuating, sharp, and puritanical, goes to church only five times on Sunday, but not to be approached as a good physician, especially in children's diseases; Fergusson, need we say, the *beau ideal* of a surgeon, simple, kind, and gentlemanlike, without humbug; Bransby Cooper the same; Babington, Addison, and Watson, the great pillars of medicine in England, without whom it would all tumble to the ground; Copland, not much known, but indefatigable, like the " busy bee," improving " each shining hour," &c.; at Bartholomew's, Lloyd, one of the " illustrious unknown," preferred by his friends to poor Sam Cooper as surgeon to that institution; Paget, the rival for Skey's place; and Skey, adored and envied by every one: these all, no doubt, will be found in time among our " representative men"—when some connecting influence is discovered to bring together all the good men in London now sadly distracted —when nepotism, practising chemists, and genteel starvation are at an end—when the College of Surgeons, like the Icthyosaurus or Dinornis is reconstructed and remodelled—when the College of Physicians is no longer like a set of genteel catacombs, but common sense and proper professional thinking the rule of life most tolerated and valued.—*Dublin Medical Press.*

***

LEPROSY IN NORWAY.

[WE find in one of the religious papers a letter dated Bergen, Norway, Sept. 20, 1852, addressed to the Rev. Dr. Wainwright, of New York, and containing an account of the leprosy as seen by the writer in that

country. The late volumes of this Journal have contained descriptions
of this ancient disease as it now exists in Syria and Palestine, and the
letter alluded to is a suitable accompaniment to them. We therefore
copy it in full, with the regret, however, that we are unable to give the
name of the writer.]

It will probably surprise you to learn that the Oriental leprosy, as described by Moses and healed by our Saviour, exists at this moment in
Norway. It is not an hour since I have seen over a hundred cases of this
frightful and loathsome disease, which is here exactly the same that you
found at Nablous and elsewhere in Palestine, and described in your
" Pathways and Abiding Places of our Lord." This disease formerly
existed in England and France, whence it was finally extirpated by the
most severe and tyrannical regulations, such as can never be enforced in
our day and country. Every person, without exception, that was afflicted with leprosy, was brought into a public " leprosy house," and, as the
disease is not contagious but hereditary, it was thus almost, if not entirely,
rooted out of those countries. It was originally brought into France by
pilgrims, who had intermarried in Palestine ; and, in the ninth century,
it was carried into Norway, after the excursions of the Northmen into Nor-
mandy ; for these countries seem to have been more closely connected
in ancient times than in our own.

That the disease has been imported is evident, from the fact that it
chiefly exists upon the Western Coast, bordering upon the North Sea, and
extends along the whole line of it, from the Naze to the North Cape.
After more than eight centuries, however, it has begun to penetrate in-
land, by the deep fiords and gulfes which sometimes indent the Western
Coast of Norway, for a distance of between one and two hundred miles.
It is now sometimes found far in the interior, but never in the Eastern
part of this country, nor in Sweden. Iceland was entirely depopulated by
the plague, and recolonized from Norway, and there the disease exists.

The government have at length taken the matter in hand, and in addition to a " leprosy house," which has existed for five hundred years, and
now contains over five hundred and thirty-five patients, they have recently built a hospital, *the first that the world ever knew* for the cure of leprosy. It has been only three years in operation, under the management
of Dr. Daniellssen ; and this gentleman believes that he has succeeded
in curing lepers, the first that have ever been cured by medical means.
He has analyzed the blood of the diseased persons, and finds it to contain too much albumen and fibrin matter, and of course directs his efforts to the removal of the excess. He has published a scientific work,
with plates, in the French and Danish languages. The institution is well
provided with fresh and sea water, and vapor baths.

I have to-day seen a number of his patients whom he considers nearly
cured, and those who have been sent home are going on well. He estimates the whole number in Norway at three thousand, and says it is increasing, and would have been much larger but for the character of the
country. I have just travelled across Norway, and it is one great mountain or rock, with fruitful crevices rather than valleys, not *one hundredth*

part of the whole surface being under cultivation ; it is by far the most thinly inhabited country I ever visited. The people dwell so far apart, that the disease has spread itself but slowly. Yet the increase has aroused the Storthing, or Norwegian Congress, to grant 35,000 species ($37,000) toward building a third hospital in Bergen. This is a véry large sum for a country like Norway, and the results of Dr. Daniellssen's experiments are looked for with the greatest anxiety, as the disease is considered a great national calamity.

But the point to which I wish to call attention is this. In some places on the Western coast of Norway the number of lepers among the people is nearly one in fifty, and it is precisely from the Western coast *that the increasing emigration to America takes place.* Dr. Daniellssen says that he is certain that the disease will show itself among these emigrants ; for he knows leprous individuals who have gone to the United States, and one in particular, quite recently, whom he endeavored in vain to dissuade, and in whom the disease was only beginning to appear. Now, though it is never contagious, it is always, and without fail, hereditary, and if there is the least spot in either of the parents, it is absolutely certain to appear in the descendants, though, like other hereditary affections, it often passes over one generation. Owing to our larger and increasing population, it will spread much more rapidly in America, and may become a prevalent disease in our Western States. But as yet it is comparatively in our own power ; for most of the Norwegians are settled together, and almost every case might now be found.

ON THE INFLUENCE OF POSTURE IN THE TREATMENT OF EPILEPSY.

BY MARSHALL HALL, M.D., F.R.S.

We have only to raise one hand and arm high above the head, and allow the other to hang down, for a minute or two, and then bring the hands together and compare the syncopal condition of the former with the apoplectic condition of the latter, to form an idea of the influence of posture in the treatment of diseases consisting of affections of the circulation, especially that of the head.

I believe ordinary syncope may pass into fatal sinking if the raised posture be continued.

I believe that simple apoplexy may become deeper and deeper, simply from the opposite course of retaining the patient in the recumbent position.

Sleep, which is a sub-apoplexy, may pass into epilepsy or apoplexy, solely from the fact of a recumbent position. As a preventive of epilepsy and apoplexy during sleep, it is of the utmost moment that the patient should habitually repose with the head and shoulders much raised. For this purpose both bed and mattress should be raised by means of a bed chair, or triangular cushion, and the patient be prevented from gliding down in the bed by means of a firm bolster, four inches in diameter, placed under the sheet, under the front of the ischia. The trunk should be raised to an angle of 45 deg. or 50 deg.

In this manner the encephalon will be less oppressed with blood, the sleep will be lighter, the disposition to epilepsy or apoplexy will be diminished. This should be the patient's habit during the rest of life.

There are two other circumstances in which attention to posture is most important.

The *first* is the condition of the patient after certain fits of epilepsy, the respiration being impeded by rattles in the throat. The posture should be much raised ; but besides this, it should not be such that the saliva may *fall* into the fauces. The stupor and insensibility prevent the patient from swallowing. The saliva, therefore, if a just position be not adopted, accumulates and falls into the fauces, and a throat-rattle and dyspnœa, painful to witness, and dangerous to life, are the consequences. The posture of the patient should be such as to allow the saliva to flow out of the corner of the mouth. In one case such a change of posture relieved the patient immediately.

The *second* case requiring extreme attention to the posture of the patient is that of *syncopal epilepsy*, or that form of epilepsy in which there is ghastly pallor of the countenance and other signs of syncopal affection. The patient should be placed with the head *low*. If this be not done, the syncope may be speedily fatal, an event which actually occurred in an interesting case a few days only ago.

The patient was none other than Ann Ross, on whom Mr. Anderson had performed the operation of tracheotomy. Her fits had changed from those of the epilepsia *laryngea* to the abortive form. The reader may remember that the patient's age was thirty-six ; that her case was hereditary, her father having been epileptic ; and inveterate, her fits having recurred during twenty-four years ; and that she herself was thin and pallid. She was seized with syncopal epilepsy ; was laid on the bed and expected to recover as formerly ; was left ; and was at length found to have expired ! A low position and proper attention might have saved the poor creature's life.

I need scarcely observe, that what I have said of epilepsy applies to many other diseases. It is the *principle* of position which I wish to enforce ; a principle, the importance of which I believe to be still greater and still more extensive in application than is generally imagined.—*London Lancet.*

THE BOSTON MEDICAL AND SURGICAL JOURNAL.

BOSTON, FEBRUARY 9, 1853.

Institutions for Idiots.—Philanthropy never lacks for objects over which to spread its broad mantle, in Christian countries. The insane, the maimed, the halt and blind, the orphan, and decrepid age, are provided for by the broad-cast charity of the world, notwithstanding the popular doctrine that it is a hard-hearted and selfish one. But there was one neglected class, whose claims either escaped observation, or have always been unwillingly recognized, till a humble individual in the Alpine fastnesses of Switzerland, whose mind embraces thoughts as grand as the mountain scenery by which he is surrounded, developed a new idea, and idiots began to have their wrongs unfolded, their neglected condition narrated, their feeble bodies cared for, and their imperfect glimmerings of reason guided by his genius. This was but an experiment, but it is now acknowledged to have been successful, and idiots are hereafter, while civilization endures, to have their share of the world's sympathies and bounty. Dr. Guggenbuhl, of Adenburg, on the top of a vast mountain, three thousand feet above Interlaken, and under the frowning brow of the Joun Frau—a snow bank towering to the sky — is quietly carrying on the laborious occupation of developing the feeble intellect of idiots. He seeks no applause, covets no renown, and yet distant nations relate his achievements for humanity. All other schools organized for the instruction of this unfortunate class of children, either in Europe or America, are but imitations.

This brings us to the consideration of an often propounded question, what is doing in New England, or the United States in general, for idiots? Massachusetts appropriates, annually, a specific sum for carrying on a course of systematic discipline and instruction ; and New York State has organized a State Institution for the same very benevolent purpose. Beyond these, we have no knowledge of any public efforts, in this direction. There is one private asylum, under the care of Dr. Brown, at Barre, Mass., distinguished for its good order and training, at which parents and guardians may place unfortunate children of this description, with the certainty of having them kindly treated.

An important query, in connection with this subject, deserves attention. Is there any period when a pupil can leave the idiot school and return home, so elevated and instructed, that his habits of cleanliness and deportment may be considered permanently established, and a course of personal industry and propriety expected? Our own observations, made on a visit to Dr. Guggenbuhl's establishment, led us to the conclusion that in the most favorable cases, the children require the vigilant attentions of instructers, to keep them up to a point of propriety necessary to make them tolerable in a family. An institution, therefore, should rather be designed for their constant home, than as a hospital for cure or a temporary residence. No efforts, however well directed or persistent, can change the organization of the cranium, or create in the brain organs which are missing. The process of developing suspended powers is a tedious one, and the laws by which it is accomplished seem to be imperfectly known. Still, since nothing is really impossible in regard to the progress of knowledge, subsequent ages may greatly advance upon the present limited attainments of physiologists and phrenologists, in the management of idiots.

With these views, it strikes us that it would be an act of sterling benevolence, and in accordance with Christian legislation, to have State Asylums for these unfortunates. The number of idiots in Massachusetts is much larger than is generally suspected, and many of them have poor parents, who are unable to provide for their every-day necessities. A public establishment would ensure comfort and order, and some degree of moral culture, and relieve those who are not able to bear the burden of maintaining them. If the incurable insane are thus furnished a home for life, it is equally imperative that idiotic children should be looked after. A house and grounds, somewhere in the interior, would not be expensive, and the propriety of the step would hardly be questioned even by the sturdiest political grumblers in the land.

Longevity.—Some men live longer than others who are exposed to the same circle of influences, and whose bodies are nourished by the same kind of food. Neither regimen, therefore, nor the mental or physical activity of individuals, can alone very essentially modify the length of days of any one. The world abounds with persons who have battled with the elements, with poverty, hunger and oppression, and are still fighting their way in extreme old age, vigorous as ever. Donald McDonald, at the age of one hundred and seven, some years since, was sent to the House of Correction, in Boston, for being quarrelsome and a drunkard. And yet we are accustomed to speak of the hardships that abridge life. On the other hand, thousands who walk with the utmost propriety, violating neither physical nor statute laws, die long before reaching their three score and ten years. The quakers, in their extreme moderation and subjection of the passions, are selected as eminent examples of long life, the result of personal training in virtue, temperance, and honesty. But longevity is not exclusively their lot. On the deserts of Arabia, near the borders of Palestine, old, dried-up specimens of humanity are numerous, who have smoked, drank strong coffee, and played the robber, yet have passed through more than one hundred and twenty years, without a day of indisposition, without the loss of a tooth, a dimness of the eye, or an abatement, as it was said of Moses, of their natural forces. Where, then, shall the medical philosopher look for the causes of longevity, or those of premature death ?

Carpenter's Physiology.—The new and enlarged edition of this work gains upon the reader at every fresh perusal. Limited as man's acquaintance is with the laws of life, it is both gratifying and instructive to contemplate, in a work like this, the immense labor achieved, and the knowledge gained, by modern physiologists. They have narrowly studied each and every function within their ken, and so closely interpreted nature, that if they have failed on some points, in others nothing has escaped them. The nervous system is now the field for exploration. Those slender white threads, creeping along the muscles ; the spinal cord ; and, lastly, the brain, even with the flood of light that has been thrown upon its organization, still put the anatomist at defiance, and perplex the physiologist, notwithstanding the aid derived from microscopical research. Dr. Carpenter is in no way behind the age, and his book certainly embraces all that is really known as physiological truth. Rich as our libraries are in researches connected with physiology, this colossal volume from the Philadelphia press should be added.

Introduction to Clinical Medicine.—A small volume, embracing six lectures, on the method of examining patients ; percussion and auscultation ; the use of the microscope, and the diagnosis of the skin, by John Hughes Bennett, M.D. &c., Professor of the Institutes of Medicine in the University of Edinburgh, has been received direct from the Scotland publishers, Messrs. Southerland & Knox. This is the second edition, improved, which we trust will be published here, because it is precisely the kind of work to be purchased. There are some good wood engravings, which very much assist the student in his examinations and explorations. It would be an idle expenditure of time to comment on any production from the pen of a man like Dr. Bennett, whose reputation needs no props in any country where medicine is taught. When a treatise has been the subject of examination by us, we like to inform the reader where copies of it may be had, especially if it possesses the weight of character and utility which belongs to this; but, unfortunately for the profession, Dr. Bennett's work is not yet to be had in America, though it should be reprinted by some of the enterprising houses engaged in medical printing.

Medical Miscellany. — George Cleney lately died near Germantown, Ohio, at the age of 108 years and 17 days.—A new medical college edifice has been commenced at Charleston, S. C.—Dr. S. Hume, of Lancaster, Pa., who died lately, bequeathed $2000 towards erecting an asylum for the reformation of drunkards.—Louis Derby died at New Orleans, at the age of 120 years, on the 2d of Jan. He was a native of Africa.—A strange disease is reported to be doing the work of death at Galena, Illinois, and at Dubuque, Iowa.—Dr. John S. Butler, physician of the Retreat for the Insane, at Hartford Conn., sailed recently for Europe, being in ill health, and unable to attend to his official duties.—Dr. Redfield has been lecturing in New York on physiognomy, with illustrations.—According to the official returns, twenty-six hundred and fifty persons died of cholera at St. Jago, Cuba, in October, November and December last, out of a population of 30.000 to 35,000 souls. During the height of the pestilence, a terrible earthquake occurred, which destroyed many of the best buildings in the city.—The New York Tribune says that David E. Buss, the young medical student who was stabbed by his room-mate and fellow-student, Wm. Erwin, on Tuesday afternoon, still lies in a critical situation at his boarding-house. The difficulty is said to have grown out of a dispute relative to the ingredients necessary to the compounding of a certain medicine.—Dr. Geo. W. Kittredge, of N. H. is nominated for Congress in that State.— The Suffolk District Medical Society continues to meet the last Saturday of each month, in Boston, at the Masonic Temple.—The cholera was raging dreadfully at the last accounts from Persia. One thousand deaths occurred daily at Tauris.—A homœopathic hospital is to be opened in London.— The Legislature of Alabama has passed a law requiring all homœopathic practitioners of that state to possess a diploma from a homœopathic college, — or they will not be considered regulars. — The deaths in London for the week ending Dec. 11th, were 1012 — only two of them by small-pox.

MARRIED,—Samuel Fulton, M D., of Pontiac, Michigan, to Miss H. C. Fisher.

DIED,—At Astoria, N Y., Dr. Junius Smith, the first to introduce the growing of tea in America. He was a man of great energy and enterprise.—At New York, Walter Jardine, Esq., an English surgeon, by suicide, growing out of extreme poverty and destitution, 35.—Dr. Charles Chandler, of Andover. Vt., 81—At Charleston, S C., of yellow fever, Dr. John A. Cleveland. —Mr. Alex. Walker, the ingenious author of a work on the "Nervous System," and others on "Beauty," "Woman," "Intermarriage," &c., which displayed much original research, died at an advanced age at Leith, on Tuesday, December 7th.—At Old Aberdeen, Dr. Rodrick M'Leod, late one of the physicians of St. George's Hospital.

Deaths in Boston—for the week ending Saturday noon, Feb. 5th, 91 —Males, 35—females, 56. Inflammation of bowels, 3—congestion of the brain, 1—consumption, 20—convulsions, 2—croup, 4—cancer, 1—dropsy, 1—dropsy in head, 3—debility, 1—infantile diseases, 6—puerperal, 2 —erysipelas, 1—typhus fever, 1—typhoid do., 2—scarlet do., 21—hooping cough, 1—hemorrhage, 1—disease of the heart, 1—inflammation of the lungs, 7—congestion of the lungs, 1—disease of the liver, 1—marasmus. 3—old age, 2—pleurisy, 1—scrofula, 2—teething, 1—worms, 1.
Under 5 years, 44—between 5 and 20 years, 15—between 20 and 40 years, 16—between 40 and 60 years, 8—over 60 years, 8. Born in the United States, 74—Ireland, 15—British Provinces, 1—Germany, 1.

Veratrum Viride, as an Arterial Sedative. — Dr. W. C. Norwood, of Cokesbury, S. C , has been very successful in the use of the American hellebone in various affections requiring a diminution of the heart's action. Two extracts are given below, from a paper of his lately published.

"Called, in February, 1847, to see a son of Mrs. T., laboring under a violent attack of pneumonia, we put him on the use of veratrum viride every three hours. Although 12 years of age, his general slender health and deformed chest, having been severely afflicted with asthma, induced us to commence with a very small dose, that we might avoid any drastic effect of the remedy. The first portion given was two drops, to be increased one drop every portion until the slightest nausea was experienced, then to lessen or discontinue the remedy, as the case might require. On taking the third or fourth portion, Mrs. T. discovered that he was getting very pale, that the skin was cool and moist, and pain scarcely felt only on taking a full inspiration. The slowness of the pulse and the pallor and coolness of the surface alarmed her, and she sent for us. We found him pale, cool, moist, and with a pulse beating 35, full and distinct. When put on the tincture, in the morning. his pulse was 120 to 125, skin hot and dry, frequent and labored breathing, pain severe, great thirst. In the short space of twelve or fifteen hours the symptoms were subdued, and by continuing the tincture in doses of from two to three and four drops, there was no renewal of the symptoms."

"In 1850 we first entered on a trial of the tincture of veratrum viride in the treatment of typhoid fever. It was due to our patients and to justice that we should proceed with caution. We accordingly, at first, gave it in mild and moderately severe cases, avoiding its use at first in all cases of unusual severity and malignancy. We first used it in the case of a negro boy of Mrs. W., which was uncomplicated and yielded readily. When called, on the third day of the disease, the bowels had been moved sufficiently by a cathartic of calomel, followed by repeated portions of camphorated Dover's powder, without abatement of the symptoms. The skin was hot and dry, great thirst, severe pain in the forehead; the eyes dull, heavy and ecchymosed; tongue covered in the centre with a dark, thin fur, tip and edges very red and dry; pulse 127, small, soft and with quickness in the stroke. that indicated greater frequency than really existed. The patient was ordered a 6 drop dose, to be increased till nausea or vomiting occurred. By mistake the dose was not increased. After continuing the treatment twelve hours. there being no abatement in the symptoms, we were notified of the fact and wrote to increase until an impression was made, and that we would see the patient in twelve hours. During the absence of the messenger, Mrs. W. discovered that the dose was to be increased, and did so, and when this reached eight drops there was free vomiting, with a subsidence of all febrile symptoms, the severe pain in the head excepted. At the expiration of twelve hours, we found the boy with a skin cool and moist, thirst materially abated, and the pulse reduced to fifty-six beats. A blister was applied to relieve the unmitigated pain in the head, and the veratrum viride was continued four days without any return of the symptoms."—*Southern Med. Journal.*

Loose Sleeves of Ladies.—A celebrated German physician is about to publish, in Berlin, a scientific condemnation of the present loose sleeves worn by the ladies. He proves that they promote rheumatism and all kinds of complaints, and recommends a return to the long and close sleeves of a former period.

THE

BOSTON MEDICAL AND SURGICAL JOURNAL.

Vol. XLVIII.   Wednesday, February 16, 1853.   No. 3.

CLIMATE OF ITALY IN RELATION TO PULMONARY CONSUMPTION.

[Dr. T. H. Burgess is the author of a work recently published in London, on the "Climate of Italy in relation to Pulmonary Consumption, with remarks on the Influence of Foreign Climates upon Invalids." Although intended for English readers, Dr. Burgess's book relates to a subject which is full of interest to people of other countries, especially to those residing in northern climates. As regards a change of residence for consumptive patients, from New England to our own southern States, the subject has been often and ably discussed in previous volumes of this Journal; and we doubt not many of our readers would be glad to know also the opinion of competent English writers respecting a removal of the same class of invalids from England to the more sunny and genial clime of Italy. The following article on this topic constitutes a review of the work above alluded to, and is copied entire from the Edinburgh Monthly Journal of Medical Science.—Ed.]

The object Dr. Burgess has proposed to himself in this volume, is to point out, that all those places supposed to be favorable for consumptive people in Italy are in point of fact injurious; that the idea of their being beneficial is a popular delusion, and that it is much better to visit some of the sheltered places in our own country, than with a view of seeking health, really find a grave in foreign climes. He says:

"The rapid and extensive variations of temperature observed in the Italian climate—the absolute necessity to consumptive invalids of changing their place of residence as the seasons change—the fatigue, discomfort and risk, attendant upon every such change—and the mania for sight-seeing in cold churches and galleries, which no invalid can overcome, have frequently, during my sojourn in Italy, suggested to me the following reflections:—

"1. Has not Nature adapted the constitution of man to his hereditary climate?

"2. Is it consistent with Nature's laws and operations, that, a person born in England, and attacked by consumption, can be cured by a foreign climate, in every characteristic opposite to his own?

"3. Why should a warm climate be preferred to a cold one, if the temperature be equable? the mortality from consumption being less in the latter than in the former.

3

" 4. A revolution must take place in the system of every consumptive invalid who goes to Italy, before he can become acclimated ; and how many must sink under the probationary process, from fatigue and exhaustion ?

" 5. If a phthisical patient derives benefit from a foreign climate, he should never leave it ; for it is obvious, if he returns to his native climate, his constitution will be again changed or remodelled, and he is then rendered obnoxious to the same physical causes which originally produced his complaint.

" 6. The rapid variations and extensive range of temperature peculiar to warm climates greatly counterbalance their alleged good effects.

" 7. It is more in accordance with Nature's laws to believe that when *change* is necessary in cases of consumption, a modification of the climate in which the patient and his ancestors were born and reared, or, in other words, *change of air in the same climate*, by removing from one locality to another, more appropriate to the patient's condition, will effect greater good than any violent transition to warm countries."— Pp. 22–24.

In our own opinion, nothing is more difficult than for a medical man practising in this country to arrive at just notions concerning the sanative influence of a foreign climate in cases of pulmonary consumption. He may read books on the subject generally ; he may study monographs on the especial advantages of particular places, and he may further converse with sensible men who have practised there, without being in any degree more enlightened. As a general rule, every local practitioner speaks highly of the superior merits of his own place of residence. He is ready to give you a list of the most extraordinary recoveries. He instances the cases of Lord this and Lady that, who, on their arrival, were in the worst possible condition, and who, during their sojourn in his locality, even surprised *him* by their rapid recovery. In short, when listening to these accounts, we feel astonished that any case of phthisis should die, did not all such practitioners, in reply to a straightforward question, acknowledge that deaths notwithstanding were very common, and that, after all, these remarkable cases were the exception and not the rule. The real questions to be answered, in reference to the sanative influence of climate, are—1st. What is the proportion of cases in which an arrest of the disease takes place, as determined by a strict diagnosis, the stage of the disorder, and the age and general strength of the patient ? 2d. Are such arrests more frequent in foreign countries than they are at home ? So far as we are aware, no series of facts exists capable of satisfying us on these points. On the other hand, is it not certain that if a phthisical person recovers his bodily strength in Madeira or Italy, the benefit is at once ascribed to the influence of climate ; whereas, if the same thing happens at home, the case is considered one of bronchitis, or at all events its phthisical character is denied ? Yet it has of late become sufficiently evident, that, with proper care and treatment, phthisis may be arrested in this country much more frequently than was formerly supposed ; and we have no reason to believe that such arrestment is more common in Madeira, Egypt or Italy, than it is in Edinburgh or London. It may then fairly be asked —Whether the practice, which has so long prevailed, of sending consumptive patients abroad is beneficial or not? Dr. Burgess unhesitatingly pronounces in the negative, and argues as follows :—

" If we contemplate the climate theory through the appropriate medium of the natural history of creation, we shall find that the argument is also in our favor. We may seek in vain along the entire range of organized existence for an example of diseased animals being benefited by removal from a warm to a cold, or from a cold to a warm country. There appears nothing in the book of Nature so violently inconsistent. The fishes which inhabit the waters of the British Islands will not thrive in the Arctic seas, nor those of the latter in the ocean of the tropics. The birds of the primeval forests of America generally die in this country, unless reared like hot-house plants ; and so with the wild animals which live and flourish in the jungles of Asia or the scorching deserts of Africa.

" Man, although endowed in a remarkable degree, and more so than any other animal, with the faculty of enduring such unnatural transitions, nevertheless becomes sensible of their injurious results. For familiar illustrations of this influence, we have only to look to the broken-down constitutions of our Indian officers, or to the emaciated frame of the shivering Hindoo who sweeps the crossings of the streets of London. The child of the European, although born in India, must be sent home in early life to the climate of his ancestors, or to one closely resembling it, in order to escape incurable disease, if not premature death. Again, the offspring of Asiatics born in this country pine and dwindle into one or other of the twin cachexiæ—scrofula and consumption, and if the individual survives, lives in a state of passive existence, stunted in growth, and incapable of enduring fatigue. If such extreme changes of climate prove obnoxious to the health of individuals having naturally a sound constitution, how are we to expect persons in a state of organic disease to be thereby benefited? In fact, view the subject in whatever way we may, we must eventually arrive at the natural and rational conclusion, that Nature has adapted the constitution of man to the climate of his ancestors. The accident of birth does not constitute the title to any given climate. The natural climate of man is that in which not only he himself was born, but likewise his blood relations for several generations. This is his natural climate, as well in health as when his constitution is broken down by positive disease, or unhinged by long-continued neglect of the common rules of hygiene.

" *Change of air in his own climate,* or removal to one nearly approaching to it, is the natural indication, and will effect whatever good climate can effect in consumption."—Pp. 19–21.

Our own experience is on the whole hostile to the propriety of sending phthisical patients abroad in search of health. We have now met with many consumptive individuals who, so long as they remained at home, continued in a satisfactory condition, enjoyed life, and carried on their usual occupations in comfort ; but who, seized with an unconquerable desire of completely getting well, through the agency of a warm climate, have gone to Italy, and died most miserably. Such cases have been so frequent with us, as to have given rise to a feeling of great scepticism as to the utility of expatriating such persons—a feeling which would have become absolute, were it not counterbalanced by a conviction engendered by foreign travel, and dependent on what may be called personal sensation, rather than actual experience of any beneficial result obtained by others. We allude to that exhilarating feeling which the traveller experiences in the south of France, or the borders of the Mediterranean, caused by the clear atmosphere, balmy air and luxuriant landscape. He who has felt that delightful sensation, and paid attention to its influence on his own bodily powers, will not easily abandon the idea that such influence, if rightly directed to the relief of certain morbid conditions, must have some effect. We believe that such a feeling insensibly constitutes the real basis of all our belief concerning the good effects of climate; and as we still think, notwithstanding all Dr. Burgess has said, that, in certain cases, it is really beneficial, it may be worth while to inquire why it often fails, and why it sometimes succeeds.

Supposing, then, that residence or travel in certain foreign countries may be beneficial in particular cases, and the chief argument in its favor are the sensations to which we have alluded, it cannot be denied that many fallacies are liable to enter into our reasonings. For instance, it does not follow that the same elastic feeling experienced by a healthy, vigorous individual on the mountain-side, on the sea-shore, or in the beautiful valley, should be felt by a debilitated, worn-out person in a similar situation. Nor is it reasonable to suppose that the qualities of mind, power of exertion, and consciousness of bodily strength—all of which are elements in the production of the feeling alluded to—should be alike in the two cases. Hence, while some persons may be benefited, and the nutritive powers stimulated under such circumstances, others will feel languor, depression of spirits, or increased fatigue, and find themselves much worse. The difficulty, therefore, is to discriminate between these two classes of persons—a difficulty which defies all general rules, dependent as it is not only on the stage of the disease and bodily strength of the individual at the time, but also on his peculiar constitution, habits, general excitability, powers of imagination, and cultivation of mind. Hence, before sending patients abroad, all these points must be anxiously considered; and even then the whole will resolve itself into the fact, which can only be determined by experiment, whether, upon actual trial, they feel better or worse.

We believe, however, that in most cases the change is at first beneficial, and that it would be to a considerable extent permanent, were it not for another fallacy which extensively prevails. We allude to the idea that the climate itself has a sanative tendency, and that the breathing this or that air is like taking so much medicine, and ought to do good *per se*. Now it should be considered, that the best climate is only useful as a means of taking exercise, and promoting the nutritive functions, without exposure to those drawbacks which are more or less common at home. It is by regarding exercise as necessary to securing active digestion that its importance as a therapeutic agent becomes obvious in phthisis, and any locality which will enable the sensitive invalid to go out daily on foot, horseback, or in a carriage, without the chance of meeting cold winds or showers of rain, must possess an advantage over one where these occurrences are common. Now all accounts agree in representing Madeira, and some other places, as more favored in this respect than even the best localities in England—and if so, they may, in the sense referred to, be more. beneficial as places of residence.

In searching for such benefits in a foreign climate, the patient has to sacrifice the occupations he may be accustomed to at home, and the society of his friends. But if this can be done without inconvenience, and without causing mental depression or a sense of *ennui*, it may even be advantageous. Mental impressions must not be overlooked. Then he will experience a great difference between the comforts of an English residence and those in a foreign house, which, to the healthy traveller, are often annoying, and to the invalid are injurious. In Rome Dr. Burgess says the streets are built to exclude, as much as possible, the rays of the sun, and in winter are as damp and cold as rain and frost can make them. And then he adds, " What a difference between the warm carpet, the snug elbow-chair, and the blazing coal fire of an English winter evening, and the stone stair-cases, marble floors and starving casements of an Italian house !"

It is well pointed out by Dr. Burgess, that those who go to the large Italian cities are exposed to other dangers connected with the desire of seeing celebrated places, works of art, churches, vaults, &c., which induce great bodily fatigue, and often chill the body by long exposure to damp air, or from standing on cold marble floors. He says : —

" It has often occurred to me, while observing the habits of consumptive patients when in Italy, that a description of the *climate*, of old ruins, cold churches, empty palaces, long picture galleries, and other places favorable for the collection of stagnant air, but where invalids notoriously pass a great portion of their time, would be much more useful and appropriate than any elaborate account of the external or. natural climate of the country which the most minute and careful observation could afford. It matters little how pure the atmosphere may be in reality, if the air the patient breathes for so many hours each day is impregnated with noxious exhalations, as it must be in the majority of instances, while he is admiring the bronzes, pictures, and statues, of the cathedral, or trying to decipher half-worn inscriptions on the mouldering walls of some ruin or dungeon.

" The attractions of the basilica of Saint Mark, a church which has not its parallel in the world, are certainly of no ordinary kind. The mosaics, sculptures, basso-relievos, and arabesques, with which it is profusely ornamented, together with the gilded arched roofs, the pavement of jasper and porphyry, the five hundred columns of black, white and variegated marble, of bronze, alabaster, vert-antique, and serpentine, are irresistible to the foreign invalid, who soon finds his way thither. and passes hours fatiguing his frame, gazing at the marvels of the building, standing on its cold and sunken floor ; for the piles underneath have given way in many places, and hence he breathes an air damp and impure.

" The Ducal Palace, close by, has also various attractions, and.I doubt whether the masterpieces of the greatest painters Venice has pro-duced, with which the ceilings and walls of the different apartments are adorned, are so eagerly sought after as the Piombi and the Pozzi, the latter being the dungeon cells in the vaults of the Palace, over which the boats on the canal pass, and with whose history so many tales of horror are connected.   These horrible dens are still dismal and damp, although the walls are boarded to prevent the humidity from penetrating."—Pp. 106, 107.

" In the renowned capital of Tuscany, wandering amongst its splen-did, but cold and damp churches, its palaces and picture galleries, many an English invalid annually hastens his end ; and it not unfrequently happens here, as in other cities of the south, that the places most fre-quented, and possessing the greatest attractions, are of circumscribed di-mensions and badly ventilated.   For instance, visit the far-famed *Tri-buna*, of an afternoon in autumn, and there you will find, in a small octa-gon chamber, like a moderate-sized boudoir, containing the most valuable gems of antiquity, and some of the finest paintings in existence, a crowd of eager spectators, even including invalids, jostling each other from want of room, gazing for hours together upon the immortal works of art around, whilst breathing all the time a heated, confined and impure at-mosphere.   An observer will not remain long before his attention is arrested by the ominous short, dry, jerking cough, and on looking round he is sure to see the same stereotyped picture of the ' English disease,' so painfully familiar to travellers throughout Italy, supported on the arm of an attendant, staring at the marble statue ' that enchants the world,' which often seems more alive than the gazing invalid."—Pp. 134, 135.

Again he points out that in Rome—

" The rank and luxuriant grass, weeds and wild flowers—the Flora of the Coliseum—which grow in profusion all over the amphitheatre, and the moist and stagnant air of the place, combine in forming a noxious atmosphere, the evil effects of which are soon experienced by strangers, whether invalid or robust, who pass any time there.   I have frequently observed invalids wandering about this vast ruin for hours, and with the aid of a guide climbing over the different stages of the mouldering walls to catch the effect produced by the variety of views which are renewed at each arcade.   At night, and by moonlight, is the favorite time for visiting the Coliseum, in order to see the effect of light and shade, with the endless details of ruins thus shown.   No consump-tive patient who is able to drive to the spot, and to crawl over the walls, ever omits such moonlight visits !   One might suppose that an individual in bad health would choose a more cheerful scene—at least one less significant of his own condition ; but it may be, perhaps, that ruins console each other."—Pp. 175, 176.

Another evil of large continental cities consists in the attractions of fashion, so that the young can seldom resist the late evening parties, the dance or public amusements, when flushed with excitement or ex-ertion, they return to their homes late at night, exposed to the chill air, the injurious effect of which is augmented by the previous heat and foul air of crowded assemblies. All such irregularities and every kind of over-fatigue are more than enough to counterbalance the supposed good effects of climate. Hence places of quietude, offering no temptations to gaiety, and possessing only natural advantages of scenery and the gentle stimulus of a clear atmosphere, mild temperature, and cheerful society, are the best.

Another fallacy is the idea that warmth is the agent which, in such cases, does good ; and people talk of a warm climate as synonymous with a healthy climate in such cases. But unaccustomed warmth is most relaxing, and tends, instead of checking, to occasion increased development of the tubercular exudation. Nothing is more common in this country than to observe how phthisical patients get worse on the approach of sultry weather in summer, and how comparatively better they are in winter, so long as they avoid exposure to cold winds. In fact, it is not a warm climate which is sought for by the invalid, but a temperate climate during the winter, in a more southern country than England. As summer approaches, many parts of the British Isles are infinitely preferable.

It follows, from all the information we have been able to collect, that that climate is best which will enable the phthisical patient to pass a few hours every day in the open air, without exposure to cold or vicissitudes of temperature on the one hand, or excessive heat on the other. Wherever such a favored locality may be found during the winter months, its advantages should be considered as dependent on exercise, and on the stimulus given to the nutritive functions, rather than to its influence on the lungs directly. It is a matter also of great importance to remember, that the comforts of home, a well-arranged diet, general hygienic rules, and a proper treatment, are as necessary in Madeira, Italy, Spain or Egypt, as they are in Edinburgh. Lastly, we will venture to say, that the good effects of a foreign climate have been greatly exaggerated ; and to all of our readers who feel interested in the matter, we cannot do better in proof of it than recommend the perusal of Dr. Burgess's well-written and agreeable volume.

M. RICORD'S LETTERS UPON SYPHILIS.

Addressed to the Editor of L'Union Medicale—Translated from the French by D. D. SLADE, M.D., Boston, and communicated for the Boston Medical and Surgical Journal.

SEVENTEENTH LETTER.

MY DEAR FRIEND,—I think that I have done justice to the monkeys ; for the present, I shall not occupy myself any more with them. If later, it can be proved to me, that they can contract anything but what I have told you, I shall be found always ready to acknowledge it. Until then, I do not see any motives to change my opinion. In waiting, let us return to the poor human species, to whom, at the present day, no one contests the claim to the verole as an inalienable right.

However, before going farther, permit me, after all that I have said to you, and perhaps even by reason of what could be recently said, to establish the following proposition, which appears to me to be impossible to overturn :

The chancre (primary ulcer) at the period of progress or of specific *statu quo*, is the only source of the syphilitic virus (morbid inoculable poison).

I have already told you in what conditions the virulent pus ought to be, in order to act; you know, also, the conditions in which the parts ought to be, in order to undergo the action of it. Let us now study the effects of this action ; in other words, the pathogeny of the chancre. This subject is a serious one, but a little dry. I depend upon all your good will, to follow my developments. Please to look for no other interest than that of the question itself.

If we make a puncture under the epidermis, with a lancet charged with virulent pus, this puncture, which ought scarcely to bleed, soon grows red, becomes prominent, and its summit is raised up by the serosity, which soon becomes turbid in order to take on afterwards the characters of pus.

Thus, puncture, redness, papule already surrounded with an areola, vesicle, vesico-pustule, and finally pustule ; such is the series, the constant succession of phenomena produced by inoculation. All this follows without interruption, without any arrest, from one hour to the other, from one day to another ; it is a pathological riband, which is constantly unrolling in order to arrive at a regular and inevitable term, that is, to the production of a pustule of ecthyma, the most perfect, and of the best possible type.

This pustule is often depressed at its summit, even umbilicated at the point which corresponds to the puncture, and upon which we perceive most generally a little drop of dried blood. If the pustule is not broken, the pus which has formed, dries up, and gives rise to a conical, brown, greenish or blackish crust. This crust tends to increase at its base ; for it covers an ulceration, the circumference of which tends itself to increase. In this increase of the ulceration under the crust, the epidermis of the areola which surrounds it and the border, is successively raised up by the suppuration ; this latter in its turn dries, in order to form a new disk of crust, while a new areola is formed at its circumference, and so on.

Tell me, without ceremony, if I am sufficiently clear in this description ; it is of great importance to me to be well understood.

The red circle (the areola) which borders the crust, is ordinarily tumefied, and encloses it as the rim of a watch encloses the glass—only, as there is here an increasing ulceration, and always new pus produced, and as the circumference of the crust is always less hard than its centre, this crust is not generally very adherent. Sometimes the crust is formed early ; at other times the pustule remains in the purulent state during a time more or less long. This pustule sometimes does not acquire a very great volume ; often it has at its commencement only the size of a lentil ; at a later period its surface might equal that of a five-cent piece and even that of a franc ; but it is not rare to see it acquire dimensions much more considerable.

The pustule offers, then, those transitions which we observe so often in other forms, and which give to it the aspect of rupia, either before the formation of the crust or when the crust is formed. There is only here, as sometimes in rupia, a difference of volume. If we break the pustule the second or third day in those cases of quick evolution; or if we break it at a later period in the ordinary cases; or if the crust is detached, we find beneath an ulceration occupying all the thickness of the skin, perfectly rounded, with the borders cut perpendicularly, as if it had been made with a punch. The borders of this ulceration, slightly separated from the adjacent parts, tumefied, serrated, and turned back, remain surrounded by the red areola which constitutes the margin of it; they are covered by a diphtheritic layer, a special adherent pyogenic membrane. The surface of the ulceration secretes a sanious, sero-sanious pus, often reddish, and charged with organic detritus; this is the virulent inoculable pus. When we cleanse this surface, we find a diphtheritic layer more pronounced than that of the borders, and which is also constituted by a special pyogenic membrane, of a greyish color, of a lardaceous aspect, and which cannot be detached. Moreover, the bottom of the ulceration reposes upon a base more or less thick, more or less engorged, according to the progress which the ulceration is to pursue—a progress especially determined by the character of the *soil* in which the *syphilitic grain* has been sown.

The ulceration which I have just described, and which has followed an increasing progress, may arrest itself at the extent which I have already indicated, or persist a long time—a month, six weeks and more, or continue to increase in order to take on larger dimensions, and to present also important modifications.

In the numerous inoculations which I have made, things have always happened regularly, thus:—An incessant evolution starting from the puncture; constant production of an ecthyma, the ulcerating bottom of which, presents in its turn, above all, the classical and typical characteristics of the chancre; ulceration with a *tendency to increase,* or remaining in a special *statu quo.*

You already see, my friend, that the artificial inoculation overthrows all that we have been accustomed to teach and to repeat to each other for ages past; you see it break the physiologism of Broussais; you also see it reduce to its proper value the doctrine of the *physiologic contagion* of a more recent date. And first, can the theory of incubation sustain itself in presence of what inoculation produces, and of those results which you can repeat every day; for, remark, it is not a unique, exceptional fact that I relate to you, but there are masses of identical facts always giving place to the same phenomena, and of which every body has the proof in their hands.

The *electric, expansive mode* of Bru; it is no longer possible to believe that the syphilitic virus penetrates the economy like lightning, that it is a shock from the individual infecting, to the individual infected. The chancre, the primitive ulcer, is no more the result of a *shock in return.* We cannot admit, at the present day, unless we are blind, that the virulent pus traverses our tissues by a solution of continuity or other wise, in order to infect first the entire economy, to hide itself at a distance, in order to return afterwards upon its steps to *hatch* in the *nest* where it had been first placed.

Special grain, the syphilitic virus, grows where it has been sown ; *particular ferment*, it is those parts which it immediately touches that enter first into fermentation. All this takes place, as we have already said, more or less quickly, according to the disposition of the soil, according to the fermentable aptitude—but all this takes place strictly, absolutely, in a point at first very circumscribed, which we shall contrive perhaps to limit bye and bye.

The non-existence of a period of incubation, a fact so evident, so true and so logical, is not yet, however, accepted ; the contrary prejudices have been of too long standing not to have the force of law, or to be easily overthrown. Those who, notwithstanding, sustain the incubation, and who believe that the virulence of syphilis is compromised if it does not exist, have made me a primary objection ; they say to me, if you obtain instantaneous and uninterrupted effects by artificial inoculation ; if you have observed only a local evolution ; if you have been struck by an apparent silence of the organism, and if you have perceived nothing which explains a general participation in the syphilitic drama, it is because you operate upon an organism already impregnated, injected ; you inoculate patients, and those patients are already inoculated.

This objection, you see, enters into the famous theory of *virulent bottles.* I have already refuted it ; I have told you what we ought to think of this opinion as respects wounds, injuries and operations made upon syphilitic subjects. I cannot help returning to it ; permit me to refer you to what I have already stated upon this subject. But I have another answer to make to this objection, besides the experiments practised upon the patients themselves. I shall answer this by the experiments made from sick individuals to healthy ones, and I shall invoke especially the recent inoculations practised upon man upon the occasion of the inoculation of the monkeys. Well, in these cases the results of the inoculation have been identical with those which I have just described to you ; that is to say, an immediate action, an uninterrupted evolution, and production of the ecthymatous pustule.

But does artificial inoculation always give rise to this uninterrupted series of phenomena ? Are there not circumstances, in which, between the inoculation and the manifestation of the symptoms, there will be a period of rest, of sluggishness, as in the inoculation of the vaccine virus ? In the contagion by the ordinary way, does there not always seem to be a time sufficiently long between the action of the cause and the manifestation of the effects ?

Yes, without doubt, and these are the cases which can justify and legitimise in some sort the theory of incubation. But when we take the pains to examine these facts with attention, we see that they have been badly appreciated. I shall try to reduce them to their true value, and to bring them back to the laws before established.

I have already said that these cases have never happened to me, in my numerous experiments, always publicly made. This arises evidently from the uniformity of the proceedings which I have employed. My honorable colleague, M. Puche, who has experimented as much as myself, and perhaps still more, has only once or twice seen these accidents manifest themselves, at the second or third day after the puncture. All those who have studied the inoculation of syphilis, know that when it does not succeed immediately, it is because it is negative.

However, we can understand that a too superficial puncture, that the virulent pus placed upon surfaces scarcely denuded, would require a longer time in order to affect the part, and in order that the effects should be produced. Here is what I have observed upon M. Robert de Welz. A first puncture very superficial, which produced no effects the first day, so that there was something which might resemble incubation. But the second puncture, which I made myself upon him, followed the regular course. The partisans of the influence of the general state would answer me, what of that? The first puncture had a slow development, because the organism was not yet impregnated. The effects of the second puncture have been rapid, on the contrary, because then the virus had invaded the entire economy. That is very well, I shall answer, but here is something which slightly deranges this beautiful theory; it is that M. de Welz had a third puncture made, which being too superficial like the first, has given like that, only tardy results.

Here is the key to incubation, my dear friend. We understand very well, without its help, how in the contagion by the ordinary methods, virulent pus placed upon surfaces more or less denuded, and consequently fitted to receive more or less quickly the virulent action, are affected more or less quickly, and give place to a morbid action more or less rapid. We know, and observation teaches us every day, and the experiments of M. Cullerier demonstrate it in an irrefragable manner, that the virulent pus can remain in contact with healthy surfaces without altering them, and without being altered itself; but we know also that surfaces constantly bathed by the virulent pus, acrid and irritating, excoriating before being specific—we know that these surfaces end by becoming eroded, and by being placed by this pus itself in the conditions necessary to the inoculation taking effect.

This sort of vesication might require a time more or less long to be produced, before the special effects appear, and simulate incubation. For example, some virulent pus is collected in a fold of the vulva, of the vagina, of the prepuce, in the interior of a follicle; it is not till a longer or shorter period after the pus shall have been thus placed, that passing through the successive action that I have just shown, it arrives at the effects of incubation. There is nothing herein which is *plausible;* it is physical and material; it is what the observation *de visû* demonstrates every day to the eyes which know how to see. How many patients there are who think themselves at first only affected by a balano-posthitis, and in whom we see chancres produce themselves, in a longer or shorter time. Add to this the carelessness of patients, the absence of all observation of what concerns them, a circumstance so common in practice, and which causes them to take for *incu-*

bation the time which has passed between the exposure to the cause, and its apparent manifestations. Under these circumstances, you will see for the chancre, as for the blennorrhagia, the explanation of these pretended incubations of an elasticity of duration so considerable, that they vary between hours, weeks, and even months.

You see that I enter more and more into the substance of these important and grave syphilographic questions. In my next letter I shall treat of the different forms which the chancre can assume.

May your good will, and that of your honored readers, still accompany me. This is for me the most valuable encouragement.

Yours, &c.,   RICORD.

RESUSCITATION OF A DEAD CHILD..

BY M. M. RODGERS, M.D.

[Communicated for the Boston Medical and Surgical Journal.]

Two months ago I was called to attend Mrs. —— in labor, under the charge of an English midwife. Labor had been slowly progressing for twelve hours, when the expulsive power of the uterus had become exhausted. On examination, I found one leg of the child protruding from the vulva, as far as the knee ; it was cold and purple. With some difficulty I gradually returned it, found the other foot, and secured both and retained them, while I endeavored to excite expulsive pains by decoction of ergot, black pepper, friction over the abdomen and warm applications to the breasts. The pains were only slightly increased ; I however made gentle traction on the feet in concert with the feeble pains, at the same time endeavoring, but without effect, to rotate the body, so as to change the position of the head. The child was large, and pressure on the umbilical cord could not be prevented. The body was delivered, leaving the face in the sacrum and the occiput behind the pubis.

The pulsations of the cord were still regular but feeble, and soon ceased entirely. The extremities soon became cold, and afterwards the body. The head was delivered forty minutes after the body, and soon became cold. The placenta was delivered in two or three minutes after the head, and, together with the child, immersed in warm water. No animal heat remained—no pulsations, and no respiration had ever been performed. Here, then, was, to all appearance, a dead child. I resolved to make an effort, by artificial respiration, to restore vitality. I proceeded in the following manner. I first closed the nostrils with one hand, then fixed my mouth upon that of the child, and slowly filled the lungs from my own—then, with the other hand, pressed gently upon the abdomen, diaphragm and chest, so as to expel the air as much as possible. I continued in this way for half an hour, when a feeble pulsation of the heart was perceptible to the hand. The pulsations continued at the rate of eight or ten in a minute, while artificial respiration was continued, but ceased altogether soon after it was discontinued. At this point it seemed as if I was balancing the little being between life and death on my own breath, and that by an effort of my will I could send him, breathing and palpitating, into life and light, or let the vital spark go out in darkness and death. Three quarters of an hour after artificial respiration v.as commenced, a single gasping, convulsive inspiration occurred, with no signs of an expiration. Two or three minutes afterwards, another inspiration ; and in fifteen minutes they increased to three in a minute, without expiration. A slight arterial blush now appeared on the face. Inflation continued five minutes longer, when an expiration followed the inspirations. A cold douche was now applied to the body, alternately with the warm bath. Artificial respiration was continued at intervals for twenty minutes, when the respiration became regular, and the body red and warm. The child was now wrapped in warm woolen cloth ; and in one hour and a half from the commencement of the experiment, cried loudly and made strong muscular motions. It has remained well ever since.

What doses this case prove in relation to the motive power of the blood, and the vitalizing agency of oxygen ? I have given the facts of an experiment, which should be more often made in similar cases. Whatever theory such a case may sustain, if the experiment can sometimes save life, the important end is attained.

Rochester, N. Y., February, 1853.

Note.—The note regarding a specific remedy for scald head, from Dr. Rodgers, was received, and will be made use of in an appropriate manner.—Ed.

THE MOTIVE POWER OF THE CIRCULATION.

BY EMMA WILLARD.

[Communicated for the Boston Med. and Surg. Journal.]

" The new theory of the motive power of the circulation (the Willardian) though defended with much skill and talent, has, as yet, failed to be established, simply for want of sufficient evidence to prove it, or facts to demonstrate it, and is now either asleep or dead."—M. M. Frisselle, *Rockville, Conn.* (See Journal, 2d inst.)

Neither " asleep " nor " dead," is the theory of the circulation by respiration ; but it is in full, healthy and vigorous life.

Suppose that after Pythagoras had demonstrated the 47th, and pronounced the Q. E. D., his hearers had failed, audibly, to acknowledge their conviction ; would that be sufficient evidence that the theorem had failed for want of proof ? And if one of the number should afterwards adduce his own silence and that of his companions as a failure of evidence on the part of the discoverer—what then ?

The Boston Medical and Surgical Journal—to its praise be it said— has taken, on this discussion, the honorable ground of an impartial liberality. Dr. Cartwright, formerly President of the Medical Society of Mississippi, while yet a resident of Natchez, was convinced by a work on " the Motive Power," &c., that the theory it contained was true. Becoming a resident of New Orleans, he proceeded to test the theory before he made public his convictions. The great experiment followed, in which he brought an alligator to life—operating on the principles of the theory—after he had been an hour apparently dead. His announcement that the theory had hereby been proved beyond a doubt, was made in this Journal, Jan. 7th, 1852, in a letter directed to me. The letters of Dr. Dowler and Prof. Forshey, eye-witnesses, verifying the great alligator experiment, were herein published shortly after; as were from time to time long and able articles from Dr. Cartwright, throwing new light and adding new proofs; and occasionally we had aid from other quarters. Witness the decided and no non-committal letter of one of the most learned and able physicians of Pennsylvania, Dr. Hiester, of Reading. Articles have also been published in the Journal contenining both the theory and its author; which when they contained what was deemed of any weight in reference to the principles in dispute, have been answered. But whenever any article has borne the disingenuous guise of seeking to destroy the theory, while it contemptuously ignored it, such article has drawn forth no comment. The subject, with minds of the first order, is now well understood.

Meanwhile there arose last summer, in New Orleans, strong opposition to the theory, headed by two eminent physicians, Drs. Dowler and Ely. Dr. Ely wrote and published an able article against it; and Dr. Dowler had one prepared for the press to prove that the alligator might be resuscitated as well by appliances to the nerves as to the lungs. Dr. Cartwright sent to General Jackson's battle-ground and procured a live alligator, which was brought to New Orleans, making the second of that race to which science owes it, that their lives have been sacrificed. through the instrumentality of a great and generous man, to prove the truth of this theory; and in the second, as well as the first instance, the point in question was proved. Dr. Dowler and Dr. Ely, and those of the opposition, skilful as they were in whatever pertains to the nerves, could not restore vitality and circulation otherwise than by respiration. The first experiment proved that restoration from apparent death could be effected by respiration, artificial though it was; the second proved, that nothing else but respiration could effect it. Dr. Dowler could not gainsay the proof, and he suppressed his prepared essay.

But Dr. Ely's was already printed. It was much praised, and there it stood unanswered. And what then? I approach the subject with awe. Cholera prostrated his infant son, and physicians were called to his side, who in this recent contest were of his opinion. Their prescriptions failed. The child ceased to breathe; and they left the father alone with the breathless body. Prejudice now struggled with natural affection, and he said, if Dr. Cartwright resuscitated a lifeless alligator, why may not I, by the same means, resuscitate my child? He made the attempt, and the babe returned to life! And he went forth, like a nobly honest man, and proclaimed what he had effected by operating upon the principles of that theory against which he had so recently written, though erroneously as he had discovered. All these facts appear in the Boston Medical and Surgical Journal, though as they are not brought together they may have failed to make their proper impression. The case of the resuscitation of Dr. Ely's child was detailed in a letter from Dr. Cartwright to me, herein published, Sept. 1, 1852. Then as late as Oct. 6th, I replied through the Journal, and brought forward the case of Dr. Ely's child to show that what I had, in 1849, stated in my work on " Respiration," to have been effected in some of the worst cases of cholera, while the patients were yet breathing, was less incredible than this restoration by the father of his breathless child.

If any reader shall be disposed sarcastically to inquire whether, in the opening allusion to Pythagoras, is meant a reference either to myself or to Dr. Cartwright, it may be said, not necessarily to either ; for standing in idea with Dr. Ely and his child, we may say—behold ! a greater than Pythagoras is here.

THE BOSTON MEDICAL AND SURGICAL JOURNAL.

BOSTON, FEBRUARY 16, 1853.

" To the Memory of Morton." —Such is the dedicatory epigraph of a quarto volume that will attract the sympathies and stimulate the curiosity of all medical men to whom the scientific deeds of the lamented Dr. Morton are familiar. The *Prospectus* alone has reached us, but the following title promises well : — " Types of Mankind : or, Ethnological Researches, based upon the Ancient Monuments, Paintings, Sculptures, and Crania of Races, and upon their Natural, Geographical, Philological, and Biblical History. By J. C. Nott, M.D., Mobile, Alabama, and Geo. R. Gliddon, formerly U. S. Consul at Cairo." So does the proposed Introduction — "The late Samuel George Morton, M.D., President of the Academy of Natural Sciences at Philadelphia ; Author of *Crania Americana* and *Crania Ægyptiaca*, etc., etc., etc. His scientific life, with especial reference to his achievements in Anthropology — founded upon his works, correspondence and *inedited manuscripts ;* the whole of the latter, through the kindness of his family, being temporarily in the possession of the authors of the present volume."

The work will be illustrated by above two hundred wood cuts, besides some lithographic plates, and will cover the entire ground of human history, from the remotest monumental epochs to the present year : the discoveries at Memphis and Meroe, at Nineveh, Babylon, and Persepolis, no less than those on our own continent, inclusive. In size, form and style, the book will be similar to volume 1st of Smithsonian Contributions to Science ; and it is to be published in the present year at the subscription price of $5, payable on its delivery. Already, we learn from Mr. Gliddon, more than three hundred of the required four hundred signatures have been received, between N. Orleans and Boston ; and among them, a goodly number of the eminent names of our city. Messrs. W. D. Ticknor & Co. have undertaken the agency, and from them prospectuses and subscription lists can be obtained.

The object of the authors is to fill up the vacuum created in ethnological sciences through Dr. Morton's death, by supplying the great results of his studies during a quarter of a century, the publication of which his demise arrested. Dr. Nott, of Mobile, one of the most distinguished practitioners of our country, conducts the physiological, anatomical, and natural-historical departments. The monumental and archæological portions are supplied by Mr. Gliddon. We feel confidence in the men; and have no hesitation in promising to the medical profession of the United States, a performance nationally honorable, and to science in every way important. We trust that many of our readers will aid the enterprise with their names and influence.

As the work advances, the Journal will notify its progress. On its appearance, we shall discuss its merits.

Occupational Influences on Health. — Dr. Josiah Curtis, of Boston, known in connection with the able reports on births, marriages and deaths, annually published under the authority of the Commonwealth of Massachusetts, is preparing a work on the influences of occupation on health and longevity. He has the ground quite to himself, and, from his eminent qualifications and the nature of his studies of late years, a curious and useful book may reasonably be expected. The author need not pass through many streets of this compact metropolis, to discover extraordinary agents at work in shortening the days of the multitude. Fresh air, open space, and good food, are all admirable topics for philanthropists to discourse upon; but how few in cities ever obtain all of them to the extent required for the enjoyment of perfect health? Some reside in garrets, elevated but often crowded; while others wither in damp, unwholesome cellars. Some are dressed in lawn, and others in rags. Profligates break down iron constitutions by excesses, and some die by starvation. There are great extremes, also, in manufacturing establishments, in the shops of artizans, and in the close dry good stores on the lines of great town thoroughfares, producing certain effects on individuals, some of them shortening the span of human existence, but few of them contributing to its prolongation. Dr. Curtis will analyze all conditions of society in regard to health, and give us the results of his investigations.

Philosophy of Mysterious Agents.—Two numbers of the five promised to the public, on the "Philosophy of Mysterious Agents, Humane and Mundane, or the Dymanic Laws and the Relations of Man, embracing the Natural Philosophy of Phenomena styled Spiritual Manifestations," by E. C. Rogers, have been received. In giving an opinion in reference to the writings of Dr. Rogers, we must bear testimony to his profound attainments. In the labyrinths of deep psychological research, he is a match for any body. Where other men would give up in despair, he plays round like a leviathan in his native element, and sees things with a clear vision, which no one else, without his mental organization and culture, could discover. He is strong in a kind of knowledge that demands the exercise of the highest forms of intellectual endowment, and therefore is in danger of writing beyond the comprehension of those he is most desirous of instructing. It is one of the misfortunes to which great minds are incident, that they over-estimate the capacities of others; and because the world makes no progress in the particular direction they sometimes indicate, it is erroneously imputed to an unwillingness to be influenced by new truths, when the simple fact is, the lessons proposed for instruction are beyond their grasp. Now Dr. Rogers has fallen into the common mistake of men of his guage, by shooting over the heads of the people, instead of strewing the fruits of his extraordinary researches gently at their feet, where they could be picked up by only stooping. Yet we have rarely examined a more logically constructed argument, or a series of propositions so orderly. Dr. Rogers has patience, energy and reason, which is not the case with all those for whose instruction he writes. When two or three more of the proposed numbers are published, we shall return to the consideration of the subject.

Outlines of General Pathology. — Under the title of Medical Essays, most of the chapters, composing a thin octavo with the above title, appeared at intervals in the St. Louis Medical and Surgical Journal. In their present form, they appeared at St. Louis in 1851; but it may be considered fresh in this market, as we have never seen a copy till within a few weeks. The author is M. L. Linton, M.D., of the department of theory and practice in the University of St. Louis, and in every sense a venerable teacher of a science that has a high rank in the domain of human knowledge. It is difficult to say or do anything remarkable, new or strange in medicine, in these days of universal light; but it is always acceptable to have truth presented, even if heard before—and especially if, by repetition, human sufferings are abridged, and happiness promoted by it. Dr. Linton is neither behind the age, nor has he run so far in advance of other minds, as to create apprehension for the stability of favorite notions in regard to pathology. With admirable good sense, and an accurate estimate of the powers of life, he has placed himself, by this volume, in a position to be remembered with respect and thankfulness by each successive race of practitioners in the West. This treatise will be a starting point, an epoch to reckon from, in all future disquisitions in the same field of exploration. On the whole, we think his wisdom is to be applauded for writing a small instead of a large work. Knowledge in a nutshell, and especially that which refers to medicine, is decidedly popular with medical men, many of whom can only snatch, from an active practice, ten minutes a day for reading.

Diseases produced by Lead Pipes.—A report presented to the American Medical Association, by Horatio Adams, M.D., of Waltham, Mass., embraces the subject of "action of water on lead pipes, and the diseases proceeding from it." When we completed reading the report, the first thought was, that "there is death in the pot" wherever these pipes are laid. But experience in the city of Boston does not yet warrant the conclusion. The report is a full collection of illustrative cases, showing that a variety of maladies are positively produced by the action of lead—and six thousand to one might be produced, in all cities having public waterworks, to show that no injury arises from potable water running through leaden tubes. Doctors are strangely disagreeing upon this subject. We are convinced that there is truth in all the statements; but in the meanwhile, the multitude are no sufferers, and pipes remain uncleansed, however alarming the facts.

The Stethoscope and Virginia Gazette.—We gave notice, a few weeks since, of a new Medical Journal to be published at Richmond, Va. The above is the title of the monthly journal of medicine which has been issued in the same city for the last two years, the first number of the third volume being out and now lying before us.   The editor, in his " salutatory," expresses strong confidence in the continued patronage of the profession, and, to use his own words, expects to " live forever."   The Stethoscope is ably conducted, and we hope the editor will not be disappointed in his expectations.

Female Physicians.—In connection with the novelty of educating women for the profession of medicine, is that of conferring degrees on them.   One of the last official acts of the Female Medical College of Pennsylvania, was to confer the honorary degree of M.D. on Miss Harriet K. Hunt, of Boston.   This lady is no every-day body.   She demands her rights, and is determined to have them too.   While paying taxes into the treasurer's office, in this city, last season, Dr. Hunt handed over the money, under a protest that must have made the treasurer's ears tingle.   Female physicians seem to be on the increase among us, and establishing circles of good practice, in spite of the jeers, inuendoes and ridicule of us lords of creation.   Believing they have certain privileges in common with the other sex in a civilized country, they begin to knock at the doors of close medical corporations, and demand to be received as fellows in good fellowship.   They persist in the declaration that they are regulars to the letter, and the only boon they ask of the organized fraternity of physicians, is to be thus recognized—be eligible to office—and, in short, allowed to participate in the ups and downs incident to such relations.   What the medical societies and schools will do with their claims, is beginning to perplex the wise ones.   It is not a matter to be laughed down, as readily as was at first anticipated.   The serious inroads made by female physicians in obstetrical business, one of the essential branches of income to a majority of well-established practitioners, makes it natural enough to inquire what course it is best to pursue?   All the female medical colleges have charters from the same sources from which our own emanate, and the law is no respecter of persons, whether dressed in tights or bloomers, in affairs purely scientific and intellectual.   State societies doubtless have it in their power either to admit them, if they can show that they are properly educated, or reject them *sans ceremonie.*   If the institutions are closed against their admission, then the public sympathy will assuredly be a shield for their protection, and we shall be denounced as a band of jealous monopolists.   With regard to the question of what the ladies themselves claim in this matter, Miss Dr. Hunt omits no opportunity of answering it ; and those who have a curiosity to know the arguments she ingeniously advances in support of the claims of the sisterhood to a medical position, may have the whole by simply making the request.

Homœopathic Provings.—One of the new subjects with which the infinitesimal periodicals are now teeming, is presented to the world under the name of *provings.*   The articles devoted to it are stupid at best, and spun out to such extreme lengths that a very devout disciple might possibly forget the title by the time he had come to the end.   It is an ingenious method of filling up pages, but it is quite ridiculous to suppose they are read by even the most learned of the new school.   By the side of these make-weights, the wordy papers on potencies, about which the homœopathic journals have been ardently engaged, are quite in place, since one is as good as the other, and neither of them are worth the trouble of reading.

Dublin Medical Press.—The Dublin Medical Press is a small but spirit-ed quarto sheet, issued weekly, and abounding in that kind of intelligence which the profession most desire. The sayings and doings· of surgeons and physicians at hospital cliniques, and society reports, are much like the same kind of matter in the London Lancet ; but the main feature, and the one of greatest interest, is its local medical news.

What to Observe in Medical Cases. — A useful manual, this, under the auspices of the London Medical Society of Observation, and republished by Messrs. Blanchard & Lea, Philadelphia. It teaches what to observe at the bed-side, and after death. A synoptical analysis will appear when we have had time for a thorough examination of its pages.

Boylston Medical Prizes.—The committee upon the Boylston medical prize dissertations for this year have made the following awards. A first prize, to James O. Noyes, of Boston, for a dissertation on " The minute anatomy of the blood ;" a second, to Nathan P. Rice, for a dissertation on " Foreign bodies in the air passages."

Transactions of the American Medical Association—Report on Hernia. —The report of the Transactions of the Association at its last meeting has not been received at this office, although issued from the press at Phila-delphia some weeks since. Separate editions of some of the reports have come to hand from the authors, and among them that on Hernia, portions of which we intend to copy.

Medical Miscellany.—In a subscription for a new hospital, a few days since, Mr. William Astor put down his name for thirteen thousand dollars, and an anonymous subscription of ten thousand dollars was made.—Dr. Mar-shall Hall is expected to visit this country, from England.—A late steamer brings intelligence of the death of Dr. Pereria. His works on dietetics and general medicine, and his Materia Medica and Therapeutics, rank among the most valuable. — The ship Ticonderoga, from Liverpool for Australia, put into Port Philip Bay on the 3d of November, with 200 pas-sengers sick of the cholera. 120 passengers had been previously buried at sea. The Ticonderoga belongs, we believe, to New York.—Dr. John C. Warren has resigned his situation as visiting surgeon of the Massachu-setts General Hospital, having served for a period of thirty-six years. Dr. Samuel Cabot has been chosen by the Trustees to fill the vacancy.

MARRIED,—At Louisville, Ky., Dr. M. P. Breckinridge to Miss Lucy, only daughter of Col. S. H Long, U. S Army —At the Hermitage, Tenn , 25th ult., John Marshall Lawrence, M.D., to Miss Rachael, only daughter of Andrew Jackson, Esq.

DIED,—At Derry, N. H., 4th inst., Dr James Crombie, formerly of Francestown, N. H.—At Cambridge, 7th inst., Benjamin D. Bartlett, M D , 63.

Deaths in Boston—for the week ending Saturday noon, Feb. 12th, 76 —Males, 35—females, 41. Abscess, 1—accidental, 2 —apoplexy, 2—Bright's disease, 1—inflammation of bowels, 1—congestion of the brain, 1—disease of the brain, 1—consumption, 15—convulsions, 2—croup, 2—cancer, 1—dropsy, 1—dropsy in head, 4—drowned, 1—infantile diseases, 7—typhus or ship fever, 1—scarlet do., 13—gangrene, 1—homicide, 1—disease of the heart, 1—inflammation of the lungs, 6— marasmus, 3—measles, 1—purpura, 1—rheumatism, 1—teething, 3—ulcer, 1—unknown, 1.
Under 5 years, 40—between 5 and 20 years, 10—between 20 and 40 years, 12—between 40 and 60 years, 10—over 60 years, 4. Born in the United States, 54—Ireland, 20—British Provinces, 2. The above includes 6 deaths in the city institutions.

Dr. Wood's Treatment of Scarlet Fever. — By Prof. J. H. BENNETT, Edinburgh.—The most recent system of treatment which has been brought forward is that recommended by Dr. Andrew Wood ; and I notice it in deference to the great experience that gentleman has acquired from his position as physician to Heriot's Hospital and other educational establishments in this city, which have been attacked by numerous epidemics of the disease. He considers that the most efficient and safe method of treatment consists in acting powerfully on the skin, with a view of thereby assisting nature to eliminate the scarlatinal poison from the system. As ordinary diaphoretics frequently fail, he has recourse to the following method : — Several common beer bottles, containing very hot water, are placed in long worsted stockings, or long narrow flannel bags, wrung out of water as hot as can be borne. These are to be laid alongside the patient, but not in contact with the skin. One on each side, and one between the legs, will generally be sufficient ; but more may be used if deemed necessary. The patient is to lie between the blankets (the head of course being outside) during the application of the bottles, and for several hours afterwards. In the course of from ten minutes to a half an hour, the patient is thrown into a most profuse perspiration, when the stockings may be removed. In mild cases, the effect is easily kept up by means of draughts of cold water, and if necessary, by the use of two drachm doses of sp. mindereri every two hours. In severe cases, where the pulse is very rapid — the beats running into each other — where the eruption is either absent or only partial, or of a dusky purplish hue — where the surface is cold — where there is sickness or tendency to diarrhœa — where the throat is aphthous or ulcerated, and the cervical glands swollen, then he follows up the use of the vapor-bath by four or five grain doses of carbonate of ammonia, repeated every three or four hours. Should this be vomited, then brandy may be given in doses proportioned to the age of the patients. Carbonate of ammonia he considers to act beneficially : 1st, by supporting the powers of life ; 2d, by assisting the development of the eruption ; and, 3d, by acting on the skin and kidneys. Where the vapor-bath was used early in the disease, and its use continued daily, or twice or thrice a day, according to circumstances, he has found that the chance of severe sore throat was greatly obviated. In regard to supervening dropsy, he considers that, by the use of the vapor-bath, with the other necessary precautions as to exposure, diet, etc., its recurrence is rendered much more rare. In the treatment of the dropsical cases, it was also very useful, and even might be trusted to entirely in some cases. Dr. Wood also condemns all depleting treatment. and even purgatives during the first ten days, as not only not required, but positively dangerous, as tending to interfere with the development of the eruption. In the latter stages, as well as in the dropsy, however, he thinks purgatives are often beneficial.

The general plan of this treatment appears to be so far rational that its object is to hurry forward the disease by applying damp heat to the skin, and by thus assisting nature to make her operations more perfect than they might otherwise be. In other words, by rendering the febrile eruption more complete, diminish the risk of its leaving behind it a tendency to subsequent disease. Whether this plan as a whole will, in practice, prove more extensively beneficial than any other, can only be determined by an extensive trial and careful comparison of the results.—*Monthly Journal of Medical Science.*

THE

BOSTON MEDICAL AND SURGICAL JOURNAL.

VOL. XLVIII.   WEDNESDAY, FEBRUARY 23, 1853.   No. 4.

THE PHILOSOPHY OF MEDICAL SCIENCE,

Considered with special reference to Dr. Elisha Bartlett's " Essay on the Philosophy of Medical Science."

A BOYLSTON PRIZE* ESSAY, BY E. LEIGH, M.D., TOWNSEND, MASS.

> " I *fear* he has got hold of his pitcher by the *wrong* handle."
> *Altered from* J. J. BECCHER, *as quoted by* DR. BARTLETT.

[Communicated for the Boston Medical and Surgical Journal.]

WE can hardly place too high an estimate upon the value of a sound philosophy of medical science. No one will deny this statement. Even those who contend most earnestly for " observation " and the strictest adherence to facts, will give to it their full assent. Though they will have no philosophy *in* science, they will insist upon their peculiar philosophy *of* science.

Indeed it is most obvious that the very shape the science will assume in the mind of the physician, or in the treatise of the medical writer, will be conformed to his views of its true nature and proper elements; so that, to the mature scientific physician, a sound philosophy of his science is of fundamental importance.

To the student in medicine, also, it is of no less consequence. The whole character and course of his studies will be shaped by it. Indeed *some* philosophy of science, either true or false, he *will* have, for no mind can be employed in the study of science without it. And a sound philosophy he will need, and will feel the need of at the outset, if he has had any experience in the study of other sciences. He will wish to know what he has before him. He will wish to have some general idea of the ground upon which he is about to tread. He will desire to ascend some eminence from which he can take a general survey of the country he is about to explore, and learn something of its general character and prominent features, before he descends to examine it in detail. In this way he will be prepared to proceed in the right direction, to make the most rapid progress, and prosecute his investigations in the wisest and most successful manner.

The very title, therefore, of **Dr. Bartlett's** work will at once attract

* Awarded by the Committee of the Boylston Medical Society, January, 1849.

4

the attention of the scientific physician, and of the reflecting student. The volume itself he will find to be one, in which he must necessarily take a deep interest. The perusal of it cannot fail to afford him pleasure, to give him valuable instruction, and furnish him food for thought. There is a charm in the style in which it is written, a beauty and freshness about it, a clearness, precision and vigor in its language, that is truly refreshing as we turn to it from our ordinary medical reading. There is a sincerity and earnestness in the author's manner, an ardent devotion to the cause he has espoused, that at once takes captive the mind of the reader. Moreover, the error he is combating, the error of substituting mere theories, hypotheses, assumptions and speculations in the place of facts and truth, is one of the gravest character—one which has exerted a pernicious influence upon our science from the earliest ages—one which is venerable for its antiquity, and carries with it the influence of great and honored names, and still maintains a strong hold upon the minds of men, though some of its more prominent developments are of recent date, and are only looked upon with ridicule or contempt. The cause he has espoused, the cause of fact and truth against theory and false doctrines, the cause of observation against speculative fancies, of true science against science falsely so called, must ever enlist the sympathies and engage the attention of truly scientific minds. He has done his work, too, in many respects, in such a masterly manner, that we involuntarily entertain for him more than the respect which his professional standing and reputation would demand ; we feel that we are sitting at the feet of a master in science.

But with all our admiration of the author's abilities, of the vigor of thought, and beauty and freshness of style which his work exhibits, with all our sympathy with the cause he has espoused, with all our readiness to unite with him in excluding from the domain of science all speculative fancies, and unfounded assumptions, we cannot receive the philosophy he has thought necessary to adopt in order to secure this end. It is not the true philosophy which fact and reason teach.

The common idea of the philosophy of science is doubtless the true one. In accordance with this idea of it, science embraces,

I. Certain *Primary Truths*, or fundamental principles, upon which all its reasonings are based. These belong to each of the sciences in common with all the others. Two of the more important, only, need be mentioned here. One is the " principle or law of causation," that " every beginning or change of existence has a cause." The other is " the principle or law of uniformity," that " matter and mind have uniform and fixed laws," that " all the processes of nature take place in accordance with uniform and permanent laws."

II. Science embraces also certain *ascertained and classified Facts* (or, as Dr. Bartlett calls them, phenomena and their relationships), some of them ascertained by observation directly—others ascertained by reasoning from previously known facts and established principles.

III. But, above all, science embraces certain *General Ideas, Truths* and *Principles*, which the thinking, reasoning mind arrives at by studying the facts that have been ascertained and classified.

Of these threefold elements does science, absolute science, consist. Take away the first, the primary truths, and the whole fabric of science is overthrown, its observations and its reasoning are worthless, its facts and its truths are gone. Take away the second, the facts, and there are no means of arriving at its truths, the whole structure and its very materials are wanting, there is nothing to be seen but the everlasting foundations. Take away the third, the truths and ideas of science, and you leave the solid foundations, surrounded by a rich supply of well-selected and well-assorted materials; but the noble structure, the beautiful living temple of science, is not there.

The second class of these threefold elements—the facts—are often, in themselves considered, of great interest and importance. But their chief value lies in the truths and general principles to which they direct the mind, and which can be fairly deduced from them. It is in these general ideas, these scientific truths, these large and comprehensive principles, that science especially consists. Take them away, and you leave only a mere naked skeleton of material facts, beautifully formed and arranged, perhaps, but lifeless, powerless, inert. It is the mind, in the exercise of its higher powers, that gives to facts their significance, and, by working among them and upon them after they have been collected and arranged, draws forth and holds up to view those ideas, truths and principles, which constitute science in its highest and noblest sense, and make it the living, efficient, all-pervading thing it is.

But the philosophy of the work which has been referred to, in its attempt to banish theories and speculations from science, has left no place for its truths and principles; it has at once taken away the foundations and removed the superstructure, leaving only a limited collection of well-arranged, and well-classified materials. It admits into science nothing but " observed facts." No other fact however clearly proved, no idea of science however clearly discerned, no principle of science however well established, no scientific truth however well known, no doctrine however sound, can gain admittance. Nothing can enter but mere facts ; and each of these must enter by itself, through one of the five senses ; and then poor pitiable reason is allowed to look at it, see what it looks like, and put it in its place by the side of others like it—that is all ! This is absolutely all the author allows science to consist of. He makes it a mere cabinet of such dead material facts as the five senses are able to pick up on the surface of things.

Such a philosophy he never could have dreamed of, had he not been, either misled by the dogmas of the grossest materialism ; or, what is more probable, blinded by his ardor to demolish speculative theories. As it is, he has set up an hypothesis against all hypotheses ; a theory against all theories ; an assumption against all assumptions ; a mere speculation against all speculations ; a false doctrine by which to annihilate all other false doctrines. For such in reality is his philosophy ; it is hypothesis, theory, assumption, speculation, false doctrine. His leading doctrine, " that all science consists exclusively in phenomena and their relationships classified and arranged," is so far from consisting of " phenomena and their relationships," that it is not even based upon them, or deduced from them ; it is neither the result of observation nor the deduction of reason ; but is a mere assumption, a speculative doctrine contrary to both.

The term "relationship" which he uses, if understood in its widest sense, might, perhaps, include the truths and principles of science. But he does not permit us so to understand him. He is too great a master of perspicuous language for that. Indeed, for him thus to use the word, would be,.to defeat his own object, and to leavé open the very loophole for the entrance of speculative theories into science, which he is so anxious to close. But he himself tells us his meaning clearly. Throughout his work he expressly excludes all truths and principles from science, endeavoring to reduce them all to the category of *phenomena*. Besides, all his relationships are *observed* relationships ; and, as appears from his remarks upon marble (pp. 12–16), are only phenomena of a particular kind, compound phenomena—phenomena observed between related substances, such phenomena as are observed when sulphuric acid acts upon marble, or a piece of marble falls to the ground. The facts observed respecting the "sensible properties" and "intimate composition" of this substance, he calls its "phenomena ;" and the facts observed in regard to its geographical and geological distribution, and when it is brought into chemical and physical relations to other substances, he calls "relationships." Here, his phenomena are what is observed in the marble itself, when examined alone, apart from other things ; and his relationships are the phenomena observed when the marble is considered in connection with and acting upon other objects. They are, after all, only observed facts or phenomena. Indeed when speaking (p. 25) of the "phenomena or relationships" of polarized light, he makes the two words synonymous. But whatever he may mean by "relationships," he means something that is observed, and he does *not* mean any truths or principles that the mind acquires by thinking and reasoning upon and studying those facts which have been ascertained and classified. And inasmuch as all his relationships thus appear to be phenomena, and the word phenomenon in itself signifies something that appears, something that is observed—the two words, "observed," and "relationship," in his statement of his principles are superfluous, and his theory may be reduced to this simple form—"All science consists exclusively in phenomena."

But such an examination of the author's expressions is perhaps unnecessary. The language in which he states his theory is so clear, so precise, so positive, so often repeated, that it is impossible to mistake his meaning. The favoring eye of a friend, admiring his peculiar excellencies and approving his general object without strictly scrutinizing the method by which he has sought to secure it, might perhaps overlook this at first. But even that friendly eye on being directed to this point, could not fail to see it through the transparent language of the author, lying there, as it does, in all the distinctness of outline which his clear intellect has given it.

The following are some of his strong and clear statements of his theory.

After referring (page 7) to the "common feeling" that facts do not constitute the whole science, but are only the foundation—the basis—upon which it rests, or the materials of which it is constructed, he affirms, on the contrary, that "The science *is in the facts and their relationships classified and arranged, and in nothing else."* They "constitute in themselves and alone the science and the whole science to which they belong. The science, thus constituted, is, so far, complete. No process of inductive reasoning or any other reasoning, no act of the mind, can add anything to what has already been done. The only reasoning that has anything to do with the matter consists simply in the act of arranging and classifying the phenomena and their relationships, according to their differences, their resemblances, or their identity." He says of the phenomena of gravitation (p. 9), They *are* the science *in themselves, wholly and absolutely.* When all the phenomena "have been ascertained and classified, the science is complete; it is finished; there is nothing more to be done, nothing can be added to it by any subsequent process of reasoning or act of the mind."

With this language, and this theory, contrast the following language of Professor Agassiz. As the lecture* in which it occurs has never been published, this passage of the report of it has been shown to him, and has received his full assent as expressing his views. Indeed it is undoubtedly a strictly verbatim report of the words spoken by him, and it is only one instance of many in which he has expressed the same views. He says :—

"But how are we to proceed to trace a law? to investigate general views from isolated facts? It is an operation which has many and great difficulties. Trace isolated facts, and from isolated facts arrive at ideas. Derive thoughts from facts. From actual facts, from material things, derive thoughts. That is the condition; that is the aim, which we should have before our minds. Form thoughts from material facts, and form new thoughts from the combination of well-known facts, and constantly improve in our thoughts, by investigating the same long-known facts. It is not simply by adding new facts to the stock of knowledge, which we already possess, that we improve in our knowledge. From well-known facts, from generally-known facts, from facts which are known to everybody, there is new knowledge to be derived, provided we think deep enough, and we think high enough of what we see, to deduce something new from old, well-known things."

It would seem unnecessary to go further after such an expression of his views by Professor Agassiz. He tells us, not that the science is in the facts, that they constitute in themselves the whole of it, that all that reason has to do is to arrange the phenomena, that no reasoning, no act of the mind can add anything to the arranged facts; but he tells us that there are *general views* to be sought and proved by investigation, that there are *ideas* to be arrived at, that there are *thoughts* to be derived from the facts, and that this should be our great *aim*—to form *thoughts* from material facts—and to *improve* in our thoughts by investigating—that there is *new knowledge* to be derived from facts which

* Delivered before the Tremont Medical School.

have been long known and classified, by *thinking deep* and *thinking high*, and that by such thinking we may *deduce something new* from them.

Here certainly is something more than facts, and more excellent than they. Here is something of a higher nature added to the facts, by the thinking mind. Here is work, and noble work for the mind to engage in among the classified facts. This is the true view of the philosophy of science, and is one worthy of its elevated character, and of the glorious faculties of the soul which are employed upon it. The authority of Professor Agassiz upon such a question cannot be disputed. So far as authority goes, none higher can be found. We have here all that can be desired in the opinion of one who has done most for science, who has drunk most deeply of its spirit, who is most thoroughly imbued with its true philosophy.

[To be continued.]

REMOVAL OF OVARIAN TUMOR.

BY D. M'RUER, M.D., BANGOR, ME.

[Communicated for the Boston Medical and Surgical Journal.]

Mrs. Frances Rafferty, of this city, aged 28 years, of delicate frame and constitution, was delivered of her third child in the month of October, 1851, by a perfectly natural labor. About one month after her confinement, she began to complain of a severe but transient pain in the left iliac region. Upon examination of her case at that time, an unnatural fulness and tenderness was perceived, which in a few weeks presented all the features of a regularly-defined tumor. From its location and the absence of functional disturbance of any of the adjacent organs, it was diagnosed to be ovarian. The increase of the tumor from this time was rapid, so much so, that about the 20th of December, 1852, her abdomen was more distended than it had ever been during any of her pregnancies ; and as the tumor had evidently become partly fluid, it was pierced by a trocar, and eleven quarts of thick, dark-colored fluid drawn off. This afforded but temporary relief, for in less than a month her abdomen had more than regained its former size. An operation for the entire removal of the tumor was *again* proposed, and consented to by the patient and her friends, who were convinced that she could live but a short time without radical relief. So great was the pressure upon the other cavities, that the utero-rectal wall of the vagina was protruded through the *labia* to such a degree as to present a tumor as large as an infant's head.

On the 20th of January the tumor was removed through an incision extending nearly from the ensiform cartilage of the sternum to the pubis. It was found necessary, from the great bulk of the tumor, to remove its fluid contents, amounting to eleven quarts, before extracting the solid part, which was found to consist of two globular masses of scirrhus infiltrated with pus, each weighing about three pounds, and connected by a dense fibrous sac of sufficient capacity to contain the amount of fluid mentioned. The following are the weights of the whole diseased mass, as accurately as could be ascertained, for a large quantity of the fluid part escaped without being measured:—Scirrhous mass, 8 lbs.; fluid (11 qts.), 22 lbs. Total, 30 lbs. If we add to this the amount of fluid previously removed (11 quarts), making 52 lbs., it will more than equal one half of her present weight.

The tumor was attached to the body by the broad ligaments, and adhered to the omentum; much of the latter it was found necessary to cut, exposing a number of vessels which were principally secured by slender cat-gut ligatures, and the whole returned into the abdomen. Its principal attachment was pierced through its centre by a double strong silk ligature, and each half secured by itself, and the ends allowed to hang from the lower extremity of the wound.

During the operation the patient was kept under the full influence of chloroform, and she was perfectly unconscious of all the proceedings, until the wound was being closed with sutures. The operation was followed by no unpleasant symptoms, and her recovery has been steadily progressive. The wound is entirely healed, and she now sits up more than half of the day. She has a keen relish for food, and no vestige of disease apparently remains, the prolapsed parts having returned to their normal position.

The operator was ably assisted by Drs. Dickinson, Morison and Field, of this city.

February 10*th,* 1853.

CASE OF HÆMOPTYSIS.

BY I. F. GALLOUPE, M.D., LYNN, MASS.

[Communicated for the Boston Medical and Surgical Journal.]

THE subject of this case is a woman about 20 years of age; has been married a year, and is now (Dec. 5th) in the fourth month of her first pregnancy. For a year before the illness I am now going to describe, she had suffered more or less from a " hacking cough " and night sweats; was thin in flesh, and of a slender constitution.

On Sunday evening, Dec. 5th, she remarked that she felt unusually well; her cough was gone and appetite much improved. She retired to bed and went to sleep, but awoke suddenly about 12 o'clock with blood pouring in a torrent from the mouth and nostrils, and soon after began to vomit. I was called immediately, and found her laboring under great difficulty of breathing, accompanied by a loud gurgling, which could be heard distinctly at a distance of thirty feet; coughing and spitting blood incessantly. The skin was pale and cool, the countenance anxious, and the pulse fluttering. At about 1 o'clock re-action began to take place, the skin soon became hot, pulse 108 and quite full, severe headache. At 2 o'clock the dyspnœa became less, and the cough ceased altogether. The quantity of blood which had been raised was about two pints.

Monday, at 9 o'clock, A.M., the patient began to cough again with violence, and spit blood, and soon after vomited. The dyspnœa was very great. This attack lasted until about 12 o'clock, when she became easy. The quantity of blood lost was four ounces. At 6 o'clock, P.M., hemorrhage occurred again, with the same train of symptoms as before, and continued half an hour, during which time three ounces of blood were expelled. This evening the patient had two dejections from the bowels, chiefly blood. She had a comfortable night and some sleep.

Friday.—With the exception of an occasional cough, with spitting of blood, the patient has been comfortable since Monday. At 11 o'clock, A.M., the hemorrhage, with its retinue of symptoms, appear-ed again, and continued about an hour. A similar attack occurred at 2 o'clock, P.M., another at 6 o'clock, and another at 8 o'clock. During the last attack (which continued two hours) no florid blood was seen, but a large number of firm, stringy coagula, appearing as if they came from the smaller bronchi. From Monday to Friday, or during the time which the hæmoptysis was comparatively trifling, large quantities of blood were discharged from the bladder, mixed with the urine. All the urine passed during that time was bloody ; and when the patient was attacked with bleeding from the lungs again on Friday, the urine became of a pale color, and of course unmixed with blood.

Saturday the patient was comfortable through the day. She coughed about once every fifteen minutes on the average, and then raised a little florid blood. The urine was bloody ; she slept some during the follow-ing night, but towards morning the cough increased somewhat ; and af-ter raising some fresh blood, she coughed up some dark-colored coagula. The pulse ranged from 120 to 140.

Sunday.—She continued much the same as the day before, until mid-night (precisely one week from the first attack), when she had another, and (as yet) her last attack of hæmoptysis. Not much florid blood was raised at this time, but for an hour she coughed up tough coagula as fast as an attendant could pick them out of her throat with the fingers. There was great prostration—the pulse was small and intermittent, and beat 140 times per minute.

I preserved the largest coagulum that I could find. It measured four inches in length, and five lines in diameter at the large end ; it had a large number of bifid branches, the whole resembling in shape a minia-ture tree.

From this time she slowly improved until she was able to move about the house without assistance, and to ride out in pleasant weather, in which condition she remains at present.

Upon inquiry I found that the hemorrhage commenced at precisely the time the patient would have menstruated had she not been pregnant. The hemorrhage continued just a week (the length of her menstrual pe-riod) without intermission, alternately from the lungs and bladder. These facts suggest the idea that it was connected in some way with men-struation.

Another point of interest is the enormous quantity of blood lost without proving speedily fatal.

January 10*th*, 1853.

SUCCESSFUL TREATMENT OF OPIUM EATERS.

To the Editor of the Boston Medical and Surgical Journal.

Sir,—When Superintendent of the Maine Insane Hospital, a few years since, a lady, aged 58 years, came under my care on account of a confirmed habit of eating opium or its preparations. She contracted the habit six years previous, in a hospital in your State, where she was treated for insanity. It had become so confirmed, that when unable to procure the article, the whole family were annoyed by her lamentations much of the night.

She was put on such an allowance of sulph. of morphine and sulph. quiniæ in solution, as kept her quiet. The medicine was administered three times a-day. The quinine was continued without diminution for four months, and the morphine so gradually diminished as to be wholly left out at that period. The quinine was continued, in diminishing quantity, two months longer, when she ceased to take either. She remained still six months, to prevent the possibility of obtaining an opiate. She has remained well ever since, and has no wish for the medicine.

Case II.—A gentleman, aged 65 years, for ten years had had an increasing ulcer on the lower part of the right leg, with varicose veins extending to the groin. When I first saw him the ulcer occupied the whole surface of the leg for eight inches above the ankle. To mitigate his sufferings, he had used opium to such an amount that the last year three pounds of the drug were eaten. Four ounces were his allowance per month. At this time he was prostrated so as to render his recovery beyond the hope of his friends.

I advised and made the amputation of the thigh. The cure was favorable ; but the use of opium undiminished.

In consultation with the attending physician, in January, of 1852, three months after the amputation, it was agreed (the patient consenting) that sulph. of morphine, equivalent to one ounce of opium, and twenty grains of sulph. quiniæ, should be dissolved in f ℥ xss. of water, with a few drops of sulph. acid, as the allowance the first week, in half-ounce doses, three in a day. Each succeeding week, all things the same, except a very trifling diminution of the sulph. of morphine.

The entire success of the plan is shown in the following extract from a letter received two days since.

" I am the daughter of the man whose leg you amputated some more than a year since. Father's health is perfectly good ; his weight is about 200 pounds. He got through with his medicine to wean him from opium, last July. We had a pretty hard struggle at the last, but we conquered."

I am aware of the difficulty, in private practice, of insuring perseverance, but the above cases are valuable as showing what may be done. Yours, &c.

JAMES BATES.

Kendall's Mills (Me.), February, 1853.

To the Editor of the Boston Medical and Surgical Journal.

DEAR SIR,—Dyspeptic invalids often put the inquiry to you, doubtless, as they do to other physicians—" Will it do me any good to take the Oxygenated Bitters?" I propose to make a suggestion as to the class of patients who are benefited by this popular nostrum, and to state what I suppose to be the cause of its usefulness. If in doing this, I can withdraw it, even in the minds of a few, from the list of the secret agencies of hocus-pocus, and transfer it to that of comprehended therapeutic remedies, acting upon rational principles, something will be done, worth, at least, the trouble of tracing these lines.

There is a large class of dyspeptic patients who suffer greatly with depression of spirits. They generally have the dark and dingy look of the face which indicates functional derangement of the liver. They are usually emaciated, nervous, hypochondriacal, fearing consumption. They are irritable in temper, seem incapable of exerting themselves, and are exhausted by an excessive secretion of urea. The urine of such persons is always acid, and *loaded with crystals of oxalate of lime.*

I find among the numerous persons I am treating for diseases of the air-passages, that many of them suffer with depression of spirits; and these all have a deposit of oxalate of lime in the urine. This fact, which has been observed by others, has been explained by supposing that the imperfect oxygenation of carbon in inflamed respiratory organs, is vicariously effected in the capillaries of the kidneys—oxalic acid ($C_2 O_2$) instead of carbonic acid ($C O_2$) being the result.

There is another class of persons who suffer much from the oxalic diathesis. It consists of lawyers, clergymen, statesmen; and, in general, those who labor hard mentally with but little bodily exercise, and who have a great weight of care resting upon them.

The crystals of oxalate of lime are octahedral in form; and, in the field of a good microscope, are beautiful objects of inspection. To obtain them, take a portion of urina sanguinis, and let it stand till a deposit takes place. Pour off the upper portion of the urine; put a part of the remainder in a watch-glass, and gently heat it over a lamp. The heat will cause a deposit of the crystals.

The proper treatment of the form of disease here described—a treatment to which it generally yields—is the following:—A careful regulation of the diet, and out-door exercise, with the use of small doses of blue pill, and nitric acid, or nitro-hydrochloric acid (which is better), mixed with the compound infusion of gentian.

The main part of the treatment is the acid; and I am confident—though I am not aware that any chemical analysis has been made—that the " Oxygenated Bitters " are composed chiefly either of nitric acid, or nitro-hydrochloric acid in the form of aqua regia. It is this principal component, I have little doubt, which has given this nostrum its success in the form of dyspepsia here spoken of, and which has brought so many certificates to the proprietors from that class of persons, including

statesmen and others, whom I have mentioned as having oxalate of
lime in their urine.   IRA WARREN.

Winter Place, Boston, February, 1853.

PERMANENT CURE OF REDUCIBLE HERNIA.

[THE Report of a Committee of the American Medical Association,
consisting of Drs. Geo. Hayward, J. Mason Warren, and S. Parkman,
all of Boston, on the treatment of hernia, is contained in the last published Transactions of the Association. As it relates to an important
class of surgical cases, which every practitioner is liable to be called on
to treat, and coming as it does from a committee well qualified to impart information on the subject, we copy a large part of it into our
pages. After referring to the answers to their published inquiries, which
were received by them from only seven members of the profession, the
report proceeds—]

While the Committee would express their grateful acknowledgments
to the individuals who have made the communications that have just been
referred to, they at the same time do not feel that all the information
has in this way been obtained that the Association have a right to expect. They have, therefore, looked to other sources in addition, to aid
them in the preparation of their report ; and they will now state, as
briefly as they can, what has been done in relation to the radical cure of
reducible hernia, and the opinions they have formed on the subject.

It is hardly necessary to go into a detailed history of the various methods that have been employed for the last eighteen hundred years for
the permanent cure of reducible hernia. A very interesting and condensed account of them may be found in a dissertation, by Henry Bry-
ant, M.D., of Boston, on "The Radical Cure of Inguinal Hernia,"
published during the present year, and for which the Boylston Prize
was awarded to the author in the year 1847.

All the operations that have been practised for this purpose, till within the last fifty years, have been of a severe character ; some of them
dangerous, and in many instances death has been the consequence.
Cauterization, ligature, sutures, excision of a *part* or the *whole* of the
sac, and *castration,* were the principal operative methods in use for eighteen hundred years. The object of all of them was to obliterate or contract the neck of the sac, and thus prevent the protrusion of any of the
abdominal contents.

    *   *   *   *   *   *   *   *   *

The severity, danger, and frequent failure of these operations, at
length caused all of them to be abandoned ; and Mr. Lawrence said
with great justice, in his treatise on hernia, more than five-and-thirty
years ago :—" Since the enlarged state of the tendinous opening is not
removed by the processes adopted for a radical cure ; since a recurrence
of the disorder is not prevented, we may assert without hesitation that
these operations do not afford any greater chance of complete relief, than
the employment of a truss."

The Committee will next inquire whether any of the numerous methods that have from time time, since that period, been suggested and put in practice, have been attended with a greater degree of success. They will not go into a minute detail of all of them, but will present such a general view as will, they trust, make apparent the ground on which their opinions rest.

It should be remarked that none of the modern operations for the radical cure of hernia are as severe as the worst of the older ones of which we have already spoken ; though some of them, it must be admitted, are very objectionable on this account.

It should also be observed that the mere fact that so many have been suggested and tried, and that none of them have been received with a great degree of favor, or, if so, that they have not retained it for any considerable length of time, is strong presumptive evidence that there is either an inherent difficulty in the nature of the infirmity that is intended to be removed by them, or that the means of accomplishing it have not yet been discovered.

It is well known that most of these operations have been devised for the radical cure of inguinal hernia, as this is the most frequent form, and the one which is, on the whole, productive of the greatest inconvenience. The object has been to close either wholly or in part the neck of the sac, òr plug up, without contracting, the tendinous opening through which the hernia escapes. It has been attempted to accomplish both these in various ways.

In some operations that have been performed for omental hernia, whether strangulated or merely irreducible, a portion of the omentum has sometimes been left in the inguinal canal, under the belief that the adhesions which it would form with the surrounding parts would prevent any future protrusion. Several surgeons have reported cases as successfully treated in this way ; but it is not stated for how long a time the patients enjoyed this immunity, and it cannot therefore be known whether the cure was permanent.

One of the Committee is able to state a case which came under his own observation, which, in his opinion, has an important bearing on this point. A healthy young man underwent an operation for irreducible omental hernia. All the omentum beyond the external ring was cut off; the inguinal canal was plugged up by the omentum, which was closely adherent to it ; and it was remarked at the time that the patient would never probably be troubled with hernia again. Within two years of that period, he was obliged to submit to an operation for strangulated enterocele on the same side. The very circumstance that was supposed to be sufficient to relieve him permanently was probably the cause why the hernia could not be returned by taxis.

It has been attempted to close the external ring by forcing the testicle into it, and then bringing on such a degree of inflammation as would be likely to retain it there by the effusion of fibrin. Sometimes this has been done without making an incision in the integuments, and at others the testicle has previously been laid bare.

This operation is certainly not admissible. It is unsafe ; it is not probable that the testicle could be kept either at the external ring or within the inguinal canal; if it could, it would, no doubt, be a source of great inconvenience and irritation, and in addition to all this, it would not, in all probability, prevent the return of the hernia, but would, on the contrary, rather facilitate it.

It has been attempted also to close the external ring and inguinal canal by means of the hernial sac. This operation has been done by Petit and Garengeot. The sac is first exposed; a portion of it is then crowded into the inguinal canal, under the expectation that adhesions would be formed between them sufficiently strong to prevent any subsequent descent of the hernia. This method is, perhaps, less objectionable than the preceding one, on the score of danger to the patient, though by no means entirely free from it, but is not any more likely to effect a cure. There is no reason to believe that it is performed by any one at the present day.

M. Gerdy has practised an operation, which consists in crowding the integuments into the inguinal canal, and removing the cuticle from them by means of caustic alkali. This is what has been called by the French "invagination by the integuments." Some modifications of this method have been suggested by M. Leroy and M. Signorini, but from what we have been able to learn, we do not deem it of sufficient importance to give any detailed account of it.

M. Velpeau states that he performed it once unsuccessfully; that it had been done by M. Gerdy upon thirty patients; and that, though many of them seemed for a time to have been cured, a sufficiently long period had not elapsed to enable any one to speak with confidence of the ultimate result. He also adds that he had seen three of the persons who had been thus operated on, and who thought for some time after the operation that they were cured, in all of whom the trouble had returned precisely as it was before.

The truth seems to be that the adhesions which may be formed between the integuments and the interior of the canal are not very firm, and that, though they may for a time prevent the descent of the hernia, yet, as they are gradually absorbed, no resistance is at length offered to it.

M. Velpeau observes that, though it is not actually a dangerous operation, there is some risk of wounding the epigastric artery, and there is some reason, too, to fear severe phlegmonous inflammation or fatal peritonitis.

M. Belma's operation attracted for a time some degree of attention, as it was less severe than that of M. Gerdy, and would, it was at first thought, be in all probability more successful. His first method consisted in introducing a small pouch of goldbeater's skin into the upper part of the hernial sac. This was followed by an effusion of fibrin, which, he supposed, would, together with the goldbeater's skin, become organized, and the two sides of the sac being firmly glued together must necessarily prevent any subsequent protrusion of the abdominal contents.

He afterwards modified his operation, because he found that his success did not equal his expectations. This he attributed to a deficiency of inflammation; and with a view of increasing this, he introduced into the neck of the sac, as near the external ring as possible, small rolls of gelatine covered with goldbeater's skin. There is no reason to believe that the result of this proceeding was any more favorable than that of the other. The operation has fallen into disuse. M. Velpeau says that the hernia returned more frequently after it than it did after that of M. Gerdy.

Dr. Jameson, of Baltimore, has given a description of an autoplastic operation which he performed on a female for crural hernia. The Committee have not seen the original account of the case, but have derived their knowledge of it from the statements that have been made in the works of others.

The sac was laid open, and the crural ring was filled up by a portion of the integuments, which were cut into a proper form and inverted. This was confined in its situation by sutures. Adhesion is said to have taken place, and the patient was regarded as cured.

Admitting that there was no danger in the operation, it is certainly not probable that any union would take place between the integuments and the ring that would be permanent; on the contrary, it can hardly be doubted that the fibrin effused in the first instance would be gradually absorbed, and that a protrusion of some of the abdominal contents would ere long again take place.

It is believed that this operation has not been repeated; or, if it has, the result, so far as we know, has not been made public. This fact would perhaps justify the inference that the relief obtained by the patient on whom Dr. Jameson operated was not permanent; otherwise, it would be difficult to explain why a similar operation should not have been adopted in other instances.

M. Graefe has described a very barbarous mode he took to bring on inflammation in the inguinal canal, with a view to the radical cure of hernia. It has no advantage over the old and justly-reprobated operation of the excision of the sac, while it is almost as severe, and far more dangerous. It consists in laying bare the neck of the sac at the external ring, cutting it off at that place, and then introducing a piece of lint, smeared with some stimulating ointment, into the inguinal canal, carrying it up to the internal ring, or even beyond. 'One end of a piece of string is to be tied around the lint, and the other end is brought out at the wound. When suppuration is well established, the lint becomes loose and can be readily withdrawn. This is said to take place usually in three or four days, and the amount of inflammation that is induced would be sufficient, it was thought, to prevent any future descent of the hernia.

This operation has been performed, it is said, with success in a few cases; a result certainly not to be looked for, and the expectation of which would not justify any man, who had a proper regard for human life and his own reputation, to repeat it.

The introduction of a seton has been recommended as a likely means of closing the neck of the sac. It has been advised to keep it in till suppuration comes on, and then withdraw a part of the threads daily, till all of them are removed. It was supposed that in this way adhesion might be produced between the opposite sides of the sac.

It is not probable, from what we know of its effects in hydrocele, that this would succeed; and it is much more probable that it would bring on such a degree of inflammation in the peritoneum as would terminate in death. From what is known of the laws of inflammation, there is much more reason to suppose that the suppurative process rather than the adhesive would be induced by this long-continued irritation ; so that, while the patient would be exposed to great hazard, he would have but a small chance of a cure.

M. Bonnet, an eminent surgeon of Lyons, has attempted to close the neck of the sac by exciting inflammation in another way. From two or four pins, with double the number of small pieces of cork, are all the instruments that are required for his operation. The contents of the hernial sac having been returned, a pin which has been passed through one of the pieces of cork is then pushed through the integuments and the neck of the sac, as near as possible to the external ring, care being taken not to wound the spermatic cord. The pin is then brought out on the opposite side, and the point is carried through another piece of cork. Another pin is then introduced in the same way. Two are usually all that are necessary ; but occasionally one or more additional ones may be required. The point of the pin which projects from the cork is seized with a small pair of pliers, and bent over so as to bring the opposite sides. of the sac into close contact. This is done to all the pins, and this process is repeated from day to day, till it is thought a sufficient degree of inflammation is produced to cause adhesion. When this has taken place, the pins should be removed, and this is usually in from six to twelve days.

M. Mayor, of Lausanne, has modified this operation by using needles instead of pins, carrying in this way ligatures through the neck of the sac, which are afterwards tied over pieces of sponge. These can be tightened as much and as often as may be thought necessary to produce the desired effect. The number of ligatures required for this purpose must depend on the size of the hernial sac.

These operations are not attended with much danger, and are by no means difficult to perform. At the same time they offer but little prospect of a successful result. They are insufficient for the purpose for which they are intended. They do not obstruct in any degree the inguinal canal, and even when most successful, they only partially close the neck of the sac.

For these reasons, probably, if not for others, they have fallen entirely into disuse, not being resorted to even by the inventors of them.

[To be concluded next week.]

THE BOSTON MEDICAL AND SURGICAL JOURNAL.

BOSTON, FEBRUARY 23, 1853.

Comparative Anatomy.—Important as the dissection of the lower animals is to a correct knowledge of the anatomy of man, it has never been a popular branch of study in the medical schools of the United States. Natural history is a favorite with a majority of medical men, and is studied as far as their professional engagements will permit ; but it so happens that they have not added as much to the domain of knowledge in that fascinating pursuit as they might and should have accomplished, simply because the very foundation of all durable progress in that direction must consist in knowing the anatomical relations which one creature bears to another, and in this they are not generally proficients. There never was a better opportunity than at the present moment for ambitious students to rise to a lofty position as naturalists, by giving an undivided attention to comparative anatomy. An American work, the result of personal researches on our own soil, by an enthusiastic and diligent inquirer into the structure of animals, would be hailed with delight. In the medical colleges, where the demonstrations are sometimes intolerably stupid, a little variation from the hum-drum routine of a daily display of human muscles, the names of which, unfortunately, are not unfrequently represented as being quite as important as the organs themselves, by a few lessons on the organization of dogs, horses, birds, reptiles and fishes, would immensely relieve the dull tedium. But what is most needed, is a treatise, under the influence of a name that would create a little enthusiasm in a pursuit that is full of interest. The study of comparative anatomy wonderfully modifies the erroneous idea that the Creator has alone been mindful of man. True, man is the superior animal, if animal he is ; but the mechanism of an insect or an infusorial mite, too small for recognition by the unaided eye, exhibits the transcendent skill as well as care of Omnipotence, in providing for them tubes, cords, and vital apparatus, with organs of sense perhaps as keen as our own. Comparative anatomy enlarges the sphere of thought ; it cannot be otherwise in the case of one who delights in studying the beautiful forms in which life is exhibited. Further still, it humbles us, by showing our relationship to the whole chain of animal organizations, whether agreeable or repulsive, and also presents such a flood of evidence of the superintending care of God over all his works, that he must be insensible indeed, who does not adore the Being who sustains and controls the whole.

Incentives to Study.—Dr. Lawson, of the Medical College of Ohio, took for his subject, in an introductory address on opening the thirty-third annual course of medical lectures in the institution of which he is a prominent member, *the incentives, means and reward of study.* He has been too long in the field, as a writer, to be disturbed by criticisms, were any one disposed to make them ; and besides, it would require something more than ordinary critical acumen to detect a careless expression, a crude thought, an unphilosophical suggestion, or a literary mistake, in a paper from his pen. Dr. Lawson makes the feathers fly on touching homœopathy. Mysticism loses all its attractive traits under his withering stroke. The incentives to study are poetically portrayed, and are excellently well set forth.

Boston Lunatic Hospital. — On account of mislaying the report of this hospital, a word in relation to it is deferred to this late day. There are no striking features in the organization of the establishment for insane paupers, at South Boston, demanding a notice. The medical superintendent represents the necessity for further accommodations. From 1840 to 1852, 820 patients were admitted ; 584 were discharged ; 62 were more or less improved ; 266 recovered, and 244 remain. Foreigners are the principal inmates. The physician has presented a good, though brief report. In more respects than one, it is a model, and might be advantageously imitated by those indefatigable persons who, in reporting their official doings, never know when to stop.

Blanchard & Lea's Medical Catalogue.—Under the cognomen of *Medical Advertiser*, these Napoleons of publishers have distributed a list of those fine editions of theirs which we all covet. It is an interesting document, though the paper is rather coarse, and the type too fine for the fathers of physic to read, even with glasses. Why don't the booksellers affix the prices in the margin of their catalogues ? It would immensely oblige many who would become speedy customers, had they any data to proceed upon touching the cost of books. This is indeed a consideration with those who earn their money as the country practitioners do, by a course of fatigue, night and day, quite incomprehensible to city physicians in white gloves and patent leather shoes. As we are often consulted by letter writers respecting the prices of volumes, we have reason to believe it would oblige the fraternity at large, if the simple improvement of the cash prices were added to catalogues and advertisements.

Philadelphia College of Physicians. — The Quarterly Summary emanating from the respectable body above named has long been a favorite with us ; and like the Irishman who longed for an annual crop of potatoes twice a year, we wish this Quarterly were issued once a month. A leader in the last number, is a memoir of the late distinguished and extensively lamented Dr. Samuel George Morton, with a fine miniature engraving. The memoir is drawn up by the accomplished Dr. Geo. B. Wood, of Philadelphia. It is ably written, by one who ranks high as a scholar, and who was the personal friend of the deceased. It cannot be abridged, nor should it be, if it could, as the beauty of the sketch would suffer materially. Dr. Wood has a style quite his own—smooth, plain, expressive and often elegant. Of the other articles in this number, the one on yeast in diabetes possesses much interest, and we recommend it to the special reading of the profession. The disease puts almost all medication at bay ; but it is possible that a principle has been detected, in the new treatment, that may lead to very important therapeutic results. Remarks on the bites of venomous serpents, with cases, are exciting. The rapidity with which the poison is conducted from the foreign extremity of a finger to the axilla, is perfectly amazing.

Periods for Repeating Doses of Medicine.—Notwithstanding the unwillingness of one medical journalist to admit Dr. Tully's ability to produce anything good in his new Pharmacologia, we have discovered some excellent suggestions already, although the author has scarcely advanced beyond the preamble to the body of the work. On the 142d page, No. 3, Dr. Tully has taken hold of the bull by the horns, in the matter of piece-mealing doses, which is an arbitrary custom with many practitioners, without any regard to fixed laws or principles. A physician orders certain powders, for example—one of which is to be taken every three or four hours; but if he were closely questioned and compelled to assign a philosophical reason for the mechanical course so often adopted, let the malady be what it may, it would be a perplexing question to answer. The theory influencing his mind, is probably this—that the medicinal power of a dose is presumed to have been expended, or nearly so, when the next is given, and thus it is like shovelling coals under the boiler to keep the steam up to a working point. Dr. Tully remarks, that " it is to a great extent the custom among physicians to have a certain set period for the repetition of doses of almost all medicines which they employ, whatever may be the case; a period having no exact, but only an accidental reference to the duration of the effects of medicines, and the nature and character of the cases in which they are employed. The consequence of this method of practice is, that the proportion of cases of chronic disease, in which any benefit is derived from medication, is so small, that the practitioner soon becomes a perfect sceptic in regard to the medicinal efficacy of most of those remedial agents which are ordinarily employed in chronic diseases; and he therefore expunges most of them from his materia medica, or employs them as placebos merely; and he is likewise liable to become sceptical in regard to the efficacy, and, indeed, utility, of all medical treatment in any chronic case." Here is room for reflection. The timing of doses must necessarily influence the condition of the patient. Too much, too often, or an excess, growing out of the mechanical course of ordering nurses beforehand how to proceed with the pills, decoctions and drops, involves consequences of the highest import. The success of treatment may be vastly more influenced by watching the pulse, than in numbering hours on the dial. Dr. Tully has made a suggestion that will perhaps considerably agitate medical circles hereafter.

Professorial Qualifications. —On the 175th page of the Pharmacology, the author asserts that he has repeatedly known literary and scientific men, who had never read a page of medicine, make application to the non-medical corporations of our colleges for medical professorships, apparently without the least consciousness that they could not fill them as well as the best practical physicians. He further observes, "I have been informed that the department of materia medica was taught in this way in one of our colleges, for a considerable time. With such instructers, Flower's advertisement of his Mississippi Fever Tonic, and Kendall & Co.'s advertisement of Electrical Febrifuge, or Speed's Fever Tonic, would be as high authority as Pereira, Stephenson and Churchill, Woodville, Cullen or Louis." Strange revolutions await a coming age, explanatory of the manner in which certain great men became great—not through their intellectual acquirements, but by the easier process of having friends at court.

Female Medical College of Pennsylvania.—The following is a list of the graduates of this College at the Commencement, Jan. 27, 1853, with the subjects of their theses :

Hannah W. Ellis, Philadelphia, Parturition. Henrietta W. Johnson, New York city, Functions of the Skin. Annan N. S. Anderson, Bristol, Pa., General Physiology. Charlotte G. Adams, Boston, Mass., De Effectis Lactationis Nimia. Julia A. Beverly, Providence, R. I., Ferrum. Margaret Richardson, Philadelphia, Phthisis Pulmonalis. Almira L. Fowler, New York city, Relations of Body and Mind. Maria Minnis, New York, Medical Jurisprudence. Augusta R. Montgomery, New York, Medical Education of Women.

American Medical Society.—Under the General Act of the State of N. York of 1848, the American Medical Society has just been chartered in the City of New York, with authority to establish a National College, National Hospital, Library, and an Anatomical Museum. The following gentlemen have been elected as officers for the present year : President, Wooster Beach, M.D. ; 1st Vice President, Wm. Turner, M.D. ; 2d Vice President, J. L. Van Doren, M.D. ; Recording Secretary, E. Whitney, M.D. ; Corresponding Secretary, J. Coleman, M.D. ; Treasurer, J. D. L. Zender, M.D.

It is evident enough, from an examination of the foregoing names, what the character of the institution will be. A charter was by no means necessary.

Medical Miscellany.—A compound solar microscope has recently been commenced in the city of New York, by Professor J. Hinds, formerly of Salem, N. Y., capable of magnifying objects 17,450,000 times. — M. Reybard has taken the Argenteuil prize for a treatise on the most practically useful improvements in the treatment of urinary diseases ; which prize, by the accumulation of an ancient fund, in 1852 was £480.—Inoculation for syphilis, a most insane idea, has been denounced in Paris by the Academy. — Health insurance companies, which were exceedingly active hereabouts a year ago, have finally all disappeared. The public discovered that the managers and officers were sure of their salaries.—Suicides are increasing in France. Those in fear of the attentions of the government, pop out of the way of the police without apology.—The second number of Dr. Griswold's Esculapian is published.—Fifty arguments in favor of sustaining and enforcing the Massachusetts Anti-Liquor Law, by Rev. Rufus W. Clark, are widely circulated. He says, from estimates carefully made, there are 400.000 drunkards in the United States, who, with the moderate drinkers, pour down their throats 60,000,000 gallons of ardent spirits annually !

To CORRESPONDENTS.— A paper on the treatment of Uterine Displacements at the South, and a notice of the death of the late Dr. Colby, of New Hampshire, have been received.

DIED,—At Princeton, Dr. Warren Partridge, 55.—At Guilford, Maryland, Dr. Benj. Gale, 102. In Paris, Dr. Baird, by suicide. — In the interior of Australia, Dr. Leichardt, the celebrated traveller, murdered by the natives.

Deaths in Boston—for the week ending Saturday noon, Feb. 19th, 78 —Males. 36—females, 42. Accidental, 1—inflammation of the bowels, 3—congestion of the brain, 1—consumption, 20 —convulsions, 1—croup, 7—dropsy in the head, 2—infantile diseases,5—puerperal, 1—epilepsy, 1 —erysipelas, 1—fever, 3—typhus fever, 1—scarlet do., 7—hooping cough, 5—hemorrhage, 1— homicide, 1—inflammation, 1—intemperance, 1—influenza, 1 — inflammation of the lungs, 3— marasmus, 3—old age, 1—pleurisy, 1— rheumatism, 1—teething, 3—tumor, 1—ulcer, 1.

Under 5 years, 36—between 5 and 20 years, 7—between 20 and 40 years, 17—between 40 and 60 years, 12—over 60 years, 6. Born in the United States, 57 — Ireland, 19 — Germany, 2. The above includes 3 deaths in the city institutions.

Opium Eating.—Dr. D. J. McGowan, of the Hospital at Ningpo, China, in his report for 1852, writes as follows respecting the treatment of that class of persons who have been so unfortunate as to contract the habit of taking opium to excess. A report of the treatment of similar cases will be found in to-day's Journal, communicated by Dr. Bates, of Maine.

" The most interesting part of my labors in a moral, if not professional point of view, has been the treatment of opium patients, several hundreds of whom are living witnesses to the success of the means employed for their relief. Not a few of these are of several years standing ; men too, who are occupied all day in labor requiring great muscular activity, and from whom every vestige of the characteristic features of the opium victim has been effaced. Some, whose vital powers were nearly exhausted, are now stalwart chair-bearers, disenthralled from the deadly vice, and once more in the enjoyment of existence. This success has been mainly owing to the stringent conditions with which they are made to comply in order to their reception as patients. Only the most resolute, or those who, impoverished by the expensive vice, are outcasts, and destitute alike of means of procuring the drug, and even the necessaries of life ; persons who have no other resource, and to whom existence is a burden, are found willing to submit to the ordeal. No opiate is ever administered to assuage the agony which the immediate and total deprivation of the charming stimulus occasions, except Dover's powder, which is given to check the wasting diarrhœa, an inevitable sequence of absence from opium in the habitual smoker. The agony of the poor creatures is indescribable ; yet animated by hope on one side, and terrified at the prospect of an early and miserable death on the other, a majority of them endure it all, until a natural appetite for wholesome nourishment is excited, when they may be considered safe. During this period they are sustained by various stimulants. It is quite possible to effect the cure of an opium-smoker by administering opiates in doses gradually reduced, which is the method pursued by native practitioners ; but persons who have been relieved of the habit in this manner, are prone to relapse, making their condition more hopeless than ever."

Tenacity of Life. — On Monday, Jan. 17th, at Wells, Me., a farmer slipped from his hay mow into the barn floor, and in his descent fell upon the point of a hay puller, which entered his abdomen and passed through his back. Thus impaled on a wooden stake, the sufferer lay on the floor in agony which may be imagined, but not described, for about an hour. He was then removed, as soon as discovered, to his house ; and two neighbors went on the railroad in a hand car to South Berwick, nine miles, and returned with Dr. Trafton, of that village, who was obliged to cut and make incisions in the sufferer (who is a fleshy man, weighing about two hundred pounds) to the extent of six inches, before the rude instrument could be extracted from his body. He accomplished it, however, and dressed his wounds ; and on Tuesday morning, the patient was quite comfortable.

Boletus Laricis, or White Agaric, as a Purgative.—Dr. Wm. M. Mc-Pheeters has tried some experiments with the Boletus Laricis, which, though notnumerous enough to determine its value as a cathartic, are sufficient to justify more extended experiments. The Boletus Laricis grows abundantly in the Rocky Mountains. It is a fungus on the white pine of that region.—*St. Louis Med. and Surg. Journal.*

THE

BOSTON MEDICAL AND SURGICAL JOURNAL.

VOL. XLVIII.　　　WEDNESDAY, MARCH 2, 1853.　　　No. 5.

THE PHILOSOPHY OF MEDICAL SCIENCE.

BY E. LEIGH, M.D., TOWNSEND, MASS.

[Continued from page 74.]

BUT let us examine some points in Dr. Bartlett's theory more in detail.

I. As already noticed, it excludes from science all its fundamental principles, or primary truths. There can be no doubt that he excludes them.
They are not phenomena, they are not even generalized phenomena;
nay, more, they are not even the deductions of reason from ascertained phenomena. They are primary truths lying at the foundation of all reasoning and observation. They are truths discerned by the mind in the exercise of its higher powers of " original suggestion," as Reid, Stewart,
Brown, and some of our most distinguished American philosophers, express it; or of the " pure reason," as Kant, Cousin, and the Continental
philosophers generally, and Coleridge, and some American philosophers,
express it. Cudworth and Locke expressed the same view, in other words,
though it is not in accordance with the leading views of Locke's philosophy. However much philosophers may differ on other points, whatever obscurity and mist may hang over other parts of their philosophy,
however wild many of their speculations may be; on this point, viz.,
that these " primary truths," together with certain " primitive ideas,"
are not observed by the senses, and are not deduced by the reasoning
power, but are directly discerned by the mind in the use of an intellectual vision which it has for such truth, in the exercise of its higher
power of intuitive perception, or original suggestion—that the pure reason has an eye that can see them directly, the moment they are brought
within the range of its vision—on *this* point they are all agreed, they
are all clear and definite in their statements, and their views receive the
ready assent of sound, thinking minds. It is only such philosophers as
Hobbes, Hume, Gassendi, Mill and Compte, and Condillac, who hold a
contrary opinion. Now all such primary truths, which are not observed
phenomena, which are not phenomena in any sense, are, of course, excluded from science by Dr. Bartlett's theory.

But, inasmuch as he has referred to some of these truths (pp. 26 and
79), to the principle that " every change has a cause " ; that everything
peculiar in the cause involves a corresponding peculiarity in the effect;
that everything peculiar in the effect, implies a corresponding pecu-

5

liarity in the cause ; and that the phenomena and processes of nature are uniform and invariable ; since he has referred to these fundamental principles, and admitted them as " universal and necessary,"* and seems to regard them as antecedent to science and essential to it, but not included in it, we will not dispute this point with him.   If he chooses to use the term " science " in a more limited sense, as embracing only the phenomena observed, and the facts and truths and ideas arrived at by the thinking, reasoning mind, by the aid of these phenomena, and these primary truths, so be it.

Still, these fundamental principles, being essential to science, being inseparably connected with all its observations and all its reasoning, it would seem most fitting, in a broad and comprehensive view of the philosophy of science, to include them among its proper and essential elements, as elements so essential, that without them science could not exist. Geometry does not discard its axioms, why then should the science of life discard its fundamental principles.

But we cannot consent to go farther, and limit science to mere phenomena, banishing all facts proved by reasoning, and all the ideas, truths and principles which constitute its higher elements.

This leads to the second point, that

II. Dr. Bartlett's theory excludes all those facts which are not observed directly, but are proved and conclusively proved by reasoning ; and moreover leaves no room for the employment of the reasoning faculty.

This lies on the very face of his theory, being one of its principal features.   He maintains expressly that no fact in science can be proved by reasoning, but must be observed by itself if known at all.   His proposition is, that " these facts, phenomena and events, with their relations, can be ascertained only in one way, and that is, by observation, or experience.   They cannot be deduced or inferred from any other facts, phenomena, events or relationships, by any process of reasoning, independent of observation or experience."   He says, again (p. 17), " Each distinct and peculiar relationship can be ascertained in one only way, by one only method, that of observation of the relationship itself."   In other places (pp. 10, 75, 76), he maintains, that " Each separate class or series of phenomena or relationship must be observed by itself," " that a knowledge of one class cannot be deduced or inferred from the knowledge of any other class, by any process of reasoning."

Now there can be no doubt that there are some facts which cannot be proved by certain other particular facts.   He has cited a large number of such instances.   And this is the only proof he has brought, of the correctness of this part of his theory.   He has shown conclusively that

---

* His remark in this connection (p. 27), that " all exceptions to this invariableness and uniformity are apparent only, and not real," is a very just one.   But his subsequent remark, " that the old saying, so constantly and blindly repeated, ' that the exception proves the rule,' is as destitute of truth as it is of meaning," is *not* just.   The " exception," though only apparent, does prove the rule.   Did not the rule exist, the exception would never be made, would never be thought of.   Were there no true coin, there never would be counterfeits.   Counterfeits prove the existence of true coin.   Exceptions (though apparent only) prove the rule.   Viewed in this, its true light, the old proverb is full of significance.

some facts cannot be proved from *some* other facts (as, for instance, that the structure of the heart does not show the nature of the blood (p. 81 at bottom) ; and that is all he has shown.

But in the preceding and in many similar statements of his theory on this point, he means more than this, though he has proved no more.

He starts with the idea, that there are certain classes or series of things so like each other, that in observing one or one hundred of them, you actually observe the whole series at once ; that each and all the individual facts in the series are observed in a lump in that one observation. Exactly as certain theologians are supposed to have believed, and perhaps some of them did believe, that each and all the individuals of the human race sinned together in that one sin of Adam. The cases are exactly parallel on the point in question, and one is just about as true as the other. However, assuming this idea (for it is a mere assumption), our author is able to bend the facts of nature to his theory, by which, in order to exclude speculation, he would exclude all reasoning from science, and allow the mind only to observe phenomena, to see their resemblances, and differences, and put those which are alike together in proper order, in all which no true process of reasoning is involved. He does not take the true view of the case, that by means of a certain number of classified phenomena, the human mind in the exercise of its reasoning faculty, and by a genuine process of reasoning—of true inductive reasoning, from particulars to the general truth—is enabled to ascend from the material facts to the truth, the general truth implied in those facts and proved by them, though it embraces all other similar facts which are yet unobserved ; and then, from this general truth thus proved by reasoning, the mind descends again by a genuine process of reasoning, though in a reverse direction, from the general truth to the particular fact, and can arrive at any one of the facts coming under that general truth, if necessary. Such a fact thus known, is a proved fact, not an observed one, and this is the character of the body of facts known to science ; it is comparatively very few of them that have been observed—or rather, science chiefly consists in the general truths, which have been proved, and are ready to be applied to any particular fact when needed.

Instead of taking this correct view of the case our author has chosen, in consistency with his theory of " observation," to scatter to the winds all these reasoning processes and their results, to banish from science those truths and principles in which its glory and life and power and practical value consist, and reduce the whole to an act of observation, an act of seeing a whole class of facts at once, while looking at one of them. But this idea is an absurd one. We may indeed know a particular fact on finding it to be a logical consequence of a general truth proved from some other fact ; but we do not observe the one in the other. Just as a man (to extend our theological illustration) may commit sin in consequence of a general course of things, resulting from a previous sin of another person, as of Adam ; but he does not sin in the sin of that person, he must sin himself if he sin at all. And a phenomenon must be observed itself, if it be observed at all.

The facts, however, that we are now considering, are not observed in any way ; they are proved by a regular course of reasoning, and in every case the mind must pass through this course of reasoning, even though it dart through it with the rapidity of the lightning's flash.   Genius, even, is not freed from this law.   Goethe and Newton were obliged to arrive at truth by this method.   A single fact, it is true, was sufficient for them, where a hundred would be needed by a common mind.   With the keen eye of genius they were able to discern the truth when millions of facts had not revealed it to inferior minds.   And probably they arrived at it in a moment.   The reasoning process was gone through by their minds in an instant, though for the first time, as rapidly and with as great facility as the mind of the most rapid pianist passes through its processes after having gone over them a thousand times.   When Newton saw the apple fall, when Goethe saw the vertebrate form in the skull of the deer—the law of gravitation, and the law of the structure of vertebrated animals, may have flashed into their minds in an instant. But the law of uniformity was the conductor by which the electric truth entered.   There is a powerful attraction between such minds and truth ; but the dazzling splendor of its instantaneous and brilliant results, should not blind our eyes to the mode in which the results are obtained. Their minds must move along the road which God has created for every mind to move in.   They must pass through the inductive process, they must go in the path through which the law of uniformity leads them. The same process which other minds have gone through, to confirm their results, that same process their minds went through when they first attained them.   The truth was then proved to their minds by reasoning, though even *they* did not dare to place it in the temple of science, till they had confirmed their result by many and varied repetitions of the same reasoning process.   And they having led the way, thousands' of minds have followed in their footsteps, each for itself verifying their results.

But to return to the theory of our author.   While he, in his peculiar way, admits that all the facts of any one class may be ascertained, from the actual observation of a few of them, he denies that the facts of any other class can be thus ascertained without being specially observed by themselves.   " Each class of phenomena can be ascertained only by direct observation of the phenomena themselves."   Physiology cannot be deduced from anatomy—nor can pathology be deduced from physiology —nor can we ascend thence to therapeutics.   Each class of facts must be observed by itself.   Nay, each particular species of facts in each of these several departments must be observed separately.   When we get down to those lower classes, those particular species of facts which are so exactly alike, that in seeing one we see all, something may be done. But above this, our previous observation is of no avail in aiding us to arrive at any knowledge of facts which have not yet come under our eye. ·

But, while each particular species of fact has its peculiarities, are there not also resemblances between the different species which enable us to arrange them in various genera ? and these genera again, in various orders ? and so on up to wider, more general, more comprehensive divisions? And is not here a sufficient foundation for reasoning from one class to another? Are there not also relations of cause and effect which enable us to reason in another way from one class to another?

It is not denied that there must be special observations in each department of our science, and in each class of facts, some to confirm the results of our reasoning (which must always be done where it is possible), and others to ascertain facts that reasoning cannot reach. Each class of facts has its peculiarities which require separate observation, unless we can reach them by reasoning from cause to effect, and *vice versa*. But there are such relations between the different classes of facts, and between the several departments of our science, that our knowledge of one department is in a great degree dependent upon our knowledge of the others, and much of our knowledge could never be attained in any other way. It is useless to follow our author through his long array of facts and argument on this point. It does not reach the question. Because some things cannot be proved from a particular class of facts, it does not follow that nothing can be proved from it. It is also useless to cite many instances. They are innumerable, and only a few obvious ones need be alluded to. Any one who has read the late investigations into the minute structure of the kidneys—of the manner, for instance, in which the tubuli uriniferæ and the bloodvessels come together in those wonderful corpuscles of Malpighi, should be slow to admit that nothing has been thereby added to our knowledge of the functions of that organ, even though the precise mode in which urine is secreted there, and the reason why urine rather than bile or any other fluid is secreted, is not known, and very likely never will be. But setting *this* aside, does our knowledge of the function of the kidney in no measure depend upon our knowledge of its anatomical relations? and upon its similarity in structure to other secreting organs? Take this anatomical knowledge away from us, and what should we know of the functions of this organ? By the aid of these anatomical facts we know that it *must* be the organ that secretes urine, and not the bladder or the ureters, or the supra-renal capsules. By reasoning from these facts, we know that the urine must be secreted in the kidney; but we never caught that organ in the act. No eye ever saw it in the exercise of its function. The well-known fact in regard to the proper function of this organ is a proved fact, and not an observed fact. The same is true of other organs. Even where we can see an organ in the exercise of its peculiar function, it is probable that our knowledge of it depends chiefly upon reasoning from its anatomical structure and relations. We know more and understand more of the function of the heart from our knowledge of its anatomy, than we do from its thumping against the walls of the chest, from the beating of the pulse, or the spouting of the divided arteries. And even those of us who have looked upon its curious movement, as seen in the opened thorax of a living animal, know very little more of its function than those who never saw it. Though, as our author says, the structure of the heart throws no light upon the nature of the blood, it does throw a flood of light upon the character and mode of its own function.   But perhaps we get a little light respecting the functions of the blood, from another source, from its own structure or constitution as revealed by the microscope and by chemical reägents.

Not to enter further into particulars, what should we know of the functions of the vesiculæ seminales, of the olfactory lobes, of the different parts of the internal ear, of the corpora quadrigemina, indeed of almost every organ or part of an organ in the body, if our knowledge of their anatomical structure and relations were taken from us.   Is it not true that a large portion of the whole circle of our physiological knowledge is more or less dependent upon anatomy and reasoning, instead of being, as our author maintains, absolutely and entirely independent of both.   He has taken the wrong view of the matter, he has " got hold of his pitcher by the wrong handle."   In regard to therapeutics, it would be easy to show that the treatment of disease by our wisest and best physicians depends in a very great measure upon reasoning from cause to effect.   There is very little specific treatment in the whole round of practice.

With reference to his exclusion of reasoning from science, it may be asked, what becomes of the method of reasoning by exclusion, by which we ascertain the character of a particular tumor, for example, by determining that it is not this, or that, or the other kind, thus excluding, one after another, the various forms of this disease, till we get to the right one, and thence arrive at the conclusion that it must be that particular form of tumor, because it can be no other.   This is legitimate reasoning, and is in constant use.   But is the fact thus arrived at, an *observed* fact ?   If so, it must be observed by *not observing !*—" *lucus a non lucendo.*"

It will be noticed that (pp. 79 and 87) the author has felt obliged to refer to the aid we derive in science from the " law of uniformity," and the " law of causation."   But in doing this, he does not modify his theory, or recede from his position, " that the only reasoning there is in science consists simply in the act of arranging and classifying."   This is strange enough.   Will the author tell us what process of reasoning there is that does not consist in the application of such laws as these, or some modification of them, to the facts of science ?   He has thus unintentionally, and contrary to his theory, admitted into science all the known processes of reasoning.

Let the mind take these laws and with them walk forth among the facts of science, and it will have work enough to do, and room enough and opportunity enough for the full exercise of all its reasoning powers. The author has admitted here all that could be asked, if he will only carry out his admissions to their full extent, and modify or remodel his philosophy so as to give reason its full scope and proper place in science, and allow it to bring with it all those facts, truths, and principles, which cannot be observed, though they can be most conclusively proved.   Of the power of reasoning, it has been well said that it " appears to have been given us in compassion to our weakness, that we may acquire knowledge which otherwise would not be within our reach.   It brings to light the great principles and hidden truths of nature, it gives grand and comprehensive views which could not otherwise be obtained, and invests men and external things and events, in their origin and in their consequences, with a new character."

[To be continued.]

M. RICORD'S LETTERS UPON SYPHILIS.

Addressed to the Editor of L'Union Medicale—Translated from the French by D. D. Slade, M.D., Boston, and communicated for the Boston Medical and Surgical Journal.

EIGHTEENTH LETTER.

My Dear Friend,—In the positive inoculations, things always occur as I have told you in my last letter. When the inoculation fails, the puncture becomes a little irritated, but this soon disappears.

However, without depriving inoculation of anything which is established, we must recognize that there is for syphilis, as for the variola, and for vaccine, *false pustules*. Their existence, if the examination is superficial, might lead to error. My learned colleague M. Puche, confesses now, with a good grace, that he has been thus deceived by *false pustules*, when he formerly practised inoculations with muco-pus furnished by balano-posthitis. Thus, he does not attach to-day the same value as formerly, to the facts contained in the *memoiré* which he has published upon this subject ; he has studied these facts better, and they have for him changed their signification. You ought to understand that I should not have committed the impropriety of speaking thus, if I was not formally authorized by M. Puche himself. My critics, then, who have made much ado about the inoculations of the muco-pus, of the balano-posthitis non-ulcerated ; who have made use of them as a weapon against my doctrines ; who wish to prove by them that the chancre alone does not furnish inoculable pus, and that the blennorrhagia which is inoculated could not well be ulcerous—these critics can no longer make use of this argument without the new verification which its author believes indispensable. These false pustules are but little developed ; most commonly they are only simple bullous elevations, beneath which, we find a superficial vesication of the skin. Here, there is not that boring of the skin, as if done by a punch, like what is observed in true inoculation. In some very rare cases, deeper inflammation might appear and produce something analogous to the furuncle. But even in these cases, the progress is always very rapid, the duration slight, from three to five or six days at most, and the healing follows also very quickly without the intervention of any treatment.

However it may be, I have said, and I persist in saying, that when the inoculation has succeeded, it is always by a pustule that the chancre commences ; this is what is incontestable, and which can be re-produced at will and with certainty.

However, the writers upon syphilis, who have ranged among the primitive accidents so many phenomena which ought not to hold place among them, might have well placed here this ecthyma developed under the conditions that I have already marked out to you.

It is true that our learned colleague M. Cazenave says that the ec-

thyma may be sometimes primitive. He even cites in his treatise
upon syphilitic eruptions, a very beautiful example of primitive ecthyma
of the lip, the direct and immediate consequence of contagion. But
what M. Cazenave says of this case, for me so frequent and common,
proves to me exactly that neither Biett nor himself have known either
the true nature or the essence of this accident. Read again that passage of M. Cazenave, and you will be convinced that he does not consider, in this particular case, the ecthyma as being only a period of the
chancre. For him, the ecthyma which he calls *primitive*, is always a
syphilitic eruption ; that is to say, the product of a general infection, constitutional—in a word, what I call *secondary symptoms.* But in order
to establish that the ecthyma is always the result of a previous general
infection, although this might be the only isolated accident by which the
syphilis commences ; in order to confound the chancre with ecthymatous commencement, the true primitive ecthyma, *contagious, inoculable*,
with the constitutional secondary ecthyma; M. Cazenave, after having
so well said that this accident could be the first and only result of the
contagion which, " apart from the influence of the virus, has need, in
order to be developed, of finding particular conditions," conditions which
finally are those *which necessitate the inoculation of the primitive accident ;* M. Cazenave, I say, wishing, against his own principles, to place
ecthyma among syphilitic eruptions, gives as examples of primary pustular eruptions, two observations where this accident was perfectly secondary, and regularly preceded by a primary accident upon the fingers.

This error is very common among those individuals who do not know
all the varieties of the chancre. Did not this happen to one of our
unhappy colleagues to whom M. Cazenave makes allusion ? Has he
not been considered as having undergone a constitutional infection,
d'emblée, and as having offered an example of primary pustular eruptions ? And yet this unfortunate colleague had had a chancre upon
one of the fingers of his right hand, a chancre followed later by an enlargement of the glands about the elbow, in the desired and regular
order of secondary accidents. All this I have myself established, and
also my learned friend M. Nélaton. It is true that a person who has
not a very great experience with venereal maladies, although he had
written much upon the subject, and who knew of the ulcerations upon
the finger, has pretended that there was nothing there but an *anatomical* tubercle, which had given passage to the virus without becoming
inoculated. I much fear that the brain of this person has given passage to this fine story without becoming inoculated in passing, with a little probability and good sense.

I have not yet finished with the primary ecthyma. You who read
all—sometimes from duty, often from taste, and always with profit to
those who read you in their turn—you ought to be surprised to see in
a *manual* upon syphilitic maladies, that the learned author, whom we
both hold in high esteem, admitted the possibility of the production of
a pustule by artificial inoculation, but not otherwise. In effect, M. Gibert denies absolutely that the non-inoculated chancre can commence
by a pustule ; he assures us that it is through an error of diagnosis

that this period of chancre has been admitted. I believe that you already see upon what side the error ought to be. If you admit, I say to M. Gibert, that a pustule can be produced by the point of a lancet : agree that it does not require a great effort of imagination to find in the processes of ordinary contagion something which may act in the same manner, such as a nail, a hair, &c., without making account of other circumstances, of which you in your quality of physician, ought to receive the lewd and shameful confessions.

You see how the most distinguished observers are nevertheless subject to error. Assuredly M. Cazenave and M. Gibert know as well as I what an ecthyma is, and yet how is it that they insist in referring it always to a general state, and that they deny the existence of it as a product of chancre ? Why ? because that theory throws too often a deceitful gauze between the observer and the matter of observation ; because that it does not suffice, as another observer has just told us, to pass ten years in a venereal hospital in order to see well all that takes place there ; because, alas! there are eyes which always look and which never see.

I ask pardon, my friend, for having so long occupied myself with the particular form of the chancre. Since I have done so, it is in my opinion time, at last, to come out from this *parrot's talk*, which always gives, without variation, the same characters to the primitive accident, as if it was immutable and eternal in its form. Nothing is more false and more contrary, to the observation of every day than this doctrine. The primary accident, on the contrary, presents numerous varieties either at its commencement, during its course, or later. Permit me to recall here what observation and experience have taught me.

In the most common cases, chancre commences by a superficial or deep ulceration *d'emblée*. The primary ulcer does not always destroy all the thickness of a mucous membrane or of the skin. Thus upon the semi-mucous membrane of the gland and of the prepuce, the ulceration may be sufficiently superficial to lead to the belief of an ulcerated balano-posthitis, and to justify certain successes in inoculation.

The ulcer *d'emblée* is produced, then, if the virulent pus has been placed upon a surface recently denuded, upon a bleeding wound, or, what is more difficult and consequently more rare, upon a wound in suppuration. Again, we see sometimes, and this has been disputed by those who are in the habit of disputing everything, the chancre commence under the form of an abscess. Thus, the bites of leeches which become inoculated, it is true, often offer an ecthymatous form ; and it also happens that the virulent pus inoculates also the bottom of the bite without inoculating the borders of it ; these could then become united, and enclose, so to speak, the virus which has inoculated the bottom, and this bottom then gives rise to a little virulent abscess of the sub-cutaneous cellular tissue, which when it opens, or when it is opened, presents a chancrous foyer. The fistulous tracks of the virulent pus in the sub-cutaneous or sub-mucous cellular tissue give rise to the same phenomenon.

All this is the true result of common practice and observation in my wards of the Venereal Hospital. I well know that in this theory so simple respecting abscess—as a form and as a primary period of chancre, an argument has been sought for, in favor of the existence of the bubo d'emblée, an existence which I do not admit, and which appears a contradiction in my doctrine. But I shall return, by-and-by, to these buboes d'emblée, and in such a way as, I hope, to satisfy my opponents.

However it may be as respects these different varieties in the commencement of chancre, they have no influence upon the ulterior form which these ulcerations will take.

This point has its importance; it becomes connected with the unity or the plurality of the syphilitic virus, a question yet sufficiently obscure, or rather obscured by the vagueness and the want of precision in facts. Here is what I can say as regards myself :—

When the inoculation is made upon the patient himself, the commencement of the chancre being always similar, the ulceration which follows the inoculation takes finally the form, and offers the same varieties, as the first accident which furnished the inoculable pus. Thus, if it is from a phagedenic chancre that the pus has been taken, the ulceration will take on the phagedenic character; if from an indurated chancre, the ulceration will become indurated, &c. Here is what my own experience has shown me. But in the inoculations which have been made from infected individuals to healthy ones, have things always passed thus? We know nothing, for in the inoculations which have thus been practised by other experimenters, they have taken note neither of the form of the accident from which the pus was taken, nor of the form of the accident which has been produced; they have been contented with saying, chancre on one side, chancre on the other, without any detailed description; so that definitely these inoculations could not be of any great assistance in the elucidation of the question.

In common observation we find that one form in an individual can produce a different form in another. But as we are never strictly sure of the source from which the infection has been taken, we can dispute the results; we can suppose that the individual who has a different form, could have taken it from another source, than that which he accuses. The results of the last inoculations which have just been made from individuals infected to those who are healthy, counterbalance and cannot serve either for or against. In the observation of M. de Welz, the pus was furnished by a non-indurated chancre, and his chancres were not indurated, which circumstance in his case might depend upon a want of aptitude. In the case of the inoculation upon the interne of the Hospital du Midi, the chancre became indurated, and yet the pus with which he was inoculated ought to come from a primary non-indurated ulcer, considering the conditions of the anterior constitutional syphilis under the influence of which the patient labored.

You see, my friend, that this question of the plurality of the virus, so clearly drawn by certain English physicians, is far from being resolved. Until now, we have always the right of believing in the existence of only one virus; it appears always rational to admit that the chancre, under given circumstances, and which can be determined in advance, commencing always in the same manner, depends upon an identical cause, the ulterior effects of which are determined by conditions in which the individual is found, upon whom they are developed. In effect, the great varieties which the primary ulcer presents at the period of progress, which are formed more or less quick, and which can be thus summed up—simple chancres ; inflammatory chancres with decided gangrenous tendency ; phagedenic chancres ; indurated chancres—appear to find the reasons of their existence in secondary causes beyond the specific cause. I do not here give a lecture ; I do not write a book upon special pathology ; consequently I cannot enter into too long details. But, in order to justify my propositions, let me recall some of the assisting causes which give to the chancre such or such a physiognomy, such or such a turn or course.

For example, observation shows what the abuse of alcoholic drinks produces, particularly in hot weather. The most simple chancres under their influence become rapidly inflammatory, and the inflammation in certain regions, as about the genital organs, in a cellular tissue which becomes œdematous so easily, arrives very quickly at gangrene. The action of alcohol in these cases, of which the English have given us such fine examples, is so pronounced that we could call these ulcers " *œno-phagedeniques.*"

As to the other varieties of phagedenic chancres—pultaceous, diphtheritic, serpigenous, &c.—we often find the cause of them in certain hygienic conditions, unhealthy habitations, bad nourishment, want of cleanliness ; in the unseasonable employment and abuse of rancid mercurial ointment in the dressings ; in certain diathetic conditions, tubercles, scrofula, herpetic condition, scurvy, and frequently in the different conditions which favor the production of hospital gangrene. Let us add to this, as we shall see later, the influence of a former syphilitic diathesis.

However, the conditions most interesting to understand, those which constitute almost in themselves the verole, are those which preside over the *induration of the chancre.*

But the *indurated chancre* being one of the important points of the doctrine which I maintain, and which these letters are intended to defend, you will permit me to make it the subject of my next letter.

Yours, &c.   RICORD.

DR. JOHN C. COLBY, OF FRANCONIA, N. H.

[Extract from an Address delivered before the White Mountain Medical Society, at Littleton, Jan. 26, 1853, and communicated for the Boston Medical and Surgical Journal.]

BY ADAMS MOORE, M.D.

SINCE the last semi-annual meeting of our Society, some of us have been called to perform the solemn duty of making a post-mortem examination of the body of one of our members, John Calvin Colby, M.D. He was not one of our oldest members ; he had hardly completed the term of middle age ; he had just entered upon his fiftieth year of life, and the twenty-fifth year of his professional duties, when, without notice, as it were, he was removed from this to a higher state of existence.

Three days before his death he was active in the duties of his profession. He was always active, always unwearied in his attendance upon his patients, and quick to mark the changing features of their diseases. He shared largely in the confidence of his acquaintance ; and no community could feel more bereaved, by the death of one man, than the town of Franconia felt when bereft of Dr. Colby.

In all outward appearance, no man of his years had a better prospect of reaching old age. The sudden termination of that prospect produced a shock that was overwhelming to his family, and spread a sadness and gloom over the region of his professional labors.

The manner of his death was unusual. I am not aware that any death of the kind has ever occurred within the observation of any of us. It was from active hæmorrhage from the stomach. The blood issued from an artery opened by a small ulcer.

Andral, the French pathologist, said that " such cases are extremely rare, and not more than five or six well-authenticated cases are to be found on record."

Dr. Geo. Burrows, the writer of the various articles on hæmorrhage from the different organs, in the " Library of Practical Medicine," quotes a few cases from English physicians. One of them is from Dr. Carswell's work on the " Elementary forms of disease." It was a case of fatal bleeding from the stomach, on account of an opening of the coronary artery by an ulcer. The scars of several others, that had healed, were found on the coat of the stomach. No suggestion was made as to the cause of the disease. It shows one important fact, which is, the occasional healing of ulcers of the stomach.

Another of these was noticed by Dr. Latham, in a patient who came under his care, while connected with one of the English Hospitals. The subject of it was a middle-aged man, who admitted that he was in the habitual use of alcoholic drinks. For the last two years, he had felt frequent pains across the lower part of his chest ; often vomited his food ; had palpitations of the heart, constipation of the bowels, and a pale and dusky countenance. Two days before Dr. Latham saw him, he was seized with giddiness and faintness, and vomited two quarts of blood. He lived three days longer, and each day had more or less vomiting and purging of blood. Upon the post-mortem examination, there was found a small excavated ulcer, with hardened edges, at the lesser arch of the stomach. In the base of this ulcer were seen the orifices of two or three branches of the coronary artery laid open by ulceration.

One other case, in the same hospital, was recorded, where the ulcer extended through the coats of the stomach, into the pancreas, and opened a branch of the splenic artery, from which fatal hæmorrhage ensued.

Dr. Colby had often spoken of being conscious of an adhesion of his lungs, which so appeared on the examination of his chest. The right lobe of the lungs adhered to the diaphragm and pleura of the ribs to a very considerable extent, and the left lobe was slightly adherent to the diaphragm. These adhesions were the result of a pleurisy more than twenty-five years ago.

The stomach contained a coagulum of blood, completely moulded to its form, of the bulk of three pints or more, with a small quantity of dark fluid, commingled with the natural secretions of the organ. The coats of the stomach were pale, and its vessels bloodless. On the posterior portion of the inner coat of the stomach, two and one half inches from its upper orifice, was an excavated ulcer of the size of an English shilling, with its edge on one side considerably elevated, and indurated, and in its base two openings quite through its coats. One of these was of the size of a buck-shot, where the open point of an artery was visible. The other perforation was of half that size. The diseased portion of the stomach adhered to the diaphragm, so as to prevent any escape of its fluid contents.

In stature, Dr. Colby was full six feet. When young, he was slim. At the time of his death his weight was over two hundred pounds. His temperament was strongly marked as sanguine. He rigidly abstained from alcoholic beverages. He always had a good appetite for food. His digestive powers were strong, and he ate freely of all the luxuries of the table, including raw apples, and drank freely of strong coffee. Formerly he chewed and smoked tobacco, which he ceased to use about ten years ago, since which time he grew more and more corpulent every year.

For the last year or more he had been subject to occasional paroxysms of pain at the lower part of the chest, more frequently after eating, and in the recumbent position.

On Friday, Dec. 3d, 1852, he travelled in his carriage about fifteen miles. On that day he felt some fullness about the stomach, and passed some blood from his bowels. He had the same symptoms the next day, and did business only at or near his office. Early on Sunday morning, the 5th, he was seized with vomiting, and ejected a large quantity of blood, both coagulated and fluid, followed by faintness if he attempted to rise. Pulse in the forenoon about 100; in the afternoon less frequent, and the patient felt much more comfortable. On Monday morning he arose, felt a good appetite for food, and partook of some chicken. At 5 o'clock in the afternoon, he vomited largely of blood, and again at 11 o'clock, the same evening. He was restless and faint until 1 o'clock next morning, when he slept, and remained quiet until about 5 o'clock in the afternoon, when he again vomited largely as before. He did not vomit again, but gradually sank, and died at half past 5 o'clock next morning.

Of the professional standing of Dr. Colby, in the estimation of the community where he was known, I cannot speak in too high terms of praise. Great confidence was placed in him. His people have no hope of finding a physician to fill his place. If he had foibles or faults (and where shall we find the physician who has none), they were few and small in the eyes of his friends, compared with the excellent traits of his character as a man, a christian and a physician.

By his professional brethren he could not be regarded as a man of great science, or a great master of medical books, but all accorded to him the reputation of a great practitioner of medicine. He studied his cases well, so far as could be done by his own powers of observation and reflection. I often met him in the sick-room, many times in cases of difficulty and doubt, and always found he had a large fund of experience to draw upon. His powers of perception, of arrangement, and of communication, were remarkably good.

PERMANENT CURE OF REDUCIBLE HERNIA.

[Continued from page 83.]

ACUPUNCTURE has been tried to a very considerable extent both in Europe and this country. Two or three rows of punctures were made through the integuments and the neck of the sac, just below the external ring, with a common needle of the ordinary size, or an acupuncture needle prepared for the purpose. There is no reason to believe that any permanent good effect has been produced in this way, and it is not probable that any one tries this method at the present time with the expectation of producing by it a radical cure of hernia.

The same may no doubt be said of the *scarification of the inguinal canal,* as practised by M. Velpeau a few times, and the sub-cutaneous *scarification of the neck of the sac,* as performed by M. Guerin. Besides the utter inefficiency of these operations, there is, especially in the former, some danger of wounding the epigastric artery.

The operation by *injection* has been done in two ways. In one, the neck of the hernial sac is previously laid open, and the fluid then thrown in ; and, in the other, it is introduced by the sub-cutaneous method. The first is the operation as performed by M. Velpeau, and the other that of Dr. Pancoast, of Philadelphia.

M. Velpeau was evidently dissatisfied with all the operations that had been performed for the radical cure of reducible inguinal hernia ; but he was unwilling to believe that no remedy could be found for it. The success which so often followed the operation for hydrocele by injection, led him to think that a similar course might produce the same results in the treatment of reducible hernia.

He accordingly performed the operation on the first favorable case that presented. An incision of an inch in length was made just below the external ring down to the neck of the sac ; this was opened with a bistoury, and a mixture of six drachms of tincture of iodine in three ounces of water was thrown in. An assistant compressed the inguinal canal, so as to prevent the fluid from coming in contact with the peritoneum above the ring. After the injection had been pushed around the various parts of the sac, it was allowed to escape through the canula. No unpleasant symptoms followed ; but the final result of the experiment has not, as far as we know, been made public.

M. Velpeau does not seem to have much confidence in the operation, and it is understood that he does not continue to perform it at the present day. He has probably learned that something more than the mere closure by the process of adhesion of the neck of the sac is necessary for the radical care of hernia. The fibrin that is effused will in most cases be soon absorbed, so that the barrier which had been relied on to prevent the descent of the hernia will be entirely removed.

About the same time, Dr. Pancoast performed the operation which is described in his work on " Operative Surgery." The hernial sac, its contents having been previously returned, was punctured with a small trocar passed through a canula. Having ascertained that the instrument was fairly in the sac, by the freedom with which it could be moved about, the point of it was then directed upwards so as to scarify the internal surface of the upper part of the sac. The trocar was then withdrawn, and half a drachm of the tincture of iodine, or an equal quantity of the tincture of cantharides, was thrown in slowly by means of a small syringe fitted to the canula. The canula was then withdrawn, and a compress was applied just above the external ring, and the pad of the truss, which had been on before the operation, was brought down over the compress.

This operation was performed in thirteen cases, in one of which only were there any symptoms of serious inflammation, and these readily yielded to leeches and fomentations. On some of these patients a single operation was performed, and on others, in whom the sac was large, several were required. All of them were evidently benefited at the time, but whether a radical cure was effected in any instance could not be ascertained, as nothing was known of the patients after a few months from the time of the operation. Whether Dr. Pancoast continues to practise it, we are unable to say.

This method has, in the opinion of the Committee, all the advantages of that of M. Velpeau, while it avoids in a great degree the danger of peritoneal inflammation, to which patients are exposed by his mode. When the hernial sac is laid open, there is, of course, a direct communication between the abdominal cavity and the external wound. This alone would be likely to excite inflammation, and if, in addition, a part of the peritoneum is subjected to the action of an irritating fluid, there is reason to fear that the inflammatory process would not be limited to the sac, but that fatal peritonitis would be the consequence.

Admitting that these operations accomplished all that they were designed to do, it does not follow, by any means, that they would in every instance produce a radical cure. All that they could effect, if successful, would be to close the neck of the sac, without contracting the tendinous opening or ring. Sir Astley Cooper very truly says—" that, although the original sac may be completely shut at its mouth by adhesion or perfect contraction, it is possible that another sac may be formed contiguous to the first." It fact, it is well known that sometimes the hernia has recurred, after the whole of the original sac has been removed. Contracting or even closing the neck of the sac is evidently then not enough ; " something more," says Mr. Lawrence, " is required ; we want a remedy that should contract the tendinous opening; for while that remains preternaturally large, a new protrusion is a highly probable occurrence."

This has been attempted in two ways. The first is by scarification of the external ring in inguinal hernia, and the other is by means of sutures. The first of these is quite an old operation. Heister says that —·" Some surgeons scarify the ring of the abdomen, or aperture through which the intestine prolapsed, together with the skin, in order to render the cicatrix more firm ; by which means many have been cured of these ruptures, especially if they continue to wear a proper bandage for a considerable time afterwards. But I think that the operation may succeed better in infants than in adults."

It is perhaps enough to say, with regard to this method, that it has been occasionally tried from time to time, for more than a hundred years, without a sufficient degree of success to gain the confidence of surgeons ; and it is not to be overlooked that the danger of wounding the epigastric artery is no inconsiderable one ; enough at any rate to deter all but the most expert from attempting to perform it.

[The length of the articles in the preceding pages prevents the insertion, this week, of the concluding part of the report on hernia.]

THE BOSTON MEDICAL AND SURGICAL JOURNAL.

BOSTON, MARCH 2, 1853.

Beauties and Deformities of Tobacco-Using. — A formidable array of medical as well as clerical talent has been gradually collecting in New England, within the last few years, against the use of tobacco. While one party sets forth its demoralizing tendencies, the other pours in broadsides of double-shotted arguments to prove its destructive effects upon health. Whether the consumer smokes, chews or snuffs, it is all the same to the great school of reformers, for they give no quarter to a man who in their opinion has no mercy on himself. Dr. L. B. Coles, a fellow of the Mass. Med. Society and of the Boston Medical Association, has been laboring indefatigably, for some years, to revolutionize the public sentiment in respect to the habitual use of tobacco. Before us is a revised edition of a book from his pen, bearing the title of *Beauties and Deformities of Tobacco-Using*—in which the author pleads, with undiminished ardor, against the use of the vile weed. Dr. Coles has exhausted all the usual arguments in sustaining his positions, so that were we ever so much inclined to give him assistance, there is nothing left for us to say, without resorting to his own tropes and striking figures. We may say, however, that we hope the leaven which he has sown is operating favorably, and that the next generation will grow up without the odor of tobacco in their garments. There is no prospect of the present hardened race, if the actual consumption of Havana cigars and the best cavendish is any criterion of the inveteracy of the habit. We are certainly a smoking, chewing people. Our intense nervous activity finds some imagined relief in this exercise of the jaws ; and as for health, it is not of the least consequence, the country being full of patent remedies for all kinds of diseases. There was a period in the history of Massachusetts, a State that has always been celebrated for legislating upon every thing, when no person could chew tobacco without a license from one of the Judges of a court—and his honor was restricted from granting it, without the certificate of a physician that it was necessary to the health of the applicant. Moral suasion is now the power that is brought into requisition, but it acts too tardily and too feebly to correct the evil. The age of bronze, of iron and of gold, may be considered to have passed by, and we are now living, as it were, in the age of tobacco. What an epoch to reckon from ! Smoke and fume seem to gather round our heads as we write. Imagination, like the Witch of Endor, calls up the ghastly, saffron-colored wretches who have died by inches, holding on to the pipe-stem. And yet tobacco smokers are the terror of railroad corporations and public-house keepers all over the country. " *No smoking here,*" is universally posted on the walls of depots, and incorporated into all travelling regulations. The tobacco man is haunted at every nook and corner of society ; but he remains obdurate, still smoking and chewing, and we fear he will continue in his evil ways till he reads Dr. Cole's expose of his last earthly condition ! It is a sad picture, but a true one. We believe, with Dr. Coles, that the less any one has to do with tobacco, the better he will find himself in the end. With these considerations, we recommend his " Beauties and Deformities of Tobacco-Using," to the special cognizance of those unfortunates for whom it was designed.

Scalds.—The popular belief that cold flour is a good remedy for scalds, has been often verified of late. The relief is almost instantaneous. Plunge the limb, if scalded, into a pan of flour. Simply dredging the burned surface, answers the same purpose ; and it is not improbable that a burn would be benefited by the same treatment. One of the latest testimonials in favor of the flour, is the following, which was taken from a respectable exchange paper.

" While at the supper table, a child, which was seated in its mother's lap, suddenly grasped hold of a cupful of hot tea, severely scalding its left hand and arm. I immediately brought a pan of flour and plunged the arm in it, covering entirely the parts scalded with the flour. The effect was truly remarkable ; the pain was gone instantly. I then bandaged the arm loosely, applying plenty of flour next to the skin, and on the following morning there was not the least sign that the arm had been scalded, neither did the child suffer the least pain after the application of the flour."

Prevalence of Smallpox.—With a positive preventive, the world has seldom been more severely afflicted with that most loathsome of all diseases, smallpox, than at the present moment. It is customary in almost every place to defer vaccination till smallpox is at the door. On the four great continents, it is now scourging the inhabitants in its most terrific forms; but the people will not generally avail themselves of the sure preventive. At Zanzibar and the regions about, at the last advices, the disease was mowing down every age and sex. "The entire population, with the exception of the Europeans, paid their tribute to the terrible scourge, the germ of which was brought from Muscat by a vessel of the Imaum. In the Persian Gulf and in that of Oman, where cholera had already raged, thousands of victims have succumbed. The disease has spread with frightful rapidity, not only along the eastern coast of Africa, but also in the interior of that continent."

Provisional Callus in Fractured Bones. — Dr. F. H. Hamilton's new views on this subject, in a pamphlet form, from the pages of the Buffalo Medical Journal for February, have been received. Dr. H. is an instructive writer on surgery, and is equally distinguished for a tact in teaching that branch of the profession. Although we have no space to copy any part of this essay, we cannot refrain from recommending the study of our friend's able performance to surgical operators. The opinions of a skilful, close observer, on a subject so important as the fracture and re-union of bones, cannot be otherwise than profitable to all young beginners ; and in this instance, the old will find themselves profited.

Reports of Births, Marriages and Deaths in Boston, for 1852. — This document, by the City Registrar of Boston, Artemas Simonds, Esq., contains the requisite tabular statements concerning the vital statistics of our city during another year. It is prepared with the faithfulness characteristic of the registry department under its present management. We have space, this week, for only a few of the sums total of the different abstracts. There were registerd, during the year, 5,308 births—viz., 2,651 males, and 2,657 females. These were children of 1,681 American fathers, and 1,733 American mothers ; and of 3.479 fathers and 3,451 mothers of foreign nativity—the birth places of 96 fathers and 72 mothers being unknown. Certificates of marriage were issued to 2,877 couples, and 2,686 marriages were recorded. The deaths registered were 3,736 ; 1,902 males and 1,834 females—1,568 being of American and 2,168 of foreign origin. Of the interments during the past year, it is gratifying to find that 2,177 of the 3,736 who died in Boston, were buried out of the city.

Motorpathy. — A new book, heralding a new theory, has originated at Rochester, N. Y., having the following title—" *Exposition of Motorpathy : a new system of curing disease, by statuminating, vitalizing motion.* By H. Halsted, M.D. These are hard terms for a new disciple to articulate. Eleven chapters of the above-named work are devoted to the consideration of uterine diseases, all of which appear to yield readily to the statuminating process. An irresistible mass of evidence is introduced in illustration of the value of motorpathy in the treatment of females who have been received at the discoverer's institution, known as Halsted Hall. The kind of medication in practice there, as nearly as can be gathered from the volume under consideration, does not differ essentially from methods perfectly understood throughout Christendom. "Among these therapeutic agents, that part of motorpathic treatment given personally, which is a process of statuminating vitalization, stands at the head. Diet, the use of water, magnetism, dry-cupping and various modes of exercise, and medication by external application, are resorted to, when the occasion demands, as aids to a more speedy realization of the objects proposed." Although the work is well written, and the author, we should think, might safely be called a literary man, it is difficult for the reader to divest himself of the suspicion that the plan contemplated by its publication is simply the circulation of an advertisement, to drum up customers for Halsted Hall.

Veratrum Viride — *Typhoid Fever of the South.* Mr. Editor. — We do not like to be a fault-finder, nor do we repudiate any thing without a fair trial, but we think writers in promulgating the virtues of any new agent, should keep upon the line of medical knowledge, and not wander into the mists of untenable sophisms and vague speculations. These remarks are elicited by reading an article in your issue of Feb. 9th, extracted from the South. Med. and Surg. Journal, by Dr. W. C. Norwood, of South Carolina, upon the virtues of Veratrum. Dr. Norwood is a clever man ; we appreciate his zeal, sympathize in his misfortunes, and admire his energy ; but we beg leave most respectfully to dissent from his opinion with regard to veratrum in Typhoid Fever ; and we believe that in this position, we are sustained by at least three fourths of southern practitioners, who are men of practical experience and extensive observation. That veratrum will control arterial excitement, we believe nobody south denies ; but that it is applicable to uncomplicated Typhoid Fever, as a general remedy, or that it will cure it, very few think. The nature and character of Typhoid Fever, it appears to us, must ever preclude the use of veratrum as a general agent, in its simple forms. If Typhoid Fever was only an excited state of the *heart* and *arteries*, then, we readily grant, veratrum would cure it ; but as long as pathology teaches us different lessons, we must search for another remedy. We do not by any means conceive, that veratrum will cure Typhoid Fever, Pneumonia, or other febrile affections, merely because it will curb the velocity of the circulatory apparatus. Digitalis is an arterial sedative, but nobody pretends to claim for it curative powers in Typhoid Fever, Pneumonia, or fevers generally. While we admit veratrum is an arterial sedative, we do not consider it a curative agent in southern Typhoid Fever, but only an adjuvant of doubtful and hazardous powers, in its influence and effect. There is a form of cardiac disease, following Typhoid Fever in its convalescence, in which we have prescribed veratrum with magic results. We believe it goes well in southern Pneumonia, and in cardiac affections of a sthenic character ; but in simple Typhoid Fever characterized by nervous mobility, we regard it not only a questionable but a *peculiarly dangerous agent.*

Should these remarks reach the eye of Dr. Norwood, we beg him to believe us a friend ; we admire his medicine for its real virtues, but fear the misguided opinions of others, who are as honest as ourselves, but not tempered in *"veratric"* zeal, will cause much odium to be cast upon the preparation by attributing to it panaceal powers which can never be realized. In conclusion, we reiterate, if veratrum will cure southern Typhoid Fever, the physicians of the South have mistaken its pathological character ; and autopsal results, as well as perspective causes, are dead letters in science. "SOUTHERNER."

P. S. We refer the reader to Dr. Pendleton's cases, Dr. Wickes' notes, and others, in the Charleston Review and Nelson's Lancet. These cases, to us, would satisfy any candid man.

MARRIED,—In Charlestown, Feb. 17th, Dr. J. C. Dorr, of Stoneham, to Miss A. Malvina Flint, of Charlestown.

Deaths in Boston—for the week ending Saturday noon, Feb. 26th, 78.—Males, 37—females, 41. Disease of the brain, 2—congestion of the brain, 2—consumption, 17—convulsions, 2—croup, 4—cyanosis, 1—dysentery, 1—dropsy, 4—drowned, 1—infantile diseases, 3—puerperal, 2—erysipelas, 1—typhoid fever, 1—scarlet do., 7—fracture, 1—hooping cough, 2—disease of the heart, 6—disease of the kidney, 3—inflammation of the lungs, 9—disease of liver, 1—marasmus, 1—old age, 2—peritonitis, 1—palsy, 1—pleurisy, 1—rheumatism, 1—teething, 1. Under 5 years, 27—between 5 and 20 years. 11—between 20 and 40 years, 21—between 40 and 60 years, 11—over 60 years, 8. Born in the United States, 54—Ireland, 19—England, 2—Scotland, 1—Br. Provinces, 1—Denmark, 1.

Prizes Awarded by the Academy of Sciences of Paris. — These very important encouragements to the laborers in the field of medical science, were awarded at the meeting of the 20th of December, 1852. Among the authors who were rewarded, we notice—Dr. Budge (an English physician) and Dr. Waller, of Bonn, for physiological researches ; M. Lebert, for his work on cancer, and the curable affections confounded with cancer ; M. Davaine, for his memoir on the paralysis of the seventh pair of nerves on both sides ; and on the influence of the facial nerves upon the movements of the soft palate, the pharnyx, and the tongue ; M. Bretonneau, for having introduced the operation of tracheotomy in croup ; and M. Trousseau, for having improved and simplified the same operation. M. Niepce also obtained a prize for his researches on cretinism ; and M. Renault, professor at the Veterinary School of Alfort, had a prize allotted to him for his investigations, both practical and experimental, on the effect produced by the ingestion of virulent matter into the digestive canal of man, or the domestic animals. M. Renault has found that the virulent fluids have no influence on the intestinal tract of domestic animals, and that their flesh does not, by such ingestion, become unwholesome.—*London Lancet.*

The Medical Profession in Paris. — The Medical Directory of Paris, published by *L'Union Médicale*, gives the following numbers as to our Parisian brethren. Doctors of medicine and of surgery, 1337 ; officiers de santé (an inferior grade), 179 ; pharmaciens, 423 ; midwives, 277. From the 1st of January, 1851, to 31st December, 1852, there died in Paris 39 doctors of medicine ; in the two previous years 64 had died. In the year just elapsed, 88 new practitioners set up in the capital. This year's list contains 15 medical men less than the last. The Directory also gives the numbers in the districts surrounding Paris, and from these statements it would appear that there is a great disproportion between doctors and patients. There are in fact less than 500 inhabitants for one medical man ; and when it is considered how many of these apply to public institutions, very little is left for individual practitioners. *L'Union Médicale* warns young men from settling in Paris, as the exuberance of professional men is enormous.— *Ibid.*

Dr. Drake's Work on the Diseases of the Interior Valley of North America. — We are happy to learn that Dr. Drake had prepared a considerable portion of the second volume of this great work, and that it is the desire and intention of his family that the portion so prepared should not be lost to the Profession. It is to be revised by a competent person, and printed as soon as possible.—*Southern Med. and Surg. Journal.*

Ligatures of Large Arteries, by Prof. Roux.—M. Roux, the Nestor of French Surgery, occasionally furnishes the statistics of his extensive experience. In a paper communicated to the Chirurgical Society we find that he has ligated the popliteal artery once, the femoral 46 times, the brachial 20 times, the carotid 6 times, the axillary 4 times, the subclavian 3 times, and the external iliac twice—making 82 operations. — *Ibid.*

The new building for the London Hospital for diseases of the chest, Liverpool street, Finsbury, is hastening to completion, and it is said will be opened in June.

THE

BOSTON MEDICAL AND SURGICAL JOURNAL.

VOL. XLVIII.   WEDNESDAY, MARCH 9, 1853.   No. 6.

REPORT ON THE PERMANENT CURE OF REDUCIBLE HERNIA.

[Concluded from page 104.]

THE operation of closing the external ring by means of sutures is, we believe, quite a recent one. It is proposed by Thomas Wood, M.D., of Cincinnati, who states that he has performed it in three cases with success. His paper on the subject may be found in the last volume of the Transactions of this Association. It is certainly entitled to great consideration, not only from the importance of the subject, but from the candid manner in which he has treated it.

He says that his "experience is too limited to warrant him in saying much in its favor, but he cannot refrain from expressing the opinion that it offers to the ruptured patient a better prospect of a 'radical cure' than any operation before proposed."

He thinks that all the preceding operations have failed, because, from the nature of the texture concerned in them, the adhesions have not been sufficiently strong to prevent the descent of the hernia, and he founds his expectations of success from his method on the following considerations :—"Tendons," he says, "when wounded, will unite again by a formation similar to their original structure."

"Tendon is a permanent, unyielding tissue, seldom ruptured by the strongest exertions of the body.

"If we can close the external ring by a tendinous growth, we may effect a 'radical cure of hernia.'"

We do not deem it necessary to go into the details of the operation ; for these, we refer to the author's paper. But we would remark that it is by no means certain that tendons, when wounded, are united by a similar substance. Much light has been thrown on this point within the last few years by the numerous cases in which tenotomy has been performed, and the Committee think that they are justified in saying, that it has been ascertained that the divided edges of tendons are united by a substance less resisting, more elastic, and not so firm as the original texture of the tendon.

But although this operation may not be found on further trial to be more successful than that of the scarification of the ring, yet, as it proposes to accomplish what has never been effected in any other way, viz., the con-

6

traction of the tendinous opening, it certainly, on this account, if no other, merits the careful consideration of the profession.

An operation similar to that of Dr. Pancoast, if not precisely the same, has been performed to a considerable extent in the neighborhood in which your Committee reside. Many persons, it is said, have been cured by it; but we have not met with any one of them who has felt that the truss could be safely laid aside. In one instance which has come to our knowledge, an individual submitted to the operation and thought himself cured. In a few months after, he gave up his truss, supposing that compression was no longer required, but in eighteen months from that time the hernia returned.

It is not pretended, however, that a cure may never be effected by this method, when all the circumstances of the case are favorable. It may happen, sometimes, when the hernia is small and recent, and when the patient is in good health and young, or has not passed the middle age of life; and it may, too, be of great advantage in some cases in which the hernia could not be kept up by the truss alone, as this operation would be likely to cause an abundant effusion of fibrine in and about the neck of the sac.

Two of your Committee have had some personal knowledge of it; the results of their observation and experience will be found at the end of this report. [See "Transactions," vol. v.]

It is an unquestioned fact that reducible hernia is often cured in young subjects. It may be accomplished in them by various means; but it should not be thence inferred that the same course would uniformly produce like effects in adults.

It may be remarked that, in children, any method which can prevent the protrusion of the hernia for a year or more will, in all probability, produce a permanent cure. If the aperture through which the contents of the sac must pass can in any way be prevented from enlarging, while the viscera of the abdomen are increasing in size, it is obvious that a great length of time would not be required to render an escape of any of the abdominal organs difficult, if not altogether impracticable. We see familiar examples of this daily in umbilical hernia, which is brought on so often in infancy by hooping cough and various other causes. *Compression*, it is well known, will, in all such cases, if carefully practised, in a comparatively short period produce a radical cure; and it is a valuable agent in the management of reducible hernia at every period of life. It has been used from the time of Celsus to the present, and it has not unfrequently succeeded in producing the desired result. It is usually applied at the present day by means of trusses. Great improvement has of late years been made in their construction. It cannot be doubted that an instrument of this kind, when nicely adjusted, so as to cause no pain or inconvenience, and at the same time to compress the neck of the sac, may, if used for a considerable length of time, prevent in many cases the subsequent protrusion of the hernia.

It is well known that pressure upon a serous membrane, when carried to a certain extent, will cause an effusion of fibrine on its inner surface, and it was from a knowledge of this fact that, in former times, the method of treating aneurism by compression was adopted. This mode often succeeded in producing a radical cure, by closing the artery leading to the aneurismal sac. The practice has been revived with great confidence within the last few years, and the results hitherto have been equal to the expectations of its advocates.

In the treatment of hernia in this way, it is of the utmost importance that protrusion should not be allowed to take place at any time ; " for if the hernia once descends during the wearing of the truss," as Sir Astley Cooper well remarks, " the cure must be considered as re-commencing from that moment." The truss, therefore, should be worn by night as well as by day.

It is important, also, that while the pressure is sufficient to prevent the descent of any of the abdominal contents, it should not be enough to cause any considerable degree of inflammation. This would not only require the truss to be laid aside altogether, but it would also stop entirely the effusion of fibrine. In inguinal hernia the pad should be so placed as to compress the inguinal canal ; and at the same time great care should be taken to avoid pressing the spermatic cord against the pubis.

A radical cure will not be effected in this way, unless the compression is continued for a length of time. It cannot be reasonably looked for in an adult in less than two years from the time the truss is first worn ; and it can hardly be expected at all in persons after the middle age of life, who are afflicted with a direct inguinal hernia of long standing. At the same time, more benefit is derived from compression in such cases than from anything else, and persons in this situation are not safe without it.

The Committee beg leave to offer the following opinions as the result at which they have arrived after a careful examination of the subject committed to them.

I. That there is no surgical operation at present known which can be relied on with confidence, to produce in all instances, or even in a large proportion of cases, a radical cure of reducible hernia.

II. That they regard the operation of injection by the sub-cutaneous method as the safest and best. This will probably in some cases produce a permanent cure, and in many others will afford great relief.

III. That compression, when properly employed, is, in the present state of our knowledge, the most likely means of effecting a radical cure in the greatest number of cases.

All of which is respectfully submitted, by

GEO. HAYWARD,
J. MASON WARREN, } *Committee.*
S. PARKMAN,

ULCER OF THE STOMACH.

[THE report in last week's Journal, by Dr. Moore, of the case of the late Dr. J. C. Colby, of New Hampshire, whose death was caused by an ulcer of the stomach, renders the insertion of the following remarks on this affection, with the details of a case in hospital practice, appropriate, and the reader will find them interesting and practically useful. They are taken from a late number of the London Lancet, where they constitute a portion of the weekly "Mirror" of the practice of the London Hospitals—this extract referring particularly to King's College Hospital, under the care of Dr. Budd.—ED.]

The diagnosis of gastric affections is sometimes easy, and at other times fraught with difficulties of no trifling kind. The ordinary derangements of the stomach brought on by a superabundance or an improper kind of food, symptomatic irritability, deficiency of chemical action, muscular debility, &c., are pretty easily recognized and treated. But affections of another class—viz., chronic inflammation, ulceration, and cancer, present groups of symptoms which have so much analogy with each other, that it is often a puzzling problem to give a decided opinion as to the actual nature of the disease.

Pain, loss of appetite, vomiting, hæmatemesis, and flatulency, are generally present, with more or less intensity, in the affections to which we have just alluded; but it would appear, from the statistics which have been made public, and from our own experience, that the common ulcer of the stomach is more seldom met with than either chronic inflammation or carcinoma of the gastric cavity. As far as hospital practice is concerned, we are bound to say that we have noticed more cases of simple ulcer of the stomach in Dr. Budd's wards than in any other institution, and we hope to serve a useful purpose by pointing out the treatment which Dr. Budd adopts in these cases—viz., the avoidance of all irritating substances, and the use of boiled flour and milk for ordinary nourishment. The course thus pursued is in complete harmony with the methods usually employed for favoring the cicatrization of ulcers situated on the surface; for soothing applications, except in cases of very languid and indolent ulcers, are, in general, the most likely to benefit the patient. It is highly probable, that in this way Dr. Budd has succeeded more than once in procuring the healing of ulcers of the stomach; and it would perhaps be well, whenever ulceration of the mucous membrane of other portions of the alimentary canal is suspected, that the above-mentioned facts be kept in view, for it may be supposed that such emollient applications might sometimes be more beneficial than preparations of opium or other sedatives. Nor need the diagnosis of these affections be strictly correct, for adopting the farinaceous diet cannot fail to be of much use, both in carcinoma and chronic inflammation without ulceration.

Some doubts have been raised as to the actual cicatrization of ulcers of the stomach; but autopsies have clearly revealed the existence of such cicatrices, though these are perhaps as rare as cicatrized vomicæ in the lungs. It is worthy of notice, that pressure on the epigastric region does not generally give severe pain over a circumscribed spot, and that it is thus somewhat difficult, in most instances, to say where the ulcer is actually situated; and it certainly may now and then happen that chronic inflammation with exudation of blood, may be confounded with ulceration and lesion of some arterial or venous branch.

We feel the more inclined to put the following case on record, as it presented the more striking symptoms of the two affections which we have just named. Most of our readers will most probably side with Dr. Budd, and consider the case as a *bona fide* instance of ulcer of the stomach. The details of the case were obtained from the notes of Mr. Marchant, one of Dr. Budd's clinical clerks.

William F———, a bricklayer, aged 40 years, was admitted October 12, 1852, under the care of Dr. Budd. The patient always enjoyed good health until about eight years ago, when he began to suffer from pain in the head and limbs; he then for a few days vomited his food, and noticed that it was tinged with blood. Soon after these symptoms had shown themselves, he brought up (as he says) seventy-two ounces of blood, of a very dark color. The man is of intemperate habits, but does not recollect whether he had been drinking to excess a short time previous to this latter attack. No pain after the ingestion of solid food was at that time experienced, nor had actual and copious vomiting of the contents of the stomach taken place until about a week before the occurrence of hæmatemesis. The patient was at this period laid up for about ten weeks, and during the subsequent eight years had, up to the day of his admission, only four attacks of sanguineous vomiting, each to the amount of about six ounces of blood. The latter was on these occasions very fluid, and of dark color; and the vomiting used to occur after a fit of coughing, though the blood never came with the sputa.

Up to nine days before admission, the patient had experienced no pain in the stomach, and no difficulty of taking food; but he now began to complain of headache, uneasiness in the bowels, slight cough, and loss of appetite. Solid food was occasionally rejected, but not streaked with blood. The gastric pain was always increased upon taking aliments of a consistent kind; and the suffering seemed to extend from the middle of the stomach to the pyloric extremity. The patient stated that he felt very weak in the afternoon of the day on which he was admitted, and vomited (according to his calculation) between three and four pints of dark coagulated blood. He thereupon became very faint, and was brought to this hospital.

His state on admission is thus described:—Extremely pallid, lips blanched, lightness and giddiness of the head, with great pain in that organ, and flashes of light before the eyes. The uneasiness over the epigastrium, and to the left of that region, has diminished, but the part still feels sore. There has been no vomiting of blood since admission, nor any rejection of food. The bowels are confined, and the patient says he has never noticed any blood in his stools. No rest at night, and great pain on pressure on the right side of the linea alba, as far as the level of the umbilicus. Liver not enlarged. On auscultation of the heart, slight systolic roughness is heard at the apex; pulmonary sounds normal.

Dr. Budd diagnosed ulcer of the stomach, and ordered ice to be sucked, and the food to consist of boiled milk and flour. The progress was extremely slow for a few days, but no other attacks of hæmatemesis took place.

Six days after admission, Dr. Budd prescribed three grains of citrate of iron to be taken three times a-day. Four days afterwards a blister was applied to the pit of the stomach ; this relieved the tightness felt in that locality. No vomiting had taken place, but the bowels were relaxed, and the patient still felt giddy. There was also some pain in the loins and right flank, but the patient rested better at night, and the food was taken with pleasure.

Up to the fortieth day after admission, the patient remained extremely weak and giddy, he had severe pain across the umbilicus, and the bowels were often relaxed, though the diet was chiefly composed of flour, oatmeal, arrowroot and milk.

At this period Dr. Budd prescribed an astringent chalk mixture, which caused the looseness to cease. The symptoms became a little mitigated on the fifty-first day. The man was then allowed a slice of meat, and had again an astringent mixture.

A week after this, there was still tenesmus, giddiness and slight diarrhœa, when Dr. Budd ordered a mixture of bismuth, magnesia and morphia. This gave some relief; but on the sixty-first day the patient was taken with violent sickness and purging, the matters vomited being very sour and green. He now took effervescent draughts, and a mixture composed of opium, catechu, chalk and logwood, the bismuth being at the same time continued. The symptoms were now effectually controlled, and Dr. Budd then gave creosote and opium in small doses.

The sickness returned, however, in a few days ; the epigastrium became very tender on pressure, especially after meals ; and the headache continued very severe. The creosote was now omitted, a blister applied to the pit of the stomach, and a combination of chalk, bismuth and morphia ordered.

From this time the patient began to improve ; the sickness did not recur ; the pain after meals diminished ; and tenderness on pressure over the epigastrium gave way. A nourishing diet was now prescribed, and the man was discharged at his own request, ten weeks after admission, warned by Dr. Budd to refrain from all stimulating and intoxicating liquors.

Here is a good instance of the degree of irritability which may be induced by one or more ulcers of the stomach. The farinaceous food, used for the first few weeks, certainly contributed much in diminishing the distress ; but as soon as a less exclusive diet was allowed, and preparations of steel ordered, the same train of symptoms as had characterized the first period of the case suddenly re-appeared. Bismuth, magnesia and morphia, form a combination which answered admirably, and which is of great value in these cases, whether there be simply chronic inflammation or actual ulceration. Dr. Budd advised the patient to avoid stimulating aliments, and to refrain from the use of intoxicating liquors ; just on the same principle, we presume, as a surgeon warns a patient on the eve of being discharged with a newly-cicatrized tegumentary ulcer, to shield the delicate structure from violence, or the contact of irritating substances. We sincerely hope that Dr. Budd's advice will be followed, and that his patient will not put himself under the necessity of again applying for assistance at this institution.

THE PHILOSOPHY OF MEDICAL SCIENCE.

BY E. LEIGH, M.D., TOWNSEND, MASS.

[Concluded from page 95.]

III. But the great vice of this theory is, that it excludes from science all its ideas, thoughts, truths and principles, leaving nothing but an array of lifeless material facts.

The author notices the common belief that there are general laws and principles in science, and tries to make them bend to his theory, by calling them "generalized phenomena," and making them only a peculiar kind of phenomena; a sort of general phenomena, which are observed, when one or two of the particular phenomena are observed— a sort of "original sin," which comes into being the moment the first particular act of sin is committed, and at once extends to all the individuals of the race. He says (p. 29) his "object is to show that all laws or principles of science consist merely in these constant and invariable phenomena and relationships." He says truly enough that a law is not a power lying back of the phenomena; but he does not say, what is equally true, that a law is a general truth proved by the facts, and not a general phenomenon observed in the facts. He says (p. 148), " a law is not an element superadded to the facts by an act of reasoning, it *consists in the phenomena* and their relationships, and is *identical* with them." "The law or principle [p. 175] is not a creature of the reason "; "it does *not* consist in any intellectual deduction, as it is termed, from the phenomena." " There are no principles [p. 220] which have any legitimate right to this character, excepting those which *consist exclusively in* these *details* themselves."

It is not necessary to argue this point here. It has already been sufficiently considered incidentally in other connections. Besides, if any mind does not of itself perceive that a general truth of science is something different from the phenomena and details themselves, and of a far higher and nobler character, argument will do that mind no good; · and if it does perceive this, argument is superfluous. Professor Agassiz, in the passage already quoted, speaks of ideas, thoughts, and general views deduced from facts; and in another place he has said, " it is not sufficient to know what the facts are, it is our task to *understand* them "; and in another place, he says, it is his object " to show how to investigate isolated facts, and to *deduce general conclusions* from them; how to arrive at general views from the actual study."

And though this point is so important, it will only be necessary to add to what has already been said, that there are in science general *ideas*, arrived at by the mind by the study of collected and arranged facts; as the idea of a vertebra. This is not a *vertebra*, nor a whole collection of vertebræ, nor anything observed, but an *idea* arrived at by the mind after comparing a whole series of arranged and classified vertebræ, and studying and thinking upon them.

Then there are general *truths*, deduced by reasoning from particular facts; as the truth that the whole bony skeleton of man is constructed on the plan of a series of vertebræ; the truth that the wing of birds, and the fin of fishes, are constructed on the same plan with the human arm.

Then there are other truths, more general, more comprehensive, deduced from the lower classes of truths; a sort of *genera* and *orders* of truths, deduced from a comparison and study of all the *species* of truth; as this, that all vertebrated animals are constructed upon the plan of a series of vertebræ variously modified and developed; till we arrive at the still more comprehensive truth that the whole animal kingdom is constructed upon one great plan, variously modified and applied to the exigencies of each particular division, order, genus and species, with admirable skill and wonderful intelligence. Now, to call these scientific truths, the details themselves—to make them identical with the observed phenomena, is too ridiculous to admit of the seriousnsss of argument.

Having now considered this theory of science somewhat in detail, it may be well to notice one or two applications of it which the author has made.

He says (p. 219, &c.) "it is the diligent searcher after facts who makes the acceptable offering on the altar of science; that the question is, What have you done? What have you seen? What new phenomena and relationships have you discovered? or, What old one have you rendered more intelligible and positive than it was before?" If we do anything for science, we must do it by discovering new phenomena, and making clearer and more positive the old ones (or else by "pointing out the only true method of reaching this knowledge"—that is, by framing a Philosophy of Science). He says, "the *fact-hunter*, as he has been sneeringly called, provided he is only a *fact-finder*, and a *fact-analyzer*, is the only true contributor to the advancement and the improvement of medical science." And what he means by *analyzing* facts, he has already told us; it is merely to look at them, see their resemblances and differences, and put like and like together.

Now I will only contrast with this, another passage from Prof. Agassiz.

He says, "Making discoveries has been the object envied by all those who have devoted themselves to science. But I think the time is past when it was desirable for any scientific man to make discoveries." "The names of the great men in science are never connected with discoveries"; and he refers to Cuvier and Humboldt, as instances. "They," he says, "have traced phenomena, and followed up their results, and that is why their results are so important, and why they have obtained such an influence upon science." As he said in the passage before quoted, they "took the old facts already known, and compared them, and studied them, and *reasoned* upon them, and *thought* deep and thought high, till they had *deduced* new knowledge from them, till they had arrived at great ideas, thoughts, general truths, which have renovated science, and given it a new aspect." No doubt making discoveries is an excellent and important method of improving science; but it is by no means the only method, and taking it as recommended in connection with this theory, it is certainly a very inferior one. There is a more excellent way, which the distinguished naturalist referred to has taught and exemplified.

Our author has much to say (p. 206, &c.) of " impartial observation," of being free from scientific prejudice ; he would have the " acute and circumspect " observer " indifferent " as to the result of his investigations, so as not to be the interested seeker for certain particular phenomena which he wishes to find.

It is very true that in science, and everywhere, a careful guard should be set against prejudice, that the mind be not warped or blinded by it, and that no previously-formed opinions, or previously-ascertained facts, should be permitted to sway our judgment in its estimate of new phenomena. We must hold our minds ever ready to see the facts as they are, however different they may be from what we expect or desire to find. We must not permit ourselves to be the one-sided advocates of any supposed truth, or fact. But, that we must go forth to observe the phenomena of nature with no ideas previously gained of what we may expect to find, with no supposed truths suggested and rendered probable by previously-observed facts ; that we should go forth and pick up facts just as we find them, good, bad and indifferent, without looking for particular facts which we expect to find, and wish to find, as the author's remarks upon this point, and his theory, require us to do, is not true. It is impossible. The human mind can't do it, at least if it has any love for the science it is pursuing. It is undesirable. The mind cannot investigate with zeal and perseverance and success, unless its feelings are warmly enlisted in the object of its investigation. It is unwise. It is not the method pursued by the most eminent men in science.

Professor Agassiz, speaking of discoveries made by observations which have no special object in view, says—" But what can we gain by such discoveries ? Very little. Progress in science can be made by such accidental discoveries, but it is not a steady progress. Steady, continuous, and constant progress can be made only by tracing, *with a view*, certain phenomena." And again, " The true method of investigation is to trace serial phenomena, to trace facts one after another in a series which point at once, by the very series which has been formed by facts, to further facts to which we have to look."

This was the method pursued by Newton in his observations, by means of which, and by his reasoning upon the observed facts, he demonstrated to the world the great truth of gravitation, which he had already arrived at from witnessing the fall of an apple. Was Newton thus impartial and indifferent, when completing that series of *arguments*, rather than observations, by which he demonstrated that the moon is attracted in a certain manner towards the earth as she moves in her orbit ? The contrary is too well known to be related.

It was by this method that the great naturalists proceeded who followed out the idea that Goethe and Oken had arrived at, respecting the vertebrated structure of the skull. And as they went on examining skull after skull, did they not expect to find the evidence of this vertebrated structure ? Would they not have been disappointed if the facts had proved otherwise ?

It is this method Prof. Agassiz is pursuing, in demonstrating his brilliant idea of the classification of the animal kingdom according to embryonic development; an idea, a truth, a principle, that will give new life and a new character to the whole science of zoölogy, if it does not pour some of its vivifying rays upon the kindred sciences.   And when he has looked at the embryos of mammals, of birds, of reptiles, to see if the organs of locomotion are webbed in the earliest stages of development, as he expected to find them, has he been indifferent?   Has he not found what he *wished* to find?   Especially when he looked for the second time to verify what he had before imperfectly seen in the robin's foot.   He himself has said, in private conversation, " that the study of science is of great service in enabling a man to *master his passions ;* for, when we are pursuing an investigation and look for a certain phenomenon and do not find it, but find that nature conducts herself contrary to what we expected, we are disposed to be *angry* with nature " (this was his word, and it was accompanied by a significant and earnest gesture) " for not doing as we wished her to.   But it is of no use, we must submit, and let nature do as she pleases."   This is a significant comment upon our author's theory of the right mode of observing facts. It is not by banishing passion from the breast of the scientific observer, but by furnishing him with the means and motives to control it, that he will remove or abate the evils he so justly deplores.

Our whole examination of the subject, up to this point, has been conducted with reference to absolute science, in its strictest sense, consisting of fundamental principles that are self-evident, of facts that are certainly known by observation or conclusively proved by reasoning, and of those ideas, truths, principles, and doctrines of science, that are also known with absolute certainty, being most fully proved.

But what is to be done with the hosts of facts that are but partially known? and with the many truths in the highest degree probable but not yet fully proved?   They certainly constitute no small part of science, and of medical science in particular, where observation is attended with so many difficulties and uncertainties, and we are obliged to be so cautious how we reason from our observations.   Are they all to be banished utterly?   According to our author's theory, they must be.   But they certainly form no small portion of science as it is commonly understood.   Some, very many of them, are in the highest degree probable, almost certain ; and others are known and proved with various degrees of probability.   They certainly ought to have, they do have, their proper place in science ; and medical science, at least in some of its departments, would be in a pitiable plight without them.   But they must keep their proper place, till such time as they can take a higher stand, and they must even bear upon their foreheads the mark of their inferior condition, till they can be emancipated from their uncertain state, and take their stand among the certainties of science.

Again, there are theories more or less probable, there are hypotheses more or less rational.   All these are to be allowed their due importance. They have done a great deal for science, and have still much more to do. She cannot easily get along without them ; but their true character must always be kept in view, and they must be dealt with and used accordingly.   While they remain theories and hypotheses, they are not to be admitted "in full and regular standing" into absolute science. They are to be "used, as not abusing them."

Dr. Bartlett has in one place alluded to the imperfection of science. It is necessarily imperfect. Such, human science must ever be. There is imperfection in the mind itself; its intellectual powers are limited; its moral proportions are deranged; and hence its very observations are imperfect; its reasonings are imperfect. But it is believed that most of the evils which our author deplores and would remove from science by banishing reasoning and its products and making science to consist of mere phenomena, are not owing, as he supposes, to mere "gratuitous assumption" and "hypothesis"; that they are not theories which have been coined in the secret chambers of the mind, and speculations which it has wrought out from the creations of its own fancy. This might be said of much of the philosophy of the dark ages, when Aristotle (and not Plato, as Dr. Bartlett, p. 223, erroneously* supposes) reigned in the schools. But it cannot be said of the false notions which have more recently infested medical science. The source of these errors is generally in imperfect observation. They arise, as errors usually arise, not so much from bad reasoning as from bad premises. It is the observations that are generally at fault in medicine. In this science, observation is peculiarly difficult. The phenomena, their relations, the true causes, the actual effects, are so various and so complicated and often so exceedingly difficult to ascertain with accuracy, that a sound judgment and peculiar discrimination are required in the observer. It is owing to a deficiency *here*—to a want of sound judgment and clear discrimination in the observation of facts, rather than to any waywardness of intellect in reasoning from them—that so much trash, so much error, so much folly, so much false doctrine, has crept into medical science and surrounded it with so many absurd theories that would rival its claims. The ridiculous errors of the homœopathists result mainly from their miserable observations. The materia medica of Hahnemann is not so much a book of false theories, it is made up (if I mistake not) almost wholly of the details of observations;† but *what* observations! It is in this way that errors find their way into science, and round about it, and gain currency. The very nostrums that are advertised in our newspapers and vended in our drug-shops gain currency by their pretended cures. If any false theory is attached to them, it is merely to satisfy the demand of the mind for something that is rational; the main reliance of those interested in their sale is upon the thousand cures, each duly certified, which they can report. It is only a twelve month since a Thomsonian professor of an Ohio university, in a lecture in this city, stated that he should report the details of some 150 successive cases of typhoid fever, all *cured* by the power of lobelia and Cayenne pepper! This is *observation* with a vengeance. It is upon observation, such as it is, that most of these follies rest. Here is the real difficulty. And the only remedy for it is to be found in a sound judgment and clear discrimination in the observer,

---

* The philosophy of Plato has been revived only within a few years. It was the Aristotelian philosophy as it existed in the schools that Bacon demolished.
† See pages 37 and 38 of this Journal, for a specimen of these "observed phenomena."

which will direct his eye to the right facts, and enable him to perceive their real value.   It is undoubtedly this that gives Louis his eminence as an observer, more than any " system of observation," or any disuse of his reasoning faculties.   But men *will* observe badly, in spite of all Dr. Bartlett or any one else can do.   There are intrinsic difficulties and obstacles in the case, and there are incapacities in the minds of the observers, which he cannot remove.   And a great portion of the evil must be submitted to.   In this as well as in many other respects, we must submit to the necessity—doubtless a wise arrangement of our Creator—of living for the present in an imperfect world.   But it is well to know the real seat of the difficulty, if only to avoid any fruitless efforts to remove it.   At all events, these defective observations, and the false theories and doctrines deduced from them, cannot be prevented, cannot be removed, by banishing reasoning and its processes and results from science.   To do this is to swing madly a two-edged sword, which hews down friend as well as foe.   It is to blow up the ship with all that is in it, to prevent it from falling into the hands of the enemy. Or, to use our author's own motto, He " trusts he has got hold of his pitcher by the right handle " ; but it is to be feared he has got hold of a handle too low, too near the bottom; and by his bold and vigorous grasp of this *wrong* handle, he has upset it, and spilled out the *higher* and more precious portion of its contents, containing all the *active principles*, which had been extracted from the remaining portion, and has left only the inert and worthless dregs.

Dr. Bartlett's object is a noble one, and he has advanced many noble sentiments and important truths in his book.   It is true that science must stick close to facts ; it is true that its laws and principles are not powers and agencies lying back of facts ; it is true that nature must be studied, and interrogated and investigated in her own broad fields, and not within the four walls of the study ; it is true, that there are some facts which cannot be proved by some others, and that each department of science and each class of facts requires its own special observations ; it is true that reason alone cannot do everything in science ; it is true that false doctrines, gratuitous assumptions, and fanciful theories and hypotheses, must be banished from science ; it is true that its facts and truths must be known and proved.   And in maintaining these truths and contending against these errors, we will join him with the whole heart and soul.   He has, in the main, taken the right side in the contest, but he has chosen his ground most unfortunately.   Fighting in a noble cause, which must, of itself, secure final victory to its champions ; bringing into the field the finest array of chosen troops, and provided with all the materiel necessary to successful warfare, he has chosen to give battle upon ground upon which he cannot gain the victory, and from which he must eventually be driven.   He has only been able to display his strength and show on which standard victory must finally rest.   He has planted his artillery in a position where it is exposed to a raking and destructive fire, while it is unable to play with effect upon the weak points of the fortress of error he would level with the ground.

Or (if we look at it, not with reference to the errors he has failed to demolish, but with reference to the science he has unintentionally annihilated by a false theory, so far as a false theory can be said to do this), in his effort to drive from the Temple of Science the ridiculous theories, absurd hypotheses, and false doctrines, which have desecrated its altars, he not only drives away those rational hypotheses which have ever been allowed to occupy a humble place near its entrance, to introduce those who are entitled to admission, till they themselves, perhaps, may be allowed to enter with honor ; but he removes from it every fact however well-known, or proved, if it has not come under the eye of the observer ; and above all, he does not allow a single niche to remain for any of the sublimest truths and soundest principles that have ever received the homage of the worshippers ; he leaves nothing but the bare walls around which is arrayed a collection of phenomena. The temple is transformed into a mere cabinet of phenomena. The collection may be large and full and extend to every department of science, and may be most perfectly classified in all its various relations. But that is all. There they lie upon the shelves, a lifeless collection of mere phenomena ; the ideas, the truths, the principles, to which they point, and which give them all their life, significance and power, are gone. It is a *Temple* no more ; and the Divinity is gone, unable any longer to dwell in it.

SOUTHERN OBSTETRICY—UTERINE DISPLACEMENTS.

To the Editor of the Boston Medical and Surgical Journal.

Dear Sir,—But little has been done for southern obstetricy ; and such has been the backwardness of the fraternity, that little has not been appreciated ; but as we belong to the class of progressive democrats in medicine, we say here go again, upon our favorite motto, " *truth without fear.*" We have recently read the valuable essays of Drs. Collins and Coale upon obstetrics, in your Journal. The former has a just regard for the speculum—a means of diagnosis in uterine disease, chaste in its application, unpainful, and correct in delineating pathological facts, but too little used in southern obstetricy. The essay of Dr. Coale, we regard an excellent contribution in the direction of a class of affections which are pregnant with interest and imperfectly understood by many practitioners. We wish we had more such productions ; the article confers credit upon the author, and we trust he will not forget us, when he distributes his pamphlet. While reading a number of Dr. Coale's treatise, we were forcibly reminded of a remark of Prof. Channing, of Boston, which had made an indelible impression upon our mind—*that uncomplicated prolapsus was not as common as suspected.* We have long been convinced of the truth and force of Prof. Channing's opinion, and we are glad one so distinguished in obstetric science has assumed the position. The practice of obstetrics in the South is followed by two classes or colors, white and black. We feel convinced the obstetric practice of the South is mainly done by the country practitioners, and those in our villages who belong to the same in fact. The country is rural, settled with an agricultural population, residing in a large majority of cases upon their farms, with white and black families of various dimensions, varying from five, ten, twenty and thirty, to forty, fifty, seventy, to an hundred and more. Among these families are a great number of black females, who from their avocation of laborers, in carrying weighty substances, corn-pulling, ploughing, &c., would naturally be presumed to have falling of the womb in many instances ; yet, strange to tell, it is rather an unusual occurrence among them. We have done a heavy practice in obstetrics. We have seen much uterine disease of almost every grade. We have noted our cases, and upon a review of them, we incline to the opinion, *that simple prolapsus of an uncomplicated character, is an accident of rare supervention in this section of the South.* The negress is a creature of an intuitive superstition, and she often imagines her " *body* " down ; but the merest digital examination will detect her error, though something must be done to pacify her fears, and you must assure her you have re-placed her " body," and enjoin ablution and rest a day or so, which accomplishes the cure. We would not by any means say, the negress never has prolapsus, for some of the worst and most intractable cases of procidentia we have ever seen among any class, have been among them ; and as a general rule, when you find such a case, it is only palliatively relieved, for reasons we may mention hereafter.

The white lady of the South, as far as we are advised, is decidedly more subject to prolapsus than the negress. This may be owing to her manner of life, in dressing, dieting, &c. ; but in the country, invigorated as all colors are by a pure atmosphere and addicted to physical exercise, the prolapse of the uterus is far from being frequent. About our cities the deformity may be oftener seen, or about our larger towns ; but we know nothing of either from personal experience, consequently cannot speak knowingly. Of *country matters* we can speak, and that from the *record.* This *prolapsus* question has been a hobby for many a pretender to secure fame, and scores of women South have been injected per vaginam with sulph. zinc., nit. arg. *et id omne genus,* to their serious detriment, for the mal-position of an organ from which they never suffered. Any man, with a thimblefull of brains, who will put himself to the trouble to examine the anatomical situation of the womb, will see, at a glance, that the organ, in its normal and physiological conditions, is not easily prolapsed, at least not with the facility once supposed. We admit real *prolapsus* is too common, but it can never be modified until we have a radical change in our mental and physical education South. But at the same time, we protest against referring every little uneasy sensation in the hypogastric region to uterine descension. It is high time we were awaking from this unprofitable and unmeaning slumber, with regard to female affections. We need and urge more investigation into their pathology and therapeutics ; and the day is approaching, we opine, when their diagnosis will be more definite, and the treatment decidedly more rational and curative. Then, and not until then, will we have less of falling of the womb, abdominal supporters, pessaries, and *crawling out of the bed headforemost and down to re-place it.* God speed the time for the benefit of our *wives* and *daughters.*

But although we protest against the abuse of the term *prolapsus,* and think it a comparatively rare affection in country practice here, we are well aware there are other forms of uterine disease, which are often in existence and seldom recognized; such as local congestion of the *cervix,* &c., to which we shall invite attention hereafter. In the treatment of *prolapus,* we wish we had time to dilate. Suffice it to say, we eschew all pessaries, as worse than useless, for reasons which to our mind are clear, and we think it would be better for the ladies at large if the *pattern of the pessary* was extinct in toto. We know that in this, and upon the prolapsus question, we will be controverted; but when by southern men, we ask for the record, and shall not submit to be considered incorrect upon the vague and uncertain scintillations of memory, or because this man, that man, or the other man, did not have the same luck, or see the same phenomena. We consider one recorded fact worth a thousand negative suppositions.

The whole profession is under obligation to Dr. Channing for his bold assumption of a clear ground, which should have, long since, been occupied. We have given our opinion of its truth South, upon our personal observation. Others may deny it; but other matters are apt to secure more attention South from physicians, than their books and diary. Few keep the latter; hence they only speak from memory, and consequently their opinions must generally be liberally allowed for. As a class of practitioners, our medical men are *bold* and *safe,* but as observers and the recorders of their observations, they are lethargic. Many of them do more practice than they think, while many again do none, and never think any one else does any. We keep a record of our cases, and know it correct, and are not willing to have our opinion confounded upon this question, only by a record, and then we are satisfied; for we set up no claim to infallibility. Respectfully and truly,

Thompson, Geo., Feb. 9, 1853. H. A. Ramsay, M.D.

OPERATION FOR HYDROCELE.

To the Editor of the Boston Medical and Surgical Journal.

Dear Sir,—I have the pleasure to forward to you for publication what I believe to be a new method of curing hydrocele of the tunica vaginalis testis, without tapping. I have adopted this practice for some time, and in a great many cases, with invariable success, but have delayed giving you this account till I had become perfectly satisfied of its being a radical cure by a relapse of the hydrocele not having occurred in any case. The following is one of the cases :—

Mr. John Norwood, a native of England, but for some time a resident of this city, about a year ago applied to me for advice. He was afflicted with hydrocele of several years' standing. He had been under the care of several physicians, who tapped him freely, but only gave him temporary relief, as the water invariably accumulated after they had resorted to all the remedies usually adopted in such cases.

On examining him I found the scrotum indicated all the symptoms of hydrocele of the tunica vaginalis testis. My mode of treatment was as follows :—I scarified the tumor all over with a lancet, and then applied fomentations of the lupus humulus as hot as they could be borne, and repeated them as often as they became cool. I kept the bowels open with mild cathartics, and administered diuretics freely as a drink. Under this treatment, followed up for about three weeks, the tumor gradually subsided, till a perfect and radical cure was effected. He is now well, no relapse or accumulation of water having since occurred. Hoping the profession will make trial of this simple treatment, and with equal success,   I remain yours respectfully,   J. X. CHABERT, M.D. *No.* 431 *Grand st., New York, March* 1, 1853.

THE BOSTON MEDICAL AND SURGICAL JOURNAL.

BOSTON, MARCH 9, 1853.

The Esculapian.—We have already alluded more than once to the new periodical of Dr. Griswold, of New York, and expressed our best wishes for its success. The following letter from Dr. G. presents some of the claims that the work has upon the patronage of physicians, which are deserving of attention, especially by those of the profession who have doubts of the expediency of preparing works of this kind for the public.

"The third number of the 'Esculapian' will be published by the time this can reach your readers, and will likely enough fail to satisfy those of our profession who are disposed to inquire of me 'why do you undertake to publish such a paper ?' I will attempt to answer why. My professional experience for the last ten years has been somewhat varied, and extended over a pretty wide field, and I may say it has been peculiar, inasmuch as it has revealed to me, as few have the opportunity of seeing, the poisoned weapons and the hands that hurl them, which are constantly being thrust at, not only the men, but the principles of our art. These means are not either feeble or effeminate alone—they are as powerful and work as rapidly as the steam press; and are controlled by shrewd men who know of nothing *good* but what makes money—this is their standard in all things. These vampires thrive ; and it has become a proverb, that to make money out of medicine, it becomes necessary to set up an opposition to the 'regular profession.' A man said to me the other day — 'Doctor, if you wish to *succeed*, you must advocate some of the popular notions in medicine.' 'How succeed ?' I asked. 'Why, *make money* '! 'Thank God,' I answered. 'I have a better success in view.' He looked at me in astonishment ; the idea was incomprehensible to him. Who will deny but that this is one of the powerful influences which fill our land with charlatans. 'Our opponents make money, we scarcely live,' say thousands, and soon they are off, enrolled in the ranks of money-makers in medicine. It is humiliating to acknowledge that men educated at all in the truth-inspiring principles of our science, could ever sell them for pieces of silver. But popular sentiment sustains them, and if they 'succeed,' they are sure of a popular reward.

"Take the press and money, or the two united in one, and we have the greatest human power over mankind ; and these two, or the mighty one, is at its busy work against us. It will not do to say that there is no help for it, simply because it has always been so to a greater or less extent. We, or our profession, has ever trusted too much to the benevolent aims which lie at the foundation of our calling ; but justice and truth were never sustained upon merit alone, and the Church of Christ would have fallen long ere this without defence. Why, then, should we let *truth* battle single-handed in medicine, when our aid would render it more effectual. The time has come when an effort must be made to establish in the popular mind a correct opinion concerning the nature and designs of our art. It will not do to leave the field to these speculators in human blood ; we might as well trust a man's safety among wolves, simply on the ground that he is a Christian.

" I have undertaken what few would dare attempt, and I trust at least to have the credit of so doing, more from a love of the principles of my chosen calling, than any hope of pecuniary reward ; for the last would argue a weakness of judgment, and belie my practice, which has ever been to heed the call of the sick to do them good, rather than for pay.

" I have never been more sanguine than now, that there is need, and would be a demand for such a paper as the 'Esculapian' is intended to be—I say 'intended,' for its design is but imperfectly developed yet. All that is required, is for it to be known ; and I fully believe that henceforth there will never be a time without a popular paper for the people emanating from our profession, although mine may die and be forgotten.

" If any differ with me as to the general character of the ' Esculapian,' I can only say, help me to make it better by advice, contributions to its columns, or subscription list, and I will thankfully receive either, and appropriate the same according to the best of my judgment. It must be remembered, however, that the ' Esculapian' is for the people, and it will not do to adapt it to educated, or professional taste. There are enough who have already been made acquainted with our paper, who would gladly aid it in its work if they were fully sure of its stability, and that it would never degenerate to fulfil a mean end. To these queries, I can only pledge my devotion to the profession I love more than any thing else on earth, and my assurances of life and health. Of course if I fail to secure the necessary patronage to sustain it, it will end with the year. No class can promote its success as well as physicians, and if they fail me I shall have the ' principles' of our calling alone to urge me to my labors. I am already assured that this will not be the case, for it is not now. Yet the enterprise requires further aid, to warrant an enlargement which I greatly desire.   C. D. GRISWOLD.

108 *Nassau st., New York.*

Dental Science and the Dental Journals. — After an examination of the Journals of Dentistry for the past year, we are constrained, as an act of justice to the fraternity, to say. that the amount of original matter they have contained, and most of it of sterling value, shows that the dental profession of the United States have not been surpassed in their literary efforts by any body of professionals among us. With other periodicals it is allowable to copy extensively from contemporaries ; but the dental editors rarely transfer a page from another Journal. Whether they will be able to continue this course interminably, admits of a question. At present there are no signs of exhaustion. Among the Journals of which we speak, and distinguished for independence, literary merit and genuine science, is the American Journal, a quarterly, conducted by Drs. Harris and Handy, of Baltimore. Place it in any institution, or before the best minds in the country, and it will command respect and confidence. Instead of being jealous of the growing fame of these publications, which deal largely in physiological inquiries, and to some extent supply acceptable reading for medical men, we are proud of their success, and omit no proper opportunity of presenting their claims to the patronage of the public.

Hydatids of the Liver.—An account of a successful operation and cure, effected by J. Edward Webber, M.D., having first appeared in the New York Medical Times, and now issued in a pamphlet, is really a thrilling narrative. Dr. Webber shows by his works that he understands the profession in which he labors. The account, detailing the condition of the patient from the time he placed himself under Dr. Webber's care, till he was discharged, well, would be studied with interest by every medical man. No doubt the pamphlet might be procured by addressing the author, 173 West 26th street, New York.

Fergusson's Surgery. — When a book reaches its fourth edition, it is pretty conclusive proof that it is a valuable one and in demand. Such is the case in regard to Fergusson's eminently practical system of surgery, with its 393 illustrations. Messrs. Blanchard & Lea, of Philadelphia, have bestowed their usual care upon the typography. This is from the third London enlarged edition, and consequently as perfect as the author could make it up to October last. We have no disposition to repeat the commendatory observations heretofore made in respect to this production. The author is known and esteemed, and his writings are authority. Those who purchase this latest edition will have the worth of their money.

Invalids at the South. — All that had been anticipated from the mildness of the climate in and about Aiken, S. C., has been realized the present winter, by northern invalids. It has been rather more rainy than usual there, some of the time, which operated unfavorably for ladies, depriving them of the amount of exercise necessary to keep the body in a healthful condition. Those, however, who have had an opportunity to study the effects of the climate, and to compare their own condition while in New England with their present vigor, are decidedly of the opinion that there is more hope of restoration by residing south, than in taking medicine at home. We are solicitous to hear from our learned correspondent, Dr. Burnett, who is passing his second season in the bland and balmy region which he has described in this Journal with the judgment of a philosopher and the enthusiasm of a poet.

Orthopedic Institution of Bamberg. — One of the most celebrated, if not the best orthopedic establishment in Europe, is supposed to be the one located in the town of Bamberg, which lies in the centre of Germany, and is sheltered by hills clothed in the richest verdure and surrounded with gardens and orchards. Bamberg is only two miles from Nuremberg. From London to Bamberg, by way of Ostend, Cologne, &c., we may travel in three days. While the patient is having his or her malformations remedied, lessons are given in French, German and Italian, and children are taught all the necessary branches of an education, besides music; and all this, including board, washing and attendance, for forty-two pounds a year. A person could not reside any where else abroad, and have such educational advantages, for twice that sum. The proprietor of the institution is Mr. Wildberger, whose faithfulness, integrity and capacity are certified to by some of the most distinguished physicians on the continent. American families going out to Europe with invalid children or friends, might derive very important relief from establishing them a while at Bamberg. With a view to putting medical gentlemen inclined to travel, on the track of the model orthopedic school of the old world, this short notice has been given. Of the various plans resorted to there for overcoming congenital and incidental lameness, it would be difficult to particularize. The institution is conducted on acknowledged scientific principles, and has the entire confidence of the medical profession, the people and the magistrates of the region round about, who are vigilant sentinels in respect to the rights and treatment of foreign travellers.

Medical School of Harvard University. — At the semi-annual examination held on the second of March, 1853, the following candidates were examined and approved for the Medical Degree.

Elisha Barber, *Medway.* Subject of Thesis, Erysipelas.

George Albert Blake, A. B., *Raymond, N. H.* Proportion.

Elisha Chenery, *North Livermore, Me.* Inflammation.

Ephraim Xenophon Giebner, *Franklin, Pa.* Pathology of Inflammation.

Edw'd Hitchcock, Jr., A.M., *Amherst.* The Geological Causes of Disease.

John Furness Jarvis, A. B., *Boston.* The Influence of the Mind in causing and curing Disease.

Francis Rufus Caleb Kittredge. *Waltham.* Apoplexy.

Graham Marr. *Simcoe, Canada W.* Intermittent Fever.

James Oscar Noyes, A. B., *Boston.* De Gangliis et Tubulis Nervosis.

Erasmus Allington Pond, *Franklin.* Alcohol and Fusel Oil.

Pitkin Boltwood Rice, *Wilbraham.* Pericarditis.

Lewis Edward Simons, *Chester, Vt.* Scarlatina.

Alfred Augustus Stocker, *Cambridge.* Chorea.

Tyler Thayer. Wounds.

John Danvir Walshe, *Cork, Ireland.* Dysentery.

John Colby York, *South Boston.* Scarlatina.

Edward Payson Abbe, A. B. was examined and approved at a special meeting of the Faculty held Aug. 19th, 1852.

Boston, March 4th, 1853. O. W. HOLMES, *Dean.*

Mortality of Lowell. — The bill of mortality of the city of Lowell for the last year, prepared by the City Physician, Dr. Joseph Spalding, has been published. The whole number of deaths was 604, of which 150 were by consumption. In 1851 the deaths were 629, and 138 by consumption. Of the deaths last year, 291 were males, and 314 females. Estimating the population of Lowell at 35,000 (33,388 in 1850), the deaths in 1852 were 1 in 58, or 1.73 per cent.

Deaths in Boston—for the week ending Saturday noon, March 5th, 83 —Males 32—females, 51. Accidental, 2—apoplexy, 1—inflammation of the brain, 1—disease of the brain, 2—burned, 3—consumption, 22—convulsions, 2—croup, 5—diarrhœa, 1—dropsy, 3—dropsy in head, 2—infantile diseases, 4—puerperal, 2—scarlet fever, 6—hemorrhage, 1—disease of the heart, 4—inflammation of the lungs, 7—disease of liver, 1—marasmus, 2—old age, 3—peritonitis, 1—scrofula, 1—spine disease, 1—teething, 4—unknown, 1—worms, 1.

Under 5 years, 31—between 5 and 20 years. 14—between 20 and 40 years, 19—between 40 and 60 years, 7—over 60 years, 12. Born in the United States, 59—Ireland, 21—England, 2—Germany, 1. The above includes 5 deaths in the ...

Foreign Substance in the Lung. — Dr. Crisp exhibited to the Medical Society of London, on the 22d of January last, the seed of a sugar-apple, which had remained ten months in a child's lung, and was then suddenly expelled. The particulars of the case were supplied by Mr. Reece, formerly of Barbadoes : — " Rebecca Jane, aged two years and one month, daughter of Thomas D——, a respectable colored man (carpenter) of Christ Church parish, Barbadoes, in playing with a seed of the sugar-apple, contrived to let it slip down her throat. This happened on the 19th June, 1840. The child suffered great agony, as might be expected, for the seed could by no means be ejected. Her sleep was irregular, and broken by convulsive jerks. She could not bear to be held in any other than a vertical position ; in the arms all day ; propped up during the night ; frequently coughed up small clots of blood. She was removed by her father to Bridge Town, and became an object of intense interest to the medical men of the island, one of whom, Dr. Bovell, declared from the first (by means of auscultation) that the seed was lodged in the left lung. Things continued in this way until 10th April, 1841, when the child suddenly gulped up the seed, which was found to be enveloped in a yellow mass of some gelatinous stuff, oval in shape, and indeed not unlike the cocoon of the silk-worm. I removed the stuff, and washed the seed, which I send to you." Dr. Crisp said the seed was three-fifths of an inch long, and about the same in circumference ; its exterior surface resembled that of a tamarind-stone. He thought the case of great practical interest, and it was also one of rare occurrence in so young a child. There were numerous cases on record of extraneous bodies in the air-passages, but they had generally occurred in adults, or in children from six to twelve years of age. Nature often managed these matters better than the surgeon or physician ; and it was not improbable, judging from recorded cases, that if tracheotomy had been performed in this instance, the result would have been unfavorable. A case bearing some resemblance to this was related by Mr. Travers, jr., in the *Medico-Chirurgical Transactions.* A girl, aged six, had a cherry-stone in the bronchus. From the urgency of the symptoms, Mr. Travers was induced to perform tracheotomy on the nineteenth day after the accident. The stone was not found ; the wound healed, and on the ninety-sixth day the stone was expelled with a tablespoonful of pus.—*London Lancet.*

Sale of Poisons by Druggists, Apothecaries and others in the United States. — The Committee to whom the above subject was referred at the late Pharmaceutical Convention are desirous of getting all information on the subject they can obtain, and will feel under obligations for contributions to that end from apothecaries, etc., residing any where within the United States. The special facts wanted are, 1st, whether any State or municipal law exists regulating the sale of poisons ; 2d, if so, how it works; 3d, if not, does any voluntary conservative action have place among druggists and apothecaries, and if so, how far ; 4th, to what extent do grocers and general shop-keepers retail arsenic and other poisons used for destroying animal life. Any communications may be addressed to " W. Procter, jr., Philadelphia," Chairman of that Committee, or to Messrs. Dr. Philbrick, of Boston, Alexander Duval, of Richmond, Va., or G. D. Coggeshall, of New York, and its other members. — *American Journal of Pharmacy.*

The Faculty of Medicine of Montpellier have sent M. Dupré, one of the professors, to Paris, to congratulate the Emperor upon his accession to the throne.

THE

BOSTON MEDICAL AND SURGICAL JOURNAL.

Vol. XLVIII. Wednesday, March 16, 1853. No. 7.

THE WEATHER AND MORTALITY IN LONDON AND THE METROPOLITAN DISTRICTS IN THE YEAR 1852.

JANUARY.—The mean reading of the barometer (at the level of the sea) was 29.769 in. ; being 0.174 below its average. The temperature of the air, 42° F.; being 6¼° above the average of 80 years. The degree of humidity was 85, complete saturation being represented by 100. The daily range of temperature was 11.4° ; being 2¾° too great. Rain fell to the depth of 3.6 in. ; the average for this month is 1.8 in. The average number of deaths daily was 155, or 4798 in the month ; the expected number, based upon the calculation of the previous ten years, corrected for increase of population, was 5442—so that the state of public health was good.

February.—Barometer, 30.044 in. ; a little above its average. Temperature of the air, 40.8° F. ; exceeding its average by 2.6°. Degree of humidity, 88 ; the same as its average value. Daily range of temperature was 12.2° ; exceeding its average by 1.8°. Rain fell to the depth of 9-10ths of an inch only. The average number of deaths daily, 147, or 4264 in the month ; being 555 less than the average, corrected for increase of population.

March.—Barometer, 30.184 in. ; about ¼ of an inch above its average. Temperature, 41.3° ; being near its average. Degree of humidity, 81, being a little below its average. Daily range of temperature, 18.6 ; being 5 degrees too great. The fall of rain was 0.2 in. ; being 1.4 in. below its average. The number of deaths daily was 172, or 5335 in the month ; exceeding the average by 228. This great increase was attributable to the decrease of temperature, and great difference of temperature during the day. An increase of more than 100 deaths took place in the first week of March, when the temperature was 36° only.

April.—Barometer, 20.122 in. ; exceeding its average by nearly ¼ of an inch. Temperature, 45.9° ; being about its average value. Degree of humidity, 76. The daily range of temperature was 24° ; between 7.4 degrees greater than its average value. Rain fell to the depth of 5-10ths of an inch. The number of deaths daily was 156, or 4691 in the month ; the corrected average number was 4392—showing an excess of 299, and which took place within the first three weeks of the month. After this time an increase of temperature took place, and an improvement was shortly afterwards observable in the public health. The meteorological conditions of this month, as well as of the preceding were greatly-increased pressure and a relatively low temperature compared with those of the preceding months, a great range of temperature, and much less rain than usual.

May.—Barometer, 29.963 in. ; the same as its average value. Temperature, 51.5° ; exceeding its average by 1°. Degree of humidity, 77. The daily range of the temperature was 18.6 deg. ; the average being about the same. The fall of rain during the month was 1.9 in. ; being that of the average nearly. The number of deaths daily was 137, or 4254 in the month ; corrected average, 4347.

June.—Barometer, 29.737 in. ; being below its average by about $\frac{1}{4}$ in. Temperature, 56.1° ; being 2° too low. The degree of humidity the same as its average, 77. The daily range of the temperature was 17.1° ; being 3.1° too small. Rain fell to the depth of 4.6 in. ; being more than double its average amount. The number of deaths daily was 135, or 4060 in the month ; and the corrected average number, 4227.

July.—Barometer, 30.034 in. ; being rather above its average value. Temperature, 66.6° ; exceeding its average by 5$\frac{1}{4}$°. The degree of humidity was 73 ; being 6 below its average. The daily range of temperature was 24.9 ; exceeding its average value by 6$\frac{1}{4}$°. Rain fell to the depth of 2.3 in. ; being about the same as the average. The number of deaths daily was 136, or 4147 during the month ; while the corrected average was 4796. The temperature varied considerably during the month, and so did the deaths at different periods. In the week ending the 3d July (whose mean temperature was 1 degree in defect) the number of deaths was 987 ; in that ending the 10th (whose mean temperature was 9° in excess), the number was 1080.

August.—Barometer, 29.826 in. ; being 0.148 in. below its average. Temperature, 62.1° ; being 0.6° above its average. Degree of humidity, 73 ; its average being 82. The daily range of the temperature was the same as its average, being 17.9°. Rain fell to the depth of 4$\frac{1}{2}$ in. The number of deaths daily was 150, or 4668 during the month ; while the corrected average was 4748. The temperature at the beginning of the month was high, and 1124 persons died in the first week. Many of these deaths were attributable to bad sewerage, a fruitful source of mortality in hot weather.

September.—Barometer, 29.916 in. ; exceeding its average by 1-10th of an inch. Temperature, 56.8° ; exceeding its average by half a degree. Degree of humidity was 77. Daily range of temperature was 17.4 ; the same as its average amount. The average number of deaths daily was 146, or 4359 in the month ; the expected number being 5023.

October.—Barometer, 29.864 in. ; slightly above the average. Temperature, 47.9° ; being 1.4° below the average. Degree of humidity, 80 ; its average being 86. The daily range of the temperature was 14.6° ; exceeding its average by 1.3°. Rain fell to the depth of 3.8 in. Average number of deaths daily was 153, or 4720 in the month ; the corrected average being 4617. This excess of deaths took place for the most part in the second week, the temperature of which was 2° below its average; that of the preceding week having been 6° below its average.

November.—Barometer, 29.642 in. ; being ¼ of an inch below its average. Temperature was 48.9° ; being 6½° too great. Degree of humidity was 83 ; being 6 too small. The daily range of temperature was 10.4° ; being 0.3° too small. The fall of rain during the month was 6 in.; which was 3.7 in. above the average. The number of deaths daily was 138, or 4129 in the month ; the expected number being 4912. The mortality during the first two weeks of the month was above its average, but on the third week it was much less.

December.—Barometer, 29.758 in. ; being 0.282 in. below the average. The temperature was 47.6 ; exceeding its average value by 8.8°. The degree of humidity was 79 ; being 10 below its average. The daily range of temperature was 9.7° ; exceeding its average by 0.8°. Rain fell to the depth of 2.2 in. The number of deaths daily was 148, or 4597 during the month ; while the corrected average was 5791 —1194 less than the average. The temperature of the months November and December was very high, the pressure was low, the degree of humidity was low, and the fall of rain was in excess.

The number of deaths in the year was 54,022 ; being about 4000 less than the calculated number.

The mean temperature of the year was 50.6° ; being 2.2° above the average.

The mean reading of the barometer for the year was 29.905 in.; being 0.046 in. below its average.

Rain fell to the depth of 34.4 inches.

REMEDY FOR INFANTILE ASPHYXIA.

BY W. P. JONES, M.D., NASHVILLE, TENN.

ONE pleasant afternoon, not long ago, I was sitting quietly in my office, when my cogitations were interrupted by the hasty steps of a large, fresh, Yankee-looking gentleman, who said his wife was suffering very much, and wanted a doctor. I followed him, and on the way was informed by the husband of the sufferer that he had only been married a few days—an interesting patient, thought I, and probably quickened my steps. On arriving at the house, I was conducted into the room, where I soon became apprehensive that the woman, though just married, was absolutely in childbirth, and that my services as accoucheur would be brought into immediate requisition. After making the usual examination, and becoming thoroughly satisfied that my conjecture was well founded, and that it was the first presentation, I sat down to await the issue, and was not long detained ; for immediately very severe pain supervened, and a fœtus was expelled ; without, however, any other vital indication than bodily warmth, and very feeble, almost indistinct, circulation in the cord.

The ordinary means, such as stimulating baths, inflating the lungs, friction, &c., were used, probably a half hour or more, without any apparently beneficial effect. At this crisis, the father (or man who should have been), entered the room, bearing upon his breath the odor of alcohol. I called to him, and told him to come and apply his lips to those of the child, and gently blow into its mouth. He looked astonished, and exclaimed—What, me, sir ! Yes, sir, said I, you are just the man, come on. He did so. He inflated the lungs, and I expelled the air repeatedly ; and together we at length succeeded in resuscitating the child, which I am constrained to regard as wholly attributable to the stimulus of the alcoholic inspiration. It is at any rate worthy of a trial, after the ordinary means have failed ; and in the absence of a drunken husband, we suggest that the accoucheur inhale the vapor of alcohol, or spirits of camphor, immediately previous to inflating the lungs of the child.— *Southern Journal of the Medical and Physical Sciences.*

STRICTURE OF ŒSOPHAGUS.

BY WILLIAM JOHNSON, M.D.

AMONG the many ills to which flesh is heir, strictures of those canals which are lined by the mucous membrane, are far from being the least interesting, whether considered with respect to the sufferings both mental and physical, which they produce, or the imminent danger to which they often subject the unfortunate individuals, who are the victims of their visitation. Memory recalls many cases illustrative of these truths, particularly two fatal cases of stricture of the œsophagus, which occurred in this region of country since my settlement here. The first case I did not myself see, but had the relation from his widow. He died a few weeks after my settlement. He was young, but absolutely starved to death, after protracted sufferings, in full consciousness of his dreadful condition. The other case I saw but once, and that a short period previous to her death. She, too, died from inanition. Prof. Dorsey, in his Surgery, relates a case of stricture of the œsophagus, where the post-mortem examination revealed an almost entire obliteration of the canal ; a probe could scarcely pass through the strictured part. Velpeau and other writers cite cases of complete obliteration of the passage.

It is not my purpose to enter into speculation, as to the causes of these affections, whether they be owing to ulceration in some portion of these canals, producing narrowing by the contraction of their cicatrices in healing, or congestion and infiltration in the adjacent tissues while the ulcerative process is still going on, or whether simple spasmodic action be prominent in their production. But any light which can be thrown upon this subject by the record of individual cases, is due to the medical public, and it is under an imperative sense of duty that I am induced to present the following case of stricture of the œsophagus.

I was consulted, the 23d of last July, by M—— C——, aged about 22 years, on account of stricture of the œsophagus. Her attention was called to it, about two years since. She was eating a piece of pickled cucumber, and was choked, and still more so very shortly afterwards, in eating a pear. Since then the disease has been gradually increasing.

Early in her disease, she could swallow nothing but liquid articles, or
solid food very thoroughly masticated, and swallowed in very minute
portions at a time.   In fact, for some considerable time back, she has
avoided taking any solid food ; particularly animal, it choking her even
when well masticated, and swallowed in minute portions—liquid food
sometimes does the same.   She became very much alarmed, in consequence of the arrest of a very small cherry stone in her œsophagus, about
the 30th of June last.   She was eating a cherry, and the stone accidentally
slipped into the œsophagus, and produced the greatest distress by being
arrested there.   She resides about two miles from me.   In my absence
my son speedily saw her.   He directed a solution of tartarized antimony
to be held in her mouth ; it produced great nausea, and in an effort to
vomit the stone was ejected.   This patient is anemic, probably from
insufficient nutrition..   Her appetite for food is good, but she is unable to
take sufficient nourishment.   The catamenia are regular.   Ocular inspection of the fauces elicited nothing abnormal.

As tentative measures, I put her for a short time on tinct. ferri chlor.,
iodid. potas., and applied an epispastic to the throat.   The difficulty of
deglutition was not in any degree relieved by these means.   I now resorted to the bougie.   My bougies were prepared by saturating strips of
muslin in melted beeswax, and when cold, cutting those pieces in such
shape, as when rolled up tight they would be gently tapering.   They
were made of various sizes, from five eighths of an inch to one inch and
seven eighths in circumference.   I commenced by introducing the smaller
sized, and found difficulty in passing these, but the difficulty rapidly gave
way, and in a few weeks I passed the larger sized with ease.   The size
that I used for the greatest length of time was one inch and three eighths
in circumference.   I finally passed very readily those of an inch and
seven eighths in circumference.

The stricture I found to be situated some inches below the termination
of the pharynx.   I passed the bougie some inches below the stricture,
which did not appear to occupy a very large extent of surface.   A
sense of resistance at the stricture in passing the instrument through it,
was experienced.   After passing it a few times, most decided relief was
obtained by the patient.   She visited my office nearly every alternate
day, for three months, and the bougie was introduced at every visit,
either by myself or my son.

The sense of suffocation, produced by the presence of the bougie in
the œsophagus, was very distressing to the patient, and she could bear it
but a short time at each introduction.   I generally passed it twice or
three times at every visit which she paid me, which was much facilitated
by covering it well with glycerine.

In using the instrument, I departed from the directions given by Velpeau.   He advises depressing the tongue with a spoon-handle or other
instrument.   This I did not find necessary, and he says nothing about
throwing the patient's head far back, which I found very important.   My
method of introducing the instrument was, to have the patient supported
by an assistant standing behind her.   The assistant was directed to bring
the patient's head far back, so as to render the passage from the mouth

into the throat as straight as possible ; the instrument would then, by a very slight curve in it, readily pass down into the œsophagus. Its introduction was rendered easier by the patient protruding her tongue (which she could do with ease) from her mouth. The patient experienced no pain from the operation ; nothing but the strangulation above spoken of.

The improvement in this case was decided, from almost the first introduction of the bougie, until I pronounced her cured. I suggested, however, at parting with her, that it would be advisable to have the instrument passed occasionally into the œsophagus, but she found herself so completely relieved that she did not return, and I learn that she remains well, and has married since. Her mother stated, but two or three days since, that she swallows her food with perfect ease ; the bougie has not been introduced since October last—nearly four months.

Remarks.—The chief point of interest in this case is, the rapidity with which it yielded to treatment. The case I would constrast with one related by Dr. Jameson, of Baltimore, in the 29th No., vol. iii., of the Medical Recorder, Jan., 1825, edited by Samuel Calhoun, M.D., of Philadelphia. The doctor's case is a very interesting one, and will pay well for the perusal. Dr. Jameson passed ivory balls of different sizes, attached to a stem, upon which they were secured, nearly every day for ten months, before he considered the patient cured. My patient was cured by the bougie passed every alternate day for three months. Whether this result was owing to the different kinds of instruments employed, or to my case being a less serious one, I do not pretend to decide. Dr. Jameson's patient, too, was a female, but more advanced in life than mine ; his being about 40 years of age, and his case, too, was of two years' standing. For more than a fortnight he did not succeed in obtaining any advantages : but by indomitable perseverance, obtained complete success. His patient was one year under treatment. These two cases, in addition to others, give ground for encouragemnt in persevering attempts to dilate strictures ; and it may yet be found that well-directed manipulation may obviate the necessity for resorting to the caustic in the management of these cases.—*New Jersey Medical Reporter.*

M. RICORD'S LETTERS UPON SYPHILIS.

Addressed to the Editor of L'Union Medicale—Translated from the French by D. D. SLADY, M.D., Boston, and communicated for the Boston Medical and Surgical Journal.

NINETEENTH LETTER.

MY DEAR FRIEND,—If I made myself well understood in my last letter, you must believe that although experimentation has not yet demonstrated in an incontestable manner the unity of the syphilitic virus, I admitted nevertheless this unity ; that I did not seek the difference of the primary effects of this virus in its greater or less activity and acrimony, as some writers on syphilis have done ; that I sought for these effects, on the contrary, in the individual conditions of the persons who were to undergo the action of them ; in such a way as, that, in spite of some

observations of Bell, and of some analogous cases, that we still sometimes meet with in practice, and in which there is only a simple coincidence, we cannot conclude from the form and the gravity of the primary accident of an individual as to the form and gravity of the malady
of the person who communicated it to him; and that, in fine, we can
no longer at the present day, say to a patient, as we formerly said—if
your malady is a serious one, it is because the person who communicated
it to you was very much diseased; for very often it is the contrary which
we observe.

This law of the unity of virus being laid down, I am going to occupy myself, as I promised you in my last letter, with the most important variety of chancre; the *indurated chancre.*

The knowledge of the induration, of that condition which certain primitive ulcers take on, is not a new thing; some pretend that we can
even find the traces of it in Galien, which does not astonish me the
least in the world, I who believe in the antiquity of the verole. What
is certain, is, that after the great epidemic of the fifteenth century, some
of the first writers upon syphilis observe and note upon this remarkable
symptom; above all it did not escape the observation of Jean de Vigo,
who has other claims upon our esteem besides the invention of his famous plaster.

However, you know that it is to Hunter that we have given the honors
of the discovery of the indurated chancre; this symptom has even received the name of the great physiologist. The Hunterian chancre, in
fact, is no other than the indurated chancre. And yet Hunter scarcely
glances at this subject; you recollect what he says—" the chancre has
generally a thickened base, and although the common inflammation extends much beyond, yet the specific inflammation is limited to this
base." But, as you see, Hunter does not make of this thickening of
the base a constant condition; and he is right, for the greatest number
of primary ulcers do not present this peculiarity. Neither does he
make it a condition of the constitutional infection; a grave and inexplicable omission, for a man of the sagacity and of the instinct of divina-
tion of Hunter.

The writers upon syphilis who came after Hunter, even Bell, with his
comparison of a *split pea*, did not recognize all the value of induration.

Since Bell, a greater portion of the other syphilitic writers have not
paid attention to this symptom.

M. Lagneau, in his treatise, does not appear to give to this any importance; however, to do him this justice, he has recognized, as Bell
and others, that the chancre can have a pustular period; but apart from
this, you will be struck like myself with that kind of confusion which
characterizes him, between the chancre which he calls *primary,* and those
which he calls *secondary.* In all cases, the induration is of no account
for him.

As to M. Cazenave, " whose work, wholly circumstantial, and which
we cannot take for serious," and whose courteous expressions which
he recently makes use of towards me, I return, in order not to keep
anything which belongs to him; as to M. Cazenave, you know his manner

of appreciating the primary accidents. It is truly beyond belief. Never-theless, are there for M. Cazenave any primary accidents, besides the *infecting act* ? For him, in fact, the other accidents are all either *pri-mitive secondary,* or *secondary primitive.* Rid yourself of these, if you can, in spite of all the esprit of which you daily give proofs. In all cases, the induration, that capital phenomenon, does not appear to exist *upon the other side of the water,* as Lisfranc, of vigorous memory, would have remarked.

And yet, who can to-day misconstrue the importance of this phe-nomenon ? They have eyes which do not see, who suffer this to pass as null and void, after all that I have done, after the judicious observa-tions of the wise professor Thiry of Brussels, of my pupil and friend M. Diday of Lyons, of M. Marchal (de Calvi), of my learned friend and too benevolent partisan M. Venot of Bordeaux, of Messrs. Acton and Meric of London, of my learned colleagues MM. Puche and Cul-lérier ; in fine, after the observations of my patients themselves in the hospital, whose education, made during twenty years, leaves few chances for the inattentive physician to commit errors.

The induration which can line the chancres and border them, merit-ing all the attention of the practitioner, permit me to study it with care. All the chancres do not become indurated ; at the present day most cer-tainly it is only the smallest number ; and if my doctrines are true, this number will go on always diminishing.

But what is the individual cause—the necessary ulterior condition, in the insertion of the virus, which causes the chancre to become indu-rated. Therein is one of the most interesting problems which the study of syphilis can present ; and the solution of it is also one of the most difficult to obtain. I have, however, the pretension to have discovered one of the unknown principles. When we ask of age the cause of in-duration, age answers nothing. Sex, temperament, hygienic habits, also say nothing. Nor do the anterior or accompanying maladies, foreign to syphilis, any more than the special medications undergone by the patients, come to enlighten you. Until the present, then, we are obliged to con-fine ourselves to the common explanation that you know—that is to say, to aptitudes and idiosyncrasies. In fine, we find that in certain indi-viduals, a first chancre does not become indurated, while a second does, and those that they can contract afterwards do not become indurated.

Where, then, is the cause of this mysterious and singular condition ? One of the causes of these differences, passed until now unperceived, let us search for, my friend, in the laws of venereal diseases, so general and so constant ; let us search for it in the analogies so great, which exist between the variola, the vaccine and the verole. We are upon the track.

The vaccine, for example, may fail at the first trial ; this will be through the want of an aptitude of which we are ignorant ; but if it succeeds, the ulterior want of success in the new vaccinations is explained ; the diathetic effect of the first vaccination is not yet exhausted ; a lapse of time is necessary, which modern observation tends the more and more to fix precisely, to render the organism fit for a new vaccinal im-pregnation.

Well, here is a capital fact in syphilogeny, a fact that a long experience has come to demonstrate to me, a fact which has been equally observed by two men that I love always to cite, MM. Puche and Diday. It is that

General rule, a patient who has once had an indurated chancre, will not have another.

As for the vaccine, so for the variola, it is probable that this law will present exceptions. I should add that it is even desirable that it should present them, for this would prove that we can succeed in destroying the syphilitic diathesis. Beyond all doubt these exceptions are more rare for syphilis, for MM. Puche, Diday and myself have yet to search in them unexceptional proofs. It is, that when there is an indurated chancre, there is necessarily *constitutional verole*. With the induration, the syphilitic *disposition*, as Hunter called it, is acquired. The *syphilitic* temperament, as I formerly called it, and as I have since repeated, is established. Finally, there is a diathetic state, a special particular disposition, in virtue of which future manifestations will develop themselves. Disposition, temperament, diathesis, which we do not double, or treble, any more than we treble the analogous disposition in the vaccinia.

The indurated chancre is to the verole, what the *true* variolic pustule is to the variola; what the *true* vaccinal pustule is to the vaccinia.

The *non-indurated* chancre is the false pustule; it is a *false* vaccine.

Herein, my friend, is an admirable law; a law which causes the verole to enter into the general rules of virulent affections; a law which dominates over the study of syphilis, as variolic and vaccinal inoculations dominate over the history of variola; a law which satisfies the mind, and which quiets it in safety, after a painful and fastidious voyage in the midst of deceiving hypotheses and of falsifying theories; a law which arithmetic, so much outraged in its first rule by one of your old correspondents, will serve to establish in spite of him, since in order to have a real amount he will add up similar values.

But I am not now charged with the special education of the pupil *de province* of your honored correspondent; with teaching him to distinguish the difference which exists between a diathesis and the manifestations which this diathesis can produce; the difference between the diathesis properly called, and the cachexy, to all which things I shall without doubt have the opportunity to revert, and upon which I fear that this poor pupil has ideas a little clouded. For the moment let him know, and he will pardon me for this magisterial locution, that the diathesis acquired by the patient who has submitted himself to the infection prevents a new chancre which he may contract from becoming indurated, and that this kind of immunity against this form of chancre—that is to say, against a new general infection—ought also to transmit itself by way of heredity. From this can be understood what I said just now; this disposition transmitted might well have an influence upon the diminution of indurated chancres, and consequently upon the diminution of constitutional veroles. Therein is also a curious study for the verole and the vaccina. This idea, sprung from my school, has been well studied in a remarkable thesis sustained by a· distinguished pupil of **Val-de-Grace**, whose name I do not for the moment call to mind.

Thus, then, the non-induration of the chancres that a patient might contract at different epochs, after having had an indurated chancre, is a primary proof, easy to verify by the statistics of the *unicité*—neologism of which I am not culpable—the *unicité* of the syphilitic diathesis; the *unicité* implicitly admitted by Hunter, since he has said that we could prevent the disposition from being established, but that it could not be destroyed once that it was established ; *unicité* of diathesis which **M.** Cazenave did not suspect to have proclaimed after us, when he wrote in his *treatise upon syphilitic eruptions* " that he does not know if we have ever succeeded in destroying the syphilitic temperament."

Truly, in good physiology M. Cazenave would not admit a double sanguine, bilious temperament, &c.; in good pathology he would no more admit a double glanders, double variola, one or a triple hydrophobia. The *non bis in idem* is also in this connection a pathological law ; I hope to expose it in all its light, in studying the evolution of constitutional accidents.

These points of doctrine established upon the etiology of induration, let us study this phenomenon at its time of appearance, its seat, its peculiar symptoms, its nature and its course, to arrive at last at the exposition of its consequences.

Such will be, dear friend, the important subject of my next letter.

Yours,   RICORD.

OPERATION FOR HÆMATOCELE.

[Communicated for the Boston Medical and Surgical Journal).]

J. C. called on me some time in June, with an injury of the testicle caused by a fall. The injury had been done some four or five months before I saw the patient. At the time he called on me, the tumor appeared to be spheroidal ; its longest diameter was four inches, and its shortest two and a half. It was quite hard, opaque and insensible to pressure (that is, pressure did not cause pain). When the injury was first done, there was considerable pain, and great tenderness for some days. The patient says it swelled considerably at first, and then increased gradually till I saw it. I commenced a course of treatment to produce absorption. I used suspensory bandages for some time, which gave temporary relief; but at last all the means employed failed, and the pain was so great he could not attend to his business. About the first of February I proposed its removal, to which he readily consented, as the pain was insupportable, though pressure of the tumor did not increase the pain. With the assistance of Drs. Robinson and Prescott, I removed the tumor after the patient had been sufficiently etherized—a brisk cathartic having been given the day previous. The tumor weighed $17\frac{1}{2}$ oz., and on cutting it open we found the tunica vaginalis testis greatly thickened from chronic inflammation. The testicle lay in the posterior part of the tumor, very much atrophied from long-continued pressure. It was changed in structure, it being gelatinous, and filled with dark grumous blood, and so soft that it was easily broken between the thumb and finger. The sac, or tunica vaginalis, which was about one third of an inch in thickness, was filled with a fibrinous substance of a darkish color, and about the consistency of cheese curd. This tumor appears to be what is called a hæmatocele, originally an effusion of blood into the tunica vaginalis testis, and the chronic inflammation produced the various changes described.

The operation has produced perfect relief. After its performance the patient was confined to his bed for a fortnight. During the first week there was some constipation, nausea and vomiting. The former yielded to warm enemata, and the latter to small doses of morphine. The patient is now well and about his business. Yours most truly,

Rockland, Me., March, 1853.   Israel N. Smith, M.D.

SOUTHERN OBSTETRICY—DR. FELDER'S CASES OF ADHERENT PLACENTA.

To the Editor of the Boston Medical and Surgical Journal.

Sir,—It has appeared to me that obstetricians have never been sufficiently definite in demonstrating the various forms of *adherent placenta.* Hence, we propose to offer a few suggestions upon two cases which we see reported in the South Carolina Medical Journal, by Dr. W. L. Felder, of Sumter, S. C., and tranferred to the Nashville Med. Journal.

Adherent placenta may depend upon various causes. It may originate from inflammation, causing an *effusion of lymph,* or from induration, or it may depend upon a scirrhous or calcareous deposition. It may also arise from uterine inertia, with evident want of contractility in the longitudinal and circular fibres of the uterus, and not attributable to any previous pathological condition, but to irregular contraction, and retarded and difficult labor. The first variety of adherent placenta is dangerous, but of rare occurrence ; while the latter is of more frequent existence, and of less importance to the safety of the woman. The first depends upon a prior pathological cause, the last upon an incidental supervention at the time of childbirth. This is our definition, and we believe it clearly maintainable.

The first form of adhesion, we repeat, is not often met with ; but when we do see it, it demands extreme caution and careful manipulation. It is a form of adhesion that cannot be relieved by any therapeutic application upon the placental *mass,* or *around its margin,* as in Dr. Felder's cases, but must be met only by prudent manual dexterity. To maintain this point, we have only to refer to the pathology of the parts. Again, hemorrhage in these cases depends upon the character of the attachments. Generally, the adhesions are limited, the detachments considerable, and the hemorrhage is profuse ; when the attachment is entire, and no part of the placenta detached, then hemorrhage is light, for the mouths of the vessels are closed, unless the womb should be in a flaccid condition and bleed from other points. Adhesions dependent upon difficult, retarded, or tedious labor, or upon irregular contractions of the womb, are often mistaken for real adhesions, as all our works on obstetrics will substantiate ; but the cases are not at all similar, for the first are easily relieved by therapeutic means, such as *ergot*, and other excitants, while the last cannot be modified at all by them, so far as delivering the placenta is concerned.

It is clear, to our mind, that Dr. Felder's cases were of our second class, dependent upon *inertia* and *irregular* contraction, or the creosote would never have relieved them. In his first case, the creosote was an excellent remedy—a *uterine excitant*—and its introduction into the uterus is by no means novel. The reflex extremities of the uterine nerves wanted excitation ; failing after the birth of the child to obtain it, *quiescence, sleep,* non-contraction and hemorrhage, were the results. When the creosote was introduced, the womb responded ; the placenta passed off, and the hemorrhage ceased. Now had Dr. Felder's first case been an adherent placenta dependent upon previous pathological deposit, he would not have seen the same results. His second case is described as one of irregular contraction causing retention. Adhesion often exists in irregular contraction. But how could the doctor tell it ? From what Dr. Felder says, we suppose this case one of mere *hour-glass contraction*, with simple retention of placenta. The womb had become inert or torpid from the long duration of the constriction ; the placenta was retained, and the creosote was the agent of excitation to its normal function in childbirth—*pain.* Had this case been seen in four or five hours after parturition, we have no idea the same effects would have resulted from the remedy.

We are glad Dr. Felder has reported these cases ; they will give an impetus to a doctrine in uterine therapeutics which we have long entertained—*that applications to the intra-uterine surface are not as dangerous as supposed, but in neglecting them we often omit an important curative means in hemorrhage.* The rational plan of treating hemorrhage dependent upon placental *retention* or *adhesion,* is to extract the *placenta,* and never leave your patient until it is accomplished. In performing the operation, the greatest tenderness is essential ; caution is the hand-maid of prudence ; no rashness should be observed. The hand should be well oiled and very gently introduced. The extraction, as a general rule, should be commenced from the nearest margin to the fundus, and descend. We say this is the rational plan of treating hemorrhage dependent upon adherent placenta ; for when we extract the *placenta,* we cause *uterine contraction* and a closure of the bleeding vessels, unless some other untoward event should arise.

What we say here is applicable to every form of adherent placenta, for no man is justifiable in leaving his patient with an undelivered placenta. Adherent placenta of any grade as defined will induce uterine hemorrhage, and it is an intelligent position to suppose a removal of the cause will suspend the flow. But, says one, suppose you cant't do it ? We answer, you can do it, in a very large majority of cases. If accoucheurs would deliver the placenta immediately after birth, which is the natural suggestion, we should have fewer cases of flooding or irregular contraction of the uterus, than we now have. ˙In a long practice we scarcely ever have had a case of hemorrhage, and it is owing to the above caution, we verily think. But we do not pretend to say that every case of hemorrhage is avoidable, though we say a great majority are. We repeat it, to permit the *placenta* to remain in the uterus too long after delivery, is culpable and dangerous. We never do it, and we challenge a success with any man. If you have retained *placenta* or *adherent placenta*, deliver it ; do it *cautiously* and *prudently*, but don't fail to do it. By doing it you secure more safety to your case ; and the earlier you do it, upon prudent principles, the better. If a small piece should remain, be quiet ; promote contraction, and it will remain but a short time, and will pass off or be absorbed. If necessary, use an antiseptic enema ; but in cold weather this will not be needed, yet in warm weather it may be useful. We never like to hear of a case of retained placenta, of four, five, or seven days ; it is not only dangerous to the woman, but it is bad *midwifery*. Prudence in obstetrics is safety ; and safety consists in delivering your patient fully, before you leave. We care not what other men say, we are in favor of the immediate removal of the placenta in all cases, under ordinary circumstances. This is the way to avoid danger.

We have now given our opinions, but we force them on no one. We are no fault-finder, no medical censor, no castigator of our brethren ; we want every man to think for himself ; we shall do it, and express our thoughts fearlessly and independently, despite of collegiate dogmas or conventional mandates. With the kindest regard, and highest respect for Dr. Felder, we repeat our conviction, that in our first class of cases *creosote* is of no effect ; in the second, under some circumstances, it may do, and admirably ; but under all circumstances, other things being favorable, the proper plan of treating *adherent placenta* is to *deliver*.

 March, 1853.   " SOUTHERNER."

DISLOCATION AND REDUCTION OF HIP-JOINT BY RHEUMATISM.
[Communicated for the Boston Medical and Surgical Journal.]

M. B., aged 33 years, was attacked at the age of 16, with rheumatism of the right hip, and confined to his room and bed six months, and then recovered, and had no lameness for eight months. Was then attacked in the left hip, and confined to bed four months. Became convalescent and commenced walking about, though feeling some lameness. Took a walk one day, of two or three miles, which brought on another attack in the same hip, which resulted, in the space of two days, in dislocation of the hip upwards and outwards—the leg being shortened two inches or more, and the toe turned inwards. Soon recovered from the lameness, but with permanent shortening of the limb. Has worn a boot on this foot with a heel two inches higher than upon the other, for seventeen years. Has had no pain or lameness (but difficulty of motion) in the hip for the same space of time.

On the 24th of December last, was attacked again. The attack was

light, merely producing moderate lameness for a week or ten days, the
patient being able in the mean time to walk about with a cane. Leg
at this time commenced growing longer, and in the space of one week
was of full length—same as the other. There was no sudden jog or
motion experienced, but a gradual lengthening. The first evidence the
patient had of the lengthening of the limb, was a tripping of the heel on
attempting to walk, which impediment increased so much that he finally
removed the high heel from the boot, when he found that he had two
legs of the same length. He has now good use of his leg, and experiences no pain in the hip except on sudden motion or slipping. The
head of the femur is now evidently *in situ.* The leg is less in size than
the other.

The peculiarity in this case is the cause and cure of dislocation by
the same agent, or rather disease —rheumatism.

I have been informed of another similar case, but have obtained no
correct history of it.   Yours truly,
Wellsborough, Pa., March 8, 1853.   C. K. THOMPSON.

THE BOSTON MEDICAL AND SURGICAL JOURNAL.

BOSTON, MARCH 16, 1853.

*A Discourse on the Life, Character and Services of Daniel Drake,
M.D.*—This discourse was delivered by Prof. S. D. Gross before the Faculty and Medical Students of the University of Louisville, Ky., Jan. 27,
1853, and constitutes a pamphlet of about 90 pages. It is just such a production as might be expected from the pen of one so distinguished as is Dr.
Gross for literary and scientific attainments, and who enjoyed a long and
intimate acquaintance with the celebrated subject of his biography.
Dr. G. traces the life of the deceased, from his father's log cabin in Mays
Lick, Ky., to which the family emigrated from New Jersey in 1788 when
Daniel was 2½ years old, to its final close in Cincinnati last autumn. He relates in detail, but not with prolixity, his attendance on medical lectures
in Philadelphia, his private pupilage in Cincinnati in 1800, his marriage
in Cincinnati in 1807, his final course of lectures and graduation in Philadelphia in 1815, his professorship in the Transylvania Med. School at Lexington in 1816, his organization of the Medical College of Ohio in 1819, his
re-call to Lexington in 1823, his return to Cincinnati and establishment of a
medical journal there in 1827, his election to a professorship in Jefferson Medical College, Philadelphia, in 1830, his organization of the Medical Department of the Cincinnati College in 1835, and his subsequent acceptance
of a chair in the University of Louisville. Here he continued till 1849,
when he resigned his chair, and again accepted one in the Medical College
of Ohio, which he filled but one session. In the autumn of 1850 he was
re-called to the Louisville school, in which he remained two sessions, when
he re-entered the Ohio Medical College, " his first and last love," now re-
organized. But just at the opening of the session the hand of death was
laid upon him, and his brilliant but varied career was arrested. Dr. D. is
next spoken of as a philanthropist and a patriot. He was concerned in

the establishment of the Commercial Hospital of Ohio, the institution for the Education of the Blind, the Cincinnati Eye Infirmary, the Kentucky School for the Blind, and the Physiological Temperance Society in Louisville. He was deeply interested in the construction of the great railroad chain between the Ohio river and the tide-waters of the Carolinas and Georgia, and also in the passage of the compromise measures in 1850 in the Congress of the United States. Dr. Drake was the author of the " Picture of Cincinnati," " Essays on Medical Education, &c.." a " Practical Treatise, on Epidemic Cholera." a work on Anatomy, Physiology and Hygiene, a small volume of " Discourses," was editor twelve years of the Western Medical Journal, and finally, in 1850, issued the first volume of his 'great work on the " Principal Diseases of the Interior Valley of North America." The second volume, nearly completed when he died, will be issued the ensuing summer. Dr. Gross sketches with great fidelity and with the skill of a master the prominent traits in the character of Dr. D. He portrays his lofty ambition, nice sense of honor, unwearied industry, unflinching self-denial, warm friendship and ardent piety. We cannot refrain from quoting a few passages from the address, although so much space has already been devoted to its analysis.

" Dr. Drake was a man not of one, but of many characteristics. His very look, manner, step and gesture were characteristic; they were the outward signs of the peculiar nature within; his conversation, his voice and modes of expression were characteristic; all tending to stamp him, in the estimation and judgment of the beholder, as an extraordinary personage. But there was one feature which jutted out, prominently and conspicuously, above and beyond the rest, and which served, in an eminent degree, to distinguish him from all the men of my profession I have ever known. This was intensity, intensity of thought, of action, and of purpose. This feeling, to which he was indebted for all the success which marked his eventful career, exhibited itself in all the relations of life; in his extraordinary devotion to his family, his attachments to his friends, his unfaltering love for his profession, in his interest in the, cause of temperance, in his lectures before his pupils in the University, in his writings, his debates, and his controversies. No apathy or -lukewarmness ever entered his mind, or influenced his conduct, in any scheme which had for its object the welfare of his species, the promotion of science, or the improvement of the human intellect. His temperament was too ardent to permit him, had he otherwise felt so inclined, to be an idle and unconcerned spectator of the world around him. It was hot, and positive, like the pole of an electric battery, intense, ever restive, always doing."

" No where did this intensity exhibit itself in a more striking manner, or in a greater degree, than in the lecture room. It was here, surrounded by his pupils, that he displayed it with peculiar force and emphasis. As he spoke to them, from day to day, respecting the great truths of medical doctrine and medical science, he produced an effect upon his young disciples, such as few teachers are capable of creating. His words dropped hot and burning from his lips, as the lava falls from the burning crater; enkindling the fire of enthusiasm in his pupils, and carrying them away in total forgetfulness of everything, save the all-absorbing topic under discussion. They will never forget the ardor and animation which he infused into his discourses, however dry or uninviting the subject; how he enchained their attention, and how, by his skill and address, he lightened the tedium of the class-room. No teacher ever knew better how to enliven his auditors, at one time with glowing bursts of eloquence, at another with the sallies of wit, now with a startling pun, and anon with the recital of an' apt and amusing anecdote ; eliciting, on the one hand, their admiration for his varied intellectual riches, and, on the other, their respect and veneration for his extraordinary abilities as an expounder of the great and fundamental principles of medical science. His gestures, never graceful, and sometimes eminently awkward ; the peculiar incurvation of his body ; nay, the very *drawl* in which he frequently gave expression to his ideas ; all denoted the burning fire within, and served to impart force and vigor to every thing which he uttered from the rostrum. Of all the medical teachers whom I have ever heard, he was the most forcible and eloquent. His voice was remarkably clear and distinct, and so powerful that, when the windows of his lecture-room were open, it could be heard at a great distance. He sometimes read his discourse, but generally he ascended the rostrum without note or scrip."

"His mode of living was peculiar, and, in the opinion of the world and some of his friends, parsimonious and eccentric. Nothing, however, could have been more erroneous. The affection of his brain, which ultimately destroyed him, and to occasional attacks of which he was for many years subject, compelled him to live differently from other men. The slightest indulgence at dinner invariably brought on an attack of cerebral oppression, followed by an inability for useful mental and physical exertion ; and it was a knowledge of this fact, the result of ample experience, that induced him never to take any thing at this meal, except a cup of tea and the smallest quantity of vegetables ; frequently, indeed, nothing but a little pastry. At his breakfast and supper, however, he generally ate as hearty as any one. I allude to this subject, trivial as it may appear, and irrelevant as it may be to the true dignity of biography, because I wish to place my friend right before this community, in whose midst he lived and toiled for so many long winters. The explanation is due to his memory, to his children, and to his friends. Boarding houses and hotels were disagreeable to him ; he could find no congeniality at a public table, and in the noise and confusion of public apartments. He preferred his own room at the University, with his cracker and a cup of tea, to the most splendid table in the State. For many years he found a congenial place and a hearty welcome at the houses of his friends. It was not to save and hoard up money that he thus lived ; for no man ever spent money more liberally, no one ever had a greater contempt for it. His late associates in this University, and a few friends in this city, who alone knew him thoroughly and truly, can best appreciate the force and truth of my remarks.

"To those who are engaged in scientific, literary, and educational pursuits, or the practice of medicine, it will not be uninteresting to know that Dr. Drake was poor, and, until the last eight years of his life, pecuniarily embarrassed. It was not until after his connection with this University that he began to lay up any thing from his earnings. His medical journal only brought him into debt. The first volume of his work has sold slowly, and had not yielded him one dollar at the time of his death. Since that period his son-in-law, Alexander H. McGuffey, Esq., has received, as his literary executor, two hundred and fifty dollars as the balance to the author's credit up to that time. This sum is not more than one tenth of what he paid for the maps alone, contained in the work, and engraved at his own expense. Nothing, in fact, that Dr. Drake ever undertook was pecuniarily profitable. He was not a man of the money-making character.

He lost money by every enterprise in which he ever engaged. His aims were always so lofty, and so far removed from self, that he never thought of money, except so far as it was necessary to their accomplishment.

"But although he has not, like Cæsar, left any landed estates, villas, orchards, or vineyards to his friends and the public, he has bequeathed them, what is far more precious and enduring, a name without reproach, a bright example, and imperishable works."

Pennsylvania Hospital for the Insane.—While passing by the stately edifice of this hospital, a few days since, we thought of the humanity with which the insane are treated in our day, in the many institutions through the country, including this long-established asylum, in which the services of the medical superintendent are appreciated by an intelligent community. The report for the year 1852, now before us, shows that 197 patients were admitted, 198 discharged or died, and 215 under care at the close of the year. The total number in the hospital in 1852, was 413. No particularly new views are promulgated by Dr. Kirkbride. He has, however, exhibited very clearly and cogently the importance of a farm, garden, and workshops ; of a library, museum, reading room, and the like intellectual appliances, for the use of lunatics, and the amount of happiness they diffuse. Then follows a particular specification of the outgoes and income, the improvements, and the donations and contributions of benevolent persons in the way of books, papers, &c. &c. Total expenditures for 1852, $53,436 76. Excess of expenditures over receipts, $3,107 14. Average cost per week for each patient,$4 59. The sum expended in 1852 on free patients, was $8,592 48. From the organization of the hospital, it has had an excellent reputation. Men of character have always been its managers, who liberally sustain the medical officers in every suggestion that promises to advance the comfort and convenience of the insane confided to their care.

New York Ophthalmic Hospital.—Accompanying the first report of the surgeons, is an address by Mr. Woodhull. It appears that in about seven months, 444 patients were admitted ; 232 discharged, cured, and 66 relieved. These are the essential statistics. Were better buildings provided, the surgeons believe that a larger proportion might be cured. Men of ability are conducting the institution, and they will by and by successfully awaken an interest in the public mind that will lead to all the accommodations necessary. Life governors are made by the payment of forty dollars. Many a man might have an office by purchase, who would otherwise never be a governor, according to the prospectus ; and since their money would open the eyes of the blind, we really hope the number of aspirants for the distinction thus proffered, may be sufficient to meet all the immediate wants of the hospital. Medical strangers, when in New York, would find themselves compensated by a visit to No. 6 Stuyvesant street, between the 2d and 3d Avenues, seventeenth ward. Surgeons, Dr. David L. Rogers and Dr. Mark Stephenson.

Anæsthesia in Midwifery.—However desirable it may be to republish all the good things perpetually pouring in from the profession, the limits of the Journal quite forbid the undertaking. To give the titles, the names of writers, and a general idea of their efforts, is about as much as is possible. Henry Miller, M.D., of Louisville, Ky., who enjoys an extensive reputation as a practitioner and medical writer, is the author of a paper in the transactions of the Kentucky Medical Society for 1852, which has been sent abroad in another form, a copy of which is before us. It is on Anæsthesia in Midwifery, and the Speculum Uteri. Those at all curious or ambitious to keep pace with the progress of this particular branch of medicine, will be interested and instructed by this production. Dr. Miller's observations on the use of the speculum uteri are no every-day sayings, but the results of a careful, conscientious devotion to the welfare of his patients, and might be studied with lasting profit by young practitioners.

New Jersey Lunatic Asylum. — The annual reports of those excellent charities, the retreats for the insane, are coming in from all sections of the union. At Trenton, the State of New Jersey has located a model edifice, of which H. A. Buttolph, M.D., is physician. In 1852, according to the annual report, the receipts from all sources were $38,048 47, and the outgoes just $39 40 less. Next follows the superintendent's report, a sensible, prudent and reliable document. As in every other asylum in America, more room is required. The people are fast going mad, evidently, and perhaps the craziest and most unmanageable are still at large. Dr. B.'s remarks on mixed forms of insanity, predisposing causes, exciting causes, on the cerebellum, &c., give an insight into the character of the writer's own mind, which is eminently qualified for investigation. He is philosophical in his views, and progressive. There is no hope for a physician who is perfectly satisfied with being at rest: an energy that is never exhausted in the pursuit of means for lessening the physical or mental woes of the unfortunate, should at least characterize the medical superintendent of a hospital given up to lunatics. Dr. Buttolph exhibits the traits to command esteem wherever his views are circulated. During 1852, 121 patients were received, which, added to the 171 inmates under treatment at the commencement of the year, show that the provision which the State made for their comfort was needed.

Dr. Marshall Hall.—Of course every medical reader is familiar with the name of this distinguished English author. He is now at Washington, accompanied by his lady and son. After visiting the South, he proposes to return and travel over the West extensively, and next season visit the Eastern States. Although considerably advanced in years, Dr. Hall is a laborious student, a close observer, and may justly be called one of the most celebrated medical writers of the age. We bespeak for him the attentions of the professional brotherhood wherever his steps may be directed.

Hydropathic Treatment of Dysentery. — A subscriber in the country writes as follows respecting a case which lately came under his observation.

"A quack hydropathic doctor was called upon to attend a married woman thirty-two years old, afflicted with dysentery. His treatment was hydropathic to the extreme ; cold bath, two and three times a day, also cold injections as often, together with large draughts of water. She grew gradually worse, became much emaciated, and sent for me at the end of three weeks of the above treatment. She was literally nearly washed to death —a mere skeleton, with just enough life to remain off her bed while it was being made. She said she was sorry they (her friends) had sent for me; she expected soon to die, and she did not wish to be further tortured by medicine. I found her with every indication of extreme and general debility. I immediately gave her small powders of morphine, and quinine three times a day; a little farinaceous diet often, to be increased with her growing strength. Without any other medical treatment, in eight days from that time she became so well that she walked about a quarter of a mile to my office, and paid her bill."

Medical Miscellany.—In the March number of the American Journal of Pharmacy, there is an unusual amount of excellent matter.—The fourth annual report of the Female Med. Education Society has been published. The sum of $3.458 22 was received by the society from various sources in 1852, ending in October.—Miss Dr. Blackwell, of New York, is the author of a book called the Laws of Life—but a copy has not, to our knowledge, been seen in Boston.—Elements of the Anatomy and Physiology of the Human System, by Justin R. Loomis, will soon be published at New York, by Messrs. Cornish, Lamport & Co.—A third number of the N. Y. Esculapian has appeared.—Dr. Cornochan's article on Elephantiasis Arabum has been issued in a pamphlet form, with a plate.—Dr. J. M. Allen's lecture, at the Pennsylvania College, at the commencement of the lectures, is a plain, sensible, well written discourse.—Remarks on Osteo-Aneurism, with a case involving the condyles of the left femur, by Dr. Cornochan, the eminent surgeon, is to be had in a pamphlet, with a plate. — The sixteenth annual report of the trustees and superintendent of the Vermont Asylum for the Insane, shows a sound condition of the institution. — Dr. Flint's prize essay on variations of pitch, in percussion and respiratory sounds, and their application to physical diagnosis, has been reprinted for private distribution among the author's friends. — Flour, under the name of *patent*, having in it a mixture of supercarbonate of soda, and known as *self-rising*, is sold in large quantities by the barrel, as a superior article. It should be avoided.—A pedlar at Apalachian, N. Y., it seems, had a medical diploma to sell!—It is said that there is a physician for every 300 persons throughout the State of New York. No wonder multitudes are leaving the profession. — Bones of the skull may be fractured at birth. Three cases have been reported in Germany, and this fact should be remembered in cases where persons are accused of infanticide, in consequence of discovering the cranial bones to be broken.—Dr. Hero was the presiding officer at the eclectic medical society meeting at Syracuse, N. Y.; an appropriate cognomen for the occasion.

To Correspondents. — The following communications have been received: — An address before the Bristol District Medical Society; remarks on Dr. Tully's Materia Medica; obituary notice of Dr. C W. Chandler; the commencement of a translation of M. Valleix's lectures on Displacements of the Uterus.

Deaths in Boston—for the week ending Saturday noon, March 12th, 69 —Males. 27—females, 42. Abscess, 1—apoplexy, 1—disease of the bowels, 1—inflammation of the brain, 2—congestion of the brain, 1—disease of the brain, 2—consumption, 10—cholera infantum, 1—croup, 4—dysentery, 1—dropsy, 1—dropsy in head, 2—infantile diseases, 9—puerperal, 1—typhus fever, 1—typhoid fever, 1—scarlet fever, 8—gout, 1—gangrene, 1—disease of the heart, 3—hernia, 1—inflammation of the lungs, 2—marasmus, 2—old age, 3—palsy, 1—scrofula,, 1—teething, 4—thrush, 1— unknown, 1—worms, 1.

Under 5 years, 40 —between 5 and 20 years. 7—between 20 and 40 years, 10—between 40 and 60 years, 7—over 60 years, 5. Born in the United States, 55—Ireland, 11—England, 1— British Provinces, 1—Germany, 1. The above includes 9 deaths in the city institutions.

Massachusetts College of Pharmacy. — At the annual meeting of the Mass. College of Pharmacy, held at the rooms of the College in Masonic Temple, on Monday, March 9th, the following members were elected the officers for the ensuing year.

President, Daniel Henchman. *1st Vice President,* Thomas Restieaux. *2d Vice President,* Samuel M. Colcord. *Corresponding Secretary,* William A. Brewer. *Recording Secretary,* Henry W. Lincoln. *Treasurer,* Samuel N. Brewer. *Auditor,* Joseph Burnett. *Trustees,* Thomas Farrington, Ashel Boyden, Henry D. Fowle, Andrew Geyer, Joseph T. Brown, Samuel R. Philbrick, T. Larkin Turner, William Brown.

HENRY W. LINCOLN, *Secretary.*

Pinto Indians.—Dr. Edw. Ludlow, of New York, communicates to the Medical Times, of that city, some account of a peculiar class of aboriginal inhabitants of certain parts of Mexico, received by him from Col. A. C. Ramsey, formerly of the U. S. Army. It seems they are a race, poor and ignorant, living mostly in villages by themselves, near the city of Puebla, speaking the Aztec language, and distinguished by different colored spots on the skin of the same individual. From this last they derive their name —"Pintos," or painted people. No two of them are alike. Some have one hand black and the other white, and the face spotted gray, blue, black or white. Others have one half the face lead color, and the other half of a copper hue. Sometimes the face is all blue, again all black or red, and the body the natural Indian color. No authentic account could be obtained of this singular race of beings, nor does their disease seem to be well understood. It is probable, however, that it is merely cutaneous, and not in any degree contagious, and no more hereditary than are the habits which in a long course of years have probably given rise to it.

Rheumatic Affections at La Charité.—"We may mention," says one of the editors of the Charleston Med. Journal, in a recent letter from Paris, "the practice pursued by M. Briquet, at La Charité, of tapping a knee-joint affected with articular rheumatism, and after drawing off the fluid, injecting with much benefit, and apparently without danger, a solution of tincture of iodine. He is in the habit of treating cases of rheumatism characterized by neuralgic symptoms, irritable condition of the heart, for example, in which digitalis is not indicated, with the di-sulphate of quinine, in doses sufficient to induce and keep up its influence. We carefully watched, from day to day, cases under his care, which have recovered entirely after its employment. The theory is: the sedative influence of this tonic on the nervous and circulatory systems, when given in quantities sufficient to produce quininism."

Glycerin Ointment.—Mr. John H. Ecky, in the January No. of the Am. Journ. Pharm., publishes a formula for an ointment which he found very useful in chapped hands, lips, excoriations of skin, &c.

R Spermaceti, ℥ss.
White Wax, ℥j.
Oil Almonds, ℥ij. (f)
Glycerin, ℥j, (f)

Melt the wax and spermaceti with the oil of almonds at a moderate heat, put these into a wedgwood mortar, add the glycerin, and rub until well mixed and cold.— *South. Jour. Med. Sciences.*

THE

BOSTON MEDICAL AND SURGICAL JOURNAL.

| VOL. XLVIII. | WEDNESDAY, MARCH 23, 1853. | No. 8. |

DR. TULLY'S MATERIA MEDICA.

BY RICHARD H. SALTER, M.D.

[Communicated for the Boston Medical and Surgical Journal.]

WE are very sorry to notice, in some of our medical journals, severe and uncalled-for strictures upon the work of Dr. Tully on the Materia Medica and Therapeutics, now being issued from the press in monthly parts. We are sorry for two reasons. One is, that such strictures, unjust in themselves, may have the effect to lessen, if not entirely to take away, the patronage of the work, and so discourage those generous individuals who have taken upon themselves the responsibility of its publication. The other reason is, that the editors of these journals will regret, in the end, if the publication should go on to completion, their too hasty remarks, and be as sorry as we are that they were ever made. If these editors will let Dr. Tully get fairly into his subject before they "let fly their pop-guns," we assure them that they will have no cause to regret following the *laissez faire* plan. In the mean time, however, should they continue to send forth their extemporaneous thoughts in the same strain, they may, so far as their journals have influence, do great disservice to the cause of medical science, in the department of the materia medica and therapeutics ; especially if such remarks should discourage the patrons of the work—for it cannot go on without patronage. We will venture to add here, for we profess to have some knowledge of what Dr. Tully can do, that if the work should be completed, it will be unsurpassed in fullness and accuracy and in practical utility, by any other work, of the same sort, in the English language. We say this without intending to undervalue other works of the kind that have been already published.

We are more sorry to perceive the manner and tone of some of the strictures referred to. We will notice particularly those contained in the Buffalo Medical Journal for January of this year. The editor of this Journal founds his argument for condemning the entire labors of Dr. Tully, on this subject, which have extended through a period of more than forty years, on one point contained in the first number, viz., the "non-absorption of remedial agents," and gives us to understand that the judgment of Dr. Tully's friends is nothing near so clear and far-sighted as

8

his own ; for, he says, that Dr. Tully in maintaining this doctrine, "adopts as the basis of the materia medica, the obsolete dogma of *exclusive solidism* " * * * " and this vicious principle will render the entire work useless." We trust that the editor will understand us as speaking com-paratively, for we are far from wishing to convey the impression that he is not clear-headed or far-sighted ; nevertheless we do think that, in this instance, he has missed his mark. We simply ask him to give us a sat-isfactory reason for his statement. We are inclined to the opinion that it matters little what theory Dr. Tully holds in reference to the par-ticular subject under consideration, whether that of the solidists, the hu-moralists, or both together, provided he gives us exact and positive in-formation on the powers and therapeutic application of remedial agents. We may be more stupid than the editor, and he may be able to prove it to us ; but, for the life of us, we cannot see how the fact of Dr. Tully's holding the opinion, an "exploded" one, if you please, of the "non-absorption of remedial agents," can in any manner vitiate what he may have to say on any particular articles of the materia medica. Suppose, for illustration, that in the case of some disease, there are certain mani-fest phenomena which plainly declare certain indications ; a remedial agent is sought for and administered to fulfil these indications. Suppose the result of this to be, that the required operation is produced, and the desired effect obtained. Now the question we would ask is, whether, in order to accomplish this result, it is necessary that we should know the precise method or process by which it was obtained from the remedy used ? Does it, in truth, make any difference, in a practical point of view, whe-ther we are able or not to comprehend the *why* and the *how*, however desirable such knowledge may be.

Again, there are certain remedial agents that we call narcotics, there are others we call nervines, there are others still which we name stimu-lants. They are so designated and distinguished from certain manifest effects which they produce upon the human body, when taken into the stomach, peculiar to each respectively. A person familiar with the known powers of the remedial agents belonging to the classes above mentioned, would be able to predict, almost infallibly, in a greater or less degree, what would be the effects from their administration. In this way, in part at least, he comes to learn how to administer remedial agents for the relief of suffering. We are only speaking in a general way. For instance, there are certain narcotics called *anodynes*, certain others called *hypnotics ;* from the fact of the one assuaging pain and the other promoting or producing sleep. There are certain nervines which are said to relieve spasm, and hence called antispasmodics. There are cer-tain stimulants that are said to relieve exhaustion and faintness, and hence are called *restoratives.* Now the question recurs : if we know that such are the facts, and are sufficiently acquainted with the powers of the remedial agents, to administer them safely and judiciously, is it necessary that we should know precisely the *modus operandi* of the re-medial agent, in order to obtain the desired effect of its administration ; much less, whether it is absorbed or not into the circulation. The pos-session or the want of such knowledge cannot, so far as we can see, affect the powers of our remedial agents, nor their correct therapeutic application. We shall adhere to our opinion, however presumptuous it may seem, until the editor shall convince us to the contrary, that whether Dr. Tully holds the "dogma" of solidism or humoralism, or any other ism, the opinion of the absorption or non-absorption of remedial agents cannot in any manner affect the value of what he may have to say on the powers, remedial operative effects, and the therapeutic application of the particular articles of the materia medica.

The editor implies that the question, whatever may be its importance, is a settled one. In this, too, we think he is rather wide of the truth. It may, however, be settled somewhat after the manner of certain political matters; a kind of settlement very likely to be unsettled at any time.

Let us look at the question in another light; let us suppose Dr. Tully to be wholly wrong in his views of the non-absorption of remedial agents; that he is simply reviving an "exploded" opinion of the solidists, and that every fact he adduces in behalf of his own views amounts to nothing at all, when placed by the side of the "*mass*" of testimony sustaining the opposite opinion. Let us suppose that remedial agents are taken up into the mass of the circulation before producing their operative effects, and that they float up and down with the vital stream—yea, so thoroughly mixed with the whole that a pint of it shall hardly contain the twenty-first or even the thirtieth attenuation of a homœopathic dose—before their proper operative effect is produced; supposing all this, will this editor be so kind as to inform us what the *modus operandi* of any one remedial agent is after being received into the mass of the circulating fluid; not, we wish him plainly to understand, its obvious operative effect, but the process by which its operative effect is produced? When he shall have done this in a satisfactory manner, we will hold ourselves bound, at least, to consider the question further, if not to give up our opinion; but, until then, we must maintain that the question of solidism or humoralism, in a practical point of view, is a matter of opinion, about which different writers may hold opposite views, without in the least affecting sound principles of the materia medica and therapeutics; so long as they give us exact information in regard to the powers of remedial agents, and their most obvious therapeutic application.

Objection has been made, in some quarters, to the use Dr. Tully makes of "barbarous and long words, which nobody can pronounce and very few understand," * * * "altogether unscientific";—that is, he has adopted terms, as applied to his classification of the materia medica and to the supposed operative effects of remedial agents, that are peculiar to himself, which nobody ever employed before him and nobody will take the trouble to understand after him. It is hardly time yet to speak fully on this subject, for Dr. Tully has not published his method of classification, and in what has already been published, he has only here and there made use of terms which can give any possible color to the objection. Nevertheless, as the objection has been made, we may say, in a general way, that where there is no settled standard, or rather, perhaps, where the adopted standard is uncertain and unsatisfactory, every author has a right to be governed by his own taste and judgment; provided he uses technical terms appropriately, and gives us clear and concise definitions of what is intended by them. If one will consider the unsatisfactory and chaotic state in which medical technical terms have existed and do now 'exist, and how indiscriminately they are employed by authors and practitioners to express the same things by different terms, and different things by the same terms, and the consequent confusion of ideas as well as of things, he will, we think, be disposed to waive his objection to an attempt to give greater precision and accuracy to medical language in general, and technical language in particular. This is, we believe, what Dr. Tully intends to do; and we most heartily wish him all success. To say that Dr. Tully is "unscientific," is only to expose one's ignorance. The only apology for the objection is, that he may be too strictly scientific in the use of the language of chemistry for permanent use, for chemical nomenclatures vary with almost every new discovery, or what purports to be such. This, however, can relate to only a small part of a system of materia medica, and is not really much of an objection in itself.

To illustrate, in part, what has been said, let us take two words, very commonly used among medical practitioners in a technical sense—*prostration* and *exhaustion*. We find that physicians in common intercourse with each other use these words indiscriminately, the one for the other— and we rarely take up a modern medical book in which the author, if the words occur at all, does not use them synonymously. We might say the same of a multitude of technical terms. Now we want no more technical words than are necessary to express their objects or ideas; and if the two words, above mentioned, are synonymous, and may be used indiscriminately to express the same state or condition, it seems to us that it would be well to dispense with one of them, and so far disencumber our technical language of an unnecessary word. May it not be, however, that most medical men of our time, for some reason or other, have lost the proper use of these words? In former times these words were used by physicians, in their appropriate and distinctive sense, and there is the same reason for the distinction now as formerly, but for some reason the distinction seems to have been nearly lost sight of. The old writers understood, by the word *prostration*, that state of the system where the vital power or energy is apparently *latent;* the vital principle* being for some cause prevented from manifesting its ordinary excitability. By the word *exhaustion*, they meant that state of the system where there was apparent positive deficiency of the vital power or energy. Whether, if we knew more about the vital power, as the living energy is called, or its relative condition in the states expressed by these words,

* By our use of the expression, "vital principle," we shall probably expose ourselves to criticism We are free to say, however, that modern philosophy is at once too material and too presumptuous to perceive the true principles of the science of man, and the form that physiology should take, in order to assume its due importance, and exercise its appropriate influence. The idea of considering *life*, or the sensible principle, as consisting in the aggregate properties of matter,—a mere mental abstraction,—having no existence distinct from organization, and to be classed in the same category with the Newtonian principle of gravitation, is, to say the least, obviously absurd. We think that the ideal and spiritual are as real as the visible and the tangible; and that physiology, as the science of life or "living organism" is called, must be based on a higher philosophy of man than now obtains, before it can exert its true and proper influence.

they would be appropriate, is beside the question. We have a notion of something, when we speak of vital power, though it may be impossible to express it in terms ; so had the old writers, and they say that the two states or conditions' indicated above could with ease be detected and distinguished. The former state may be compared to an elastic spring depressed by a weight ; the latter to the same spring with its elasticity destroyed. It will be obvious, we think, to any fair-minded man, that if there is ground for the distinction, as we contend there is, it is practically of no small importance.

For further illustration of our position, we will refer to two classes of remedial agents ; for example, *Narcotics* and *Nervines.* From a careful and somewhat extensive examination of writers on the materia medica and collateral subjects, we have not been able to find one who has given a full, clear and satisfactory definition of the terms themselves, much less a satisfactory account of the operative effects of the remedial agents to which the terms are respectively applied. This shows obviously that the writers themselves possessed no distinct and clear idea what manifest operative effects were necessary to entitle a remedial agent to the name of narcotic or nervine ; and that this defective state of their knowledge rendered it impossible for them to distinguish accurately one class from the other. The term narcotic implies the idea of something that will produce torpor and stupefaction—and nearly every writer we have examined on this subject, attaches some idea of this sort to all of the remedial agents arranged under this head. In general, writers say, that narcotics affect the sensibility in some way, and induce stupefaction, insensibility ; and ultimately, when administered immoderately or excessively, they produce delirium, coma or convulsions or both. The greater part of these writers say that narcotics produce primarily a stimulant effect upon the nervous and vascular systems, and that this stimulant effect is followed by depression of the vital powers, which is supposed to be the operative effect of a narcotic proper. When they describe the particular operative effects of the remedial agents of this class, they say, in a general way, that they are narcotic, anodyne, hypnotic, stimulant, sedative—making a distinction between narcotic and sedative,—inspissant and perhaps calmative ; and these are called its physical or physiological actions. Sometimes, however, they refer the operative effect of a drug to some *act or original impulse of volition,* when it cannot be satisfactorily referred to some physiological action as it is termed. Nearly all of these terms, and others we have not mentioned, but equally *clear and expressive,* are applied to almost all of the remedial agents arranged under the class narcotics. It would seem, as far as we can judge, that writers on the materia medica take as the type of the class, some one article which combines in itself several distinct powers, and from the operative effects of this, with which, perhaps, they are most familiar, judge of the whole. To say the least, it is a very unphilosophical mode of proceeding, if it be so. But to proceed ; when they speak of the uses' or therapeutic application of these remedial agents, the following terms are very frequently employed, viz., antispasmodic, antidysenteric, febrifuge, antihysteric, antirheumatic, and many others just as _definite and expressive._ The doses and mode of administering the remedial agents of this class are not better understood ; the latter especially in respect. to combination, frequency of repetition and length of time for continuance, as adapted to different types and forms of disease. We cannot now go into particulars. We will add a few words on the class nervines.

This class is more frequently denominated antispasmodics, which, from the definition given to the term, would comprehend a greater or less number of the remedial agents of nearly every class in the materia medica. It is commonly stated that they are stimulants, or rather stimulants of the nervous system, and tonics of the nervous system, and even narcotics, and scarcely to be distinguished from them !! It is stated also by some that both narcotics and nervines are _alteratives_ (a term, by the way, conveying no distinct meaning) ; but whether it be so or not, in this instance it is grossly misapplied to express a change in the _quality_ of the _vital action_ of the nervous system. What sort of vital action can anybody predicate of the nervous system ? if none, much less can any _quality_ of action of the nerves be appreciated by any one. If no appreciable action can be predicated of the nervous system, how is it possible to ascertain whether there be increased or diminished action of that system, as the term _stimulant_ of the nervous system would seem to imply ? How inappropriate, then, is the use of such language, unless we attach different ideas to it from the generality of writers. Nevertheless, whatever that difference may be, we are persuaded that the writers who employ it would not be a little puzzled, if put to it, to define what they mean by any _quality_ of action of the nervous system, or indeed _any action_ at all.

Now we not only think, but know from actual experience and observation, that there are such remedial agents as pure or simple narcotics and nervines, and that their manifest operative effects, when administered to persons in health, may be observed, noted and determined with a degree of accuracy and precision, that, so far as we are aware, has not been obtained, as yet, by any author on the materia medica. The same may be done, also, when these agents are administered to fulfil certain indications in morbid or diseased conditions of the human system —if administered judiciously ; especially can this be done, if in addition to a clear and precise idea of the powers and operative effects of our remedial agents both in health and disease, we have also a tolerable knowledge of the true natural history of the existing disease, at least an accurate appreciation of existing symptoms—particularly in reference to the locality of their origin and peculiarity of their cause—and of those most likely to appear in the progress of the disease, so as to be able to distinguish, with a degree of certainty, between the symptoms of the disease and the operative effects our remedial agents are capable of producing. By careful and accurate observation, then, of what may be considered and understood as the manifest operative effects of simple narcotics and nervines, we are in some measure prepared to appreciate the operative effects of those remedial agents which possess two or more powers : for example, narcotic and stimulant powers ; or narcotic and alterative, or, more properly, deobstruent powers; or nervine and deobstruent powers; or narcotic, stimulant and nervine powers. Especially shall we be prepared for this, if we have clear and precise ideas of the manifest operative effects of simple stimulants and deobstruents. In order to make ourselves clearly and rightly understood, it may be well to mention, in this connection, that hydrocyanic acid, spigelia Marilandica, and hyoscyamus niger, are examples of simple narcotics; that chloric ether, moschus, coffea and vanilla aromatica, are examples of simple nervines; unless it be that chloric ether possesses also a stimulant power; but we are inclined to think that it is a simple nervine; that some of the preparations of ammonia and phosphorus are simple stimulants; that iodine and leontodon taraxacum are examples of simple deobstruents, in their primary operative effects, unless the former may also possess some moderate degree of tonic power, though no one would be justified in administering it for its tonic power alone; still this operative effect of iodine should be taken into account when administered for its deobstruent power. Opium may be taken as an example of a remedial agent producing primarily nervine, narcotic and stimulant operative effects, according to the mode of its administration, besides other operative effects unnecessary to mention in this place. Alcohol and wine are examples of remedial agents producing primarily stimulant and narcotic operative effects. Conium maculatum and digitalis purpurea are primarily narcotic and deobstruent in their operative effects.* Assafœtida is nervine and deobstruent. These statements are made on the supposition that the articles are used medicinally, with reference to their curative powers, for alcohol, opium and iodine might be so administered as to kill in a short time, but their operative effects in producing such a result are very different from what is produced when given for their remedial effects.

We could go much more into detail on these points, and others having a close relation to them, and show at large, were this the occasion for doing so, that materia medica and therapeutics are ill understood by the generality of writers on the subject, and besides, that there is a great deal of confusion, indefiniteness and uncertainty in regard to what may be considered as best understood; but we think we have said enough to make our point clear, whatever may be the opinion of others about it. If, however, any one wishes to examine the matter carefully and critically, let such an one do it in reference to any one of the remedial agents above mentioned, and examine different writers on the subject in connection with it. Take, for example, first, hydrocyanic acid; it is called a contra-stimulant, or sedative, in distinction from narcotic, and yet it is said that its primary operative effect is that of a stimulant. We shall proceed cursorily in this examination, and without much detail. 2d. Coffea Arabica is said to be a stimulant, stomachic, astringent, febrifuge, and even a cathartic; and yet its only medicinal

---

* Digitalis probably possesses also primarily emetic and cathartic powers. But the doses required to produce such effects must necessarily be so large as would render it somewhat inconvenient to the doctor and his patient, if it did not jeopardize the life of the latter; and therefore it seems to us inexpedient to use it for such purposes.

operative effect is that of a simple nervine. 3d. Vanilla is said ,to be a stimulant, and useful as such in asthenic fevers ; and yet it is only a simple nervine, and not at all adapted to fulfil any indication in asthenic fevers, or any fevers whatever, as a remedial agent. 4th. Phosphorus is said to be a tonic and refrigerant, a very curious and most ingenious combination ; and yet it is only a simple stimulant, but one of great power and well adapted to cases that nothing else would reach. 5th. Leontodon taraxacum is said to be primarily a tonic, while it is only a simple deobstruent, and a weak one too. 6th. Iodine is said to be a *special* stimulant, producing, in some unknown way, a *change in the nature or quality of vital action;* also a tonic, purgative and diuretic. What idea can one have of the powers of iodine from such language ? To speak particularly of only one of its supposed operative effects, that of a purgative, we do not deny that it may be so administered as to be the occasion of purging, yet it does not act in this way by any remedial operative effect, but by being improperly given so as to produce irritation and perhaps inflammation of the stomach and bowels. It is no more a purgative medicinally than iron filings or coarse bran. 7th. Digitalis purpurea is said to be a contra-stimulant, narcotic, stimulant and diuretic—a strange medley. It is undoubtedly a narcotic, and also *diuretic in certain cases, with proper management ;* its operative effect as diuretic being only secondary, by virtue of its primary and more general operative effect as deobstruent.

We will not proceed further in this way, for we think that even now our critic will agree with us, that there is a great deal of confusion, indefiniteness and inaccuracy in the various systems of the materia medica, arising in part, perhaps, from the misuse of terms, but more likely from the authors not possessing clear and distinct notions, and correct information of the matters treated upon. We will remark here, by the way, that remedial agents should be classed according as one or other of their primary operative effects predominate ; for instance, if the narcotic power predominates, among the narcotics, &c.

It is very common, in books of materia medica and theory and practice, to recommend particular articles of the various classes of remedial agents in particular diseases too indiscriminately, without sufficiently considering or specifying the condition of the system under the influence of disease, and the applicability of the article to that condition—as though the several articles of a class might be substituted for each other. In health, or even in case of a mild non-malignant disease, it *might* not matter much—such is the wonderful power of accommodation and recuperation possessed by the living human system ; but as a general principle it is of great consequence. It may be oftentimes the difference between life and death. How often do physicians prescribe cathartics, emetics, &c., as though it were of little consequence what article is used, provided the particular effect is obtained.

Different remedial agents of the same class differ in a greater or less degree in the peculiarity or quality of their operative effects, whether on man in health or as remedial agents. This not only obtains in regard to articles that possess more than one property or power, but also is it true of such articles as possess only one property or power. For example —spigelia Marilandica, datura stramonium and talula, hyoscyamus niger, and belladonna, are all simple narcotics, and yet each of them varies in the character of its operative effects. This will be obvious to any one who will push them so far as to produce decided narcosis. Hence may be inferred their applicability to different forms of disease, as well as to the varying shades of phenomena produced by disease in which they may be indicated, and that no one article of any single class is an integral substitute for another. In regard to many articles we think this may be clearly shown. Though, as we have said, they are not perfect substitutes for each other, they are adapted to *similar* cases ; but still, at different periods of any particular case there is often room for choice. To explain, suppose a person to be wakeful from morbid irritability and irritation—and for reasons, we might not wish to administer opium for relief; if we should give a sufficient quantity of the extract of hyoscyamus to relieve the morbid condition of irritability and irritation, sleep would probably be obtained. Now opium will produce sleep when given to a person in perfect health ; and hyoscyamus will not. Hyoscyamus promotes sleep by virtue of its narcotic power, whereby it relieves the morbid condition which produced the wakefulness, and it does this by acting directly upon the nervous system. Whatever may be said to the contrary, hyoscyamus will not assuage simple pain, of any degree of severity, if administered to any extent that would be safe, and yet it may be accomplished perfectly and safely with opium. In short, neither of these articles could possibly be a perfect substitute for the other.

From what we have already said, it can easily be inferred that we think there is some room for improvement over and above anything that exists in all the systems of materia medica and therapeutics ; for it must be acknowledged that, as they now are, they mislead the student, give origin to a great deal of false doctrine, and a great deal more of bad practice, and at length there results a want of confidence in any remedial agents whatever.

It may be asked, what has all this to do with the objection that has been made to Dr. Tully's use of language as applied to his classification and to terms descriptive of the operative effects of remedial agents. Much every way. We have endeavored, in as few words as was possible for our purpose, to make it appear, that there is a great deal of inaccuracy, confusion and uncertainty in the use made of technical terms in medicine, especially in the materia medica ; also, that there is a great deal of inaccuracy, indefiniteness and uncertainty respecting the variety of information contained in works on this subject. We refer particularly to a want of positive knowledge in regard to what is called the physiological and curative powers of our remedial agents. We have also endeavored, in a cursory way, to set forth that more accurate and definite information is possible. Now it is promised in the prospectus of Dr. Tully's publishers, that he will give us precise and positive information respecting the powers and actions of remedial agents, discriminating accurately the operative effects of the different classes, and the peculiar action of each individual article of the several classes, together with

their correct therapeutic application ; that he will be clear and precise
in his use of language in general, definite and accurate in the use of
terms in particular,—a kind of knowledge we think of vital importance,
and of which, we fear, the generality of our practitioners are lamentably
ignorant, and from which ignorance, we know of no existing work on the
same subject, whereby they may redeem themselves.   The publishers
promise, too, that Dr. Tully will give a new system of classification
founded upon principles, in a great measure, if not entirely, unlike any
that have ever yet been promulgated, and which may be adopted as a
safe practical guide, which cannot be said of any existing classification
of our remedial agents, as far as we are informed.   We have occasion
to know that the publishers will not fall short of any promises they have
made ; for Dr. Tully can, and we think will more than fulfil them.   It
is definite and precise information respecting the operative effects of remedial agents in disease as well as in health, and their correct therapeutic application, that is wanted to inspire confidence in their use ;
and even more than this is promised.   Our conclusion, then, is, that when
there is so much to gain, it is comparatively of little consequence what
terms Dr. Tully makes use of to convey the promised information—
provided they are appropriate and sufficiently distinctive.   We have no
misgivings on the subject whatever.   We are sure that the language
generally, and the terms in particular, which Dr. Tully will make use
of, will at least be comprehensible, though it may require some patient
application of mind to apprehend the variety of matters of which he
will treat.   ＼

Before concluding, we must allude to another objection to the work
of Dr. Tully, and we can do but little more than allude to it.   It is
said that Dr. Tully is "*behind the age.*"   A very important fact, if
true.   There is, however, another fact which we know to be true, and
which it might be well for the objectors to consider.   We refer to the
fact of there being in every age certain individuals who get so far in
advance of the age in which they live, that they leave all that is valuable for it or themselves behind them ; and can find no better employment than to be always carping at the common-sense views of sensible
people.   For them the past is nothing. the future everything ; they neglect the one, and never attain the other.   They make high-sounding
pretensions about their new ways—when there is no show of a beaten
path—blustering and fermenting, frightening some and cajoling others
—of no ostensible benefit to themselves, the age in which they live, nor
to the generation that succeeds them.   The only sensible remark such
people have ever been known to make, is "that the age is behind
them."   We don't mean to say that those who have made the assertion
in regard to Dr. Tully, belong to the class of persons we have indicated ;
they can decide that for themselves ; but we should like to be informed
of their reasons for making the assertion at all, and in what way they
can sustain it—for, as it stands, we have no criteria by which to combat it, and must be left to our own resources or conjectures.   We should
consider it a high compliment to have the same thing said of us, in this
age of extraordinary enlightenment, when theories in politics, religion,

medicine, and even general literature, are so refined and diluted as to transcend all common-sense views of things, as well as contradict the experience of ages. Such assertions, however, are always relative, and really have very little force ; they ought to have none, in fact, or rather, perhaps, no more than is sufficient to give the unthinking part of men an idea of the strong powers of mind, great industry and immense erudition of those who make them. However the case may be, we believe that Dr. Tully will give us something that will serve in some measure to restrain the restless and oftentimes misdirected activity of some of the pretending cultivators of medical science in our time, especially help to correct " that depraved appetite for mere medical gossip, and the frothy inanities of extemporaneous journalism," which has obtained such a head in this country at the present time ; and particularly assist to revive the taste for good, sound medical literature. This by the way. We have seen nothing, in what has been already published, that would justify the assertion in the sense in which it was intended, or in any good sense whatever. That Dr. Tully may not harmonize with all the notions and opinions on medical subjects of the present day, we will not deny ; this certainly can be no cause of discredit, and time will be necessary to determine whose opinions are most fallacious and whimsical. It is very strange, too, that any one should venture to charge Dr. Tully with being " behind the age," on a subject of which the greater part of our profession of the present day, by their own confession, are most lamentably ignorant. Ignorance confessed, however, is a most happy omen, for it is the first step to knowledge. We hope, therefore, that Dr. Tully will have a fair hearing before he shall be condemned, for he has been a most laborious student for the last forty years, an original and careful observer, with a most extensive practical experience ; and we look with confidence for the results, in part, in the work now being published.

Not wishing to be misunderstood in our remarks, particularly in the comparative commendation of the work of Dr. Tully, we repeat more fully what we said at the beginning, that we do not intend to undervalue, and certainly not to disparage at all, many excellent works now extant on the same subject. We refer particularly to Pereira, Paris and Thompson, among the English ; Barbier, Merat and De Lens, among the French. Bigelow and Dunglison must have whatever preëminence there is among the Americans at present. We trust, however, that the time is not distant when America will stand at least the equal of England and France on *this* subject, as she does on some others of general and particular science. When Dr. Tully's work shall be completed, so that it may be *studied* and duly appreciated, we confidently believe that it will not only equal the best works of the kind, but quite supersede them all.

Boston, Feb. 15th, 1853.

P. S.—Since the above was written, we have seen several very favorable notices of Dr. Tully's Materia Medica. The New York Jour-

---

* The above communication was received during the Editor's absence from the city, which will account for its late appearance in the Journal.

nal of Medicine and Surgery says—"It will add greatly to the domain of practical medicine." The New Hampshire Journal is equally favorable. Prof. Huston, of Philadelphia, has also noticed the labors of Dr. Tully very favorably. There are other equally commendatory notices that might be referred to.

OBITUARY OF CHARLES W. CHANDLER, M D., OF ANDOVER, VT.

[Communicated for the Boston Medical and Surgical Journal.]

DR. CHANDLER, the subject of this notice, was the son of John and Esther Chandler, and was born in Chester, Vt., Sept. 8th, 1771. He was the sixth child in a family of nine children, all of whom lived to a great age, the average being over 80 years. His ancestors came from Woodstock, Conn., at which place his father, John Chandler, and also his grandfather, Thomas Chandler, were born. The last-mentioned person was the first Clerk (1763) of the Proprietors of the Township of Chester, originally called *Flamstead*, and for a time *New Flamstead;* and he was the first Representative from the town of Chester in the Vermont Legislature (March 22, 1778), and for three sessions was Speaker of the House, viz., in 1778, 1779, 1780.

Dr. Chandler had no other than the ordinary advantages of education, such as were afforded by the common schools of his time. As he was born five years before the Colonies separated from the mother country, and six years before Vermont was formed into an independent State, when this region was comparatively a wilderness, it will be perceived that these advantages must have been very limited. He studied medicine for a while with his brother, Dr. Chauncy C. Chandler, of Chester, and continued his study with a physician in Cooperstown, N. Y., where he was engaged for a time in teaching school. He attended the medical lectures of Prof. Nathan Smith, at Hanover, N. H. He was twice married. First, to Nancy White, in October, 1803, by whom he had three children; and second to Mrs. Mary Larkin, in January, 1815, by whom he had two children. Twice has he been called to mourn over the sundering of the tenderest earthly relationship, and both of his sons have gone down to the grave before him. Henry, his youngest child, on whom he leaned as the staff and stay of his old age, died in 1839, at the age of 21, to the sore grief and disappointment of his father; and the oldest of his children, Wolcott C. Chandler, M.D., died in the midst of his activity and usefulness, in Natick, Mass., in 1849. Dr. Chandler's three daughters still live to mourn the death of one of the kindest of fathers and best of men.

He settled in Andover, Vt., in the year 1799, and remained there until January, 1852, being for more than half a century actively engaged in the practice of medicine in that town and the region round about. It was the profession of his choice, and one for which he was peculiarly fitted by native endowment. With a well-settled conviction of his aptitude for it, he entered it early in life, and he devoted himself to his profession with untiring energy and unabated zeal until his health and strength failed him, a little more than three years ago. In the month of December, 1849, a shock of paralysis disabled him from further active service, and gave him the first distinct admonition to set his house in order in preparation for his decease. During the period of his decline, the shadows have been gathering slowly but steadily over his pathway ; the orb of vision has been growing dim ; white blossoms have covered his head ; and all his faculties have been sinking under the weight of accumulated infirmities, until at length his body has been borne to the grave, to mingle with the dust as it was, and his spirit has returned to God who gave it.

Dr. Chandler maintained a high rank as a physician. His superior medical skill has always been acknowledged, and his practice has been extensive in all the region round about ; and no country more hilly and bleak, no climate more cold and severe, can be found in our whole land, than are presented in the field of his labors. In his early days he travelled over a large extent of territory, when the roads were very bad, both in summer and winter, and the country new ; to wit—Chester, Grafton, Windham, Londonderry, Landgrave, Peru, Weston,- Mount Holly and Ludlow. He was ever ready to go when he was called for, whether it was to the rich or the poor, by day or by night, through mud in summer or snow-drifts in winter. He travelled hundreds of miles on snow-shoes where he could not go with his horse ; and in one winter of unusual severity, he travelled in this way more than 300 miles. · He never stopped to inquire if he should be likely to get his pay, and consequently he had notes and accounts to the amount of hundreds, and, I presume, thousands of dollars, which are not worth the paper they are written on ; yet his doors were ever open, and his table spread for the weary and hungry.

He was distinguished for independence of character. This quality was connected with his athletic physical frame and vigorous constitution. A native of this severe clime, he has ever breathed its bracing air ; been inured, from his earliest youth, to toil and hardship, and performed as much hard service in his profession, perhaps, as any other man ; few, indeed, have ever performed as much. All these external circumstances and influences had nurtured in him firmness of purpose and decision of character. Entering upon his professional career at so early a period, while this whole region was but partially settled and thinly inhabited, he found the practice of medicine by no means an easy or a lucrative business. He began, indeed, in poverty. He acquired some means for prosecuting his studies by teaching school. But had he not been made of " sterner stuff" than many exquisite young men of our day, he would have failed in the outset. He was· not a man, however, to put his hand to the plough and look back. By economy,·perseverance, and fidelity to every engagement and to every duty, he succeeded in accumulating a competence of this world's goods, not only for himself and his immediate family, but also an abundance to scatter in charity among the poor and needy, who never called on him for relief to be turned empty away. His character was firm. Its type was furnished, not by the flowing river and the changing cloud, but rather by the solid rock and the sturdy oak of his native hills.

Another prominent trait in his strongly-marked character, and connected with the preceding, was his sterling integrity of purpose. Hypocrisy and dissimulation were altogether foreign to his nature. Integrity, the crowning virtue of humanity, was his crown and glory. Flattery could not seduce him from the path of conscious rectitude, nor fear intimidate him into what he believed to be wrong. This element of his character was conspicuously manifest during the anti-masonic excitement, which raged in Vermont like a pestilence. He was a Freemason, and ever consistent and unwavering in his attachment to the masonic institution, whose liberal principles and benevolent purposes were so congenial to his own generous spirit. I mention this in justice to his memory. I mention it because it affords an illustration of his character. I mention it, because his steadfast adherence to that institution, through good and through evil report, through all the stormy trials to which it was subjected, and when others, of weaker nerves, of pliable natures and easy virtue, who were susceptible to the bias of party and the contagion of popular fanaticism, gave way and betrayed their trusts, and professed or denied just as the mob of party directed, just as office and interest swayed them, was all the more honorable to him. While others were swayed by the popular gust that swept over the land, Dr. Chandler,

> " Resolved, and steady to his trust,
> Inflexible to ill and obstinately just,"

Just to his idea of right and true to his conscientious convictions, would not deny what he knew to be right and true, though the heavens should fall on his devoted head. He had the indomitable spirit of the good seraph Abdiel :—

> " Among innumerable false, unmoved,
> Unshaken, unseduced, unterrified,
> His loyalty he kept, his love, his zeal;
> Nor number, nor example, with him wrought
> To swerve from truth, or change his constant mind,
> Though single."

Another striking trait in Dr. Chandler, was humanity and benevolence. He distributed freely of his means to all who had a claim on his bounty. He was " given to hospitality." His heart and hand were open as day to melting charity. With filial piety he relieved the wants and ministered to the comfort of his father in his old age, and thus proved himself a dutiful son. He fulfilled the capital precept of christianity, " Learn first to show piety at home and to requite thy parents." He never forgot to do good and communicate wherever his services or charities might be needed. He visited the fatherless in their affliction as cheerfully and faithfully as he did those who were able to reward him for his services. The poor found in him a benefactor and friend on whom they could rely with implicit confidence. In him was realized the character of Job: " When the ear heard me, then it blessed me; and when the eye saw me, it gave witness to me; because I delivered the poor that cried, and the fatherless, and him that had none to help him. The blessing of him that was ready to perish came upon me; and I caused the widow's heart to sing for joy. I put on righteousness, and it clothed me; my judgment was as a robe and a diadem. I was eyes to the blind, and feet was I to the lame; I was a father to the poor, and the cause which I knew not I searched out."

He was remarkable for the frankness and simplicity of his manners, and for a certain kind of native unaffected humor; a humor, however, which never turned sour the milk of human kindness. No man ever had a greater dislike of affectation. He had a plain way of doing and saying things, which was direct and to the purpose. He was a man of solid, rather than showy parts. Possessing in a large degree, strong masculine common sense, he despised pedantry and all the verbal tinsel of empty pretension. The useless ostentation of learning, and the shallow pretence of the quack, whether in medicine or in religion, was what he detested. Among his brethren of the medical profession there may be those who excelled him in skill or in attainments, but I presume none ever excelled him in professional courtesy, in fidelity to his trust, in kindness and humanity. He was not faultless, "but e'en his failings leaned to virtue's side." Under a somewhat rough exterior there beat one of the noblest and most generous of hearts, and he was emphatically an honest man. He was a firm believer in christianity, and in the ultimate restoration of the whole human family to holiness and happiness. His religious faith shed a serene and holy light over the closing scene of his earthly existence, which was in keeping with the general tenor of his life, calm, trustful and happy.

He died in Ludlow, at the house of his son-in-law, Abram Adams, Esq. A few moments before he expired, as he was raised up and asked if anything could be done for his relief, he replied, " *All is well.*" In this cheerful frame he passed to the world of spirits.

North Chester, Vt., March 1st, 1853. **J. O. S.**

CHLORIC ETHER IN PUERPERAL CONVULSIONS.

To the Editor of the Boston Medical and Surgical Journal.

Sir,—The narration of the following case may be of little interest to your numerous readers, and my object in reporting it is to elicit, through the pages of your Journal, their experience with ether in the same disease.

Mrs. ———, aged 26, of light complexion, and nervo-sanguine temperament, was attended in her first confinement by Dr. G. D. Peck, Dec. 29th, 1852. Her labor, which was perfectly normal and comparatively easy, terminated in eight hours by the delivery of a healthy male child of medium size. Two or three hours prior to the termination of the labor, she made mention of pain in the supra-orbital region, but of so slight a nature as not to attract the attention of the medical attendant.

Three hours after delivery, viz., 7 o'clock, P.M., during which interval the patient remained every way comfortable, she was seized suddenly with an epileptiform convulsion. Her accoucheur was soon present, when her pulse were found but little augmented in frequency, and herself conscious during the intervals of the convulsions, of which she had three during the first hour, lasting some five minutes each. The feet were placed in warm water, iced water was applied to the head, which was above normal temperature, and of jalap gr. xxx. were administered, being the most active medicine at hand.

At 8 o'clock I was invited to see the patient with her attendant. She still answered, but hesitatingly ; exhibited some agitation, but could not remember that anything had happened ; had a wild and brilliant, but not injected eye ; pulse 120 per minute, pretty firm and quick. Twenty ounces of blood were taken from the arm, in the erect position, causing pallor and partial syncope. More cathartic medicine was given, and cold still applied to the head. Thenceforward the paroxysms, augmenting in severity, occurred at pretty regular intervals of an hour and a half each, until 2 o'clock, A.M., Dec. 30th. Meanwhile the bowels had been freely moved, aided by stimulating enemata.

At this time the convulsions occurred in such rapid succession as to merge into each other ; the face full and livid ; respiration deep and laborious ; deglutition suspended, and pulse at the wrist almost imperceptible and very rapid. It now seemed evident, after employing these active measures without avail, that life must soon terminate ; and at this critical juncture it was resolved to try the influence of anæsthesia.

The concentrated chloric ether was accordingly administered upon a napkin—slowly at first, but constantly, until the patient was brought under its influence, when the convulsions ceased entirely, and there only remained a lateral motion of the head upon the pillow, and some irregular movements of the limbs whenever allowed to escape from under its influence. The use of the ether was continued for an hour and a half, during which time all the more formidable symptoms had abated, and the patient apparently slept at intervals.

During the succeeding day she was delirious, attempting at times to rise from the bed, when the inhalation of a little ether would quiet her agitation and cause rest. In two days reason was fully restored, she having remembered nothing after the first spasm. Her convalescence has been as rapid and complete as in ordinary labors.

Northampton, March 12th, 1853.   James Dunlap, M.D.

THE BOSTON MEDICAL AND SURGICAL JOURNAL.

BOSTON, MARCH 23, 1853.

Moral Sanatory Economy.—That kind of instruction which is calculated to advance the health and morals, and therefore the happiness of the people, cannot be otherwise than valuable. As society progresses in what is usually denominated civilization, there are developed an immense train of social evils. Too often, when the mind is cultivated, the body falls into utter neglect. Many of the vices, also, of refinement, are quite as destructive and as difficult to control, as the grosser moral maladies that are supposed to belong to the lowest stratum of the community. It requires courage in our age of boasted intelligence for a single-handed man to declare the fact that there is rottenness in the bones, and that corruptions are festering in high places; to point out to individuals the sins that tend to abridge the span of their existence, and in the face of the multitude assert that disease, premature decay, and physical and moral suffering, are the positive results of those violations of law which are every day committed. Henry McCormac, M.D., of Belfast, Ireland, an author whose works are calculated to transmit his name with respect to future times, has produced something new, and more important than might at first sight be supposed. It is a popular treatise on "Moral Sanatory Economy,"—which in plain terms exhibits the more concealed vices which abound, are deplored, but have not been eradicated, or scarcely kept at bay, in Christian countries. Having the pleasure of a personal acquaintance with the learned author, and knowing the amount of influence which he exerts in his native land, it is particularly gratifying to bear witness to his standing, and declare with what earnestness and benevolence he labors to elevate and advance the race. The range of topics in this able production admits of a multitude of convincing illustrations, in the way of evidence, to show how much truth has been overlooked, even by medical moralists, but which should no longer be concealed. There are twelve chapters on the following subjects, which are elaborately argued; viz., female degradation, employment, education, household culture, criminal management, physical training, clothing, food, drink, air, drainage, and prevention of disease. In these chapters Dr. McCormac points out the sources of mental and bodily impurity, and conducts us, stage by stage, through the greatest of lazar houses, the world, indicating, at each step, the poison to be avoided, while he holds up to view the glorious results of a life of honest compliance with nature's simple demands. We scarcely know how to take leave of this important treatise. Some of the American publishers would find their account in bringing out an edition of it. It is selling rapidly in Great Britain, as it would doubtless do here.

The Milk Trade of New York.—Mr. John Mullaly, of New York, has had the courage to expose the whole system of iniquity practised by milk dealers in and about that great city. But it will not deter the consumers from giving their patronage to the same men who have imposed upon them with impunity, nor frighten the milk merchants from an established scheme of cheating. There is a degree of recklessness and determination on the part of those concerned in the milk trade, that defies the press, the physicians, and even the law. This grows out of the immense demand for milk, and the impossibility of proving who are the real rascals at the bottom of the business. In the hurly-burly of swallowing a cup of coffee at an over-crowded hotel, any white fluid that looks like milk may pass for that beverage, or at least escape a chemical analysis, though considered excessively bad in the estimation of a stranger. The poor suffer severely in consequence of the vile stuff sold them for milk. Their children are made sickly, and positive disease is often developed in them. In drinking in a supposed nourishment, what multitudes take into their stomachs diluted corruption derived from animals enfeebled by improper food and by being housed perpetually in narrow places, where they inhale an atmosphere laden with exhalations from decomposing matter. There is some good milk retailed in New York, and there may be, also, many very honest retailers. But to dilute with water, and then introduce mixtures to give the characteristic consistency, flavor and degree of richness peculiar to the unadulterated article, is admitted to be a common practice in London, and has been imitated extensively in New York. Whether we have any thing besides water in Boston milk, remains to be ascertained. The demand does not apparently warrant any extra efforts at imitation. When our population has doubled, the materials for cheating may come cheaper than country milk, and then ingenious deceptions may be expected.

We have visited the vast milk establishments of London, and retain a distinct recollection of the condition of the poor imprisoned animals (in one stable four hundred in number) that furnish milk for the multitude. Ulcerations of the liver and a diseased state of the lungs are common, where many cows are kept together in stables. Milk from animals fed on the miserable slops of a brew-house, or distillery, must be of a wretchedly poor quality to begin with—and when it passes to the retailers, it is impossible to conjecture the processes it undergoes to increase the quantity, with a view to a profit on the materials intermingled. The fresh brains of calves, sheep, pigs, &c. beaten up in a small quantity of milk and then poured into a number of gallons of the vilest combination of milk, water, &c., make a factitious fluid that actually passes for genuine milk! What the effect must be on the public health, and especially on that of children, who are by far the largest class of consumers, may be readily conjectured. Under all circumstances, it is best to dispense with city milk as much as possible, if it is the product of cows kept in town ; and in the next place, when from the country, continue to purchase of those whose honesty is a guarantee of its purity. There is no stopping place in detailing the mischief that accrues from the habitual use of poor milk. Cheating in every department of trade is certainly rife throughout the world. Either honesty does not meet with encouragement, or the heart of man is inclined to evil perpetually.

Massachusetts Lunatic Hospital. — The twentieth annual report of the trustees states that the bills for 1852, were $24,414 05. They allude to the increase of foreign lunatics, and further observe " that gross impositions are undoubtedly practised by foreign states upon the public charitable provisions of this Commonwealth." For all purposes, the expenditures were $43,878 35, in 1852. Whole number of patients admitted in 1852, 309— and in 20 years, from 1833, 4,170. There were 103 discharged well the past year ; 34 discharged improved ; 61 not improved ; 43 died ; and the whole number at the institution in 1852, 775. It is melancholy to discover in the tabular columns that 28 inmates were the victims of intemperance and 26 of masturbation ; while the multitude from unknown causes, takes in those of all conditions of insanity, thrown upon the hospital—of which little is known beyond the fact that they are lunatics. Dr. Chandler, with his usual good judgment, has offered but few comments, while he gives all the exact facts, as far as discoverable, in regard to the general health, every-day condition and mortality of the unpromising class of patients placed under his humane care.

Butler Hospital for the Insane. — This institution is under the charge of Isaac Ray, M.D., and is located at Providence, R. I. The average number of patients in 1852, was 139 1-20. One hundred and forty-five could be comfortably accommodated. From the circumstance that Dr. Ray is acknowledged as good authority in matters relating to mental alienation, his report is sought for by general readers. Physicians are not the exclusive examiners of these annual accounts of what is transacted within the walls of lunatic asylums. The community weigh the assertions, the opinions, and the facts, as they are given by medical superintendents. Dr. Ray, therefore, comes in for something more than a mere turning over of the leaves of his reports. In the present report, we have the elements of a treatise on the effects of our political system upon the mental organization of the masses. " But the mental activity which is excited directly by free institutions," says Dr. R., " is not confined to political matters. It pervades every sphere of action, every exercise of thought. The almost absolute freedom from restraint and the independence of foreign control even in opinions merely, lead to a certain hurry and impetuosity of the vital movements, and an impatience that seeks for results by extraordinary effort or superficial methods. Between the calm, steady and persevering endeavor, the adherence to routine and prescription which mark the European, and the novel, dashing career of the American, defying all rule and contrary to all precedent, what a remarkable contrast!" It is not certain where the doctor would end, were his reflections fairly elaborated ; but the inference is conclusive, that our rapidity of thought and action, and free inquiry, our bold, determined way of doing, saying and writing upon every thing, every body, and at all times, in and out of season, oftentimes leads to madness. Yet with all the gravity, consideration and deference to old saws and old customs in Europe, the asylums there are as densely peopled as ours. Dr. Ray is a man of originality, and we like his independence in striking out with boldness into the deep waters of the ocean of thought. Much more remains to be said on this interesting topic.

Medical Miscellany. — In Massachusetts the number of State paupers who are foreigners, is " eleven thousand, three hundred and twenty-one." —In 1852, 2,361 were sent to prison in Massachusetts, for intemperance.— The whole number of interments at Mount Auburn Cemetery, near Boston, since it was opened to the public, is 5,580. — Charles Willey recently died at Nottingham, N. H., at the age of 106 years.— A correspondent wishes to know what has been the experience of the profession in the use of " chloroform" (either by inhalationor given internally), in " consumption." — The city government of Boston have wisely forbidden the interment of any more bodies in the cemeteries under the churches in the city proper, and in the older burying-grounds.

To CORRESPONDENTS. — The following papers have been received, and will have an early insertion :—New Apparatus for Fracture of the Radius ; Epidemic of 1852 in Newton.

MARRIED, — At New York. John Nelson Borland, M.D., of Boston, to Madeline Gibson, of New York. — At Portsmouth, Va., Dr. W. E. Wyshan, U. S. Navy, to Mary Eliza, daughter of Dr. Thomas Williamson, U. S. N.—Joseph Comstock, M.D., to Miss Caroline E. Champlin, both of Lebanon, Conn.

DIED,—At Buffalo, N. Y., 4th inst., Dr. P. Christie, Surgeon in the U. S. Navy, 63.

Deaths in Boston for the week ending Saturday noon, March 19th, 78. Males, 47—females, 31. Apoplexy, 1— inflammation of the bowels, 1 — Bright's disease, 1— disease of brain, 2—congestion of brain, 1—consumption, 10—croup, 11 — dropsy in head, 5 — drowned, 1 — infantile diseases, 9—scarlet fever, 5—hooping cough, 2—disease of the heart, 1—inflammation of the lungs, 10—disease of the liver, 1—palsy, 1—old age, 4—peritonitis, 1—pleurisy, 1—disease of the stomach, 1—scald, 1—suicide, 1—teething, 4—tumor, 1—unknown, 1—ulcer, 1. Under 5 years, 45 — between 5 and 20 years, 8—betwen 20 and 40 years, 8—between 40 and 60 years, 7—over 60 years, 10. Born in the United States, 64—Ireland, 10—England, 1— Scotland, 1—France, 1—Germany, 1. The above includes 3 deaths in the city institutions.

Tracheotomy Performed with Success. By DR. FOSTER, *Resident Surgeon of the Charity Hospital, New Orleans.* — An Italian fruiterer, ætat. forty-five, being constantly exposed, in conducting his business, was attacked with laryngitis about the latter part of December, and on the 31st was admitted into the Charity Hospital. Complained of much pain and tenderness over the larnyx, attended with dyspnœa and asphyxia, hoarseness, inflamed fauces, etc. Was treated with tartarized antimony ; and his fauces touched with a strong solution of argent. nit. The day after his admission, the dyspnœa became intense, with aggravation of all the symptoms. Was now ordered gr. v. calomel ; morphia one sixth gr. every hour. Repeat the cauterization.

On the afternoon of same day, second after admission, there being no abatement of symptoms, to which was now added lividity of face and lips, the operation of Tracheotomy was deemed imperative, and was accordingly promptly performed by Dr. Foster, the House Surgeon. The venous hemorrhage was profuse ; but soon subsided after the trachea was opened. An " *ovate curved canula* was placed in the opening, and within this *one of smaller size,*" which can be easily removed when it becomes obstructed with mucus. On the third day both canulas were removed. Fifteen days after admission, the patient was discharged cured. — *New Orleans Medical and Surg. Journal.*

Syrup Assafœtida. — It is sometimes desirable to administer assafœtida otherwise than in pill or *per anum*, especially to juvenile patients; and consequently in the least disagreeable form possible ; for which reasons the following formula, which I have composed, to produce a syrup of the article, may be of some practical use,—R. Assafœtida ℨi. ; Aqua. ℥viss. fiat emulsio ad quem adde Sacch. Alb. ℥viij. et cum calore balnei aquoisa fiant Syrupi ℥ x. quo misi bene Ol Carui gtt. x. The whole of the assafœtida, when clean or carefully selected, can be triturated into emulsion, which should not be strained, nor should the syrup, nor the scum be removed ; as this and the sediment which is deposited, after standing some time, may be readily re-incorporated by agitation, which should be done before the use or administration of the medicine. I consider this preparation much more artistical, efficient and accurate than that of mixing the tincture with simple syrup, as it is sometimes made.—*N. York Journal of Pharmacy.*

Physicians to the Household of the Emperor of France.—Napoleon III. has organized the medical staff of his household. By an Imperial Decree of the 31st December last, the following appointments are made :—

Dr. Conneau, First Physician to his Majesty, and Chief Physician to the Household.

MM. Andral and Rayer, Physicians, with a salary of 8,000 francs.

M. de Pietra-Santa, Assistant Physician, and Secretary to the Medical Staff, salary 6,000 francs.

MM. Jobert (de Lamballe), A. H. Larrey, Surgeons, with a salary of 8,000 francs.

MM. Begin, Berard, Bouillaud, J. Cloquet, Gaultier de Claubry, Michel Levy, Louis, and Velpeau, Consulting Physicians and Surgeons.

MM. Arnal, Bonlu, L. Corvisart, Delaroque, Fleury, Longet, Tenain, and Vernois, Physicians and Surgeons, to serve quarterly, salary 6,000 francs.—*Gazette Médicale de Paris*, Jan. 15th, 1853.

THE

BOSTON MEDICAL AND SURGICAL JOURNAL.

VOL. XLVIII.   WEDNESDAY, MARCH 30, 1853.   No. 9.

To the Editor of the Boston Medical and Surgical Journal.

SIR,—I offer to your readers a translation of a series of lectures on the subject of " Displacements of the Uterus," delivered in Paris during the early part of the last year, at the " Hôpital de la Pitié," by M. Valleix, who is now giving special attention to uterine displacements, and who is well known as the author of the "Guide du Médecin—Praticien," &c. The lectures were reported for the " Union Médicale," of last year, by M. T. Gallard, principal *interne* in the department of M. Valleix.   L. PARKS, Jr., M.D.

Boston, March 11th, 1853.

DISPLACEMENTS OF THE UTERUS.

GENTLEMEN,—As I announced to you, at the commencement of these lectures, we proceed to devote several sessions to the study of displacements of the uterus—a subject, the importance of which I hardly need to point out, as you very well know that it has already been for some time the order of the day, and that the numerous discussions, to which it has given rise, are far from being terminated.

These displacements, gentlemen, are much more frequent than you would be persuaded to believe. If, in fact, you visit a hospital, where diseases of the uterus are specially attended to, you will be astonished at the great number of patients you will find affected with these complaints, which, some years since, were scarcely mentioned ; and there is assuredly not a medical or surgical clinique, of any kind, which might not present to you several cases of them.

It is not only by their frequency, that the study of these lesions is rendered interesting—a study, difficult it is true, but necessarily fruitful of results. There are many other inducements for engaging in their investigation. First, I would mention the number and variety of symptoms presented by displacements of the uterus. You will see, indeed, under what diverse aspects these symptoms, confining themselves as they do to no one point of the economy, may manifest themselves, and how great is their obstinacy, and sometimes their gravity.

There is a second consideration, no less worthy of your attention, which is, that the tendency of these diseases is not to spontaneous recovery, but, on the contrary, to self-perpetuation, and to aggravation in proportion to duration—facts you will learn from the different cases which will come before you in the course of these lectures. It is then difficult, at first, to comprehend why the study of uterine displacements has been so neglected until within a few years past, as, formerly, very few physicians were occupied with them, and the only modes of treatment devised were insufficient or purely palliative. These remarks, be it understood, gentlemen, apply particularly to displacements of the uterus in the non-pregnant state ; since the effects of displacements occurring during pregnancy had, long ago, challenged attention, and the means of remedying them had been diligently sought. The very simple reason of this is, that these effects, showing themselves suddenly, in consequence of the displacement of a voluminous uterus, give rise to an injurious compression of neighboring organs, and manifest themselves by symptoms intense in proportion to the size of the organ. There was then a necessity of devising prompt treatment for these cases, and, thence, it was impossible that the subject should not receive attention. But since, in the different circumstances of the non-pregnant condition, the axis of the womb does not ordinarily deviate in a sudden and rapid manner from its proper direction ; since, on the contrary, the progress of the disease is slow and insidious ; since the really serious symptoms do not manifest themselves till after a certain time, and, besides, are never so alarming as in cases of pregnancy, it is not astonishing that they have attracted less attention.

Further, we will remark, that this negligence we are pointing out in the study of uterine displacements applies to diseases of the uterus in general, either because the means of exploration were insufficient, or, because the lesions showing themselves rebellious to the inefficient modes of treatment with which it was in the power of the practitioner to meet them, but slight importance was attached to the knowledge of diseases which could scarcely be relieved.

When M. Recamier had introduced, and made general, the use of the speculum, more notice was taken of uterine diseases. But the invention of this instrument, which was of so great service in one respect, was rather injurious to the study of displacements. Attention was given almost entirely to affections apparent to the eye, and susceptible of direct examination ; and, by consequence, to those having their seat upon the neck of the uterus.

Now, this means of examination was insufficient to make known the numerous and varied affections, the history of which I am about to unfold to you ; since, in their diagnosis, the speculum is of no great advantage. Some, indeed, have gone so far as to deny it any utility in these cases. In this opinion, however, there is error and exaggeration. Generally speaking, the speculum is not sufficient by itself. Sometimes, it affords us no information. But, most often—as it has been in my power many times to demonstrate to those among you who visit the wards with me—it may afford a certain degree of aid. In fact, when on introducing the speculum in the direction of the vaginal axis, you do not find the cervix uteri, or, if, finding it, you disclose a portion which normally should not be in view, ought you not to suspect the organ to have deviated from its habitual direction ? This inference should have occurred to the reflection of those, who, in the early days of the use of the speculum, so often pointed out the difficulty of finding the cervix uteri, and spoke of the practice and skill necessary to the operator to enable him to seize it, when directed posteriorly towards the sacrum, or anteriorly towards the pubis. For if the cervix uteri always preserved its normal direction, this difficulty in finding it would not have been experienced, since it would have been sufficient simply to carry the speculum in the direction of the axis of the vagina. The real importance, then, of this means of investigation, has been undervalued.

Finally, there is a cause more powerful than all the foregoing, of that species of abandonment to which displacements of the uterus have been consigned, in that preconceived theories have prevailed upon this subject. It was thought that to displacements by themselves, no interest attached, and that the symptoms experienced by patients were rather to be attributed to the *engorgement** by which the former are always accompanied. Thus, the declaration of Cruveilhier—that " the displacement is nothing, the congestion is all " ! He added, also, " put an end to the one, and the other will disappear of itself." This opinion was shared by M. Dubois, and by other authors highly to be esteemed, and was based upon the following grounds (for you well know that views adopted by MM. Dubois, Cruveilhier and Bennet, must be fortified by arguments and facts of great weight) ; first, congenital displacements were found without congestion of the uterus, and unattended by any pain, by any symptom, of the nature of those we shall have occasion to observe. In the second place, cases have been seen, in which an acquired inclination of the uterus carried to a great extent occasioned no suffering, particularly when the uterus was small, and the surrounding tissues maintained their suppleness.

But these are exceptional cases, from which it behoves us much to be on our guard against drawing a too positive inference. For, on the other hand, I have been able to collect a great number of facts, the result of which is, that once the uterus is returned to its normal situation, how great soever may have been the congestion, and without anything having been done to dissipate it, there is, almost always, a relief, so great, so complete, so rapid, that it cannot be attributed to the disappearance of the congestion, since the removal of this has evidently been impossible.

As a remarkable example of this class of cases, I will cite the instance of a lady whom I lately saw. She had a retroflexion, dating back, as is to be inferred from the account furnished me, nine years. The value of this case is enhanced by the fact that during these nine years, the resources of every possible mode of treatment for congestion —bleeding, cauterization, &c.—were exhausted upon the patient. Not only did she fail of obtaining relief, but was the victim of increased suffering. About six months ago she came to consult me, when I recog-

---

* " Engorgement," as defined by Duparcque, is enlargement by congestion, hypertrophy, &c. &c.—Warrington's version, pp. 76 and 77.—TRANS.

nized the retroflexion, and commenced a course of treatment, which was interrupted by a particular circumstance. This lady lost an only daughter of the age of 14 or 15 years, and, during the first moments of her grief, gave no thought to her own illness. When, finally, treatment could be recommenced, I put in practice simply the re-placement of the uterus, with the aid of the sound. The uterus, brought into its normal position, maintained itself there for some time (as it was easy for me to ascertain by tactile examination), and immediately this patient, who, for nine years, had undergone constant distress, being unable to take a single step without suffering, and with difficulty enduring the jolts of a vehicle, felt a relief so marked, that she was able to rise and walk home without pain. After some hours, the uterus having returned to its abnormal position, the symptoms re-appeared. The next day, a new re-placement, and a new relief for the space of five or six hours. Then a re-appearance of the symptoms. After the fourth application of the sound, the relief was permanent, the pains not returning. A menstrual period arriving the next day, and the flow pursuing its regular course, the patient naturally was not examined for some time. When we, saw her again, the uterus had maintained its normal position.

This recovery is still too recent for me to feel myself sufficiently authorized to regard it as definitive. But, if it continues, it will be one case the more to add to those I have collected, in which the *application of the sound sufficed* to cure a displacement.   -

I have cited this fact simply to show you the real part played by congestion, since, in the case of this female, where the congestion was considerable, the uterus being 8½ centimetres* in depth, and necessarily preserving this size after the re-placement, it was not sufficient to produce the symptoms, all of which disappeared, at the same time with the displacement, to be re-produced when that returned. I will add that what occurred in this particular case is a matter of daily observation, and the uterus is seen to keep up, during a longer or shorter space of time, a state of congestion, which it is not (in this organ more than in any other), the work of a moment to dispel; although the symptoms may have disappeared, or nearly so, as soon as the uterus has been brought to its normal position. But this point in the history of uterine displacements being too important to be treated thus incidentally, I shall have occasion to return to it, at the proper time, when you will see the real importance, in uterine displacements, of the state of congestion—a condition of the organ which is far from being of no consequence.

[To be continued]

M. RICORD'S LETTERS UPON SYPHILIS.

Addressed to the Editor of L'Union Medicale—Translated from the French by D. D. SLADE, M.D., Boston, and communicated for the Boston Medical and Surgical Journal.

TWENTIETH LETTER.

MY DEAR FRIEND,—The indurated chancre should still be the subject of our conversation. This subject is important, but a little dry, and I need all your kind attention.

---

* About three inches and two lines.

In this variety of the primary ulcer, the form remains more regularly rounded, provided the ulcer is seated altogether upon homogeneous tissues. The borders are almost never separated from the neighboring parts. They are not always cut perpendicularly—slightly prominent, they are continuous with the base, which is hollowed out, as it were, *in the form of a little cup.* The surface of the ulceration, greyish, lardaceous, is sometimes variegated. Its centre is then of a darker tint, indented, brownish; we should say like that of a little cockade, which has caused the common name of *partridge's eye* to be sometimes given to this form.

But the induration which constitutes the principal character of this variety of chancre, at what period does it commence? What is the length of time which passes between the act by which the contagion is produced, and the first manifestation? The solution of this question is very important, for, from the moment that induration has taken place, the malady is no longer only local. I have attempted to fix this period, but it is not always easy. The patients do not ordinarily present themselves till a long time after the contagion ; and not being aware of the importance of the pathological condition of which we are here speaking, they have not noticed the commencement. What explains in the majority of cases this want of attention on the part of patients, is, that the indurated chancre is essentially indolent, of slow progress, suppurating little, that they do not perceive it till very late, and often it even passes unnoticed by them. You recollect that I have already cited to you some examples. I again speak of them, in order that you may remind those who always believe in the miracle of constitutional veroles *d'emblée.*

We are not always sure of the date of the coitus, or of the contact to which we ought to refer the chancre itself ; consequently it is very difficult to know when the induration commenced. However, in the cases where it has been possible to arrive at anything precise, it is never before the third day that the induration manifests itself. In all cases, it is always in the course of the first or second week. It would appear even certain—at least until new observations more precise come to prove the contrary—that if a chancre exists for more than three weeks without induration, it will not become indurated. Induration is a precocious phenomenon. Certain conditions can deceive and make us believe in indurations at a later period. Let us examine these.

The specific induration is not always easy to discover. Either in consequence of the ordinary contagion, or after the artificial inoculation, the infected part often becomes the seat of an inflammatory process, which Hunter called the *common inflammation,* and in which the specific induration is enchased and masked during a certain time ; so that it is only according as the simple, œdematous, sub-phlegmonous, or more plainly, inflammatory engorgement is absorbed, that the specific induration becomes marked, and is found as it were exhumed from the inflammatory atmosphere which surrounded it. Until then, the characteristics of the engorgement, whether œdematous or inflammatory, having prevailed, we cannot consider the specific induration as commencing until the moment when we begin to perceive it; and it is thus that we could believe in tardy indurations, in chancres which have not commenced to indurate until after three weeks, a month, and even longer still after the contagion.

Certain local applications, as cauterizations for instance, give rise sometimes to factitious indurations, which we can produce at various epochs, and which might deceive. These factitious indurations could even be complicated with specific indurations, and thus render them difficult to recognize. We know that the late antagonists to the virus, formerly said that they could produce a chancre similar to the Hunterian chancre, with corrosive sublimate. Similar—yes, they are right; but identical, no. In fact, with the corrosive sublimate, the chromate of potash, the liquid acetate of lead, so often employed in common practice, the hot ashes from a pipe, and sometimes simply with the nitrate of silver, we give rise to accidents so analogous to the indurated chancre, that physicians who have not a large experience with this condition, are daily deceived. It is only in consequence of errors of this kind, that we can believe that the indurated chancre is not inevitably followed by constitutional accidents.

There is another cause of error from which some writers upon syphilis have not escaped, and among others Mr. Babington, the annotator of Hunter. Some patients might preserve from a first contagion an induration, and contract afterwards upon this induration a new chancre. If we did not know well the history of the antecedents, we might believe that this last chancre had commenced with induration, and that this might be the first phenomenon of the contagion. This is a great error; the induration comes on always consecutively to the ulceration. The circumstances in which we have not taken into consideration a previous induration, due to a former contagion, could make us suppose when the patients had contracted a new chancre upon this induration, that this new chancre had in its turn become indurated; an error which might cause us to admit more exceptions to the law of *unicity* than there really are.

You know that there are some writers upon syphilis who pretend that all the primary accidents, whatever they may be, can be followed by secondary accidents, and if there is any exception, it would be in favor of blennorrhagia. Well, these writers upon syphilis admit so much the more, that the non-indurated chancres, as well as the indurated ones, can be followed by constitutional accidents. It is, then, quite important to understand how far this is true. You have already seen that common inflammation can mask the specific induration and cause us to believe in another form of chancre. It happens also, in some circumstances much more rare, that the ulceration, after having been indurated, becomes phagedenic. If, then, we have not seen the commencement of the disease, we might still be deceived, and believe in the possibility of constitutional accidents after the non-indurated phagedenic chancre.

On the other hand, the induration, without losing its immense value, does not always assume well its form; it does not constantly assume the same development; it is sometimes superficial; we must know how to search for it in order to discover it in the thickness of the skin or of a mucous membrane. It gives sometimes to the touch only the sensation of a lining of parchment. I designate this form, at the Hospital du Midi, under the name of *parchment-like induration.* The indurated chancres for this reason, are very often taken for simple excoriations, for simple cases of balano-posthitis, when they do not pass entirely unperceived; for they are superficial, on a level with the neighboring healthy parts, and sometimes even a little more prominent.

The induration ordinarily attacks all the base of the ulceration; but in some rarer cases, it affects only the borders, and is then only annular. It is with this form of indurated chancre that we might preserve the denomination of *primary annular syphilis.*

When there exists no complication, the induration is abruptly circumscribed by the healthy tissues; it is much more extended than the ulceration to which it serves as base. It is constituted by a hard nucleus, as if cartilaginous, resistent, elastic, indolent and perfectly rounded; this nucleus lifts up the ulceration above the level of the neighboring healthy parts, and constitutes then a variety of *the elevated ulcer.*

The induration presents itself sometimes under the form of a *crest* more or less prominent, when the plastic infiltration which constitutes it, does not take place in homogeneous tissues, and meets with resistance at some points, as happens at the reflexion of the prepuce in the groove at the base of the gland—a seat where, after all, we find the best characterized indurations. If we compress the skin or a mucous membrane upon an induration, these tissues grow pale, and we observe something analogous to what happens, when, in turning over the eyelid, we compress the conjunctiva upon the tarsal cartilage.

The induration is produced ordinarily in a slow and gradual manner. Sometimes it grows by jerks; in some cases it remains a long time but slightly marked, in order to take on afterwards extensive proportions. The tissues often become indurated to a great extent; I have seen the whole of the base of the gland, which appeared to have taken on a cartilaginous transformation, and which might be taken for a cancerous degeneration. One of the most curious observations in this respect, has been offered to me by a patient sent to me by Prof. Andral.

The induration, after having diminished or even disappeared, is very subject to return. It is not rare to see it then take on dimensions more considerable than it had at first.

The term of the induration is not limited. In those cases which are superficial, parchment-like, I have seen complete resolution take place, so as not to leave any traces after less than a month's duration. At other times, on the contrary, it persists during some months, and even years. The groove about the base of the gland—a region, where, as I have said, they are the most marked—is also that, where they remain the longest. Upon the gland, upon the neck of the uterus, at the vulvar circle, where it is often little marked and very difficult to appreciate, the induration disappears very quickly. It is sometimes very ephemeral in the urethra, especially in females; also in the anus, and in the vagina. We need to pay much attention in order not to be deceived. Upon the tongue, and especially upon the lips, it remains sometimes quite a long time. In all cases, when the induration commences to disappear, the ulceration has been already a long time cured. When resolution takes place, the induration undergoes some modifications ; it loses its resistance, its elasticity, it becomes, as it were, gelatinous, and finishes by leaving in the place that it occupied, a wrinkled spot, of a brown copper-colored tint.

The indurated chancre, which is less often multiple than the other varieties, and of which the specific ulcerated period is soon limited, either *sua sponte* or by the effect of art, takes on, however, under certain circumstances, sufficiently extensive dimensions. It extends itself and deepens. We might believe, then, that it was going to produce great loss of substance; well, when the cicatrization is complete, we do not often find any further traces of it, for it is the plastic exudation which has alone served as food to the phagedenism, in guarding the neighboring tissues from the progress of the ulceration. This condition, so common to the indurated chancre, is important to understand as regards the etiology of constitutional syphilis, for it is not the cicatrices which are the most numerous, nor the deepest, which prove that infection has taken place.

The specific induration is the certain absolute proof that the constitutional infection has taken place. It is the passage of the primary accident to the secondary accident. In fact, the indurated chancre is the variety which loses the quickest the principal characteristic of the primary accident, viz., the possibility of furnishing the inoculable pus. But if it always demonstrates the infection, and if its increase is in ratio with the gravity of the accidents which are to follow ; if we can consider it, pardon me the expression, as a *syphilomètre*, we can also regard it as an excellent measure of treatment ; for it is one of the accidents which ordinarily obey the best a mercurial treatment. There are, however, circumstances, under which the induration resists ; it is then, the most often, not any longer with the specific induration that we have to deal, but with an organized tissue, which has succeeded it ; that is to say, with a tissue of a fibrous nature. It is thus that I have been able to explain an induration which a patient presented to me in my wards in the Hospital du Midi, who was affected with a caries of the frontal bone, which came on thirty years after a chancre at the base of the gland, and in whom that induration persisted under the form of a well-pronounced nucleus. The difference is still very difficult to make out, in a great number of cases, between the tissue of a fibrous character and the specific induration.

The specific induration has for its anatomical seat, the thickness of the skin and the mucous membranes, the sub-cutaneous cellular tissue as well as the sub-mucous, but it would seem that the lymphatic capillary vessels should be the seat of predilection. It is in fact where the lymphatic net works are the best designated and most abundant, that the induration takes on its best form and its largest dimensions. What still comes to the support of this opinion, is the manner in which the induration extends, and is propagated. We see, then, that it is in following the lymphatic vessels, which, according as they become more voluminous, are designated in the form of cords.

As to the intimate nature of the induration, as to its essence, as to what constitutes it, organic chemistry, which has afforded us so many marvels of late years, which has, perhaps, given us too many, has as yet found nothing ; and the microscope, which .always promises, and which sometimes keeps its promises, has only yet recognized in the specific induration, fibro-plastic tissue, proportionately very abundant, but which does not differ from what we find elsewhere and in other conditions of non-specifity.   This is, at least up to the present time, the result of the researches undertaken by one of my very distinguished disciples, Mr. Acton, of England, and of those which have been since made by MM. Robin and Marchal (de Calvi) at Paris.   The same results have been obtained by our learned and industrious colleague and micographist, Dr. Lebert, to whom we are indebted for such beautiful works.

Such are, my friend, the results of my researches and of my observation upon the indurated chancre.   I simply indicate them to you here, for, as I am obliged often to repeat, I do not write a didactic work upon syphilis.   I recal only the principal points of my doctrine, upon the occasion of the objections which are still from time to time, and more or less directly addressed to me.   The developments form the subject of my oral teaching ; they are, moreover, the subject of an extended work which I am preparing, and of which these *letters*, so to speak, are only the *summary*.   From this work, I select the general principles, the essential points of the doctrine, indicating, the principal motives upon which they are based ; and this work, imperfect though it may be, has no other merit than that which the position of your readers gives it, who are no longer pupils, but learned and enlightened practitioners, and to whom these indications ought only to recal the studies and researches previously and completely made.

Yours,   RICORD.

NEW APPARATUS FOR FRACTURE OF THE RADIUS.

BY RICHARD M. HODGES, M.D., BOSTON.

[Communicated for the Boston Medical and Surgical Journal.]

THE attention of the profession having been recently called, through this Journal, to a new apparel for fractures of the lower extremity of the radius (Dr. Bond's), I am induced to offer the description of another, which, so far as I am aware, has never been made use of in this neighborhood ; and having witnessed its application and efficiency, I am able to speak of it from personal experience.

The great variety of methods recommended in treating this accident, probably arises from the loose manner in which the term " fracture of the lower extremity of the radius " is applied to all fractures of the lower *half* of this bone, the indications varying so much according as they are more or less distant from the radio-carpal articulation.   The fracture for which I wish to describe an apparel, is that which was so long confounded with dislocation of the wrist ; and to illustrate its adaptedness it will be necessary to review in a few words, the nature of this fracture and its displacement.

The radius forming nearly the whole of the upper articulating surface of the wrist-joint, the ulna being but indirectly articulated with the carpus, sustains the whole shock of a fall, is generally alone fractured, and this almost invariably at the same level ; " the principal division of the bone has always seemed to me," says Malgaigne ('Traité des Fractures, Paris, 1847, p. 605), " to occupy very nearly the same point, viz., where the compact tissue of the shaft entirely disappears to give place to the spongy tissue of the epiphysis." This point is rather less than an inch from the articular surface, varying with the age and size of the subject. The direction of the fracture is always transversal (Voillemier), and the character of the deformity is so constant, that when it takes place from a fall on the palm of the hand (the almost unique cause), it may be diagnosed across the room. Oftentimes, crepitation being so rare, this is the only means of diagnosis. This deformity arises from the following displacement. The lower fragment penetrates with its palmar edge the substance of the upper, and this with its dorsal edge the substance of the lower ; or else, the whole lower fragment covers the superior, which enters it like a wedge. The lower one inclines backward at the same time that it mounts upward, and the penetration of the upper fragment is greater on the dorsal and radial side of the wrist, owing to the direction of the force which fractures. There results a tumor on both the back and the front of the wrist, from the projection of the two fractured ends. The prominence on the back of the wrist is much greater than that on the inside ; this, together with the backward inclination of the hand, constitutes the *talon de four-chette* of M. Velpeau, the distortion of the arm, wrist and hand suggesting an ingenious comparison to the lines of curvature presented by a silver fork. There is no inclination of the fragments towards the interosseous space, for the simple reason that the fracture takes place at a point where no interosseous space exists, and the upper fragment would be an insuperable obstacle to the displacement of the lower one in this direction. The upper one might possibly be displaced in this sense when the fracture is a little higher than the classic level, but even then the irregularities of the lower fragment would be almost sure to hold it in its place, as is proved by the fact that movements of rotation given to this are communicated to the upper one in almost every case. The shortening of the radius by the mutual penetration of the fractured surfaces, makes the styloid process of the ulna more prominent than natural.

But this may project from another cause. For notwithstanding the anatomical disposition of the parts which renders the radius so peculiarly liable to suffer alone, the ulna is at times fractured, and when this happens the lower fragments tend, both by the nature of the displacement and the direction of the force, which ordinarily impinges more on the radial side of the bone, to carry the lower end of the ulna outward, and this becomes a prominent deformity, because the hand tends to abduct in following the direction of the altered obliquity of the end of the radius.

From this exposition of the nature of this fracture, it would appear that the indications are—1st, and most important, to obviate the displacement of the lower fragment of the radius backward ; 2d, when both bones are broken, to bring the styloid process of the ulna into its place ; and 3d, to restore the interosseous space between the upper fragments.

An objection to almost all the apparels in use, arises from the nature of the deformity, and their inefficiency in preventing it or maintaining the natural position of the parts. " Whether one or both bones be fractured, *the deformity exists only from the loss of parallelism between the fractured ends and the turning backward of the lower fragment. In fact, the only indication is to push this forward.* If to the backward cant of the lower fragment of the radius is joined a displacement outward of the styloid process of the ulna, with a projection inward of the upper portion of that bone, there result two new indications, viz., to push outward the ulna, whilst you endeavor to push the styloid process inward " (Malgaigne, loc. cit., p. 616). The sling of Cline, splints curved laterally, permanent extension, &c., are all powerless, and the *attelle cubitale* of Dupuytren, acting on the hand only, fails to affect the ulna.

The fracture being reduced and the parts well moulded into their proper places, the arm is enveloped loosely by a few turns of a roller. Upon the outside of the wrist, *below* the level of the line of fracture, is placed a square compress, about a quarter of an inch thick and of the same width as the wrist at this point. Along the inside of the arm is placed a graduated compress, extending from the upper third of the arm down to the line of fracture only. These being held in place, the hand is then flexed upon the arm to very nearly its utmost extent, without using force, and bandaged from just above the elbow down to the metacarpo-phalangeal articulation with a roller, starched, dextrined or not, carefully and judiciously tightened at the point of fracture, and is so maintained till its removal be advisable. The limb is placed in a sling, and thus carried, the hand flexed on the arm, till the cure is effected. Ordinarily in three weeks the apparel may be abandoned, though it may be removed at frequent intervals for inspection and bathing of the parts. If during the first few days the swelling be too great to admit of its application, it may be deferred till its subsidence, and any temporary expedient for maintaining the flexion of the hand substituted for it.

What is the operation of this mode of treatment? The substitution of a natural for an artificial splint, one that by virtue of the flexion of the hand, adjusts and confines the parts in their proper place when once restored to that position. The tendons of eight muscles, viz., the *extensor ossis metacarpi pollicis,* and *extensor primi internodii pollicis,* on the radial side of the wrist ; the *extensor carpi radialis, longior* and *brevior, extensor secundi internodii pollicis, extensor communis digitorum, extensor minimi digiti,* and the *extensor carpi ulnaris,* on the dorsum and ulnar portion of the wrist, and the posterior annular ligament, are spread out over the parts, and by the tension arising from flexion, adapt an equalized compression in a way which no artificial splint could do. Their combined action presses the lower fragment forward, and restores the backward obliquity of the radius in the most perfect manner. The *extensor carpi ulnaris*, passing through the posterior groove of the lower end of the ulna, prevents lateral and posterior displacement, and by the effort it makes to pull in a straight line, retains in position the styloid process of that bone. The graduated compress of the inside of the arm, separates the upper fragments and prevents their tendency to approach each other, whilst it assists in bringing them into parallelism with the lower. The lower fragment we have seen requires no appliance for the former purpose. The dorsal compress merely adds to the power of the extensor tendons, to keep the fragment in place and constantly pushed forward.

It remains to speak of its effect upon the subsequent use of the hand and fingers, and the degree of pain resulting from its use. The deformity it unquestionably obviates, and there is no apparel yet known which is not the source of more or less pain, unless it be Bond's, the only advantage of which is that it regards the comfort of the patient, without regarding the indications of the deformity. The apparel just described, I believe, causes as little pain as any ; the muscles and tendons are stretched in their natural direction, a position far more comfortable than the lateral bending produced by the common lateral-curved splint. For the same reason, the subsequent stiffness that must follow any treatment whatsoever, is less likely to be very great, and during the whole treatment movement of the fingers may be practised to any extent —a great advantage, not to be obtained by any of the other methods proposed. The materials of which to make the apparel are to be found anywhere, and when made, you have no irregular surfaces of splints, no angular projections, nothing but the uniform compression of a well-applied bandage, which at any time may be taken off and re-applied without trouble or assistance. Such seem to be its chief recommendations. Of course, in cases where the extremity is crushed and broken into many fragments, the result of this, as of any treatment, will be unsatisfactory, and the consolidation more or less irregular. And though inapplicable to cases of fracture higher up than the one I have spoken of, and to those exceedingly rare cases, where the displacement of the lower fragment is to the inside of the wrist instead of the outside, this method of treatment seems to fulfil all the indications in fractures such as I have above described.

The idea of this method is, I believe, of Belgian origin, and I had recently the opportunity of seeing very satisfactory evidence of its usefulness, in the wards of M. Velpeau at the Hôpital de la Charité at Paris.

No. 12 *Essex st., Boston, March,* 1853.

EXCISION OF THE TESTES.

[Prof. S. D. Gross, in his report to the State Medical Society of Kentucky, on " Improvements in Surgery," gives the following account of a singular operation performed by himself.]

A very novel case, justifying, in my opinion, excision of the testes, came under my observation in 1849. So far as my information extends, there is no account of any operation for a similar object upon record. The patient, at the time I first saw her—she had always been regarded as a girl, and had been so pronounced by the accoucheur—was three years of age, having been born on the 10th of July, 1846. At the age of 2, she began to evince the feelings and disposition of a boy ; she rejected dolls and similar articles of amusement, and became fond of boyish sports. She was well-grown, perfectly healthy, and quite fleshy ; her hair was dark and long, the eyes black, and the expression very agreeable. Upon making a careful examination, I found the external genitals in the following very singular condition. There was neither a penis nor a vagina ; but instead of the former there was a small clitoris, and instead of the latter a cul-de-sac, covered with mucous membrane. The urethra occupied the usual situation ; the nymphæ were unnaturally small; but the labia were well developed, and contained each a testis, quite as large, consistent and well shaped as they ever are in boys at this age.

It being apparent from the facts of the case that it was one of monstrosity of the genital organs, usually denominated hermaphrodism, the question at once occurred whether anything ought to be done to deprive the poor child of that part of the genital apparatus, which, if permitted to remain until the age of puberty, would be sure to be followed by sexual desire, and which might thus conduce to the formation of an unfortunate matrimonial connection. Such an alliance, it was evident, would eventuate only in chagrin, disappointment, and, probably, in disgrace. Certainly no impregnation could ever occur, and even copulation could be performed but imperfectly. I gave the subject all the consideration that I was able to bestow upon it ; I felt the responsibility of my position ; a new question, involving the happiness of my little patient and the deepest interest of her parents, was presented to me. I appealed to the records of my profession, but in vain, for a precedent. Under the circumstances, I sought the advice of a medical friend, Professor Miller, in whose wisdom and integrity I had unwavering confidence. He saw the child, and examined her ; he viewed the case, as I had done previously, in all its aspects, physiological,-legal and surgical, and his conclusion was that excision of the testes would not only be justifiable, but highly proper ; that it would be an act of kindness and humanity to the poor child to deprive it of an appendage of so useless a nature, one which might ultimately lead to the ruin of her happiness. The parents were already solicitous for an operation, and having imparted to them our decision, I no longer hesitated in regard to the course I ought to pursue.

I performed the operation of castration on the 20th of July, 1849, aided by my pupils, Dr. D. D. Thomson of this city, Dr. Greenbury Henry of Burlington, Iowa, and Dr. William H. Cobb of Cincinnati. The little patient being put under the influence of chloroform, I made a perpendicular incision into each labium down to the testis, which was then carefully separated from the surrounding parts, and detached by dividing the lower part of the spermatic cord. The arteries of the cord being secured with ligatures, the edges of the wound were brought to- gether with twisted sutures, and the child put to bed. Hardly any blood was lost during the operation. About two hours after, the labium became greatly distended and discolored ; and, upon removing the su- tures, the source of the mischief was found to be a small artery, which was immediately drawn out, and tied. No unpleasant symptoms of any kind ensued after this, and in a week the little patient was able to be up, being quite well and happy. The testes were carefully examined after removal, and were found to be perfectly formed in every respect. The spermatic cords were natural.

I have seen this child repeatedly since the operation, as her parents live only a few squares from my office, and have watched her mental and physical developments. Her parents, who are persons of obser- vation and intelligence, assure me that her disposition and habits are those of a girl ; that she takes great delight in sewing and house-work, and that she no longer indulges in riding upon sticks and other boyish exercises. Her person is well developed, and her mind uncommonly active for a child of her years.

VERATRUM VIRIDE.

THERE is considerable discussion at present going on among some of our southern practitioners in reference to the value of the *veratrum viride*, as a remedial agent. The preparation used, is Dr. Norwood's saturated tincture. The advocates of the new remedy strongly contend for its utility in various diseases, among which may be mentioned pneumonia, typhoid fever, pertussis and catarrhal fever. Dr. Branch, of South Ca- rolina, states that he has been using it for months in pneumonia as well as typhoid fever, in doses varying from three to twelve drops of the satu- rated tincture of Dr. Norwood, and he considers it as one of the most valuable discoveries of this or any other age. He always conjoined opiates or stimulants, and sometimes both, with it. Paregoric as an opiate and brandy as a stimulant were preferred. At the same time, he used the shower-bath, blisters or alteratives, as the case might require. Dr. Branch's article on this subject is found in the Charleston Medical Journal for September.

Dr. Blackburn, of Ga., also furnishes for the same Journal an article on the same subject. He says—" I have given it in pneumonia, catar- rhal fever, and pertussis, and I have never failed to reduce a morbidly- increased circulation to a healthy standard. Nor have I ever seen any unpleasant symptoms accompanying its therapeutic action, save nausea. I have given it to infants with the happiest result. I have lost only one case of pneumonia out of fifteen since I commenced relying upon the veratrum viride as a controller of the circulation."

Dr. Geo. B. Pearson testifies that " in pneumonic inflammation, whe- ther typhoid in character or synochoid, there is always increased celerity of the pulse, preternatural heat, &c. The remedy seems well calculated to fulfil the obvious indication of reducing the pulse, abating the heat, &c. Its extreme effect resembles that of lobelia."

Dr. T. T. Robertson, of Winnsboro', adds—"I also believe, that with it we can do something more than simply conduct typhoid fever through its stages, I believe we can *cure* it."

On the other hand, Dr. Pendleton was disappointed in the effects of this medicine, and does not hesitate to denounce it in round terms in the same Journal. We do not like, however, the spirit in which he does so. That " *experimentalism in medicine* " of which he so disparagingly speaks, has been the means of elevating the science and commending it to favor. Neither medicine nor any other science, is satisfied with the attainments of to-day. It stretches forward, and aided as it is by a host of noble sciences, all contributing their offerings to promote the general welfare and happiness of man, it is destined to accomplish yet greater results.

Veratrum viride is also called American hellebore, and according to Dr. Wood, Indian poke and poke root. It should not be confounded, from their common names, with the phytolacca or poke root properly. The veratrum is indigenous to the United States, growing in swamps and wet places. The root is the part used, and should be collected in the autumn. The form in which it is most usually administered is that of tincture. Of the saturated tincture from three to fifteen drops is the dose—Dr. Branch never prescribes at first more than six drops—seldom more than four—until he " arrives at the susceptibility of the patient, and increases a drop at every subsequent dose until the wished-for effect is produced, to wit, a cool surface, a pulse reduced to the desired standard as to frequency, but never diminished in volume, strength, or any other necessary quality, and here I hold it ' firm and fast ' for a few days, which generally breaks up the case."—*Southern Journal of Medical and Physical Science.*

THE BOSTON MEDICAL AND SURGICAL JOURNAL.

BOSTON. MARCH 30. 1853.

Vaccine Irregularities. — An exchange paper makes the following statement. " Dr. Tinsley — an English practitioner of long experience in Cuba, and a graduate of Paris, has discovered, in the course of his practice in cases of smallpox, that vaccine virus, after having once passed through a negro's system, becomes useless as a preventive to the white race."

For many successive years we were constantly devoted to this one branch of practice, and hundreds of colored persons in Boston were vaccinated, from whom virus was taken and afterwards inserted in other individuals. It was always found as active in its effects as when elaborated in the arm of a white patient. The experience of a multitude of practitioners, it is presumed, might be collected, to substantiate this statement;

in fact, its truth has been proved within the last two weeks in New England. At Havana, as in all other tropical regions, it is difficult to propagate the virus, from one individual to another, owing, unquestionably, to some atmospheric condition with which physicians are not familiar. During the extreme heat of July and August, we have much difficulty, even in our northern climate, in keeping vaccine virus, on account of the state of the weather, which is then analogous to the climate of Cuba. In Siam, and in the interior of Asia Minor, smallpox rages almost every year, on account of the uncertainty of the action of the vaccine virus. The absorbents are inactive, or the intense heat modifies the lymph, if it does not utterly destroy its prophylactic properties, so that scarcely one in a thousand obtains the protection which is so generally secured in Northern countries. The announcement of Dr. Tinsley's *discovery*, therefore, we consider entitled to no credit. The failure of his operations is doubtless due to climate, and not to a dark skin.

Barnstable District Medical Society. — From some unexplained cause, the Massachusetts Medical Society seems often to be placed in an anomalous position. The lawsuit in which it successfully embarked has become an old story, and now an opportunity presents for again commanding public attention. It seems that the Barnstable District Med. Society some time since censured a Boston surgeon, for having consulted with an irregular practitioner, somewhere in their region of country. This naturally gave offence. Being out of the country at the time, we know nothing of the matter beyond the action of the two societies. The Counsellors of the State society in Boston, resolved, "that the Barnstable District Medical Society should be called upon to rescind so much of its transactions as are derogatory to the character," &c., particularly the resolve beginning with the words," &c., "the doings of the said District Society on this point to be reported to the corresponding secretary of the Mass. Med. Society." Prompt as minute men, the offending branch held a meeting, and this is the first declaration. "Voted, that in the present aspect of the affair, it would be inconsistent with the truth, and unbecoming the character of this society, to comply with this request." Then follows a narrative of the offence charged, which has been made a matter of record in the archives of the Barnstable District Society. Whether the next step will be an inquiry into the contumacy of a subordinate body, for refusing to alter a record, or whether this will be the last of the affair, we are unable to say.

Practice of Medicine in Canada. — A thorough reform is contemplated by the true friends of medical science in the lower Province. The scheme of an act to regulate the practice of physic and surgery has been submitted to the profession for examination, running thus — "No person shall, after the passing of this act, receive a license from the Provincial Medical Board to practice physic, surgery or midwifery in Lower Canada, unless he shall have undergone due examination before the said board, and obtained a certificate of qualification from it," &c. With a view to obtaining the opinion of medical gentlemen, a circular of questions was addressed to each one, and such answers as they returned, touching the expediency or inexpediency of the proposed enactment, has been published by the government. Some of the replies indicate a liberal disposition — a kind of willingness to live and let live; and were they familiar with the history of medical legislation in the New England States, their own legislature would not perhaps be urged to action. While we had protection, that is, while ignorant pretenders were prevented by law from imposing upon the people, there was a constant uproar, a restlessness and a ringing of " monopoly," which died away with a repeal of all laws relating to the matter. Every one now in Massachusetts is at liberty to take medicine according to his own inclinations; and all who are employed, can compel those who employ them, to pay for their services; yet all this has not injured the standing of the well-qualified practitioners, though the irregulars of all denominations have a plenty of patronage. We are a people excessively prone to medicine taking; and those who have any new preparation, whether worthless or not, can generally find a market for it in New England.

Dr. Hughes's Lecture. — At Keokuk, in the State of Iowa, where the Indians held their powows comparatively but a few moons since, a university is located, with an endowment in lands that will give it immense resources in after ages. A school of medicine is flourishing under its wing already, and the discourse delivered at the opening of the last course of lectures, by J. C. Hughes, M.D., carries no indications on its frontlet of being delivered on the outskirts of civilization. It is a well-written, animated, production, full of excellencies, like the enterprising inhabitants by whom the author is surrounded. He appears to be as well read in Talmudic traditions, as in modern medicine; and if the Shasters are not at his tongue's end, the Mohammedan opinion that Adam was as tall as a palm tree, is to him a familiar fact. Dr. Hughes is fitted for the place. Tact is essential to success, but when combined with sterling good sense and a well-grounded preparation for instructing those who are desirous of being taught, it is powerful for good.

Prescriber's Pharmacopœia. — The third American edition, from Messrs. S. S. & Wm. Wood's press, 261 Pearl street, New York, contains some excellent additions. In the first place, it has been carefully compared with the 9th edition of the United States Dispensatory by Drs. Wood & Bache, and the formulæ altered to correspond with those received authorities. The uses of medicines, and the whole of a well-written series of instructions in respect to diet for the sick, are from the American editor, and immensely enhance the value of this portable little guide in everyday practice. Here is a miniature volume, that might almost be carried in a vest-pocket, containing a multitude of facts and suggestions, besides specifically noting the doses of all the usually prescribed remedies. It is a convenient reference in making out a prescription, when one happens to forget the name of an article, the exact quantity that may be given, &c. We cannot have too many prompters of this kind, in the practice of our profession.

Obstetric Catechism. — A small volume has been published by Messrs. Barrington & Haswell, of which Joseph Warrington, M.D. of Philadelphia, is author, called " The Obstetric Catechism; containing two thousand and forty-seven questions and answers on obstetrics proper." The work is decidedly behind the age in its typography and artistical finish, and falls far below the general appearance of Philadelphia books. There are one hundred and fifty illustrations, but these, too, are below the usual

standard of anatomical drawings. Besides these deficiencies, we are dis·
posed to object to the dialogue form of giving instruction, which may be
considered as obsolete in the estimation of scholars.   When the industrious
author appears in a new edition, he can change this style advantageously.
It is evident enough, from a perusal of the text, that Dr. Warrington is
familiar with the department of practice to which the strength of his pro-,
fessional life has been principally devoted.   From the multitude and cha·
racter of the pupils instructed by him, there can be no doubt of his high
attainments ; and he deserves a far better introduction to the medical
world than in the pages of the Catechism before us.

Maclise's Surgical Anatomy, by Piper. — Our friend Dr. Piper is the
very personification of artistic and literary industry.   He not only writes,
draws, and illustrates his own works, but he contrives to better the text of
other authors. A new edition of Maclise's Surgical Anatomy, with additions
from Bourgery, is coming out under his critical eye, published by Jewett
& Co., of Boston, and the same firm in Cleveland, Ohio.   Of course,
every one having an ounce of patriotism in his composition, will encourage a native effort of this kind, which is intended to place in the hands of
the profession a rare series of surgical plans of the human body, true to
the life, and at a price far below the original English cost.

Massachusetts Register.—Occasionally it happens that intelligence of
common interest to business people, among whom physicians are inva-
-riably to be numbered, may be propagated through the pages of this Journal, without having the exclusive odor of medicine.   No other apology
need be required, for directing the attention of the profession of Massachusetts, and perhaps those residing in other sections of New England, to the Massachusetts Register for 1853, published by Mr. George
Adams, 91 Washington st., Boston. It is such a perfect guide to everybody's
house and business — including druggists, apothecaries, surgical instrument manufacturers, as well as accounts of hospitals, dispensaries, charities, the residences of officers of all denominations, both in the public service and corporations, together with an immense amount of statistical information of all kinds—that it would be a book worth having on every
physician's office table.   It is a key to men and things in every city and
town in the Commonwealth, besides imparting incidental information over
a still larger field, always acceptable and often indispensable.   -

Organic and Physiological Chemistry.—Daniel Breed, M.D., of the U.
S. Patent office, is the translator of Dr. Carl Löwig's Principles of Organic
and Physiological Chemistry, which will be appreciated by all who cultivate that grand department of science.   It is intended for a text-book—containing not only all the old discoveries, but also all the new facts, says the preface, relating to the animal and vegetable kingdoms.   Dr. Draper, of New
York, would never have allowed it to be dedicated to himself, did he not entertain a favorable opinion of the work.   We cannot, at present, do much
more than announce its appearance. The Messrs. Hart, late Carey &
Hart, of Philadelphia, are the publishers. The volume is a good-sized
octavo, of 481 pages.   There is a strict technicality about it, that will suit
advanced students.   For mere popular study, it seems not to have been intended by the author.   Profound research and deep learning pervade every
page throughout.

The Bristol District Medical Society held its regular quarterly meeting at Taunton, March 9th ; twelve of its members were present. At this meeting were chosen officers for the ensuing year, viz : — *President*, Dr. R. M. Randall. *Vice President*, Dr. Ira Sampson. *Secretary*, Dr. Wm. Dickinson. *Librarians*, Drs. James B. Dean, Phinehas Savery. *Board of Censors*, Drs. Thaddeus Phelps, Charles Howe, James B. Dean. *Board of Counsellors*, Drs. Benoni Carpenter, J. D. Nichols, Dan King. *Delegates to American Medical Association*, Drs. William Dickinson, Thaddeus Phelps, Ira Sampson.

In connection with the customary transactions, a very able and interesting paper was read by Dr. Dan King, upon the subject of " Quackery," as it is practised *in* and *out* of the profession ; the duty of the regular practice in regard to it; the mutual duties of the members towards each other, and the reciprocal duties of physician and patient with reference thereto.

The next regular meeting will hold its session at Attleboro,' on June 8th. · Wᴵᴸᴸᴵᴀᴹ Dᴵᴄᴋᴵɴsᴏɴ, M.D., *Secretary*.

Medical Miscellany. — It seems that a reform medical college has been organized at Charlestown, over the bridge, opposite Boston. What has become of the one in Boston? — F. Tuthill, M D., of New York, is an excellent collector of medical intelligence for the newspaper press. — Six gentlemen were graduated at the new Dental College, at Syracuse, N. Y. The institution seems to have been established in strength and respectability. —A person looking at some skeletons, the other day, asked a young doctor present where he got them. He replied, ' We raised them !'—Dr. John G. Stephenson is lecturing very acceptably to large audiences at Terre-Haute, Indiana.—The Siamese Twins, accompanied by one of each of their children, are to be publicly exhibited in Boston next month, being the first of a series of exhibitions in this country and Europe—six months to be spent in the former and a year and a half in the latter.

To Cᴏʀʀᴇsᴘᴏɴᴅᴇɴᴛs,—The following communications, in addition to those previously acknowledged, have been received : — Quinine in Rheumatism ; Adulteration of Drugs; Nitrate of Silver in Dyspepsia ; Report of a Surgical Clinique of the Philadelphia College of Medicine.

Pᴏsᴛᴀɢᴇ ᴏɴ ᴛʜᴇ Mᴇᴅᴵᴄᴀʟ Jᴏᴜʀɴᴀʟ. — As some of the subscribers to this Journal appear to have misunderstood the provisions of the act of Congress of last year which apply to the postage to be paid upon the Journal, we would again state that our weekly issue can be sent to subscribers in this county, *free*; and to any part of the State, at 3 1-4 cents per quarter. When sent to any other part of the United States, the quarterly postage is 6 1-4 cents. The monthly series is sent at the rate of 4 1-2 cts. per quarter to any part of the country. In all cases, these quarterly postages must be paid in advance by subscribers at the office of delivery ; if not thus paid, the rate is much higher.

· Eʀʀᴀᴛᴀ. — In the article on "Tully's Materia Medica," in the last number of the Journal, the word *organized* should be inserted before the word matter, in the fifth line of note on page 152. On page 154, 20th line from top, after the word " diminished," insert *strength of.*

Deaths in Boston for the week ending Saturday noon, March 26th, 72. Males, 35—females, 37. Inflammation of the bowels, 2—disease of the bowels, 1 — congestion of brain, 1 — consumption, 8—convulsions, 2—croup, 3—cancer, 2—dropsy, 1—dropsy in head, 5 — infantile diseases, 4—puerperal, 1—erysipelas, 2—typhus fever, 3—typhoid fever. 1—scarlet fever, 4—homicide, 1—hooping cough, 6—hemorrhage, 1—disease of the heart, 1—inflammation of the lungs, 6—disease of the liver, 1—marasmus, 2—old age, 1—palsy, 2—pleurisy, 1—rheumatism, 2—scrofula, 1—syphilis, 1—teething, 3—unknown, 2—worms, 1.

Under 5 years, 34 — between 5 and 20 years, 8—between 20 and 40 years, 17—between 40 and 60 years, 6—over 60 years, 7. Born in the United States, 53 — Ireland, 17 — British Provinces, 1—Germany, 1. The above includes 7 deaths in the city institutions.

Vital Statistics in Kentucky. — We have before alluded to the fact that much attention has been directed in Kentucky to the subject of vital statistics. In the Transactions of the Medical Society of that State—a document which is highly honorable to the Committee of Publication — is a report by the standing committee on this subject. From it we have gleaned the following interesting items.

In the whole State, the population averages 31 persons to the square mile ; Jefferson county, the densest, has 171 — and Harlan county, the sparsest, only 6 to the square mile. The whole number of deaths for the year, ending June 1, 1852, was 15,211—being 1 in 64.46 persons, or 1.55 per cent. But the mortality varies greatly in the different counties. Arranging them in four classes — the first, comprising 18 counties, with a population of about 55 persons to the square mile, gives a mortality of 1 in 41.40, or 2 38 per cent. The highest in any one county was 1 in 25.72, or 3.83 per cent. Sixteen of these counties were visited by the cholera. The second class, of 20 counties, with a population of about 30 to the square mile, presents an average mortality of 1 in 58.92, or 1.69 per cent. The third class, 30 counties, and 29 persons to the square mile, gives a mortality of 1 in 79.16, or 1.23 per cent. One county in this class, entirely surrounded by those of the fourth or most highly-favored class, presents the anomalous condition of being wholly destitute of physicians— " no member of the profession having yet had the courage to penetrate within its borders." The fourth and last class comprises the remaining 32 counties of the State. The population is about 21 to the square mile, and the mortality was 1 in 122.35, or .81 per cent. The least mortality was 1 in 376, or .26 per cent. These last counties are generally mountainous and sterile, the population sturdy, and living in the utmost simplicity. Although the above exhibits so favorable a state of public health for the whole State, there are certain portions of it which are far otherwise. Among these is the city of Lexington, from which statistical returns have been received for the last twenty-one consecutive years, and also for the years ending the 10th of January 1818 and 1821. During the year 1817, the mortality was 1 in 90.88, or 1.10 per cent., and the births in the proportion of nearly three to one of the deaths. In 1820, the mortality was 1 in 64.71, or 1.54 per cent.; the births not enumerated. During 21 consecutive years from 1831, the whole number of deaths was 4,120, being an average mortality of 1 in 36.52, or 2.73 per cent. The births during the same period were 4,331. Only one year of these twenty-one gave as many as two births to one death. During two of these years — 1833 and 1849 — the cholera prevailed ; in the former of which the mortality was 1 in 9·70, or 10.30 per cent. In 1837 it was the least of any year — 1 in 110.79 ; and last year it was 1 in 31.84, or 3.14 per cent. The committee state, that the conclusion to which they are led by these returns is, that there has been in Lexington for some years past, an increasing mortality, the causes of which demand a thorough and prompt investigation.

Wool-Spinning Mills and the Public Health. — At this moment an investigation is being made into the state of health of those engaged in woolspinning mills, with the view of ascertaining the effects of oil as a prevention or cure of diseases, especially those of a pulmonary character. In those mills oil is extensively used, and the people engaged working there, although enduring the greatest hardships and privations, enjoy the best health,—*London Lancet.*

THE
BOSTON MEDICAL AND SURGICAL JOURNAL.

| VOL. XLVIII. | WEDNESDAY, APRIL 6, 1853. | No. 10. |

EPIDEMIC OF 1852 IN NEWTON.

BY EDWARD WARREN, M.D.

[Communicated for the Boston Medical and Surgical Journal.]

WHILE the influenza was prevailing in the winter of 1851–1852, I was called to a succession of cases, occurring at distinct intervals and in different localities, which varied in many particulars from any which I had previously seen.

CASE I.—The first case occurred Dec. 19, 1851. A young lady— who had gone to attend a female patient who was recovering from a severe attack of pleurisy, and who was also subject to eczema—was suddenly seized with chills and vomiting, accompanied with severe headache, redness of the face, and some other symptoms, which led her to suppose she had erysipelas—a very severe attack of which she had formerly experienced. She was very much depressed.

I saw her a few hours after the attack. Her countenance was very much flushed. Face but little if any swollen ; of a deep scarlet hue, something between that of scarlet fever and of erysipelas. I found her sitting in her parlor. She had violent headache, nausea, tongue thickly coated, slight sore throat, breath very foul. Pulse *slower* than natural. Voice strong and muscular, strength good. 1 directed her to go to bed, and take an emetic of ipecac., to be followed with Dover's powders. Her face to be bathed with lead-water.

Dec. 20th.—I found her greatly improved. Redness of countenance nearly gone ; headache relieved ; pulse as yesterday.

21st.—Sitting up. Redness remains only on one side of the nose. I found it only necessary to regulate her diet, and caution her against exposure or exertion. She had no return of the affection. The attack was attended, throughout the whole, with foul breath and foul perspiration.

CASE II.—The second case took place in this village, about three miles from the location of the former. Mrs. ———, a young married lady, of poor health, who had recently lost a child, and who had also been much in attendance upon a person very ill with typhoid fever, was seized in the night, after a hearty supper, with symptoms similar to those described above.

She had violent headache, nausea and retching ; with pain in the side, which she supposed to be pleuritic. She could not, however, fix the

10

spot. There was erythematous redness of the face, unattended with swelling. - Pulse *slower* than natural, skin cool and feet cold. I prescribed a blister to the side, opiates for the relief of the pain, and lead-water to the face. Her state of previous ill health led me to avoid more powerful medicine.

Dec. 11th.—Much better. Redness of the face gone. Pain in chest gone. Some pain in bowels. Pulse much as yesterday. Breathing easier. Breath and perspiration foul.

By the third day, the redness of the face was entirely gone. She became able to sit up, and in a few days was about her household avocations. My attendance ceased on the 15th. Imprudence in diet and exertion brought on another attack, more severe than the preceding, about January 1st. There was no redness of the face, and the pain was more definitely confined to the bowels.

As the symptoms were severe, and attended with vomiting, &c., I thought it best to give ipecac., which I had avoided in the first attack, in consequence of her previous impaired health. Croton oil was applied to the bowels; elixir of opium for the relief of the pain. She recovered slowly from this attack, but again relapsed from a similar cause, and finally, by her husband's desire, returned to a homœopathist whom she had formerly employed. By the most rigid enforcement of rest, and seclusion from visiters and excitement, she eventually recovered, and by spring was able to walk out.

CASE III.—The sister of the above, Mrs. ———, who had also watched with the fever patient above alluded to, and who had been in attendance upon her, now became ill. She employed the same homœopathist as her sister. On the second or third day of her attack, I was informed that she was covered with an eruption or rash, which resembled poisoning by ivy or dogwood. I believe that no name was given to the disease. She had a lingering illness and a tedious recovery.

CASE IV.—Jan. 9th, I was called to visit a child, about three quarters of a mile from the location of the last two cases. It had been suddenly seized, in the night, with what the parents regarded as symptoms of scarlet fever; violent tossing in bed; intense redness of the skin; some vomiting.

I found the whole surface covered with deep red; no sore throat; pulse languid. The child lively, and apparently not very sick. The absence of sore throat, the slowness of the pulse, and the darkish hue of the rash, led me to pronounce decidedly that it was not scarlet fever. I prescribed an emetic of ipecac, to be followed with Dover's powders. The next morning the rash was gone, and the child was well! In this case, as well as in the others which precede and follow, a roughness of the skin was left, such as succeeds ordinary attacks of erysipelas.

All these cases were sporadic, some occurring in Newton, and some in West Needham, at distances of fiom half a mile to three miles apart. Some cases now appeared in one family in Weston, distant from any of the others, and directly traceable to contagion.

In January or February, the principal of a neighboring female seminary, alter suffering for some time from influenza, had an attack of a disease which presented, as I am informed, some very obscure symptoms, but was at first considered as typhoid, and subsequently as typhus fever. He died after a fortnight's illness, and several of the young ladies in the house were attacked with severe symptoms considered as influenza.

Case V.—Miss ——— was very severely attacked at night, with symptoms of fever, violent pain in the head and back, nausea, &c. She was treated homœopathically, and in a day or two was able to come home. I found her languid, depressed, and very much in the state which some forty years ago was called slow fever; ten years subsequently, dyspepsia; and of late years, typhoid fever.

She was able to walk about house, and to ride and walk out. The only tangible symptoms were foul breath and foul perspiration, languor and depression. My principal prescription was elixir vitriol and gentle exercise in the open air. Two of her brothers were shortly after attacked in the same way. Violent headache, nausea, foul breath and foul perspiration, were the principal symptoms. They recovered without medical treatment.

Cases VI. and VII.—The mother was next attacked in a similar manner. She recovered and resumed her daily occupations, but after a week of great anxiety and exertion, about family concerns, a much more violent attack came on, and I was sent for.

Feb. 23d.—I found her sitting up in bed, moving her body backward and forward; face slightly swollen, very red, and headache intense. I prescribed an emetic, elixir vitriol as a drink, and an opiate at night.

On the succeeding night I was called to her, as she had had repeated attacks of vomiting and pain in the bowels. She and her family were greatly alarmed. After the application of a mustard poultice, and one or two doses of elixir of opium, the vomiting ceased, and she became more comfortable.

24th.—Much as yesterday; sitting up in bed; headache continues, but nausea and pain in the bowels have not returned. Is much depressed. Breath and perspiration very offensive. The face is less swollen. I prescribed the continuance of opiates for the relief of pain in the head and elsewhere, elixir vitriol in water as a drink, a laxative when required. Diet farinaceous.

This morning I was requested to prescribe for the remaining son, who was suddenly seized with all the same symptoms. I prescribed an emetic of ipecac. The next day I found him entirely relieved. He kept house for a day or two, as a matter of precaution, but had no further trouble.

Mrs. ——— after this gradually improved; her headache and the redness of the face subsided. During her convalescence, she took fifteen drops of elixir of vitriol three times a-day, and appeared to be greatly benefited by it. In the early part of her illness, it gave more immediate relief—not to the pain, but to the other unpleasant symptoms —than anything else. She subsequently expressed her conviction that she had been very dangerously ill, and stated that she had felt an entire disgust to life. She was so much convinced of the unusual character of the sickness, that she came to the conclusion that the disease which had been brought to her house from the seminary, and which had caused the death of the principal, was ship fever.

Some months after this, in November of the same year, she was attacked with a disorder of a similar character, commencing with chills and all other symptoms precisely similar. A description of this attack will be given hereafter.

I may state that in all these cases there was a want of tangible symptoms. I could find nothing to explain satisfactorily the suffering of the patient, nor his own conviction of the severity of his case.

Two cases now occurred, about a mile distant from the locality of those last mentioned, of more serious character. I doubt whether I should class them with the above. The symptoms in the onset of each, however, precisely resembled those of Case IV.

CASES VIII. and IX.—Feb. 14th. I was called to see a boy about 2 years old, supposed to have symptoms of scarlet fever. He was taken suddenly in the night with chills and vomiting. I found him covered with an erythematous flush, of rather a dark scarlet ; tongue much coated, pulse slow. *No sore throat ;* on the whole, resembling precisely, as I have said, Case No. IV. I should premise that his grandfather had an attack, Dec. 18th ; his grandmother, Dec. 24th ; and his mother, January 12th ; similar to those above described, and confining them to their beds three or four days each. A transient erythematous flush, foul breath and foul perspiration, slow pulse, headache, depression without muscular debility, were the main characteristics in each. The mother was most severely affected. She had great redness of the surface, and severe pain in the bowels, to which she had been previously subject.

In addition to his other symptoms, the boy had a stiffness of the muscles of the neck. I prescribed for him an emetic, to be followed by Dover's powders.

Feb. 15th.—More comfortable. Swallows readily, but complains of soreness upon the left side of the neck. Some swelling there. I applied solution of sal. ammoniac, in vinegar, to the neck.

16th.—Tumor has increased ; breathes badly ; very restless, with some delirium in the night. I prescribed bread and milk poultices to the neck ; Dover's powders every four hours ; and a mixture of muriatic acid with confection of roses every four hours alternately. He seemed relieved by this treatment ; the tumor pointed, and soon began to discharge, when he became at once quite easy. He continued slowly to improve, and soon became able to sit up a little, and to take broth, beef-tea, and finally a little meat. The Dover's powders were gradually omitted, but the acid continued.

In the mean time his sister, about 4 years old—a very interesting child—was attacked in a similar manner. Great redness of the whole surface of the body, foul breath and perspiration, seemed the principal symptoms, when I saw her. I found her lying upon the sofa, free from pain, and apparently but little sick. In these two cases, as in the others mentioned, the muscular strength was good and the voice natural. The first onset had been severe, but she was relieved at the time of my visit.

She continued for about three days nearly the same. On the third day she was removed into the chamber with her brother—a room about 8 feet by 10, but ventilated by an open fire-place. This evening she began to breathe badly, but still had no difficulty in swallowing.

24th.—About 3, P.M., severe croupy breathing came on, attended with great distress. I found her sitting upon her mother's knee, quite rational. She submitted very readily to an application of the solution of nitrate of silver to her throat. This was repeated two or three times, and all the usual remedies were resorted to; but to no purpose. She died about 9 o'clock the next morning.

The boy was now doing so well, that I intermitted my visits for a day or two. It had been judged expedient to remove him from the chamber, when his sister became more ill. He was carried to the lower part of the house, and not confined to one room.

On visiting him again, I found him sitting up and dressed, but more feeble than before. His nurse, with the idea of getting him on faster, had indulged his appetite too freely. The excitement and exposure of the funeral, the opening of doors, and the seeing many people, had undoubtedly an unfavorable effect. He was now in a low typhoid state. I prescribed nitrous ether, quinine, and subsequently wine; beef-tea or broth to be given at regular intervals. He was precisely in the state that occurs after scarlet fever or dysentery, where the disease has been removed, and the child literally starves to death, not from want of nourishment, but because the organs of nutrition can no longer do their duty. He died on the fourth of March.

At the time these children were attacked, there was no case of scarlet fever in the neighborhood, nor had they been exposed to it in any way that could be traced.

CASE X.—A child in a neighboring house was attacked with similar symptoms; chills, erythema, &c. I prescribed an emetic, and the next day the redness, or rash, was gone, and the child was well!

CASES XI. and XII.—In the next house, however, closely adjoining the one in which the fatal cases had occurred, three children were seized with similar symptoms. One had them very slightly; the next, a little worse; the third, an infant, severely. It had little sore throat, but a stiffness of the neck and external swelling. For the relief of this swelling, and thinking it important to promote speedy action, I prescribed a bread and milk poultice. The parents demurred. The grandmother advised the substitution of a rind of pork. The parents proposed a consultation, either with a homœopathist, or with a very respectable practitioner, not a member of the Massachusetts Medical Society. I declined, on the ground that one medical man was sufficient for the case. Dr. T——— was sent for, and very judiciously compromised matters by prescribing hog's lard for the neck; and the good old remedy of black-currant jelly, to be taken inside. The tumor, like that of surgical celebrity, touched by the dead man's hand, was instantly relieved, and, in thirty-six hours, had disappeared. The patient was long ill, but eventually recovered.

The gentleman who treated the last-mentioned case, as also a young medical amateur, who, I believe, saw the preceding fatal cases several times, expressed no doubt that the disease was scarlet fever. Whether scarlet fever or not, no other cases occurred in the neighborhood. My reason for classing it with the disorder described in the other cases, is that the eruption differed from that of scarlet fever; there was no evidence of sore throat; the swellings on the neck were entirely external; in short, the whole symptoms were those of the prevailing epidemic. I believe, too, that croup rarely succeeds scarlet fever; but croupy breathing may be the result of erysipelas.

The next case it may also be considered improper to class with the foregoing. Whether of the same genus or not, however, or whether it may be considered one of softening of the brain induced by typhoid fever several years previous, there can be little doubt that it was modified and accelerated by epidemic influence, and partook in a great degree the character of the others. The former cases I saw within a few hours after the attack, and before any medical treatment was resorted to. This one I saw much later, and cannot tell whether there was any definite onset of the symptoms, or whether the chills and erythema which attended the other attacks took place in this.

CASE.—April 10th, I was requested to visit a young lady who, I was told, was rapidly "running down." I was informed that she had an attack of typhoid fever four years since, which had nearly proved fatal. She had a very slow recovery, and had never regained her health. For some time past she had evinced an entire lassitude, and want of interest in everything, with an utter dislike to exertion of every kind. No appetite. One period she had just passed without menstruation.

She walked into the parlor where I was waiting for her; though evidently with great exertion, and unfit to be off her bed. She was of sallow complexion, and presented the symptoms noticed in Case V. There was some cough; but I found, on examination, no physical signs of pulmonary disease. The cough was slight and dry; of a nervous or irritative character. The general appearances were those of slow typhoid fever. Understanding, at first, that the cough was the principal subject of alarm, I prescribed an expectorant, and the muriate of iron as a tonic.

Upon my next visit, I found that she had an aversion to all common food, and had frequent attacks of vomiting. She had foul breath and offensive perspiration. The cough was not troublesome. She had, at times, pain in the back part of the head; and sometimes in the back. Excessively nervous and sensitive. Some fulness of the bowels.

Finding that the iron and the expectorant could not be borne, and that all food produced vomiting, I gave her an emetic of ipecac., and afterwards elixir vitriol in water. This she took for some time without difficulty. When I found her in bed, she lay upon her back, perfectly still and motionless, the knees often drawn up; never speaking voluntarily, and answering a question only after a long interval and with great apparent effort of mind; as if the organs were too sluggish to convey and to answer the efforts of the will. There was fulness of the bowels, as I have stated, but no particular *pain on pressure*, even when she complained of pain there. She rejects all common food. Either medicine or food produces vomiting. She had, also, for some successive evenings, what were described as violent " nervous " attacks ; that is to say, paroxysms of shaking violently the whole body. Sometimes I found her with her feet drawn up in bed, and a restless motion of the lower limbs.

For the soreness of the bowels, I prescribed the external application of croton oil ; a favorite prescription of my friend, Dr. Hosmer.

She manifested no improvement. Her appetite was capricious ; her mind dwelling upon what she should eat, rejecting all wholesome articles of food, but eager for whatever was denied her. Dandelions were earnestly craved for ; and when allowed, eaten for a few days with relish, but soon became disgusting. Her principal desire was, and had been for some time before I saw her, a mixture of butter and vinegar.

I was encouraged, for some time, to think that the disease might be mimetic, or sympathetic. The absence of the menses, the capricious appetite, and many other symptoms, favored the idea. A physician in full practice in Boston, to whom I stated the case, gave this opinion.

Having tried creosote to check the vomiting ; quinine, and every other remedy, calculated either to relieve the nausea or to give tone to the system, I tried Port wine and Madeira, both of which were rejected. I next resorted to brandy, which was retained (perhaps because the vomiting stage was past). Under its use she became able to bear a little nourishment. Costiveness existed through the whole course of the disease. To obviate it, I employed injections of oatmeal gruel. I presume that this answered in some degree the place of nourishment by the mouth. This method of nourishing the system, where food cannot be taken by the mouth, is well known. Brandy was taken for about a week, and apparently with good effect. She had no vomiting, bore nourishment better, but did not improve in strength.

May 18th, thirty-eight days from the time of my first visit, she evinced such signs of cerebral disease, that I requested Dr. Hosmer, of Watertown, might be sent for in consultation. He arrived in the afternoon, and made rather a rail-road visit, but agreed that the principal disease was now in the brain. He advised croton oil to the back of the neck, and continued doses of calomel or blue pill.

She was somewhat roused from her dormant state by the consultation, and anxious to know the result. She had received the idea that by proposing a consultation, I wished to abandon her case as hopeless. She seemed encouraged by the communication, that though in great danger, we did not yet consider her situation desperate. The next day she seemed a little brighter. For a week longer she continued nearly in the same state. There was torpor or hebitude of the brain ; but no aberration of intellect. The mental and the moral powers were retained, but they were torpid, as if under the effect of a narcotic. After this, she became more dull ; though neither delirium nor stupor could be said to take place. She slowly sunk, and died May 28th, ten days after my consultation with Dr. Hosmer.

It has been so little the custom, in this neighborhood, to make postmortem examinations, that in the case of a young lady like this, it was out of the question. I had no doubt in my own mind that there was softening of the brain. Disease had undoubtedly been progressing there for a long period of time. The prevailing miasm had accelerated its course.

The resemblance of this case to one of more undoubted character, occurring the present season, has been one additional reason for my describing it here. I may also state that in a post-mortem examination I made upon the body of a boy about five years since, in Boston, during the prevalence of the dysentery as an epidemic, I found the brain of the consistency of curdled milk. The attending physician mentioned to me no other symptoms, but those of disease of the bowels. Some symptoms of peculiar character had, however, occurred, within two years previous, and the mother desired me especially to examine the brain. On opening the skull, the contents, which were greatly distended, fairly splashed upon the floor, and were, as I have said, of the consistence of curdled milk. Here was a case where the patient had retained in a degree his mental faculties, and died, not of the cerebral disease, but of the reigning epidemic.

In a future number of the Journal I hope to describe the epidemic of the present season, similar to that of 1852, but in a more developed and serious form.

Were I driven to seek a name for this, I would choose that of " irritative fever," to designate a variety of a species which has nearly synonyms enough to fill a page in the Medical Journal.

Newton Lower Falls, March, 1853.

ADULTERATION OF DRUGS.

To the Editor of the Boston Medical and Surgical Journal.

SIR,—Among the various subjects brought to the consideration of the American Association, that of the adulteration of drugs is of the first importance. I believe the credit of first suggesting a national measure for the arrest of this evil, belongs to the New York College of Pharmacy. Nothing, however, was done effectually until the meeting of the American Medical Society at Baltimore, in 1848, when sundry resolutions were offered, resulting in a memorial to Congress, by which we are in possession of the existing law. Of the distinguished gentlemen prominent in bringing forward a measure so fraught with blessings to the community at large, were Dr. T. O. Edwards, of Ohio, then an eminent member of the House of Representatives, and at present a professor in one of the western colleges ; Dr. C. C. Cox, a prominent member from Maryland, formerly a professor in one of the Philadelphia colleges ; and Dr. Usher Parsons, of Rhode Island, a physician of admitted note and worth. The two last mentioned, in connection with the celebrated Dr. J. W. Francis, of New York, were made a committee to draft and report the memorial. At this lapse of time we recall, with much gratification, having had the honor of a seat in the convention, the general interest manifested in a subject, which, regarded in every point of view, was a most fitting topic for discussion in the early history of the National Society. The gentlemen previously mentioned were eloquent in vindication of the proposed action, making, in the course of their speeches, the most startling disclosures of frauds committed by the producer, foreign trader, and home manufacturer and vender.   The resolution of Dr. Cox, of Maryland, found on page 31 of the printed proceedings of 1848, while it furnishes evidence of the superior sagacity of that distinguished gentleman, points to the remedy demanded at this time in view of the frauds practised in our country.   The law affecting the imports does not reach, the adulterations practised at home.   Indeed, the closure of the channel of foreign fraud had the effect of opening new avenues of mischief in the domestic trade, and the medicines brought from abroad were subjected to every species of dilution and admixture in the wholesale drug establishments of the large cities.   Some action, looking to. the increase of this evil at home, is imperatively demanded of the Association at its approaching meeting in New York.   This subject has been already broached by one of the able committees of the Society two years ago, and we shall · do no more than suggest the mischief, leaving the *remedy* to the *doctors* of the nation.   C. R. E.

Philadelphia, March 21, 1853.

NITRATE OF SILVER IN DYSPEPSIA OR CHRONIC GASTRITIS.

To the Editor of the Boston Medical and Surgical Journal.

SIR,—During the last twenty years I have had many cases of inveterate dyspepsia or chronic gastritis.   A long course of dieting, with occasional *pro re nata* medicines, has afforded partial relief only, in many cases.   Some years ago, I used nitrate of silver and opium in cases attended by chronic diarrhœa, with success, and more recently I have used the same remedy when diarrhœa was only occasional and often absent.   From the trials I have made and the success I have obtained, I think the nitrate promises to be a very useful remedy.   My experience has not been large in the use of it as a remedy for dyspepsia ; but in a few cases, and so far as I have made trials, it has acted with the promptness and certainty of quinine in ague.   I begin with a pill containing a. quarter of a grain of nitrate of silver and a quarter of a grain of opium, administered three times a-day.   After using this quantity several days, I double the quantity of the nitrate, but not of the opium ; and when opium is contraindicated, I omit it altogether.   In some cases I gradually increase the nitrate to one grain (and even two grains in one instance) three times a-day.   The remedy certainly deserves further trial, and my design in this short communication is to call the attention of the profession to an important subject, and to request others to try the remedy and note the results.   W. A. GILLESPIE, M.D.

Louisa Co., Va., March 24, 1853.

SURGICAL CLINIC OF THE PHILADELPHIA COLLEGE OF MEDICINE.

[Communicated for the Boston Medical and Surgical Journal.]

WEDNESDAY, March 3.—This clinic, which is constantly growing in importance, presented, on the present occasion, many cases which were well calculated to evoke the skill of the officiating surgeon, Dr. Bryan, as well as to exemplify the triumph of the healing art in alleviating and removing the sufferings of humanity.

Among the cases presented to the class in attendance, were the following :—

1.—Miss M. A., Pine street, states that during the past two weeks she has suffered severe pain in left eye ; feels a great repugnance to light ; had tried various remedies, all of which were ineffectual, the pain still continuing to increase. On the evening of the 21st, this patient applying for aid at the Philadelphia Medical College, she was brought before Dr. Bryan, who, on examination, discovered several incipient ulcers of cornea. The vessels of the sclerotica surrounding the iris were turgid with blood, and the conjunctiva, through its entire extent, considerably inflamed. The diathesis of the patient and the character of the inflammation, led to the diagnosis that the case in question was one of scrofulous ophthalmia. She was directed to take, in divided doses, the following purgative. R. Sennæ, ℥ ss. ; mannæ, ℥ ij. ; magnesiæ sulphas., ℥ij., sem. anisi, Əj. ; aquæ, Oj. As a collyrium—R. Zinci sulphas., grs. iv. ; morphiæ sulph. gr. j. ; aquæ distillat., ℥ ij. Admov. ter in die. A blister was applied to the temple as a contra-irritant. This patient now states that she feels considerably relieved, and is directed to continue same treatment until next clinic day.

II.—Mr. J. B., Pine street, a young man of 17, had applied at surgical clinic, some months ago, for surgical aid. On examination a tumor was found to project from the posterior nares, which caused indistinct articulation and impeded the respiration, especially during sleep. As there was nothing indicating that the tumor was of a malignant character, its excision was undertaken and accomplished by Dr. Bryan. Some time after, the patient again applied for relief, and on examination a new fungoid growth presented itself, exceeding in magnitude that previously extirpated. It extended from the most elevated point of the septum narium to within a few lines of the epiglottis, and was a source of great distress to the patient. In attempting the excision of this new tenant, it was discovered to be highly vascular, as it bled freely during the preliminary efforts for its removal. This occurrence suggested the propriety of having recourse to a different mode of treatment, i. e., its removal by ligature. This operation was performed to-day with every prospect of ultimate success. The difficulty experienced in passing the smallest instrument, armed with a ligature, from the anterior to the posterior nares was well calculated to test the perseverance and skill of the surgeon, but art and knowledge are omnipotent and must be successful. The ordinary ear catheter was used with a double ligature, to the end of which a piece of cat-gut was attached for the purpose of getting the ligature into the mouth from the posterior nares. The loop was passed over the tumor, and the ends of the ligature fastened to the proximal extremity of the catheter, which was left in the nostril. No hæmorrhage followed, and the patient is now doing well.

III.—Mrs. J. S., 7th street. This lady had been suffering from whitlow during a period of two months. This is her first application for advice at this institution. Whether as the result of bad treatment, or inattention on the part of the patient, the ulcerative process had destroyed all the soft parts on the inner aspect of the two distal phalanges of index finger of left hand. An amputation of the defunct parts was suggested to the patient, but she feels unwilling to submit to the operation.

IV.—C. R. Russell Vagus, now sojourning in this city, states that about a year ago he fell from a considerable height, the apex of the shoulder and side of the head being the points of impact. This patient is a man of great muscular development, and required the most erudite tact of the finger to ascertain the condition of clavicle and shoulder-joint. Having applied on yesterday, and being carefully examined at that time, the leading symptoms were discovered to be, inability to elevate the arm, pain at the insertion of the deltoid muscle, and at articulation of clavicle and humerus. The absence of that deformity which attends luxation of the joint, as well as fracture of clavicle and humerus, corroborated by the touch, led to the inference that the injury amounted simply to a severe contusion of the parts. Cups were applied to the vicinity of the articulation, and four ounces of blood abstracted. To-day the mobility of the arm is considerably improved. Some febrile excitement still continuing, the patient was directed to take of magn. sulph. ℥ ss., to be repeated cras mane, and to apply a blister to the parts.

Having disposed of the other cases in attendance, Dr. Bryan next drew the attention of the class to a new instrument of his own invention, to be used for the purpose of trephining. The many instruments already devised for this purpose, are all liable to one of two objections. Either they are difficult of application, or they are dangerous to the patient. These difficulties appear to be well obviated by the instrument in question. A subject being in readiness, Dr. Bryan proceeded at once to test the value of his invention. A flap being raised from the anterior inferior angle of one of the parietal bones, the instrument was applied, and in two minutes the required circle of bone was removed, without wounding a single fibre of the dura mater. The middle meningeal artery was seen ramifying in the exposed membrane, but the arterial coats continued intact. Thus at length have we obtained an instrument* by which this operation can be executed *cito, tuto et jucunde.*

Philad. Coll. Med., March 24, 1853.　　　JOHN F. J. SULLIVAN.

QUININE IN RHEUMATISM.

To the Editor of the Boston Medical and Surgical Journal.

SIR,—While we are not disposed to deprive any man of his well-earned laurels, we are not sure it is the better policy to stand by and permit an-

---

* A cut and description of this instrument may be seen in the first of April No. of the Philadelphia Medical and Surgical Journal.

other to ride into power upon the suggestions of his brother, without giving him credit for it. We are led to these remarks from noticing in your weekly edition of the 16th inst., an extract from a letter in the Charleston Medical Review, conferring upon M. Briquet the honor, we infer, of curing rheumatism combined with cardiac disease, by full doses of quinine. If it was the design of the writer to create the impression that M. Briquet was the author, or that the treatment was even *novel*, we beg him to be undeceived. If the writer will look into Dr. Reese's Gazette for 1850 or 51 (we speak from memory), he will find a case recorded of the successful management of rheumatism by full doses of quinine, with its suggestion in cardiac disease incident to rheumatism. We laid no claim to the discovery of the remedy ; we were the first, we believe, to report it in this country, and we are the last man to permit another to steal " *our thunder,*" or bear off our laurels, before our eyes, however unimportant they may be. The first patient we cured and reported for Dr. Reese is alive yet, and living not many miles from us, and can easily be found to testify to the cure. We recollect, not many years ago, Velpeau received great praise for suggesting *copperas water* in erysipelas, when actually every old woman in the South had used it years before he ever thought of it. We say this in no disparagement to the great Parisian, whose genius we admire, and whose ability it would be the height of folly for any man to deny. But it is a fact which cannot be too strongly and forcibly reprobated, that European physicians often secure renown for things which do not justly belong to them, and we are not sure our own countrymen are not to blame for it to some extent. We do not pretend to say that we are the discoverer of the quinine treatment in rheumatism ; but we do say we have a better claim to it than M. Briquet, and we appeal to the Medical Journal referred to, to our medical brethren here, and we can maintain it by a most reputable surgeon of the United States Army from the State of South Carolina.

We hope the writer in the Charleston Review will take the matter in no unkind sense, for we act upon the square and adopt the motto—" *Let justice be done if the firmament fall.*" We do not know that it is the design of the writer to convey the impression that the remedy and the practice are novel and original with Briquet, of Paris ; but if it is, we have shown that he is laboring under an egregious error; and we can further say to him, that so far as progress in medicine is concerned— the Young Physic of the age, on this side the Savannah —it is not to be advanced " *by mousing owls to be hawked at and killed,*" particularly by transatlantic birds.   Respectfully,   H. A. Ramsay.

Thompson, Colum. Co., Geo., March 22, 1853.

BITE OF THE RATTLESNAKE.

BY THOMAS A. ATCHISON.

I was summoned in haste on the evening of the 20th of September, 1852, to see Miss R———, a young lady aged 17, living five miles in the country, who (I was informed by the messenger), while taking a stroll in company with her mother, was bitten by a rattlesnake. I arrived at half past 7 o'clock, two hours and a half after the accident. I found my patient almost moribund, pulse wavy and scarcely perceptible at the wrist, surface cold and bathed in perspiration, face swollen, with a besotted expression, mind wandering, pupils dilated, could not see, declaring it was very dark although candles were burning in the room, asked frequently if it was not raining hard, although the night was calm and clear. Upon examination, I found that the bite had been inflicted upon the instep of the left foot ; two little punctures were very perceptible, around which there was a greenish areola, with some puffiness.

Having heard of the marvellous efficacy of " spirits " in the relief of similar cases, I at once determined to give the remedy a full and fair trial. Reason and analogy sustained it. The nervous system was overwhelmed by a swift and deadly sedative poison, it must be supported by an equally powerful *diffusible* stimulant ; accordingly I gave half a glass of whiskey, which was swallowed with avidity. Meanwhile the wound was freely scarified and cupped, and the extremities placed in a hot saline bath ; twenty grains of carb. ammonia was then given, which was immediately thrown up, together with the contents of the stomach, colored a bright grass green. A common-sized glassful of whiskey was now given, the patient draining with eagerness the last drop, and begging with the energy of instinct for more ; thus a glass of whiskey and twenty grains of carb. ammonia were given alternately every half hour, until three pints of the former and eighty grains of the latter were taken ; and what is remarkable, not the slightest intoxication ensued ; on the contrary the urgent and alarming symptoms gradually gave way, warmth was restored to the surface, the pulse returned to the wrist, the mind was called back from its wanderings, and she fell into a quiet sleep, from which she awoke at 5 o'clock, A.M., complaining of intense pain in the foot shooting up the inside of the leg to the knee. Ordered morphia, one fourth grain ; fomentations of laudanum and camphor, followed by poultice of linum lini, with the effect of entire relief of pain. The following day castor oil was given to move the bowels ; from that hour she suffered no further inconvenience from the bite.

The instinctive avidity and impunity with which this delicately-nurtured young lady took so large a quantity of spirits, sufficient under ordinary circumstances to have killed a regular *habitué*, would excite astonishment, if we did not reflect that it was antagonized by the depressing effect of the poison on the nervous system.

But the most interesting feature in this case remains to be stated : Miss R———, at the time she was bitten, was the subject of well-marked hooping cough, which was then epidemic in the neighborhood ; she had had the disease about three weeks, consequently it was at its acme, but on recovering from the effects of the poison, to her great surprise and gratification her cough had disappeared also, nor did it return ; being essentially a spasmodic disease, it was swept away by the powerful impression made upon the nervous system.—*Southern Journal of the Medical and Physical Sciences.*

THE BOSTON MEDICAL AND SURGICAL JOURNAL.

BOSTON, APRIL 6, 1853.

Trials and Rewards of the Medical Profession.—That veteran of sur-gery, Dr. Mussey, who has been prominent in the professorial chair, and eminent as a practitioner, now in the full strength of advancing age, while his honors are thick upon him, has embarked in a new enterprise. The Miami Medical College, located at Cincinnati, is altogether a new creation, and Dr. M. is the main pillar in sustaining the structure, as we understand the matter in this direction. At the opening of the first lecture session, in October last, as professor of surgery, Dr. Mussey delivered a discourse on the trials and rewards of the medical profession. No person can be more familiar with these matters than himself. Pithy illustrations of the phases of a physician's every-day intercourse, give a zest to the lecture. The whims of the sick ; the ignorance of those assuming to be wise ; the stu-pidity of some, the flattery of many practitioners, and their mean subservi-ency to their inferiors for the sake of business, as pictured by him, are true to nature. The spirit and tendency of this essay are good. It recog-nizes the workings of a Divine Providence, not precisely in words, but in principle ; and there is a truthfulness in his propositions, that the under-standing acknowledges at sight. Dr. Mussey has a reputation that com-mands the respect of the best class of minds, and we hope that the frosts of age may approach him gently, and his last days be as happy as the morning and meridian of his professional career were peaceful and pros-perous.

The Mother and her Offspring.—An occasional notice of the preparation of this treatise, by Stephen Tracy. M.D., formerly of the missionary service in China, has appeared in the Journal. Within a few weeks, it came from the press of the Harpers, in New York, in a neat and acceptable form. Several publishers in Boston had the refusal of the manuscript, but declined putting it in type, imagining, no doubt, that it would not be a very saleable production. If so, then it is the third work that has been recently rejected by them, either one of which, in a money-making point of view, would have been profitable. Dr. Tracy's book, it is confidently predicted, will have an immense run. While the plan is truly professional, it is calcu-lated for popular circulation. There are twenty-three chapters, embracing the following leading topics, viz. :—indications of pregnancy ; preserva-tion of health during the period ; preparations for confinement; re-produc-tion in vegetables ; re-production in the lower animals ; re-production in human beings ; confinement ; regimen of the nursing mother ; washing and bathing infants ; dressing of infants ; clothing of infants ; nourishment of them ; wet nurses ; weaning ; diet after weaning ; sleep of infants ; exercise ; mental influences ; government and habits ; intellectual culture : diseases of pregnancy ; diseases occurring after confinement, and diseases of children. There are hundreds of subjects discussed in connection with these leading heads, comprising every condition of mother and child, through all periods of gestation, and from birth through the various stages of moral and physical training. Dr. Tracy is a charming writer. He understands what is wanted, and has the ability to meet the demand. To write on these topics, and avoid technicalities on the one hand, and any shadow of grossness or vulgarity on the other, was a difficult undertaking. As it is, no fault can be found with the book, or the pure English in which it is dressed; and a high moral tone pervades its 361 pages. Although fitted to another meridian, medical students might glean knowledge from it, that would enable them to direct and to do many things appropriately, in the commencement of practice, which often devolve upon them. These semi-professional lucubrations do not interfere with the regular province of the physician; on the contrary, if they fall under the eye of sensible, reflecting persons, the effect is to increase their confidence in the resources of legitimate medicine, and in well-educated practitioners. The diffusion of elementary physiology among the masses, is absolute death to quackery.

Opium Trade.—A new edition of a sketch of the history, extent and effects of the opium trade in India and China, by Nathan Allen, M.D., of Lowell, Mass., is now before the public. Our views have not been changed in regard to the character of this able production, since we had occasion to speak of it some months ago. Dr. Allen has concentrated an immense amount of information from reliable sources, which lays open the great moral evils of the commerce in opium. It is absolutely horrible that a Christian nation like England, can persist in such wrong doing, with a full knowledge of the misery, poverty, degradation and destruction of life that invariably follow. A synopsis of the woes that cling to opium-smokers in China, would be too formidable for re-publication in any periodical, and those who would know the extent of suffering that belongs to an habitual use of the terrible drug, as exhibited on a grand scale in those countries, are confidently referred to Dr. Allen's publication, as the source of more correct information that can be found in so small a compass, in any author in the English language. Copies may be procured at Messrs. Mussey's, Ticknor's, and Fettridge's, in Boston.

Mysterious Agents.—Dr. Rogers, the learned and persevering author of a series of numbers on the philosophy of mysterious agents, has brought out No. III. which surpasses the two first in point of interest. No man has written more profoundly on the dynamic laws and their relations to man. Some of his facts, illustrative of propositions, almost bring ghosts into the room. Dr. Drury's account of the haunted house, and what he both saw and heard, in the hamlet of Willington, seem to have afforded Dr. Rogers a strong case. Ingenious as he is, we are not wholly convinced that his views are correct. As the work progresses, it becomes fascinating to a philosophical mind. The author proposes soon to bring out a volume on witchcraft, and to possess himself of all the facts touching its existence in New England. He has been diving into the archives of the State House, and has examined the original Court papers produced on the trial of the witches at Salem. A rare and curious production may therefore be anticipated.

Cosmography.—Little as medical men may have to do, in their daily business, with a history of the earth, it is far from being beneath their notice to watch the progress of general science, and especially that noble one, astronomy. Still, we should not have gone far out of the legitimate course of our hebdomadal, to speak of a subject so vast, were it not that one of the brotherhood, a modest, retired practitioner, has suddenly surprised and delighted his acquaintances with a course of philosophical reflections on the formation of the solar system, accompanied by the promulgation of a new theory, that invests his deliberations with peculiar interest. Whenever a physician distinguishes himself in any department of knowledge, out of the common course of his orbit, he exalts the profession to which he belongs; and we have reason to be proud of the bright array of great names in the calendar of fame, that sprang from our ranks. Charles F. Winslow, M.D., of Waltham, Mass., formerly of Nantucket, and for many years a resident of the Sandwich Islands, has written a small volume, under the unobtrusive title of "Cosmography; or Philosophical Views of the Universe," that is calculated to give activity to the thoughts of one class of philosophers, the astronomers, if no others. He labors to develope and establish the theory, that repulsion is a planetary force. In the second part, the reader is presented with an analytical examination of the solar system, and the application of the theory of *repulsion* to the creation of the universe. Part third is intensely captivating, and embraces the consideration of the inequalities of the surface of the solid spheres, and the successive revolutions observed throughout the crust of the globe, as results of the alternating intensity of cosmical forces. Not daring to obtrude largely, upon purely medical readers, topics which are in no way connected with the special objects of this Journal, we shall merely announce to those of them who cultivate a taste for general science, that Dr. Winslow has secured to himself an elevated position by this publication. He demonstrates the possession of a mind capable of grasping great thoughts, and of conducting inquiries of the loftiest import.

Atlas of Pathological Histology.—If the proposed international copyright becomes a law, re-published foreign works on medicine and surgery will be vastly enhanced in price. There is not a book worth having, of European origin, that cannot be purchased in the United States, when it comes out in an American dress, very much below the prices asked abroad. Joseph Leidy, M.D., of Philadelphia, is the translator of Dr. Gottlieb Gluge's "Atlas of Pathological Histology," which appears in a beautiful form, with double columns in folio, illustrated by copperplate engravings. Messrs. Blanchard & Lea are the publishers, and of course the typography is unexceptionable. The translator says of Pathological Histology—" its importance to pathological anatomy is of the same character as normal histology is to normal anatomy; and this cannot be better represented than by referring to the great and permanent advance which physiology has made in its relation to the physical structure of the organs of the living body. Pathological anatomy also is, beyond doubt, of the highest value in medicine, for a scientific treatment of disease must necessarily depend, to a very considerable extent, upon our knowledge of material changes which are so frequently the source of those symptoms which indicate its existence." Whoever sees this finished publication, will covet it. Copies are to be had at Ticknor's, Boston.

Penn Medical College.—What kind of an institution is it? One of its professors (Emeritus), resides in London; and another in New York.

The circular announcing a Spring session in Philadelphia, was printed at Providence, R. I.! There is one grand feature in the prospectus, that might be profitably imitated by the venerables who have never acted energetically beyo'nd securing their fees. It runs thus—viz., " The sessions of the Penn College will be full of interest to their close—for the several professors will not weary the students with speculative nothings, long drawn out, merely to occupy the hours daily assigned in the continuance of a longer term." The Penn College has learned one bad trick, copied from those who are older in the field,—the sale of matriculation tickets. In claiming attention and patronage on the score of peculiar moral qualifications, it would be a capital idea to renounce the unrighteous demand of five dollars under the name of *matriculation*. It is an indirect way of sponging the students. If legally tested, we apprehend that monies, thus collected, would necessarily have to be returned. The students pay for instruction, and not for keeping buildings in repair. They are not obliged to maintain fires, pay janitors or black the boots of the faculty.

Providence (R. I.) Bill of Mortality.—An orderly arranged annual abstract of the deaths occurring in the neighboring city of Providence, for the year 1852, has been published. It gives a grand total of 914, of which 199 were by consumption. Dysentery was the disease which swept off the next highest number—75; hydrocephalus 33, and typhoid fever 29. No epidemic appears to have been recognized in the time, and the mortality may be considered as no way extraordinary.

Naval Board of Medical Examiners.—Having carefully examined thirty-four applicants, they finally selected nine, who were the best qualified, and who will be commissioned assistant surgeons, as follows,—viz.: James H. Stuart, of Pennsylvania; J. Pembroke Thom, of Virginia; John M. Browne, of New Hampshire; John. F. Taylor, of Delaware; Henry Clay Caldwell, of Virginia; Thos. J. Turner, of Pennsylvania; Wm. T. Hord, of Kentucky; Wentworth R. Richardson, of Massachusetts; A. Clarkson Smith, of Pennsylvania. Six others. already in commission, were found worthy of promotion—Wm. Lowber; P. J. Horwitz; B. Rush Mitchell; D. B. Phillips; James Hamilton; J. L. Burtt.

Lunatic Asylum in the District of Columbia. — A site for a hospital for the insane of the District of Columbia and of the army and navy, has been purchased for $25,000. It is situated about two miles south of the Capitol, and contains about 190 acres, nearly one half in a high state of cultivation. Congress appropriated $100,000 for the site and buildings, and the latter will be erected when the plans have been properly examined and approved. Dr. Charles H. Nichols has been appointed superintendent.

New York State Lunatic Asylum.—This is a mammoth institution in its external appearance. In passing by, the traveller would be led to suppose the establishment was a fortress. Imperfection seems to be apparent even in this model lunatic asylum, as the managers state that ventilation was unprovided for in its orginal construction. It is remarkable that there should have been such a large amount of money expended to make this asylum the very best in the Union, and at this late period the announce-ment be made that " *ventilation was unprovided for in the original construc-tion of the buildings.*" Sixty thousand dollars are now asked of the Le-gislature for warming and ventilation. For one year, ending December 1, 1852, the receipts from all sources were \$80,001 35 ; and the outgoes the same. Whole number of patients during that time, 825 ; and the number of applicants greater than in any previous year. Sixty were refused , and in all, 75 citizens of the State had the doors closed upon them for want of accommodations. The medical superintendent suggests the erection of another hospital for two hundred patients, of the male sex only. He ap-proves of having the sexes in distinct houses, accompanying the recom-mendation with proper and sufficient reasons. The medical report says that 156 recovered in 1852 ; 11 were much improved ; 42 improved ; 152 unimproved, and 39 died. Among the causes leading to the insanity of the inmates, 46 were made so by intemperance ; 29 by spiritual rappings and popular errors ; 23 by domestic trouble ; and 40 by masturbation. Most of the physician's report is made up of details of items that are needed to better the asylum, together with remarks on the domestic man-agement of the internal affairs of the institution.

Revalenta Arabica.—Considerable attention seems to have been given in England, to a new farinaceous compound, especially designed for the food of invalids and children, under the name of *revalenta arabica,* an agency for which has been recently established by Dr. Litchfield, at 215 Washington st., Boston. Without being at all influenced by the thousand and one certificates accompanying each package, testifying to the sovereign cures effected by it, it is sufficient to state the simple fact that the ara-bica food meets the approbation of those who have the care of the sick. Being easily digested, and highly nutritious, the demand is said to be large in Great Britain and on the continent. Dr. Litchfield would not, we think, have identified himself with a worthless preparation ; and Dr. Ure has certified that it is a pure vegetable farina, perfectly wholesome, easily digestible, and likely to promote healthy action of the stomach and bowels, and thereby to counteract dyspepsia.

Use of Quinine in the Treatment of Rheumatism.—Dr. Ramsay has shown, on another page of the Journal of to-day, that he is entitled to the credit of having used quinine in rheumatism previous to the occurrence of the cases of M. Briquet, alluded to in the Journal of the 16th ult. Those cases, however, were not the first which M. Briquet has thus treated ; as we perceive in the London Lancet of Jan. 14, 1843, a particular ac-count of this mode of treatment both by Briquet and M. Devergie of the same Hospital (St. Louis). The latter objects to the employment of larger doses than from 15 to 30 grs. per diem of the sulphate. We mention this cir-cumstance in accordance with the principle of the motto which Dr. Ramsay quotes—" *Fiat justitia ruit cœlo.*"

Monumental Stone.—A committee was raised at the last meeting of the American Medical Association, for the purpose of procuring a suitable stone, with an appropriate inscription, for insertion, in the name of the associa-tion, in the national monument to the memory of Washington, now in progress in the City of Washington. Dr. Atlee, the Chairman, has issued a circular, soliciting a subscription of one dollar from each member, to be transmitted by mail, to Jno. L. Atlee, M.D., Lancaster, Penn.

State Lunatic Asylum for Western New York. — Governor Seymour, in his message to the Legislature, recommends the erection of another Lunatic Asylum in this State, to be located in its Western portion. A bill has been brought forward in the Senate in accordance with this recommendation. The necessity for increased accommodations is very urgent and ought not be delayed. — *American Journal of Insanity.*

Medical Miscellany. — The Quarterly Review, in answer to the question — "What is man ?" says — " Chemically speaking, a man is forty-five pounds of carbon and nitrogen, diffused through five and a half pails full of water." — During the famine year of 1846 in Ireland, there were more marriages than ever before were registered in that country. — Orfila has given 8,000 francs to the Academy of Medicine for a biennial prize fund. — In the Pennsylvania Med. College, 56 recently graduated with M.D. ; at the Kentucky Med. School, 39 ; Missouri University, 26 ; St. Louis, 33 ; and at the Maryland University, 59. — A woman in the Cincinnati Hospital presents the following appearance — Her legs are enormously enlarged, being over two feet in circumference at the ancles, and her body is swollen to the shoulders in even larger proportion, being not less than ten feet girth. Her disease commenced about three years since, and has now assumed a chronic form. — In the State of Georgia there is one Medical College, with six teachers and 150 students, who pay into its treasury some $10,500. — Dr. Jedediah Miller, the lately appointed Health Commissioner of New York, has a salary of $3,500. — They are determined to have a marine hospital at Burlington, Iowa. — A new medical theorist divides all diseases into two classes, — viz., those of which the patients die, and the other from which they recover. — A revolutionary soldier 104 years old, is on a visit at Cincinnati, from Richmond, Virginia. — A charter has been granted by the Legislature of Pennsylvania, for another medical college, called Chrono-Thermal, probably to be located in Philadelphia. The people of that State understand the art of concentrating medical power and influence, by accommodating all parties and shades of applicants. — At the Philadelphia Medical College, 27 recently took the degree of M.D. At the Homœopathic, 55 ; at the Pennsylvania, 55 ; and at the Jefferson, 223. — Public health is restored at Hayti — the yellow fever having entirely disappeared.

MARRIED,—D. E. Stillman, M.D., of Dover, N. Y., to Miss E. Wadsworth.—In Boston, E. Brown Sequard, M D., of Paris, to Miss E. Fletcher.—In the Cherokee country, D. D Hitchcock, M.D., to Miss M. Worcester.—At Syracuse, N. Y., Charles N. Germaine, M.D., to Mrs. Mary J. Johnson, both of Syracuse

DIED,—In California, Dr. C. C. Abby, of Littleton, Vt. Dr. Dunkan, late member of Congress. —At Danvers, Mass., Andrew Nichols, M D., aged 70, a worthy man, and an eminent practitioner. —In Paris, M. Orfila, the celebrated chemist and toxicologist.

Deaths in Boston for the week ending Saturday noon, Arpril 2d, 80. Males, 43—females, 37. Inflammation of the bowels, 2—bronchitis, 1—congestion of brain, 1—inflammation of the brain, 2—burns and scalds, 2—cancer, 1—consumption, 10—convulsions, 1—croup, 6—dropsy, 2 —dropsy in head, 5 —drowned, 2— infantile diseases, 3—typhoid fever, 2—scarlet fever, 5—homicide, 1—hooping cough, 1—disease of the heart, 4—inflammation of the lungs, 12—marasmus, 2— old age, 6—palsy, 1—peritonitis, 1—teething, 2—tumor, 2.

Under 5 years, 36 —between 5 and 20 years, 12—between 20 and 40 years, 10—between 40 and 60 years, 11—over 60 years, 11. Born in the United States, 67 — Ireland, 9—England, 1 —Scotland, 1—Switzerland, 1—So. America, 1. The above includes 4 deaths in the city institutions.

Surgical Operation on a Turkey. — H. G. Howe, Esq., of Lawrence, Mass., describes an operation performed by himself, which may be of use to growers of poultry, and is of interest also to surgeons. One of his turkeys was noticed for several weeks to be drooping, and was found to be likely to die. On examination, the crop was noticed to be full and hard, and it was determined to open it. The creature was secured, and with a sharp razor the skin of the breast was laid back, and the crop opened, which was found nearly bursting with *dried hay,* nearly a hat full of which was taken out. With a needle and thread of fine silk the opening was carefully sewed up; the turkey was then kept quiet for a few days in a warm box, with a little soft bread soaked in milk for food, when it was allowed to run at large and soon completely recovered.

South Carolina Asylum for the Insane. — At the last session of the Legislature of South Carolina, an appropriation of $30,000 was made, for the purpose of erecting a new building or buildings for the accommodation of the insane patients in the State Institution of Columbia. In January last a committee was appointed from the Board of Regents, to report on the most serviceable manner of laying out this sum, and, from their printed report, we are glad to find that a proposition to give up the present Institution entirely, and to commence a new Hospital in the country, has been seriously entertained, although no definite action has yet been had on the subject.—*American Journal of Insanity.*

Commencement of the Female Medical College, Pennsylvania.—A large and fashionable audience graced the Musical Fund Hall, on the 27th Jan., at the commencement of this institution. The new President, Mr. Cleaveland, who is a popular principal of a female academy in our city, conferred the degrees in Latin, after reading the diploma to the successful candidates (nine in number), for its honors. The "charge" was delivered by Dr. Cornell, Professor of Physiology. He performed his difficult task most successfully, and is evidently a practised public speaker. He referred, among other things, to the acknowledged physical inferiority of the American females, and urged on the lady-graduates to seek the cause and remedy of this great evil.—*Philadelphia Med. and Surg. Journal.*

We understand the above statement respecting the reading of the diplomas to the graduates is not correct. The portion of the President's remarks which was in Latin was addressed to the officers of the College, and the diplomas were very properly left for the graduates themselves to read.

Vital Statistics of Petersburg, Va. — A writer in the Intelligencer, of Petersburg, in some remarks upon a table of deaths for nine years, prepared by him, estimates the number of deaths by consumption during that time in that city to have averaged 15 and a fraction per year, or about 1 in 533 annually of the population. This disease stands at the head, as in more northern climates, of the causes of death. Next in number comes cholera infantum—126 in nine years. Pneumonia stands next—63 deaths in the same time; and pleurisy and affections of the bowels and brain next. Old age stands 10th on the list. As in other places where cholera has prevailed, it is perceived that in Petersburg the mortality was unusually low during the year succeeding its prevalence, being less than any year of the nine.

THE

BOSTON MEDICAL AND SURGICAL JOURNAL.

VOL. XLVIII.   WEDNESDAY, APRIL 13, 1853.   No. 11.

QUACKERY—ITS CAUSES AND EFFECTS, WITH REFLECTIONS AND SUGGESTIONS.

An Address read at the Quarterly Meeting of the Bristol (Mass.) District Medical Society, held in Taunton, on the 9th of March, 1853.

BY DAN KING, M.D.

PERHAPS no subject is less interesting to a promiscuous audience, than that of medicine. To. unprofessional men its contemplation is neither entertaining nor pleasing. Its associations are of a disagreeable and repulsive character. Although the initiated view the subject in a different light, and always feel a deep interest in all that relates to the profession, yet to them almost everything connected with the subject has become a common every-day matter. It has no novelty, nothing to give it any new zest or interest. The deep-toned enthusiasm which heightens the importance and gives eclat to addresses on spirit-stirring occasions, never lends its aid to us to swell our themes or adorn our performances. We are not assembled on a 4th of July morning, surrounded with the ensigns of freedom, our bosoms burning with patriotic emotions, and our ears stunned with the loud acclamations which usher in that glorious anniversary. We are not about to welcome some proud hero, his brows already laden with glowing chaplets. We are not standing beside some towering monument, its base covering the dust of heroes, and its summit pointing the way their spirits have gone. None of these grand, exciting scenes are ours. Whoever writes or speaks upon medical subjects, must leave the regions of fancy and come down to the world of facts. Our business is with sober realities, naked truths and stubborn facts. It is not our province to divert and to please, but to exhibit truths, to expose errors and urge duties. We cannot expect, therefore, that any popular audience will be very much entertained by an address on an occasion like the present.

Those who read the Boston Medical and Surgical Journal, may perhaps recollect a short editorial article which appeared in the twentieth number of the last volume, calling the attention of its readers to the subject of quackery, and particularly to that variety which is practised by such as are sometimes called come-outers—men who turn traitors, and then set up the apology of a prompting conscience. After some pertinent remarks, the writer goes on to say—" Presuming that others have contemplated the erratic course of many a recusant brother, what course, in their opinion, can be devised to uphold the respectability of the medical profession, and preserve it from the contempt of well-directed minds?" Immediately after reading that article, I thought I would furnish the Journal with some remarks of my own upon the subject; but not having done so, I have since thrown together a few reflections and suggestions upon it, and they comprise the substance of the present discourse.

I am aware that this is a hackneyed subject; that it is more than a thrice-told tale; that it has so long and so often been made a subject of examination and inquiry, that it has lost all its novelty. But, nevertheless, it is a grave subject; its magnitude is by no means diminished, and the importance of the inquiry, "What can be done"? is every day increasing. Quackery is a demon which probably always did and always will exist, to perplex and annoy our profession and curse mankind. Empty as the air, fickle as the wind, and transitory as the phantoms of a vision, yet ever maintaining its power and accomplishing its purposes. The subject is odious enough in any view we may take of it; there is much to be blamed within and without our profession; but the usual practice of placing the whole to the account of the common people, is erroneous and unjust. The ancient Egyptians believed that every disease was the work of some aerial demon; and when the sick were suffering in consequence of their own violation of organic laws, when they were enduring the necessary result of their own acts, they sought for the cause in everything else but themselves. Some malignant star or evil genii were accused; and instead of correcting their own evil habits, as they should have done, they sought relief by endeavoring to propitiate the good and exorcise the bad spirits. They looked abroad for a cause which they might have found at home. They sought it in foreign objects, when it was within themselves; and he who supposes that the unprofessional public is justly chargeable with all the guilt of modern quackery, is little wiser than they. Reformations, like charities, should begin at home; and the people may with propriety say to us, "physician heal thyself." Yet in my present remarks I shall not confine myself to such faults as are found within our own precincts, but take the liberty to notice such as are uppermost in my mind, wherever they may belong. That tolerably well-educated physicians do sometimes become quacks and nostrum venders, is admitted; but I think it will generally be found that that class is made up of men of defective education, men of low capacities or eccentric minds, men who are better fitted for jockeys or showmen than for a learned profession, and always men whose avaricious propensities surpass all their moral sensibilities, having no ground of charity for their pretended promptings of conscience. It must be admitted, also, that there are hundreds of men in the profession, with degrees in their pockets, which they never merited; men whose mental organization, intellectual attainments, social training and moral principles, by no means qualify them for the station which they assume. They possess few or none of the necessary elements of success, and for their standing in the profession they rely almost entirely upon their parchment, which they are scarcely able to read.

Now the general character and standing of a profession is made up of the character and reputation of those who compose it. Every competent and honorable practitioner contributes towards its usefulness and respectability, and every incompetent or backsliding member helps to impair its usefulness and bring it into disrepute. Men of all ages may be found in the profession who do it no honor. They sit upon it like an incubus. Their tendency is not upward and onward, as it should be, but downward and retrograde. Like so many dead weights, they hang upon and depress it. It is so, though perhaps to a less extent, in the other professions. It is not every lawyer, admitted to the bar, who is qualified to shine as an advocate or become respected as a jurist. It is not every merchant or trader whose temper, tastes and acquirements qualify him for his business ; and those who fail to succeed in any profession or occupation, usually disparage it. Young men are often very unfortunate in their choice of a business for life. When they come to be actually engaged in a profession or occupation into which accident seems to have thrown them, they often find that it is neither what they expected nor what they want. It does not suit their condition or inclinations, and they have no ambition to contribute to its general welfare, or make themselves eminent in it. They discharge its duties poorly, or abandon it altogether. And since perfection is nowhere else to be found, it were unreasonable to expect it among physicians. In all professions, the best have only fewer faults than some others, and I do not know that ours has more than its share of the common infirmities. For this state of things I cannot conceive of any effectual remedy, and we may, perhaps, as well sit down and conclude to take the world as it is, and cast a broad veil over all the countless frailties of humanity. But the direct outrages of quacks and nostrum makers cannot be viewed in the same light. When individuals abandon the legitimate practice of medicine and engage in the manufacture of quack medicines, it is because they are strongly tempted so to do by the almost certain prospect of becoming rich by such means. They see that the confidence of the public in our profession is weak and vacillating, that reason and prudence easily give way to whims and caprice, that public opinion is unsettled as the ocean, and that established truths are no more regarded than traces in the sand which every coming wave is liable to obliterate. They see whole communities gaping for humbugs, and adopt the oft-repeated adage, viz., "The world's a cheat, and he is a fool who does not have a hand in it." They see that men are so easily cheated in nothing else as that which pertains to their health and life. They see that nothing is too absurd or ridiculous to be believed ; that mystery is more potent than reason ; that the greatest falsehoods are often taken for the greatest truths, and that the public make little distinction between the most ignorant pretender and the most learned and experienced practitioner. Whoever takes his stand in the great arena of quackery soon finds that his success depends not upon the real value of his compounds, but upon his skill in fabricating and promulgating falsehood. He has no farther use for medical science or moral principle—stratagem and fraud supply their places. Calculating upon the easy credulity of the public he becomes confident of success, and his hopes seldom fail.

Whilst scores of honest and skilful men retire from the field penny-less and disheartened, the mercenary charlatan often finds his coffers filled to overflowing. He can purchase townships, build stately mansions, give princely entertainments, and take a station in the highest ranks and among the most wealthy classes of society, and all this takes place because the influence of our profession is insufficient to prevent it. In the whole history of medicine there probably never was a time when it had less authority, and certainly there never was a time when it deserved so much, for never before did it possess such a vast amount of knowledge. No other profession requires the degree of study or mental effort. No other requires so much intellectual, moral and social training, and no other carries with it so much incidental information. Yet this profession seems to have lost all its ancient dignity ; it has far less authority now than it had in the days of Galen and Paracelsus. Medical men appear to have become inattentive to this subject, and forgotten the respect due to their calling. It is not so with the other professions. They are tenacious of all their rights, and scrupulously preserve all their prescriptive honors. The good of society requires that every profession and occupation should be duly respected in its own province ; and the more important the calling, the more necessary it is that it should receive its due regard. Take away all respect from the clergy and desecrate the pulpit, and you destroy their usefulness ; religious and moral order would come to an end ; scepticism and infidelity, in all their wild confusion, would everywhere prevail, and the darkness of chaos brood over society. If we take a view of the circuit of some eminent practitioner who has long had the confidence of all around him, we shall find very little if any quackery lurking within his borders ; his shadow terrifies and his frown banishes it ; his authority is duly regarded ; and all the puffs of newspapers and handbills, and the declarations of deceivers and their deluded votaries, are insufficient to impair public confidence in him. On the other hand, wherever educated physicians are not respected ; where quackery meets with ready success ; where the ignorant disciple of some new scheme is seen to ride slipshod over the community, there we have good reason to suspect that the present or former incumbents have been remiss, incompetent, or have committed some palpable errors, by which the profession has been disparaged.

Shakspeare tells us, " the evils that men do, live after them ; the good is often interred with their bones." It is sometimes so with physicians. An unworthy practitioner may have created and left behind him prejudices or jealousies which it will require many years to remove. Scientific medicine and quackery, like truth and falsehood, are adverse powers, and whatever promotes the one embarrasses the other. Therefore whatever adds to the respectability, the influence and authority of our profession, tends to discourage and destroy quackery. For his own sake, for the sake of his profession, and for the sake of society, every physician should take and maintain a high standing in the community. It is not enough that he is appealed to with earnestness in an hour of pain ; that he is respected in the sick-room and has authority in the nursery ; that he is the favorite of aunt Bàthsheba, uncle Jonathan and a host of others.   It is not enough that he is celebrated as an accoucheur, or eminent as a surgeon.   He must be somebody in society, apart from all professional considerations.   He should be known and respected everywhere, not merely on account of his profession, but for his general intelligence, the refinement of his manners, and his circumspect deportment.   He should be seen and heard and known in the hall and drawing-room, as well as in the chamber of the sick.   The physician, who, like some old nurse, is never wanted anywhere out of the sick-room ; who is only employed as a thing of convenience, and then set aside for further use ; who has no influence in every-day life ; whose character and conduct do not contribute towards the formation of public opinion, or public manners ; whose impress is not apparent upon the face of society—such an one has not half the influence that every good physi-· cian should have, and will be unable to do half the good that every physician should be able to do.

For a considerable time past, the public newspapers have contributed largely towards misleading and depraving the public mind.   It is a lamentable fact that three quarters of all these papers derive their principal support from the proprietors of quack medicines.   Page after page is filled with their fulsome statements, outraging common sense and doing violence to common decency, every word and syllable of which is false, and much of which the inmates of a brothel would blush to read by daylight.   Almost every apothecary keeps a full assortment of these indispensable articles, and with many it is their principal business.   Here the public are led to suppose they may always find a remedy for every disease, because such are advertised and highly recommended.   Upon this state of things the high-minded physician looks with chagrin and mortification.   The aspect is too formidable for his encounter, and he stands abashed.   He subscribes for the newspapers that are constantly pouring falsehood and pollution into the public mind, and setting his profession at naught.   He gives his patronage to the apothecary who is constantly dealing out panaceas, and who in the absence of the doctor has always something to recommend as better than any other known remedy.   In consequence of this, the invalid, instead of seeking for the most competent medical adviser, pores over newspapers and pamphlets, to find the most extraordinary catholicon ; and when he has made up his mind to try some worthless nostrum, no sound medical advice to the contrary will weigh a straw in his mind.

Now we can do little directly to correct this state of things.   Printers work for money, and will ever be ready to put in type whatever pays best, and the venders of nostrums are influenced by similar motives. Perhaps, on the whole, professional employment is not much abridged by all this ; for in general, such remedies, being improperly used, as they often are, do quite as much harm as good, and therefore we might have little cause to complain.   Yet we have good reason to complain on another account.   This course of proceeding tends to destroy public confidence in all medical means.   It gives printed lies an authority above verbal truth, and prepares the way for every new scheme in quackery. It may in time partially work its own cure. Newspaper statements are coming to be less and less regarded ; and the time may come when every reasonable man will conclude, as he may now without doing any great violence to facts, that every such newspaper is an entire falsehood. The most that we can do in this matter, is to organize and improve our profession, increase its worth, its influence and authority. By so doing we shall diminish the nostrum business and benefit the community.

One word upon the administration of medicine. This matter has, I think, been too little attended to in the practice of many physicians. Articles are often prescribed and administered in nauseous and repulsive forms, when they might be made much more agreeable, or something else much more pleasant might answer quite as well or better. Modern quackery has taken advantage of this, and now nearly every nostrum in the shops, and everything prescribed by quacks, in the shape of medicine, is either pleasant to the taste or entirely insipid ; so that the quack, rather than offer his patient a disagreeable bolus, gives him nothing but a placebo. And for this reason alone practitioners of that class are often employed, it being so easy to take their medicine. It is indeed easier to swallow a few grains of sugar of milk than a dose of wormwood, although the latter might sometimes be useful, but the former never. It is certainly a duty which every practitioner owes his patient, to make all his treatment as pleasant as possible ; and in making prescriptions, this should never be forgotten.

Another unhappy circumstance, which tends in no small degree to embarrass our profession, is the want of friendly intercourse and kindness of feeling among professional brethren. It is a lamentable fact that jealousies, envies, hatred and ill will are often secretly entertained where nothing of the kind should be allowed to exist a moment ; and if physicians reproach, backbite and dishonor one another, can they expect the public to respect them ? In the present crowded state of the profession, some appear to suppose, that in order to succeed themselves, they must ruin somebody else. This is a sad mistake ; for although an individual acting upon this idea may disturb the peace of others, and impair public confidence, yet the blow is almost certain to recoil upon its author with augmented force. No reputation surreptitiously acquired is likely to be of long duration ; and the world's experience may teach every prudent man that a persevering, upright line of conduct is the only sure road to permanent success ; that the way for an individual to rise is to build himself up by adding to his own stock of knowledge, and making himself more and more worthy of confidence and respect.

There are hundreds of men about the country, who pretend that they were once regular physicians, and practised in that way as long as their tender consciences would let them ; but having found out some new and better way, they have, out of a sense of duty, abandoned the *old* practice, as they call it, for something that is infinitely better. Now a large proportion of these pretenders are ignorant men, who have had no medical education, but being too lazy to follow their own proper occupation, have abandoned—not medicine, but their agricultural or mechanical implements, for what they erroneously imagine to be much easier, viz., the practice of quackery. But it must be acknowledged that among this nefarious class there are some who have been educated and admitted as regular members of the profession. If you learn the history of these men, you will generally find that they tried their hands awhile in the practice of their legitimate calling ; but owing to their want of perseverance, or their own unfitness or incompetence, they were not successful, and therefore abandoned an honest and honorable course for one of hypocrisy and fraud. Of all quacks, such men are the most detestable. By the common consent of all nations, when an individual becomes a traitor and takes up arms against his country, he is considered an outlaw deserving nothing better than the gallows. And is the man who abjures a calling so big with responsibility, and for the sake of money undertakes a crusade against human life, less guilty ? Although such men may and sometimes do enjoy a temporary prosperity—although they may glory in their own shame and bask in a brief summer's sun— yet the time will assuredly come when their sin will find them out, and *mene tekel* be written upon them.

[To be continued]

M. RICORD'S LETTERS UPON SYPHILIS.

Addressed to the Editor of L'Union Medicale—Translated from the French by D. D. SLADE, M.D., Boston, and communicated for the Boston Medical and Surgical Journal.

TWENTY-FIRST LETTER.

MY DEAR FRIEND,—How do the chancres heal, how do they cicatrize ? Let me say a few words to you upon this subject, which has its importance.

The period of healing is announced by the disappearance of the areola of the ulcer. Its borders become disgorged, sink, or they shelve towards the bottom, and the separation from the surrounding tissues ceases, if it has taken place. The margin becomes of a pale tint, of a greyish-pearl color, and finishes by taking on again the normal color of the neighboring tissues. The bottom becomes cleansed ; the grey, diphtheritic, lardaceous layer is at first as if transpierced with granulations, which later fill it up everywhere, and give to the ulceration a granulated aspect, and a healthy, rosy tint. The pus then becomes less abundant, creamy—*laudable*, as we can say here with justice, for it ceases to have the power of inoculating. As the parts fill up, the epidermis spreads from the circumference to the centre, and cicatrization is completed as in every wound which has suppurated, or as after every other ulceration which has no longer any cause of being one.

The *cicatrix of chancres* may be more prominent than the neighboring parts ; sometimes it is upon a level, and more frequently depressed, according to the thickness of the tissues attacked ; it is indelible in a great number of cases, while in others, it disappears completely, as often happens after an indurated chancre, or when the chancre is seated upon a mucous membrane.

But, as those who have had much experience know, the period of reparation may have its irregularities. In the serpiginous chancre, an extremity often becomes cicatrized, while the other continues to increase ; sometimes it is one side which heals, and the other ulcerates again ; frequently, in fine, the healing takes place in one or several points at the centre, while the circumference augments its unhealthy circle without ceasing. Finally, you well know, that upon certain individuals, excepting when a well-directed treatment has intervened, or when we have not understood how to repress the granulations by cauterizations, or when foolish prejudices have prevented us from doing this, these granulations become, as they say, luxuriant, vegetating, and give to the ulceration certain aspects, which have gained for it the names of *granulated, fungous, vegetating chancres.* Veritable vegetations, varied in their form, may then be produced, of an accidental epigenic tissue ; they have not, on this account, a syphilitic nature, as we shall see by-and-by.

At this period, as I have already told you, when the chancre has infected the economy, it may itself undergo a local trasformation, and finish by presenting the characters of mucous tubercles, and thus justify the opinion of those who, for want of analysis, have not understood these changes, and who have admitted that these accidents may be either primitive or secondary, and that in all cases they were contagious ; an opinion which I have already combated.

But here is a point of doctrine upon which I insist, and which I ought to recall to you ; it is that the chancre which may increase at different periods, *never relapses when once cicatrized.* If a new inoculable chancre shows itself at a later period, after complete cicatrization, we may affirm that it is the result of a new contagion.

After all that I have just told you, it is very certain that, taking into account the morality of patients, so far as we can weigh and measure it, by knowing the conditions in which they have been placed, by recalling the seat of preference of chancres, their number most frequently limited ; by knowing also how to appreciate well the different varieties and the period of progress and of the specific *statu quo,* the progress, the duration and the different aspects which they could present at the period of reparation and even after cicatrization, as also the influence more or less pronounced of the mercurial treatment, in certain cases we can arrive at an almost absolute rational diagnosis.

However, the physiognomy of the primary ulcer is ordinarily so expressive (excuse the word), at the specific period, that in seeing we recognize it. We must distrust this first impression ; it may cause us to commit indiscretions that will cost us something to repair. You have allowed me a pathological anecdote ; I make use of your permission, happy if I can distract you a little from the dryness of my preceding descriptions. One day, one of our very grave *savans* enters my office, and without any other preamble shows me a diseased organ, saying to me, what is that ? I answer at once, it is a chancre. Well! sir, it was my wife who gave it to me. Then, sir, it is not a chancre. And why not, if you please? Because, I replied, what distinguishes simple ulcerations resembling chancres from the true chancres, is the source from which we believe to have taken them. My patient was not duped by an argument, which would have sufficed for certain physicians whom you know, and contented himself with saying, with much dignity and resignation: cure me.

But the diagnosis, is it always as easy as is believed, as some of our classical authors profess ? I appeal to M. Lagneau, who has in our day so worthily represented them. Remark rather, if, in spite of all the care which he takes with it, he succeeds in distinguishing the primary chancre from what he calls, with so many others, the secondary chancre. Throw a glance again upon the synoptical and comparative table which he has made of ulcers which might be confounded with those which are caused by the syphilitic virus, and tell me if this is the case, and especially if it enables you to establish this with certainty.

Mercury, that touch-stone so infallible in the eyes of the faithful, and which has been the foundation of the division of the *true* and the *false* syphilis in England, is a deceptive reagent. It often cures non-syphilitic accidents, while it aggravates those which are so, and which are sometimes cured without anything.

How many chancres there are which are overlooked by experienced practitioners ! How many errors committed, especially in regard to the different varieties of the indurated chancre, the most dangerous of all ! Sometimes we believe them simple excoriations, sometimes we can be deceived to a degree to consider them as true cancerous degeneracies. My colleague and friend, Dr. Vitry, of Versailles, ought to recollect a patient to whom a physician of Paris was called, not to judge of the nature of his complaint, but to amputate his penis. I recognized the existence of an indurated chancre, with considerable increase of the plastic exudation, and the pills of the iodide of mercury replaced the knife.

One of our learned professors of the Faculty of Paris, who is as cognizant with syphilis as with other diseases, in the diagnosis of which he excels, ought to remember the history of a great Russian Lord whom we saw together at the house of our honored and regretted master, M. Marjolin, and in whose case he would not recognize a primary accident, because there only remained the specific induration, and because this Lord could not account for nor explain to us, how he could have contracted this accident, which shortly afterwards, as I had predicted, gave the most convincing proofs of a constitutional affection.

If you will let me, I will relate to you another little story. The nephew of Cullerier one day sent to me a fashionable writer, to ask my advice respecting an ulceration which he had upon the corona glandis ; an ulceration with an indurated base and which did not then present the characteristics of the borders, and of the base classically required in order to constitute a chancre. I did not the less recognize an ulceration with the specific characteristics of the induration which I have lately described, and with the ganglionic radiation which we shall have to study presently. Cullerier was not of my opinion, inasmuch as he had examined the two only women accused, and whom he had found healthy. The nephew did not admit the mediate contagion, nor spontaneous syphi-

lis, and as he had faith in what the patient said, he could not admit
the existence of a primary ulcer. I, who often doubt, even with the
most certain proof, and who admit all the rational ways of contagion,
remained convinced that the patient had been deceived—that he was
mistaken, or that he deceived us. In fact, six weeks had scarcely
passed before constitutional symptoms well characterized—too well, for
they were very difficult to cure—manifested themselves. But while
Cullerier was still asking himself how and why the patient had the verole, I was called to the house of a distinguished lady. I arrived, knowing neither the end nor the motive for my visit. This great lady was
mysteriously seated in her boudoir, and, in spite of the twilight that
reigned in the place, I could perceive upon her face, evidences little deceptive of a secondary affection. Doctor, she says to me, what I have
to say to you is very delicate. Wishing to cut short a painful confession, I said to her, I see what it is, Madam, and your face explains to
me sufficiently why I have the honor of being in your presence. What
do you mean? she asked, with astonishment. That you are sick, madam,
and that doubtless you require my services. Not in the least. I have
requested your visit in order that you should aid us in preserving M.
X——— (the writer who had been sent to me by Cullerier), not only
from his malady, but also from his dangerous intrigues. And here was
this lady, who took upon herself to draw me a portrait, little flattered,
of the two women whom Cullerier had examined, whom he had found
healthy, and who were, according to her, the cause of all the evil. I
had great trouble, as you may suppose, to make this lady understand
that the source from whence our poor writer had taken his trouble was
situated much nearer to me, and to obtain the confession that the pressing interest which she had for our patient had other motives than a pure
Platonic affection.

Thus it is with all of them, my dear friend; and the moral of this
anecdote is, that the men of the world never make to you full confessions; that in having relations with great ladies, or with others in whom
they have confidence, their ideas are a thousand leagues from the truth;
their suspicions do not rest upon the veritable source of their malady,
and they search for it where it does not exist.

You see, then, how difficult the diagnosis of chancre often is; and
how wrong we are to deny the existence of it, when the patients do not
aid us in discovering the source from whence they have taken it.

It is, then, because I know all the difficulties of the diagnosis in
a sufficiently large number of cases; it is because I have seen men the
most skilful, commit frequent errors, that I have said, and do still say, in
spite of the contrary opinions, that the only positive, unequivocal pathog-
nomonic characteristic of chancre at the period of progress or of specific
statu quo, is found in the pus which it secretes, and which can be inoculated; whence I conclude that *inoculation gives the most certain evidence of the specificity of the ulcer.*

I said in the work that I published in 1838, that if we ought to give
mercury in all the cases where a primary virulent accident exists, we
should be always assured of this virulence by practising in time artifi-

cial inoculation. But be assured, this operation, to which some persons might object, and which they have the right to consider as dangerous, when one does not know how to make use of it, is not necessary for practice, and I have never advised it as a general rule.

The prognosis and treatment of chancre are based upon other indications, than the virulence ; for it is the induration and its accessories, which inoculation is unfitted to make us distinguish, which foretels the future fate of the constitution, and requires the specific treatment. This is what I hope to be able to demonstrate.   Yours,   Ricord.

PROTECTION FROM SMALLPOX BY VACCINATION.

BY ZACHARY LEWIS, M.D., KING AND QUEEN CO., VA.

On the 25th of June, 1851, I was called at night to meet Dr. Robinson to see a little girl aged about 12 years of age, a daughter of Mr. E. W., deceased, who, it was said, had the measles. On entering the room, to my astonishment I found she was literally covered with the eruption of confluent smallpox.

The history of the case is this :—She had been carried to Baltimore some two or three weeks before, where she was exposed to variola infection. She returned home, however, and continued as well as usual until Wednesday, the 18th, when she was taken with a high fever, pain in the head and back, and all the symptoms, as was supposed by the family, of measles. About Saturday an eruption made its appearance on the face, arms and breast, when I considered it a genuine case of confluent smallpox. The family became greatly alarmed, as the children, several in number, together with a numerous family of negroes, had never been vaccinated. Mr. W., in his lifetime having had no confidence in the protection afforded against smallpox by the vaccine disease, never had any of his family vaccinated. We decided at once to vaccinate the whole family ; but as neither of us had matter at the time which could be relied on, it was not done till the next day.

A young lady of the family had been sleeping on the bed with the patient, and several small children were constantly in the room during the whole course of the eruptive fever (up to Wednesday night). I continued in attendance until Sunday morning, at which time my services were dispensed with.

The case terminated fatally on the next Thursday afternoon, when I was again called in to see the family who had been vaccinated. I found on examination the vaccine matter had taken most beautifully. The patients had no eruption, except the pustule on the arm, with the exception of the eldest son of Mr. W., who had a considerable number of pustules, but no more than I have seen in patients who had not been exposed to smallpox virus. He had no more fever than the rest of the children, and continued to walk about the house and yard during the whole time.

The above case is one of the many going to confirm the great and beneficent doctrine of Jenner, which, tending to avert one of the most deadly of human evils, deserves, like the doctrines of religion and liberty, the warm support and cordial acceptance of every enlightened citizen.   Although the history of vaccination is a history of its uniform and ascendant progress over all obstacles, whether of ignorance, prejudice, or avarice, there have always been those who, unwilling or unable to survey the whole subject, which ought to carry conviction to every judgment, have preferred to rely on their own limited experience of a few doubtful exceptions, and reject the boon of Jenner, rather than yield assent to a mass of evidence such as has scarcely ever been accumulated in any other department of human investigation.   The doubts, hesitancy and fears of such individuals ought not, and it is believed will not, prevent the extension and ultimate triumph of vaccination, when the variolous contagion, like the Jewish leprosy, shall cease to deform and destroy the race of man.   The dogma of Willis, " Convenet enim bomini omni soli et semel, variolis aut morbilis affici," has already ceased to be true or accepted, however true it might have been anteriorly to the researches of Jenner.

What corroboration, in fact, is necessary or possible where it is admitted, on the experience of half a century, that millions of lives have been preserved ; that variola has from some countries been wholly exterminated, and, in most parts of the globe, disarmed of its dangers and deformity ; that thousands of individuals, protected by its means, have been inoculated, and with impunity exposed to the concentrated contagion of smallpox—in fine, since the growing light of experience and philosophy teaches both reason and the senses that the doctrine of Jenner is incontrovertibly true ?   The proposition to be solved is not, whether any cause can so change the structure, irritability and sensibility of the living tissues as to incapacitate them from suffering a second impression from a similar cause, for there are no physiologists who will deny the affirmative to be true.   Mankind wish to know whether vaccina can so change the structure or properties of the tissues as to render them unsusceptible of the impressions of variola.   This is the true question in the public mind:—Shall we be safe from smallpox if we are vaccinated ?   The testimony of all Europe, Asia, Africa, and the experience of the United States, will answer, yes,   Who doubts that measles, once suffered, incapacitates that individual, in all future time, from undergoing the same pathological state ?   And yet what practitioner, of a few years' standing, has not witnessed a second attack of rubeola ?   Is not the same thing true as regards parotitis, varicella, scarlatina, &c. ?   Confessedly, these diseases have been known to attack a second, and even a third time in numerous instances, ever since they became the subjects of medical history ; and this, too, without invalidating the truth of, or preventing the public reliance on, the general rule, that an attack is only sustained once by each individual.   Jenner's immortality is due to this, that he first invented, and successfully practised, the art of substituting a mild and safe animal poison to effect that modification of the constitution which, previously, had only been produced by a harsh and often mortal one.—*Stethoscope and Virginia Medical Gazette.*

PERFORATION OF THE STOMACH.

BY EDW. GOVETT, ESQ., M.R.C.S.E.

The subject of this case was a young Irishwoman, 24 years of age, hitherto healthy, of active habits, and following the situation of a domestic servant in a private family. On the evening of Sunday, the 16th ultimo, she left her employer's house apparently in good health, having made no complaint to any one previous to her departure : but on returning home at 10 o'clock the same night, in a cab, she complained of extreme pain in the epigastric region, stating, at the same time, that she had been very sick. There was no peculiarity about the pulse, and the tongue was ordinarily clean. In the absence of obvious cause or knowledge of previous disease, I concluded that she must have eaten some indigestible substance, which had produced the symptoms above related, and accordingly prescribed at once a stimulant. Being a visiter, on the point of leaving the house for my own residence as the deceased entered, I hastily gave directions that further assistance should be obtained if she grew worse. On the following evening (Monday) I heard that she had died at about half past 1 o'clock, P.M., of that day, having previously had the professional assistance of a gentleman in the neighborhood, who found her in a state of extreme collapse, and having much the appearance of a patient in the last stage of cholera, but without the diarrhœa or cramps. Stimulants, hot-water bottles, and mustard poultices, were ordered ; but she died in about twenty minutes after his arrival, remaining sensible to the latest moment ; the entire duration of her sufferings from first to last being about eighteen hours.

At a post-mortem examination by the surgeon in attendance and myself, we found, on opening the abdomen, that the entire peritoneal covering of the cavity and its contents was in the highest state of inflammation ; large quantities of pus and lymph between the convolutions of the intestines ; the great and lesser omentum being in a shrivelled and highly-engorged and partially-agglutinated condition : in short, such was the fearful state of the abdominal viscera, that we were entirely puzzled how to account for such an enormous amount of mischief arising in so short a period, until, upon examining the stomach, the cause at once appeared, viz., a perforation of that organ, of the size of a sixpenny-piece, with smooth white edges, somewhat hardened, and nearly as even as though it had been cut out with a wadding punch. The situation was at the superior and anterior wall, and about two inches and a half from the pylorus ; the villous coat was obliterated in the neighborhood of the opening, and the vessels around it red and greatly distended ; the other parts of the lining membrane were healthy.

It appears to me that there are several points of interest in the case :

1st. The remarkably sudden appearance of the symptoms without previous derangement.

2d. The preservation of the mental powers to the last moment ; and

3d. The peculiar character of the perforation itself.

I am informed that several similar cases have occurred in the same district, and that it has been difficult to trace the disease to any evident exciting cause.—*London Lancet.*

WHAT IT IS TO BE BILIOUS.

WHEN an idea gets abroad and becomes popular, and a saying to express it becomes familiar in our mouths, it takes a long time to get either of them out.

The word *bilious* is probably used to express a greater variety of conditions, or ailments, than any other in the vocabulary of medicine, and strange as it may seem, it is very seldom used in its true sense, or to explain the condition which it implies.

To be bilious is to have a redundancy of bile—an active accumulation of this secretion from the blood by the liver, and from thence to pass into the gall-bladder; but the term is commonly used to express the contrary condition, one in which the liver is torpid in its action, and consequently the bile remains in the blood and is carried through the system, showing itself in the transparent tissues, as in the white part of the eyes, and even the skin.

In this case it is very seldom a disease, but a symptom merely of disordered function, as in fever, however slight, when the secretions are diminished, and that of the liver accordingly. The people are so frequently " bilious," that patent-medicine venders make capital of it, and advertise nearly all their nostrums for " bilious complaints," and thus they hit almost every one's case. Popular notices have been industriously propagated upon this subject by quacks, and thus they have furnished the (supposed) disease, and the remedy—like shrewd tradesmen they create a demand to promote sales.

No opinion will so readily satisfy most patients as to tell them they are " bilious "; this they think they understand, and what is more, in nine cases in ten, you will agree with them " precisely," than which nothing is more satisfactory. We are sorry to acknowledge that many physicians who do not like to talk, or have learned that it is not safe to do so, often take this method to get rid of troublesome customers. Such men are usually considered amiable and smart—amiable because they say yes to everything, and smart because they know as much as their patients. In out-western phraseology, the term bilious has quite a different signification—one which is by no means complimentary—partaking in a measure of the ancients' notions, and associated with a sour disposition and bad temper. This unhappy state of the moral man, our worthy ancestors, at an early day, ascribed to " black bile," and we are not sure but that they are entitled to the credit of being nearest right, for when the liver is torpid, the bile is darker in color and irritating to the mucous surfaces over which it passes, in proportion as it is in such cases less in quantity; and an irritable temper is no doubt often associated with this condition; and that a little super-carbonate of soda or mild aromatic will make a man amiable oftentimes, is a fact well known among physicians. The same is also true of the use of mild cathartics; hence cross children are often treated with a dose of castor oil, which removes the exciting cause.

If quacks only knew enough, it would be easy to get fortunes by making a medicine upon this principle for bad tempers, as buyers would be found in plenty, of both sexes, to provide for the usual consequences of washing-day, and cold dinners ; and thus two customers would be secured in every family where the machinery of the kitchen does not move regularly. Let our readers remember that to be bilious is to be bad tempered, and this popular ailment will soon be expunged from the calendar.—*The (New York) Esculapian.*

THE BOSTON MEDICAL AND SURGICAL JOURNAL.

BOSTON, APRIL 13, 1853.

Medical Jurisprudence of Insanity.—Messrs. Little, Brown & Co., of Boston, have recently produced the third edition of this work, by I. Ray, M.D., with additions. Though the first was thought nearly faultless, the author's subsequent experience and reflection must have considerably improved what came before the public in 1838. It would be a needless waste of time to describe the peculiar excellencies of this important treatise. Lawyers and physicians generally are quite familiar with its merits. If there are any members of either of these professions who are not so, an opportunity is now afforded of making up for lost time. In its present aspect, Dr. Ray's book is a large octavo of 520 pages, in a clear, distinct type and on good paper. No point seems to have been neglected, of the least importance, that might aid in understanding the delicate and almost infinite shades of lunacy. Idiocy, imbecility, pathological symptoms of mania, intellectual and moral mania, legal consequences of mania, dementia, febrile delirium, duration of madness, lucid intervals, simulated insanity, concealed epilepsy, suicide, somnambulism, effects of insanity on evidence, drunkenness, legal consequences, interdiction and isolation, and the duties of medical witnesses, are the heads of some of the numerous subjects ably discoursed upon in the work. The publishers deserve a generous patronage.

What is Life ?—This question was asked at the opening of an address to the candidates for degrees, at a late examination in the Medical Institution of Yale College, and answered by the learned gentleman by whom it was propounded—Benjamin Welch, M.D., one of the board of managers. So many have traversed the same path, and explained what life is, each in his own way, which very rarely corresponds with the definitions of others, that it is a difficult point to determine who is right or who is wrong. In the meanwhile, the amount of physiological facts which each one collects in the effort to establish a theory, is adding to the stock of knowledge which has been accumulating for ages ; and if no one has yet satisfactorily defined what life is, the world is the wiser for their researches. Dr. Welch lays down one proposition, that meets our individual approval, because it is plain common sense. It is this—" The first and essential law of our existence, is that of progress." There is no repose for nature, or in nature, and Dr. Welch takes a departure from that text, on which he reasons like a deep philosopher. He touches very delicately upon that old worn out topic of discussion, the connection of mind and matter, and, my his credit, owns up, as the brokers say, by plainly declaring that th

is entirely beyond our comprehension, instead of wasting strength in the
attempt to show, as many have, what never can be shown. After passing
over this mysterious connection, Dr. Welch discourses admirably on the
moral obligations of physicians, and their high destiny if they fulfil the
mission upon which they set out in life.

Clinical Phrase Book.—Montgomery Johns, M.D., became satisfied,
from experience, that it was quite convenient, if not absolutely necessary,
to have a sufficient acquaintance with the German language to interrogate
the patients whom physicians are often called upon to treat. The immense emigration to this country has filled our cities and large towns with
foreigners, whose vernacular in many cases is German, and the physician
who can speak their language makes himself very acceptable to these strangers, and has a manifest advantage over those who are unable to converse
with them. Without particularly descanting upon the value of the accomplishment of understanding the literature of Germany, whoever examines
Dr. John's Phrase Book will perceive how easy it is to master a series of
questions that may serve in other meridians besides a sick room. It is
a small duodecimo, containing a dictionary of English and German; elements of grammar, phrases, measures, weights, materia medica, and some
of almost every thing necessary to learn in order to comprehend the meaning of a German who knows nothing of English. It is a useful and acceptable publication. Messrs. Lindsay & Blakiston, Philadelphia, have
done justice to the typography.

Lectures on Life Insurance.—Moses L. Knapp, M.D., late of Iowa, is
the author of a thick, respectable-looking pamphlet, of 242 pages, devoted
to what he pleases to call the science of life insurance. A friend of ours,
who has given it a reading, comes to the conclusion, with ourselves, that it
is essentially the advertisement of a few insurance offices. Such has been
the character of the efforts in New England, to induce people to take out life
policies, that many who were inclined to view these institutions favorably,
have been disgusted, if not alarmed in regard to the security of offices
whose agents were running every where over the country. In this production of Dr. Knapp, there is not a single new idea, or an old one presented in a novel form. Facts and arguments which have become stale
from constant repetition, are reproduced, accompanied by statistical memoranda and tabular proofs. If Dr. Knapp had come out boldly and fearlessly, declaring, at the outset, just what every one will believe who reads
his lectures, that he has been well paid for this service by interested parties, quite as much of a sensation would have been made, as by his ostensible attempt to carry the point under the cloak of disinterested scientific investigation. Having been an advocate for life insurance, in offices of a high
character, whose responsibility and resources are properly guarded by the
Legislature, we shall offer nothing in objection to a fair and honorable course
of business enterprise in this line; but an opinion is extensively entertained that two thirds, at least, of all the life offices are unsound, and that
their incomes go for the support of a few presidents, secretaries and directors, instead of securing from want the families or friends of deceased individuals. We fully agree with Dr. Knapp when he says, "The companies
that are taking advantage of the public ignorance and practising decep-
tion, resorting to usages that are utterly condemned and shown in this

work to be fallacious, are the occasion of the deepest solicitude and re-
grets on the part of all persons who have examined the subject with that
careful attention it merits." Now if the publication of this book itself is
not of the same nature as some of the doings which he reprobates, the
object of its publication is wholly mistaken.

Rush Medical College.—N. S. Davis, M.D., who ably sustains the chair
of pathology and practice, at Rush Medical College, delivered a valedictory to the graduating class on the 16th of February, which has since been
published by the class. He is a good writer, earnest, sincere, and always
to the point. In this instance the address is a fine specimen of what a
farewell discourse should be. It is not so long as to weary the reader, nor
could it have been tedious to those who listened to it. Short sermons are
generally popular, and orations are never prized when they weary an
audience. Just enough in this instance was said by Dr. Davis, and consequently the fundamental truths he wished to impress on the minds of the
class, will be likely to remain.

Advertising by Physicians.—Throughout New England, and to some
extent in the other States, a steady and uninterrupted effort has long been
made by organized medical associations, to prevent the! members from advertising themselves in a way which may be considered objectionable or injurious to the honor and dignity of a liberal profession. Stringent as the
regulations for this purpose are, occasionally some one ventures to announce himself to the public. This is accomplished in two modes—first,
by withdrawing from his associates altogether; or, second, by stating,
through an appropriate medium, that he is devoted exclusively to a specialty. While those who pursue all other branches of commendable industry are allowed, by common consent, to advertise, practitioners of medicine
and surgery must be introduced to the people through the verbal representations of individuals, who of course propagate the intelligence of the
skill, attainments and other qualifications of a medical gentleman, as circumstances, gossip, or the marvellousness of a neighborhood may dictate.
One of the strong and often repeated complaints made against this prohibition, is that the officers of all medical associations have their names
heralded abroad in official notices, records, and various publications of the
societies over which they preside, which secures to them the advantages of
an advertisement. They are extensively known abroad as the prominent
members of the association to which they belong. This gives them publi-
city and patronage, while the rank and file, those who actually sustain the
burden of maintaining the institution which thus gives prominence and
distinction to one or two, are kept out of sight. Members of medical societies have been known to withdraw their connection on this account.
They could accomplish nothing, as they believed, while they remained;
and as by advertising their remedies or their experience, they could have business, they preferred the frowns of their former associates, to starvation.
When their fortunes were made, no serious objections were ever known, it
is said, to prevent their returning to the fold, on abandoning the way that
has conducted them to wealth. This is the kind of reasoning that the disaf-
fected resort to; and the success that attends many who pursue a course opposed to the law, has a tendency to make members restive under the prohibi-

tion, and to doubt whether its stringency, in forbidding almost every species of professional advertising, does not operate, on the whole, to the injury rather than the benefit of the profession. Again, it is said, that those practising a particular branch of medicine or surgery are seldom troubled by the sentinels of professional propriety, when their notices appear in the newspapers; nor is it suggested that it borders on quackery, or is an ingenious scheme for evading the no-advertising doctrine, to send professional circulars through the post-office. As this is an important subject, it might be well to have the views of the profession expressed more fully upon it than it has yet been.

Institution for Idiots.—At Barre, Mass., fine accommodations are provided for the moral and physical training of imbecile children. The locality, the conveniences, and. above all, the qualifications of those who have the daily charge of the unfortunate inmates, are eminently fitted for the purposes designed. The Barre institution is the first established in America. In some respects it is superior to Dr. Guggenbuhl's school at Interlacken. The town in which it is situated is delightful, the village particularly inviting, the society cultivated, and the air, the purity of the water, the scenery, and the immediate appointments of the buildings, all justify us in recommending Dr. Brown's establishment to the notice of parents. A report now before us, the first we remember to have seen, besides furnishing necessary information respecting the general economy of the establishment, contains comments on cases, in which individuals have risen from an extremely low mental condition, to be mindful of the proprieties of life. A regular system of instruction is unremittingly pursued, that rarely fails to accomplish happy results in developing some of the dormant faculties, while the personal condition of even very hopeless cases is bettered by perseverance. A happier home could not be found for eccentric or idiotic children. One continuous effort is operating, from the hour they enter, to implant just ideas and good habits, and promote their health and happiness. As a whole, the children constitute a large social family. Those desirous of knowing the particulars as to prices, the process of gaining admission, &c., can ascertain by addressing Geo. Brown, M.D., Barre, Mass.

Suffolk District Medical Society.—At the annual meeting of this society, held on Wednesday, 6th inst., the following gentlemen were elected officers for the ensuing year:—Dr. John Homans, *President;* Dr. Samuel Parkman, *Vice President;* Dr. John B. Alley, *Secretary;* Drs. Ephraim Buck and Silas Durkee, *Supervisors;* Dr. Wm. E. Coale, *Librarian;* Dr. N. B. Shurtleff, *Treasurer.*

The Counsellors and Censors of the State Society for Suffolk District, with one or two exceptions, were re-elected. A committee was appointed to nominate a list of delegates to the next annual meeting of the American Medical Association in New York, and report at the monthly meeting of the Society on Saturday, 30th inst.

Excision of the Testes.—A correspondent sends us the following, which he thinks might with propriety be inserted in the Journal as an *erratum.* The circumstances of the case referred to were novel, and it is not perhaps strange that there should be a difference of opinion respecting the expediency of the operation which was performed. He says—

In the article on "Excision of the Testes," in the Journal for March 30, pp. 180-182, for "she" and "her," read "he and "his." To take a child having testes, for a young Miss, is, to say the least, a mistake, which, together with the operation itself, ought to be numbered among the "corrigenda."

Medical Miscellany.—Dr. C. Graham, of Kentucky, is reputed the greatest rifle shooter in the world.—Smallpox has appeared in the vicinity of South Hero, Vt.—Four hundred and thirty-one students attended the lectures of the University of Pennsylvania, the past season.—Dr. Warren, of Boston, and Dr. Mott, of New York, have been elected members of the French Academy of Medicine.—In one of Lindsay & Blakiston's small sheet catalogues, the prices of medical books, published by them, are given in the margin—an improvement generally demanded by physicians in the interior.—Dr. Brown's case of extensive disease of the cervical vertebræ, with clinical observations on other forms of caries of the spine, has appeared in a beautifully printed pamphlet.—Dr. Hereford, of Petersburg, Va., is represented, in the Intelligencer of that city, as saying that the general bad success of physicians in the management of scarlatina, is in consequence of giving too much physic.—The Medical Society of Virginia are about memorializing the Legislature for a law of registration.—A physician states that cod-liver oil may be administered without the least disgust to a patient, by chewing and swallowing a small quantity of the roe of a smoked herring both before and after taking the spoonful of oil. A piece of sardine will answer, if herring is not palatable. The disguise is perfectly effectual.—The proceedings of the Homœopathic Medical Society of the State of New York, in 1852-3, have been published in a pamphlet.—The students of the Rush Medical College, Chicago, have presented one of the faculty, Dr. Davis, with a valuable microscope.—Smallpox has appeared at Stanwix, N. Y.—Female colleges were denounced at a meeting of divines and others, at Pittsfield, Mass., the other day. They object to these modern institutions for turning women into men.—Additional cases are reported in the late Southern Medical Journals, of the beneficial effects of the veratrum viride in the treatment of typhoid fever, typhoid pneumonia, chronic rheumatism, &c.—Dr. Nathan Allen, of Lowell, is said to be preparing an article on the abuse of opiates in Great Britain and the United States, and will thankfully receive any statements of facts from physicians and others bearing upon this subject.

MARRIED,—At Columbus, Ohio, Norman Gay, M.D., to Mrs. L. E. Neiswanger.

DIED,—Dr. Alexander Duncan, formerly a member of Congress from Cincinnati, killed by falling from a wagon—At Curacoa, W. I, James H. Adams, M.D., of yellow fever, late of New York, 31.—In New York, Dr. James Campbell, 57.—In Philadelphia, Prof. Wm. E. Horner, of the University, 60.

Deaths in Boston for the week ending Saturday noon, April 9th, 75. Males, 38—females, 37. Accident, 3—inflammation of the bowels, 1—disease of the brain, 2—bronchitis, 2—consumption, 16—convulsions, 2—cromp, 3—cancer, 1—dropsy, 2—dropsy in the head, 5—infantile diseases, 9—puerperal, 4—erysipelas, 1—typhoid fever, 2—scarlet fever, 4—hooping cough, 1—inflammation of the lungs, 8—disease of the liver, 1—marasmus, 2—old age, 1—poison, 1—rheumatism, 1—teething, 3.

Under 5 years, 40—between 5 and 20 years, 5—between 20 and 40 years, 17—between 40 and 60 years, 8—over 60 years, 5. Born in the United States, 54—Ireland, 18—England, 1—British American Provinces, 2. The above includes 8 deaths in the city institutions.

Treatment of Spontaneous Aneurism by Rest and Absolute Diet.—
Professor Bush, of Lexington, has communicated to me the particulars of
a case of spontaneous aneurism of the abdominal aorta, in which marked
relief of the symptoms seems to have followed the observance of a most
rigid diet.   The patient, Mrs. Anderson, a mid-wife, aged sixty, resides
in Madison county, Kentucky, and has led a very exposed and laborious
life for many years.   When Dr. Bush first saw her, about three months
ago, the tumor, situated just below the stomach, was about the size of a
pullet's egg, and pulsated most violently, emitting all the usual aneurismal
sounds.   The heart was involved in the trouble, laboring, and irregular in
its actions.   Believing that the case would be fatal, Dr. Bush merely advised quietude and absolute diet, barely enough of the lightest and least
stimulating articles to support life.   For a short time she grew worse, and
her physician, Dr. Evans, informed Dr. Bush that a post-mortem examination could be obtained when she died.   Not long afterwards he learned
that, under a rigid adherence to the treatment, the woman was rapidly improving, in fact, getting well, with a decided subsidence of all the local
symptoms.   "This," adds Dr. Bush, "is the whole of my experience in
spontaneous aneurism, excepting one or two cases which I have seen in
the hands of Dr. Dudley, treated in the same manner, but not of Kentucky."

The starving plan of treatment, first recommended by Valsalva, and so
happily employed by Dr. Bush in the above instance, is worthy of the serious consideration of the surgeon in all cases of spontaneous aneurism,
inaccessible to the ligature.   When properly carried out, it may not only
retard the fatal progress of the disease, but occasionally even effect a cure,
especially in the milder and more recent forms of the affection.   Valsalva's plan, as is well known, was to subject his patients to the most perfect
rest in the horizontal posture, and to diminish the quantity of food gradually, till only half a pint of soup was allowed in the morning, and a quarter of a pint in the evening, with a very small quantity of water, medicated with osteocolla, or mucilage of quinces.*   This treatment was aided,
particularly in robust subjects, by the repeated abstraction of blood.   Professor Dudley asserts that he has cured some cases simply by restricted
diet, without the use of the lancet; and a recent foreign journal mentions
several instances of a similar kind relieved by Dr. Bellingham, of Dublin.
—*Dr. Gross's Surgical Report to Kentucky State Medical Society.*

Dr. Bennet Dowler.—Our learned friend and fellow-citizen, Dr. Bennet
Dowler, whose able pen and successful research into national and anti-
quarian history have contributed, at times, so much interest to the
columns of this journal, and whose pamphlets have obtained such
general and deserved fame, has received a letter from Mr. Charles C.
Rafn, secretary of the Royal Society of Northern Antiquarians, at Copen-
hagen, of which the king of Denmark is president, informing the doctor
of their purpose to elect him a fellow of that renowned society, and commending, in the highest terms, his successful prosecution of his enlightened inquiries into science and history.—*N. O. Delta.*

Dr. Dowler's friends at the north will rejoice to hear of the merited honor conferred upon him.

---

* Cooper's Surgical Dictionary, art. aneurism.

THE.

BOSTON MEDICAL AND SURGICAL JOURNAL.

| Vol. XLVIII. | Wednesday, April 20, 1853. | No. 12. |

LECTURES OF M. VALLEIX ON DISPLACEMENTS OF THE UTERUS.

TRANSLATED FROM THE FRENCH BY L. PARKS, JR., M.D.

NUMBER II.

Gentlemen,—Having explained the reasons which have prevented uterine displacements from receiving all the attention they merit, it now becomes my duty to bear witness that they have not been *entirely* ignored by authors till within the last few years, and to lay before you the state of science upon this point.

Historic Sketch.—From all time, as I have before stated, obstetricians have, as a matter of necessity, in consequence of the severity of the symptoms, described displacements produced during pregnancy. But there is so great a difference between displacements during gestation, and those which manifest themselves in the non-pregnant state, that, as well for purposes of study as for those of treatment, these two states should be distinctly separated from each other.

M. Ameline in a very valuable thesis, containing highly useful information on the subject of anteversion, has, like ourselves, examined the history of the question, and has presented it in a very complete manner.

In order to trace the first notions on the subject of displacements of the uterus, we must go back to Hippocrates. And yet, his expressions are so vague, that the question may be entertained whether or not he really has these affections in view. I proceed to cite the principal passages in which he seems to allude to them, in order that you may judge for yourselves.

In the book " De morbis mulierum (edente Foësio, p. 153) he says, " Postquam igitur mulieri quæ nunquam peperit, menses delitescunt neque foras exitum evenire possunt, hic morbus oritur. Id autem contingit si uterorum os conclusum aut *obtortum* fuerit, aut *pudendi pars aliqua inversa*, horum enim alterum si adfuerit, neque mulier viri consuetudine fruatur. "

This phrase has been believed to refer to uterine displacements, although there are but two expressions which can justify such a supposition ; viz., " *os obtortum* " and " *aut pudendi pars aliqua inversa.*" By the first of these two expressions, he evidently designates a torsion of the cervix obstructing the flow of the menses. But, remark the vagueness of the term "*pudendi pars aliqua*"—a term applicable to any portion of the genital organs. You perceive, however, that it is the non-impregnated uterus which is in question, since, in fact, the subject under discussion is that of women who have not yet borne children.

The second passage, occurring in the book " De natura muliebri (edente Van der Linden, op. omn., v. ii., p. 161)," is a little more explicit and is thus conceived :—" Si uteri ad *medium lumborum processerint*, dolor imum ventrem habet, et crura *contrahuntur ;* et quum *alvum exonerat* dolores acutiores fiunt ; et *stercus cum vi prodit* et *urina distillat* et animo linquitur. Quum sic habuerit fistula ad vesicam alligato uteros sufflato et fomentum adhibito."

Further on, he says—" Morbo autem liberabitur ubi conceperit ; *supina etiam pedibus altioribus* decumbat ; posteà *appositas spongias* ex lumbis religato mulier os uterorum corrigat, et dirigat, et suffitum exodoratio adhibeat."

The meaning of "*ad medium lumborum processerint*" is not perfectly clear, unless allusion be made to one of those peculiar movements, which, in the opinion of the ancients, the uterus could execute in the abdominal cavity. But, when Hippocrates speaks of *severe pains in defecation* —of *frequent micturition*—I am much inclined to believe that he wishes to designate a lesion of the uterus approaching to displacement. Meanwhile, I am not quite sure that he had not rather in view the pregnant, than the non-pregnant state, and I ask myself, also, if he has not, instead of displacements, simply described an inflammation of one of the tissues in the neighborhood of the uterus. These inflammations which I have several times had occasion to mention to you in these lectures, having for their principal seat the cellular tissue about the uterus, produce the symptoms of which Hippocrates speaks. Only, these symptoms are more marked on the side of the rectum, if the seat of the inflammation is in the posterior region, whilst if it is in front, or upon the sides, it is the bladder which suffers the most. You perceive, at all events, that for these cases, whatever they may be, he proposes particular modes of treatment. I limit myself to pointing out to you, the *elevation of the lower limbs and of the pelvis*, which has also been latterly advised by Mr. Gerdy ; and the sponges which he places (he does not explain himself very categorically in this respect) behind or in front of the cervix uteri. In regard to the fumigations, I do not dwell upon them, inasmuch as they have no interest for us.

Arriving at Aetius we find a more explicit description, and one which fully satisfies us that he had recognized displacements of the uterus. In his "Tetralogy," ch. 77, he thus expresses himself—" If the inclination of the uterus takes place posteriorly or inferiorly, there follow a numbness and trouble in the lower limbs. Sometimes, even, movement is entirely impossible, or provokes insupportable pains, while constipation becomes so obstinate, that injections cannot pass the rectum except the patient kneel. Gas, even, cannot be discharged. The pains augment when the patient is seated, especially if the inclination takes place towards the pubis. The lower portion of the belly and of the hypogastrium become swollen and painful, and sometimes there is retention of urine."

After this very precise enumeration of the principal symptoms, if we could retain doubts of the nature of the affection he wishes to describe, the mechanical treatment which he proposes would dispel them, as he adds, "whatever the mode of inclination, it must at first be treated as an inflammation or exacerbation of the uterus. If the malady persists, we must *remedy the displacement.* We recommend to the midwife to introduce the *finger into the rectum,* and to place there a *bougie* as a permanent support."

This passage refers very evidently to displacements of the uterus. But it is probable that the author had in mind displacements which are produced during pregnancy, the symptoms he describes being in fact so intense that it seems scarcely possible to refer them to displacements of the non-impregnated uterus. The same inference is to be drawn from the treatment, since it is principally in the displacements which occur in pregnant women, that recourse is had to this manœuvre, which consists in replacing the uterus by means of the finger introduced into the rectum. As to the means recommended for maintaining the uterus in place, it seems to me that the word "bougie" does not perfectly translate the expression "*glandeam,*" employed by the author; and, to be more than probable that he meant to designate by that expression a *tampon* of a certain volume. I point out this fact, because the same means have been resorted to by M. Huguier in our time.

We observe, further, in relation to the species of displacement, that the symptoms described by Aetius refer particularly to *retroversion,* although, in a certain place, he describes phenomena existing on the side of the bladder and of the hypogastrium, in consequence of the inclination of the womb toward the pubis. But, is he speaking here of anteversion, or simply of the pressure exerted in front by the cervix, in consequence of the movement impressed upon it by the backward inclination of the fundus? Details are wanting to enlighten us upon this point.

Ambrose Paré has also taken up the question of abnormal positions of the uterus, but, far from teaching us anything new, he causes us, believing as he does in the migrations of the uterus within the abdomen, to fall back amid the vague notions where we found ourselves before reading the passage of Aetius which I have just cited to you. You will find the passage to which I allude in vol. 2d of his "Œuvres Complètes" (Paris, 1841, édit. Malgaigne, p. 752).

Among the authors who more recently have occupied themselves with these affections, I will cite Morgagni, who in letter 46, §16, reports a case of displacement caused by an engorgement of the liver and spleen. Then comes Levret (Journ. de Méd. de Vandermonde, 1773), who in his capacity of obstetrician occupies himself particularly with displacements during gestation, without, however, neglecting these affections in the non-pregnant state, as he is one of the first, who, since Hippocrates, has recognized the existence of retroversion in the virgin. It was at this epoch that a discussion commenced, which has continued till our time, upon the possibility of uterine displacements apart from gestation. Jahn (Sillog. oper. minor, etc.; quam curavit D. J. T. C. Schtegel, tome i., p.

612 ; cited by M. Lacroix, Ann. de la chir. franc. et étrang., tome xiii., page 420 et seq., 1845) has asserted that complete retroversion cannot exist except in pregnant women ; and other authors have supported this opinion. But, to-day, there can no longer be any doubt for those who have examined patients, and it will suffice for you to pass a few minutes in our wards, in order to establish the existence of a number of cases of uterine displacement in the non-impregnated uterus. William Schmitt (Remarques et expér. sur la rétrov. de l'utérus * * * Vienne, 1820) has reported numerous examples of them. His observations have been since cited by several authors, especially by M. Lacroix. After his paper, we find a number of works, of which it will be sufficient for me to cite the principal. These are an important treatise by M. Martin the younger, of Lyons (Mém. sur la rétrov.) ; the theses of M. Bazin (De la rétrov., 1827), and numerous articles scattered among the different treatises on obstetrics.

Thence, we enter upon a period during which these diseases have been studied in a more fitting manner, and with all the care that they merit. It is difficult, even at the present time, to add anything to the description of the symptoms which was given in 1827 by M. Ameline (Essai sur l'antéversion de l'utérus * * * *). In his thesis on anteversion, that author admits two degrees of derangement according as the uterus occupies a position entirely horizontal, or, on the contrary, lies with its fundus lower than the cervix, in such a manner that the latter being closely invested (coiffé) by the posterior *cul-de-sac* of the vagina, there may be retention of the uterine mucus, and even of the menses. Admitting fully the existence of the first degree, I must say that the second is at least extremely rare—having, for my part, never met it. I have often seen the cervix situated in the same horizontal plane as the body, having its opening directed backward, and situated high up so as to be very difficult to reach with the finger, but not more elevated than the body.

More than this, M. Ameline was the first to describe and to give its name to *anteflexion*. He also proposed the name of *retroflexion*, doubtless, however, from the expression of John (Diss. de utero retroflex, 1787), a denomination which has also passed into general use.

M. Lacroix having occasion to treat the question of uterine displacements as a subject of a thesis in a *concours*, engaged in researches which he has since continued, and the results of which he published in 1845 (loc. cit.). This work contains more numerous historical references than that of M. Ameline, and, in addition, observations borrowed from other authors. But, although the title of his book was "*anteversion and retroversion of the uterus*," he confines himself almost entirely to retroversion, a detailed description of which is followed by general remarks. Mad. Boivin and M. Dugès (Traité pratique des Maladies de l'Uterus, p. 136) have furnished interesting cases which have been borrowed by other authors. Finally, M. Hervez de Chégoin (Mém. de l'Acad. Roy. de Méd., v. ii., p. 319, 1833) has published a memoir followed by several articles, in which he treats of the different uterine deviations, and proposes a particular mode of treatment.

Such was the state of science on this subject, when, in 1843, Prof. Simpson, of Edinburgh, published his first paper treating of displacements of the uterus (Contributions to the Pathol. and Treat. of Diseases of the Uterus ; the Lond. and Edin. Monthly Journal, v. iii.). It is only very incidentally that he speaks of these diseases, because, considering the question from the most general point of view, the author is occupied chiefly with the diagnosis of diseases of the uterus, and with the employment of the sound as·a means of exploring this organ.

This work is divided into two parts, the first containing a series of propositions tending to demonstrate the utility of physical means, and of the sound in particular, for the exploration of the uterus. This part concerns us little, and will even seem to you idle. But you must recollect that Dr. Simpson practices in a country where these means of exploration were, till of late, but little used ; where even the question has been agitated of rejecting them entirely as immoral. And you are not unacquainted with the excessively warm and personal discussion which Dr. Bennet has had to sustain upon this subject. It is not then astonishing that Prof. Simpson felt obliged to commence by combating these prejudices. The second part is devoted to the description of the uterine sound, and to the demonstration of its utility. The sound that I present to you is that which he has described and employed. I do not know whether or not he has since accepted the modifications to which it has been subjected in order to reduce this excessive curvature. It is divided into inches and half inches English, and presents prominences and depressions at determinate distances, to enable the finger to recognize the length to which the sound has penetrated into the cavity of the uterus, without the necessity of withdrawing it for that purpose from the vagina. The first prominence is situated at five inches English from the point of the sound, there being between these two points a depression situated at the distance of two and a half inches from each. The utility of this instrument will be perfectly demonstrated to you, when we come to speak of the diagnosis of displacements of the uterus.

In this first paper of Prof. Simpson, there is no mention made of his instrument for the complete replacement of the uterus, nor of the radical cure of displacements. It was not till 1848 that he published a new paper "upon the frequency, the diagnosis and the treatment of retroflexion or retroversion of the non-impregnated uterus," Dublin Quarterly Journal, vol. v.). He allows no distinction between retroflexion and retroversion, which, according to him, are merely different degrees of the same disease separated by shades very slightly perceptible. I shall recur at a future time to this opinion, which has some foundation, but which I do not entirely share, because, if it be admitted to the full extent, there would be less perspicuity in the description of the diseases under consideration ; and because, on the other hand, there exists some difference in the symptoms according as there is a simple retroversion or a retroflexion, although this difference may disappear little by little and by slight shades in the series of cases which unites each of the two extremes.

A*s* to anteversion, we have only, according to Prof. Simpson, to apply to that, what has been-said upon retroversion. This might be admissible if we had regard only to the deviation of the axis of the uterus. But, the organs which may be compressed not being precisely the same in the two cases, there results often a difference in the symptoms. Without doubt, the treatment is the same, although here again in its application there are important shades of difference to seize, since if they be neglected our success may be thereby compromised.

Prof. Simpson is one of those who regard the speculum as useless in the diagnosis of uterine displacements. But, you recollect the reasons which have led us to regard this statement as too sweeping, a point to the consideration of which we shall return in another place. It is a matter of regret that this paper neither furnishes details of the observations on which it is based, nor gives the date of the first application of the pessary it describes, the latter point being important as answering any questions concerning the priority of invention.

Thus M. Velpeau apprized us in his remarks before the Académie de Médecine (discussion of 1849) that he had some fifteen years before conceived the idea of sustaining the uterus by introducing into its cavity a stem supported by a half-disc of caoutchouc, which he turned sometimes in front and sometimes behind, according as he had a retroversion or an anteversion.*

As to Prof. Simpson—he employed, in the beginning, not a half-disc, but a complete disc, supporting a similar stem which he introduced into the uterus. This disc was maintained in the vagina like a common pessary. As its introduction was difficult and embarrassing, he at first caused a joint to be constructed at the junction of the stem with the disc, in order that the whole might penetrate more easily into the vagina.

Later he renounced this contrivance in favor of another instrument with which 1 will make you acquainted hereafter.† Although I have seen in an English Journal (" On Malposition of the Unimpregnated Uterus," &c., by Thomas Lightfoot ; the Medical Times, Sept. 20th, 1851) a representation of a similar instrument attributed to M. Velpeau, I think no claim has been laid to its authorship by that professor, and that there has been some confusion in the mind of the writer of the article.

Following Dr. Simpson, many English and American physicians have given their attention to uterine displacements. I will only mention Drs: Protheroe Smith (Obstetric Record, p. 35), Beattie (Dublin Journal, 1847), Rigby (Med. Times, 1849), Samuel Edwards (Provinc. Med. and Surg. Jour., 1849), Bond (Amer. Jour. of Med. Sc., 1849), Mac Cready (Amer. Trans., 1849), Cumming (Edinb. Month. Jour., 1849), &c. These names will re-appear when we come to speak of the points which they have specially studied.

---

* The translator ventures to ask if it be not high time the maxim were generally adopted that, as far at least as the public is concerned, the *real inventor* is not he who first conceives the idea of a particular mechanism, or first undertakes experiments tending to its elaboration, but he who conducts such experiments to a successful issue, and gives the benefit of them to the world

† M. Valleix (unless I err as to the instruments to which he refers) is somewhat mistaken in stating that Prof. Simpson has renounced the pessary above described. Dr. S. still uses it, as I know from personal observation, and, I think, employs it quite as often as the second instrument alluded to in the text.—TRANS.

You recollect the discussion which took place at the Académie de Médecine, on the occasion of a paper by M. Baud, " On Displacements and Engorgements of the Uterus and their means of cure." In this discussion were engaged MM. Velpeau, Huguier, Malgaigne, Dubois, Hervez de Chégoin, Amussat, Gibert, Moreau, Roux, Jobert, Récamier, all authors who have attended with care to diseases of the uterus, and who, therefore, were qualified to elucidate the matter. Unfortunately, the question was badly stated, so that it is difficult to distinguish what place the author of the paper intended to assign to engorgements and what to displacements. The confusion in the language of the paper was re-produced in the discourses pronounced on this occasion. Since then, M. Huguier and M. Amussat have proposed special modes of treatment with which I shall make you acquainted in the course of these lessons.

Finally, we have lately had at the *Ecole de Paris* three theses on displacements of the uterus.' The first is that of M. Dufraigne (*De la retroflexion,* thèse, Paris, 1851). It contains several cases from the wards of M. Huguier at the *Hopital Beaujon.* In the second, which we owe to M. Grimaud (*De l'anteversion de la matrice,* thèse, Paris, 1852), we have a discussion of the means employed by Prof. Simpson to replace the uterus, and the modifications to which we have subjected this instrument. Lastly, the third—that of M. Piachaud of Geneva, one of the most distinguished *internes* of the Paris Hospitals, was " defended " in the month of March of the present year. Its title is " Displacements of the unimpregnated uterus" After a well-described symptomatology, founded upon some cases reported with rigorous exactness, it contains details of treatment, and an explanation of the most recent modifications, which I have engrafted upon Dr. Simpson's method of remedying displacements, with a description of the apparatus which we daily employ.

To conclude, I will remind you that in 1851 and 1852 I inserted in the " *Bulletin de Thérapeutique* " two articles describing my modifications of Prof. Simpson's instruments, as well as of the manner of using the apparatus, and that Dr. Gaussail gave in the " *Journal de Médecine de Toulouse* " (1851) a very accurate and very excellent report of lectures delivered by me at *l'Hotel Dieu de Toulouse,* and before the Société de Médecine of that city.

DR. KING'S ADDRESS ON QUACKERY—ITS CAUSES AND EFFECTS.

[Continued from page 215.]

I must notice another cause of complaint, although it is rather a delicate subject. I allude to the improper neighborhood interference with the sick. When a person is known to be confined by sickness, the neighbors generally turn out to visit him ; sometimes from motives of benevolence, and often from mere curiosity. A few, perhaps, will find their way to the parlor, and others be seated in the kitchen. Each one is big with some sage advice, which she is very desirous to deliver herself of. One of the first inquiries is, who is the doctor? If a visiter has herself employed some new quack, or seen his advertisement, she has a great curiosity to see his treatment tried, and therefore insists upon his being called ; or if her favorite is already in attendance, she must assist him by some additional prescription of her own. Every visiter must prescribe something before she will leave the premises. She has seen just such cases before, or been in a similar condition herself, and can tell what, if anything, will cure. She must examine the medicine, and inform the patient whether it will agree or disagree with his constitution, and suggest the propriety of changing the treatment if it should not cure immediately. Every new visiter has some special advice to give, until the patient and his friends are bewildered and confounded ; and unless they are people of intelligence and firmness, they are liable to be led astray. Aunt Betty and Aunt Thankful are such good neighbors, such constant visiters, so very kind, the patient and his friends would be very sorry to offend them. They will certainly be very angry if their advice is not immediately complied with. Therefore, to please these good creatures, the prescription of an experienced and skilful physician is thrown aside as soon as his back is turned, because Aunt Betty don't think it best for the patient to take such medicine, and because she knows of something better. If the patient dies, it is because the doctor knew nothing ; and if he recovers, the neighbors cured him. Such measures are often carried on so slyly as to escape the notice of the attend-' ing physician, and when he supposes that he alone has charge of the patient, some officious nurse or neighbor is superintendent and prime manager, and disposes of his prescriptions and directions as she pleases ; and when she pleases, turns him off for whom or what she prefers. This course of proceeding not only annoys and provokes the physician, but endangers the patient, and often renders abortive the best medical means. It degrades the physician to a level with the most ignorant adviser. This is a prolific fountain of mischief that seems destined never to dry up. Its bitter waters flow over this whole country, poisoning the public mind and quickening and nourishing the germs of quackery. Every new pretender is careful to get into the good graces and make sure of the services of some such satellites to herald his skill and proclaim his success. This is no small matter. It is a grave subject. The dishonor done to our profession and the evils inflicted upon society by such means, are incalculable. I allow that there are very few wellbred, refined, intelligent, considerate persons who are guilty of such conduct. I know that it is done mostly by a class of low, thoughtless persons, who instead of minding their own business, undertake the care of a whole neighborhood. I know that the most refined and discreet are the least apt to meddle in such matters ; and this circumstance, instead of helping the matter, gives the whole business to a set of low gossips, who are always on hand wherever they are countenanced.

To guard against all such interference, the physician should always be careful to give all necesssary directions as to food, drink, clothing and management of every kind, so that there may be no call for advice in any of these particulars. His directions should be given with authority, and at each returning visit he should be careful to see that every minutia has been attended to. Every officious meddler should be kindly but firmly rebuked, and the family of the patient be made to understand that the directions of an attending physician are not to be countermanded with impunity. Let the separate provinces of the physician and the nurse be well defined; and if the latter is allowed to assume the duties of the former, the physician should not be contented to come in as a partner, but surrender the whole.

Another thing which does much to degrade the profession and embarrass its members, is the universal, indiscriminate and unlimited credit which attends the practice of many physicians. The compensation is so meagre and so tardy, that physicians as a class are poor, if we except those who have acquired property by other than professional means. Such ought not to be the case. Every well-educated physician has made a large investment of capital in his preparation for practice, and when his arduous, irksome and responsible duties are required, that capital and those services ought to afford him a fair and prompt remuneration. In general, there can be no good reason why the bills of physicians should not be settled as often and as readily as the bills of grocers, butchers or tailors; and such physicians as let their bills lie year after year, without presenting them for settlement, not only injure themselves, but disparage the profession generally. The public are not so much to blame in this particular, as those physicians who set such examples and adopt such practices; and as the fault is mainly our own, so the remedy is in our own hands. If physicians generally would set themselves to work to correct this crying evil, by endeavoring to make regular settlements, they would soon find themselves better off, their services held in higher estimation, and their patients better pleased. The physician may be sufficiently charitable and indulgent, and at the same time make all reasonable and seasonable collections; but if he gives the public to understand that he considers his services of little value, he will have no reason to complain if that public adopt the same opinion. Every practitioner should endeavor to make his services really valuable, to satisfy his employers that they are so, and demand a reasonable compensation for them. If he fails to do this, he is a poor physician. It is notorious that a considerable share of the business of most physicians is never paid for; and the public appear to think that it is the bounden duty of all physicians to go at every beck and call, regardless of compensation, and whoever refuses to do so is thought to be remiss in duty and unmerciful. This mistaken notion has existed so long that it seems to have become a settled principle in public opinion, and at this time probably more than one fourth of all the medical service done in New England is never paid for at all, and some practitioners never collect one half of their charges. Consequently many a practitioner, who has labored hard all his life, leaves his family with little more than a mass of unsettled accounts, which, had they been paid as they should have been, would have made a good estate. This condition of things is very wrong. Many who never pay their physician, pay all their other debts punctually; and those who are absolutely unable to pay, should be provided for by the public. Physicians are under no more legal or moral obligations to labor for nothing, than any other class of men ; and this the public should be made distinctly to understand. With most other men, the evening of a well-spent life is rendered more comfortable by relaxation and retirement from business. The merchant or the mechanic often retires in independence, surrounded by all the comforts of life, to recline upon beds of down and enjoy that repose which the infirmities of declining years demand. Not so with the physician. The more eminent the man, the more urgent are the calls for his services. As his physical powers decline, his labors increase. Nothing but a total disability is sufficient to excuse him. And when his trembling limbs can no longer endure fatigues, watchings and privations, when he is literally worn out, he is given up and set at naught ; and though he may " still live," he is soon forgotten. Once his smile gave hope, his sadness despair ; now, " none is so poor to do him reverence." He descends to his grave unhonored and unwept. No matter how eminent or how important have been his services. No matter how many anxious days and sleepless nights he has endured in the cause of humanity. No matter how many years of unrewarded labor he has spent, standing between his patients and their last enemy. The winds of winter pass over him, and he is remembered no more. Not so with clergymen and statesmen. They are venerated in life and eulogized in death ; some friendly angel records their merits in gold, and they are embalmed in history.

I know that it is much easier to complain of evils than to find remedies for them ; and I know, also, that there are many evils which inevitably attend the profession of medicine, that no human efforts can remove. Yet there are some others which may be partially or entirely cured. It is vain to think of putting down quackery by declaring open war against it. If you attempt to overthrow it by reasoning, you will find your arguments wasted. If you attack it with invectives and sarcasm, you help to build it up by creating a sympathy for its authors. But leave the vile miscreants in their own filthiness, and take care to improve, unite and build up an educated profession, and the work is half accomplished. Nothing short of this can do it ; all other efforts are impotent.

Much would be gained by taking measures to mark more strongly and distinctly the line of separation between physicians and quacks, by showing the world the wide distance between a class of educated and honorable men, and a set of ignorant pretenders. And for this purpose, every qualified physician should become a member of some regular medical society. This should be considered an indispensable measure, which the interest and honor of the profession and the safety of society imperiously demand ; and whoever, after sufficient opportunity, refuses or neglects to do so, should be considered guilty of a dereliction of duty. I am aware that there are at the present time some good practitioners who, owing to their own carelessness, or their remote location, or some personal pique against some particular member, have neglected to unite with the regular society. All such should be kindly invited to come in. On the one hand, medical schools and medical societies should cautiously guard against the admission of incompetent or unworthy members, and on no account allow their established rules to be set aside to accommodate particular cases; and on the other hand, all proper efforts should be made to bring in every worthy practitioner. The barrier that separates scientific medicine from ignorance and imposture, should be high as the mountains and firm as adamant. It should be apparent to all observers, that there was nothing without, worthy of notice. When an individual assumes the high and responsible station of physician, and receives his professional honors, he takes upon himself obligations to the profession and to society ; he tacitly engages to regard the welfare of both. It is said that Hippocrates required all those whom he instructed, first to take a solemn oath, the principal obligations of which were to be faithful to the sick and sustain unblemished the honor of the profession. The substance of that oath should be had in perpetual recognition. Every physician should be conscious that he is not living for himself alone, but for his profession and for society.

There is a class of practitioners, most of them elderly men, who appear to suppose that they have no other obligations than those which begin and end with themselves. Each pursues his own independent course, having very litttle to do with either medical men or medical books. Their practice is fixed. It always was and always will be about the same thing. They are too wise to learn, and too old to be taught new tricks. And these are the men who make the loudest and most doleful outcries against quacks and quackery. Everything which disturbs the even tenor of their way is sure to receive their unqualified denunciation. Now of all men these have the least reason to complain of quackery. They are its very founders and supporters. Through their means it has sprung up and been sustained, and they are in a measure responsible for the whole of it. For it was to avoid them that men had recourse to quack remedies. A whole community shudders at the contemplation of a Dr. Jalap, and to escape his clutches they fly to Dr. Saccharum, or anything else. If the thing ended here, it might be of little consequence. But it is not so. Men of this stamp are taken for samples of the regular practice. This is called the old mineral system, and everything, except some nice new quackery, is supposed to be of the same sort. But this is a mistake. Those who suppose that there are few or no improvements making in scientific medicine, at the present time, and those who suppose that every new scheme is a real improvement, are alike, mistaken. Within the last half century, medicine has certainly undergone greater improvements than any other profession. A vast amount of severe labor has been bestowed upon it, both in this country and Europe. Old theories have been corrected or exploded by physiological and pathological investigations. New remedies have been discovered, and the treatment of diseases has been changed from a heroic practice to one milder, safer and more pleasant, and I think more successful. Whoever has been in practice for the last twenty years, and has not been borne along by this tide of improvement, and made wiser and better thereby, is certainly in the back ground and far behind the times. He has neglected his duty to himself, to his profession and to society, and if the public leave him where he has left himself, he will have no right to complain. Every supposed improvement, from whatever source it may have originated, has been examined and tested, and either registered and treasured up as valuable, or discarded as worthless ; so that the public may be well assured that whatever is ultimately rejected by the profession, is not worth retaining, and whoever pretends to possess any important medical knowledge that is not taught in our regular medical schools, or cannot be learned from our publications, is himself an impostor.

[To be concluded next week.]

EXPERIMENTS TO DETERMINE THE TRUTH OF MARSHALL HALL'S THEORY RESPECTING EPILEPSY.

To the Editor of the Boston Medical and Surgical Journal.

Sir,—Some time ago, I read in the New York Medical Times an extract from a letter of Dr. Marshall Hall upon the induction of simulative epilepsy of the laryngeal kind, with strychnine, and its suspension by tracheotomy. I at once determined to try the experiment upon at least ten goats. Accordingly I engaged several, having a few myself, and I herewith send you the result of the first experiment, which was made to-day. From the notes, you will see there was a failure to produce the results of Dr. Hall ; but nevertheless, I conceive his position plausible, and this experiment not a fair one ; consequently I shall continue the series, and keep you informed of the issue. I selected the goat for the experiments, from the fact, that in point of intelligence it approaches man as near as any of the animal tribe. I intend to institute a still further series of investigations in *transfusion, neurology, poisoning,* &c., of which I shall keep my brethren duly and fairly informed.

March 30th, 1853.—Present, Dr. Griffin. A young male goat, in fine health, was placed in the enclosure, and one eighth of a grain of pure and tested strychnine given him, at precisely 15 minutes before 9, A.M. In 10 minutes after the dose, evident signs of venereal excitement presented themselves. At 9 o'clock some cough supervened, with twitching of the muscles of the neck, and a tendency to run back. At 5 minutes past 9, he looked dejected, with twitching of the muscles of the neck and limbs. At 15 minutes after 9, the goat not being further affected, we gave him one eighth of a grain more of the strychnine. At 30 minutes after 9, the *priapism and tendency to run backwards were on the increase slightly.* At 45 after 9, no further increase being made, we gave him one fourth of a grain more. At this juncture he leaped through a crack in the pen, and ran off into the barley lot, very intent at grazing. The *priapism increased* in a few minutes, but the twitching was not so evident. At 55 minutes after 9, he was still grazing heartily, as if the strychnine had given him a relish for *burley ; priapism yet up.* At 20 minutes after 10, he had ate heartily, and the twitching had subsided. We haltered him and gave him one half of a grain of strychnine, and placed him in the enclosure again. In five minutes extreme *priapism and urination* appeared, with faint twitching. At 40 minutes after 10, we left him, and returned to the enclosure at 30 minutes past

11, when we found him lying very calmly and quietly in the corner of the pen, chewing his cud. At our approach he sloped through a large hole and made his escape, bidding defiance to us and our strychnine. At 1, P.M., we caught him and gave him another dose of strychnine, *a full grain.* He jumped off in the barley patch again, and while I close this article (4, P.M.), he is enjoying a delightful repast upon his vernal pasturage.

The only thing I have discovered in this trial, is the evident production of *venereal excitement—priapism,* with small muscular twitchings. That the strychnine was good, I have abundant evidence in the number of crows I have poisoned with it, and also the dead rats I have thrown out of my office this morning. But notwithstanding this failure, I have not a doubt but Dr. Hall is correct, and I shall try the experiment again and again. Respectfully, **H. A. Ramsay, M.D.**

Thompson, Geo., March 30, 1853.

THROAT INSTRUMENTS—THE LONDON LANCET.

To the Editor of the Boston Medical and Surgical Journal.

Dear Sir,—Our English progenitors on the other side the water, taken individually, I have ever regarded as the most high-minded and honorable race of men to be found ; and a well-bred English physician I have supposed incapable of any other than the exactest propriety in his intercourse with his brethren at home or abroad. In reading a brief editorial in the last London Lancet, I am pained to feel that this favorable judgment may have been too universally applied.

Under the head of "new inventions," the editors speak of various instruments for making topical applications to the throat. They first introduce and describe Dr. Horace Green's spatula and probang, which they say was manufactured for them, under Dr. Green's personal inspection (while in London we presume) by Mr. Coxeter."

They next introduce " Dr. Ira Warren's shower syringes, three in number, very neatly made, and contained in a neat case," which they describe with tolerable correctness, but they object that in their hands they are not "easily applicable in practice." "In fact," they say, "the safety of the glass syringe and the piston can only be secured by the use of both hands (!)—of which one is required for holding down the tongue."

After alluding to one or two other syringes which appear to be of little account, as they do not describe them, they say—

"Mr. Coxeter's laryngeal shower syringe [Mr. Coxeter, the reader will see from the second paragraph, is the editors' manufacturer] is by far the most convenient form in which a syringe can be used for these applications to the interior of the throat and the posterior nares. It consists of a seamless tube, composed of silver, not unlike that of a medium-sized catheter. It is curved in a form suitable to its intended uses. The distal extremity is somewhat flattened from side to side, and is perforated by fine openings, which admit of the emission of the contained

fluid in the form of a delicate shower. The proximal extremity is fitted with an elastic suction-bottle, which, by its own action, charges the
instrument with the fluid, which is then emitted by simply compressing
the bottle with the thumb. Rings are attached for holding the little instrument, and an ingenious arrangement is made, by which the quantity
of fluid ejected can be accurately regulated. The inventor says this
shower syringe possesses the advantage of applying gently, and without
friction, to an irritable surface, the remedial agent intended to be employed. It does this more generally and uniformly than the sponge,
and is entirely free from the risk to which the latter, in becoming detached from the whalebone, is liable. Our experience in the use of the
instrument entirely corresponds with this favorable report of the inventor."

If you had never before heard of either of these syringes, Mr. Editor,
you could not infer from the above that one of them had any claim
to paternity of the other, or was in any sense more entitled to consideration except on the ground of its better adaptation to the end proposed.
You would not know, from the article in the *Lancet*, Dr. Ira Warren's
residence, or even that he was an American. You will be surprised to
learn, therefore, that about the first of August, 1852, I put a neat set of
my shower syringes into a package, with one of my tonsil instruments,
and sent them as a present to the editors of the London Lancet, accompanied by a brief note, expressed in as civil terms as I could employ,
asking them to accept my small offering to the profession in England ;
and if they deemed the instruments of any value, to make them known.
Seven months have passed, and no private note has acknowledged their
reception. In the meantime, it seems, the syringes have been put into
the hands of Mr. Coxeter, their manufacturer, who has made one *on the
same principle*, merely adding an India-rubber bag to it, and nearly
spoiling it, as the reader will soon see, by his attempted improvements.
The editors then call him the "*inventor*"! saying nothing about his
having stolen it from me, or the manner in which they had abused private confidence in helping him do it.

Had these gentlemen noticed my instruments on their reception—commending to such extent as they thought proper, and objecting as their
judgment dictated ; had they then waited till Mr. Coxeter had made his
alterations, and on their completion announced that he had attempted,
and, in their judgment, effected a real *improvement* on my instrument ;
however easily their criticisms might have been set aside, no objection
could have been raised to their proceeding, much less could any im-
peachment have been brought against their motives. But to withhold
my invention seven months from the profession in England, and then
to announce it simultaneously with Mr. Coxeter's instrument, as if they
were two rival claimants, seeking, on equal terms, professional favor, was a
proceeding very like concerted fraud, based on a violation of private
confidence.

Let us now look at the two instruments. The only objection raised
against mine is, that the glass barrel and piston are not safe with those
editors, unless they use both hands ! I don't know how they would

manage to break the glass. Would they dash it against the teeth of the patient? They could not, for it is not the glass syringe, but the silver tube only, which enters the mouth. Would they crush the barrel between their fingers? I doubt their ability to do it if they would, and cannot conceive a good motive for it if they could. Would they drop it in the act of using it? I think not, unless it burned them. During the last three years I have used these syringes about nine thousand times, always with one hand, depressing the tongue with the other, and have never broken a piston or a barrel. I employ them with the same ease that I do a spoon in feeding myself, and should as soon think of applying both hands to the one as to the other. I have found no American physician who could not use them readily with one hand.

The rings which Mr. Coxeter has attached to his instrument are not original, having been long used on aural and other syringes. They would have been attached to my syringes, but that they would have increased the expense, while the instruments are quite as easily used without them.

The distal extremity of Mr. Coxeter's instrument is flattened from side to side. If the globe is retained and flattened, any mechanic can see in a moment that it cannot be as easily insinuated into the larynx as a perfect sphere. Moreover, in withdrawing it, the various projecting parts of the throat would catch upon its shoulders, and slide off with less facility than from a globe. If the sphere is wholly removed, as the cut in the Lancet seems to indicate, then the point is too sharp, and no prudent physician would risk the chances of wounding the throat by its use. In any view of the case, there seems to be no better reason for the alteration than the desire to *appear* to furnish a new instrument, while in fact it is only mine a little altered for the worse in shape.

As to the rubber bottle at the other end, it is wholly unfit for the purpose intended. Its self-acting mode of charging the instrument is alone sufficient to condem it. No sportsman who intends to bring down his game, would think of charging his piece by some self-acting machine which would be liable to draw in twice as much, or twice as little, powder as he desired. In brief, no prudent man needlessly puts anything beyond his control, which needs to be done accurately. Moreover, the rubber bag, by the action of acids, &c., would necessarily soon become intolerably foul; and no person of cleanly habits would permit a fluid to be injected from it into the throat.

I have spoken freely, for I confess to a feeling of indignation. Men who stand, like the editors of the Lancet, at the portals of professional opinion, should be men of large and liberal souls, who are disposed to give any new thought or instrument that comes to them, clear papers of "safe conduct," to travel anywhere—to fame or to oblivion, without improper molestation, and especially without a *seven months' imprisonment.*

The truth is—and there are times when it should be told—that in the construction of ships and boats, locomotives, farming implements, several kinds of machinery, surgical instruments, &c., the Americans are far in advance of the English. While it is clear that the latter are slow to

acknowledge this, I did not suppose any respectable Englishman would resort to anything unfair or deceptive, with a view to *appropriate* what belongs on this side the water.   I. WARREN.
Boston, April 13, 1853.

THE BOSTON MEDICAL AND SURGICAL JOURNAL.

BOSTON, APRIL 20, 1853.

Female Hygiene.—E. J. Tilt, M.D., of London, a good writer, whose views and teachings are of the first class, has favored the world with a book of 436 pages, under the comprehensive title of "Elements of Health and Principles of Female Hygiene." Dr. Tilt says it is intended to supply a desideratum. The health and diseases of man are as familiar topics as the stars, but no one has distinctly written on the constitution of woman and her peculiar diseases, in the manner in which he has done it. He has the ground, therefore, to himself. We cannot perceive that there is much in the work that is not known to physicians ; but there is enough in it quite new to the ladies, and sufficiently divested of scientific display to be understood by them to their advantage. Multitudes of females entertain the opinion that their own physical organization is a secret with themselves. They do not know that science has brought it within the domain of investigation. Those best informed, however, express their surprise at the amount of information collected, explanatory of their bodily construction, yet still insisting upon it, that no one but a woman can comprehend the physiological laws that govern their being. If they will put themselves in communication with the physiological researches which have been made in this matter, they will comprehend their own ignorance, and acknowledge their obligations to the profound investigations of medical men. On the subject of marriage, Dr. Tilt conveys an amount of information that will be found of great importance to women. He shows why old men should not be united to young girls, and the reasons, too, for objecting to other matrimonial connections. But besides the discussion of topics relating to the marital relations of woman, the diseases to which she is incident, and by which her thread of life is so often prematurely broken or her sufferings protracted, are faithfully described. This treatise is for the instruction of females rather than of the sterner sex ; yet it may prove serviceable to the medical practitioner, not so much from its minuteness in describing symptoms, as for the scheme of generalization which pervades its pages.

Legitimate Medicine and the Massachusetts Medical Society.—Report says that a paper is about receiving the names of petitioners, to the Mass. Medical Society, requesting the adoption of measures by which the homœopathic members of the society shall be excluded from the same ; and if such measures are not adopted, then it is stated the memorialists will themselves sever their connection with the society. Perhaps rumor may have exaggerated the determination of the dissatisfied ; but that something is contemplated, of a decisive character, in relation to the homœopathists in our state society, is generally credited. Should a strong demonstration be made to thrust them out, it is impossible to divine the condition in which all parties will find themselves when the smoke of party feeling clears up. Several estimable, highly-educated young physicians, who have complied with every demand of the University, and studied under the best masters of medicine, have abandoned every precept and principle recognized in the schools, and turned homœopathic practitioners. What is to be their destiny? Are they empirics, irregular practitioners in every sense, and therefore justly denounced by those with whom they formerly associated? This, and similar questions, will naturally arise, and they must be met without equivocation.

Organic and Physiological Chemistry.—Daniel Breed, M.D., of the U. S. Patent Office, is the translator of Dr. Carl Löwig's Principles of Organic and Physiological Chemistry, which will be appreciated by all who cultivate that grand department of science. It is intended for a text-book—containing not only all the old discoveries, but also all the new facts, says the preface, relating to the animal and vegetable kingdoms. Dr. Draper, of New York, would never have allowed it to be dedicated to himself, did he not entertain a favorable opinion of the work. We cannot at present do much more than announce its appearance. The Messrs. Hart, late Carey & Hart, of Philadelphia, are the publishers. The volume is a good sized octavo, of 481 pages. There is a strict technicality about it, that will suit advanced students. For mere popular study, it seems not to have been intended by the author. Profound research and deep learning pervade every page throughout.

Principles of Botany.—"The Principles of Botany, as exemplified in the Cryptogamia," by Hartland Coultas, is a little book, but treating of important subjects. Part first treats of the simple elementary organs of plants; the second is devoted to compound—and both are illustrated by diagrams. Any body might understand the elements of the science with this economical and plain assistant. A general mistake pervades text-books, the authors proceeding as though the pupil was as perfectly familiar with all the terms and propositions, as themselves. In this modest duodecimo, learning is truly made easy. Messrs. Lindsay & Blakiston are the publishers.

Colonial Medical Degrees.—There is an uproar among the brotherhood in Canada. The Legislature have been trying to accommodate one party, but have offended the other. They have law, but no order. A special committee, to whom was referred a bill to amend the laws relative to the practice of physic, surgery and midwifery in Lower Canada, reported. But the commotion has not been allayed. A. Hall, M.D., an able, learned member of the faculty in McGill College, has come forward with a pamphlet, addressed to the Colonial Parliament, in which he pleads with the fervency of an experienced advocate for the rights and dignity of the profession. Notwithstanding the admission that Englishmen have an inalienable right to die in any manner they please, Dr. Hall insists that the Legislature are obligated to consider the good of the whole. In other words, quacks ought not to be tolerated, even if there is a minority of fools willing to employ them. It has been found impossible thus to regulate medical practice by law in Massachusetts; and in the Canadas, it is morally certain that no act of parliament, abridging the privilege of the people in taking pretended remedies from irresponsible persons, can long be enforced. In marriage and medicine, the law is powerless beyond a certain point.

Medical Advertising.—Various matters connected with this subject are receiving increased attention at the present time. Last week a few of the reasons were alluded to, which have induced medical gentlemen, in respectable standing, to relieve themselves of the embarrassments imposed by regulations which define all advertising to be quackery. The evasions of these regulations are certainly numerous, and often ingenious, and are practised in conformity with a supposed inalienable right of introducing themselves to the public. Every order of tradesmen, merchant and mechanic, state openly in the papers what they can do, as well as what they have to sell. If nothing improbable is promised, nothing held forth that is not strictly just towards others, such notices are considered proper and are a convenience to the individuals and the public. Those in want of the personal service or wares of the advertiser, go where the service or commodity is to be had. A severe attack in the N. York Medical Gazette, on one or two Boston physicians, who are accused of having openly violated, in their advertising cards, the common code of observances recognized by an educated profession, seems to have put a new train of thoughts in motion. It will not be denied that those practising and advertising specialties have a great advantage over those who are in general practice and therefore have no standing advertisements in the daily papers or periodicals. Were a general practitioner to keep a similar notification in type, saying that he practised in cases of diseased liver—that he had given unusual attention to the treatment of typhus fever, the croup, scarlatina, &c., or the whole of them, he would be expelled from his connection with any regular medical association of which he might be a member. On the other hand, if a gentleman advertises that he is practising exclusively on the eye, the ear, throat, or confines himself especially to dropsies, not a word of reproof follows. Here is a difference which does not seem reasonable, and gives cause for complaint. A suggestion worth turning over in the mind, has been presented from a source that commands respect—although we by no means consider it a weighty argument. It is, that empirics make their fortunes by this very plan which is forbidden to the regular physician. One thing is certain—viz., that no progress is allowed in this direction. While all other interests in the world are being modified by the circumstances of the age—no deviation from the perpendicular legislation of the founders of medical fraternities, has been tolerated. If any one will have the kindness to propose a scheme to obviate the difficulties of the case, for the purpose of allaying an incipient storm, the profession might be benefited.

The " Old School" of Medicine.—Those the least qualified to speak understandingly upon medical systems, are exceedingly flippant on the subject of reform. They anathematize the " old school," as it is called, without knowing any thing of its character. And what has the " new school " accomplished ? Without including all who may claim a place in this class, it may be said of some of them, that although they were wholly unknown before they commenced selling cayenne by the drachm, instead of eating it on their corned beef, they are stirring up the elements prodigiously. With them the world is not only going wrong, but it may come to a positive stand-still if medical science is suffered to be taught in peace to respectable pupils. Breaking down and uprooting institutions which teach doctrines they cannot comprehend, is considered progression; while the huddling together of a few ambitious spirits, determined to rise on the ruin of their superiors rather than not rise at all, is called an effort at reformation. When any course of instruction for the education of physicians can be proposed, superior to the one generally adopted, there will be a willingness among physicians to receive it; but innovation and novelty are not always considered by them as real reforms.

Burlington (Vt.) Medical School.—A medical department of the University of Vermont was formerly in operation, but for causes best known to the corporation has been suspended for some years. By the following editorial announcement in the Montpelier Watchman and State Journal, it appears that the school of medicine has been revived.

" The Medical Department in this institution has been revived, and in the list of lecturers appointed we observe the names of Dr. Orren Smith of Montpelier, and Dr. S. W. Thayer of Northfield."

There will now be three medical institutions in Vermont, authorized to confer medical degrees. Whether a multiplication of these colleges in that State is desirable or beneficial, are questions that may hereafter be agitated.

Medical Miscellany.—At St. Jago, the yellow fever still sweeps its victims off with fearful rapidity. At Rio Janeiro it seems to be in perpetual activity, and by the latest advices the mortality was very severe.—A woman in Dutton. N. H., we see by the papers, gave birth to four sons at a single birth, who are all doing well.—A " medium" being lately consulted as to the character of the disease of which a person had died, spelled out *consumption;* but it turned out that he was blown up in a steamboat.—On board the steamer Blue Wing, on the Kentucky river, lately, was a mother and 12 children—6 pair of twins—from Washington county, Kentucky. She, together with her family, are about to settle in Indiana. She has been married but seven years, and is now the mother of twelve live children.—Affections of the lungs and neuralgic pains are very common at the north at present.—Mr. Wilson of Keene, N. H. is constantly improving his spinal apparatus—the finish of which is beautiful.—Dr. M. Clymer, (formerly of Philadelphia), has resigned the Chair of Institutes and Practice of Medicine in the University of New York. Dr. John A. Swett has been appointed to succeed him.

DIED,—At Danvers, Mass., Dr. Joseph Shed, 70.—At Millstone, N J., William D McKissack, M.D., æt. 60.—In Goldsboro', N. C., Samuel A. Andrews, M D, æt. 56.

Deaths in Boston for the week ending Saturday noon, April 16th, 74. Males, 38—females, 36. Accident, 1—apoplexy, 1—burns and scalds, 2—congestion of the brain, 4—consumption, 14—convulsions, 2—croup, 3—dropsy, 1—dropsy in the head, 6—infantile diseases, 9—puerperal, 1 —typhus fever, 1—scarlet fever, 7—hemorrhage. 1—hooping cough, 2—intemperance, 2—inflammation of the lungs, 6—disease of the liver, 2—marasmus, 2—mortification, 1—old age, 1—palsy, 2—pleurisy, 1—scrofula. 1—worms, 1.

Under 5 years, 39—between 5 and 20 years 5—between 20 and 40 years, 16—between 40 and 60 years, 9—over 60 years, 5. Born in the United States, 56 — Ireland, 16—England, 2. The above includes 5 deaths in the city institutions.

Medical Science.—Those who look upon medicine as an art, whose armamentarium consists solely in the drugs and chemicals of the Pharmacopœia, take but a narrow and imperfect view of the scope and objects of a science, which, rightly considered, takes cognizance of the entire apparatus of nature in its manifold relations to the health of mankind. Of what insignificant moment is the drug which the physician prescribes for an exceptional occasion of manifest disease, compared with those agents, water, air, and the elements of food, derived from the animal kingdoms, whose influence is daily and hourly acting upon the human frame! In the sense in which we understand the term medicine, and in which it has always been presented in this journal, Medicine includes Hygiene. Could we for a moment admit that the art we profess was only concerned with the cure or treatment of those obvious deviations from health which the pathologist describes, and did not embrace the wider subject of investigating the means of preserving health and ameliorating the physical condition of our fellow-creatures, then indeed we might contrast Hygiene and Medicine; we might view them as almost distinct sciences; we might, as some have done, whose limited vision is circumscribed within the contracted circle of their daily practice, restrict our attention to the relative merits of precipitated or sublimated brimstone, to the neglect of those universal agents which are constantly operating upon the health of millions.—*London Lancet.*

Cholera.—At last we are about to be rid of that scourge of the four quarters of the globe—the Cholera ; it has, we would fain believe, accomplished its work of death ; fulfilled its mission, under Providence, and departed from among us. In no part of the United States does it prevail to any extent ; it has spent its force—dried up the fountains of life in millions of subjects—swelled the bosom of the earth with its victims—made desolate the hearts and households of thousands of families, and gone forth to other climes—to other regions, to renew the contest for life or death with the sons and daughters of mortality. Cholera ! its mere name sends a thrill of horror to the heart of the brave as well as the timid ; to many it will convey sad recollections and heart-rending reminiscences, of friends, relatives and kindred, who were cut off from earth by the Great Destroyer. But why pursue the subject ? Let the past be forgotten.
Quis talia fando* * temperet à lachrymis ?
* * * animus meminisse horret, luctuque refugit ?
We trust we have seen the last of this scourge ; let us hope that it has departed from us forever!—*New Orleans Med. and Surg. Journal.*

Decease of Professor Horner.—We are pained to announce the death of the distinguished anatomist, Dr. Wm. E. Horner. He died of disease of heart. Dr. Horner held the chair of anatomy in the University of Pennsylvania, for nearly, if not quite a quarter of a century. His works on anatomy have long been recognized as standard text-books in that department of science. In his early professional life he was connected with the army, and served, during the last war with Great Britain, on the Niagara frontier. Some interesting reminiscences of this period of army service, from his pen, have lately appeared in the Philadelphia Medical Examiner. In his decease science loses one of its most distinguished votaries ; but his justly earned reputation, and many excellencies, still remain to confer honor on the American medical profession.—*Buffalo Medical Journal.*

THE

BOSTON MEDICAL AND SURGICAL JOURNAL.

VOL. XLVIII.   WEDNESDAY, APRIL 27, 1853.   No. 13.

EPIDEMIC OF 1852-53 IN NEWTON AND VICINITY.

ERYSIPELAS, MALIGNANT PUSTULE, DIFFUSE PERITONITIS, PHLEBITIS, IRRITATIVE FEVER.

BY EDWARD WARREN, M.D.

[Communicated for the Boston Medical and Surgical Journal.]

IN regard to the cases related in my last communication, I may observe that several medical gentlemen to whom I described them, stated that they had seen nothing of the kind.

I have just found the following note from Dr. John Ware, to whom I had written an account of the earlier and slighter cases. His note is so much to the point, that I hope he will excuse me for copying it. It is dated March 5, 1852. He says :—

" I can make nothing of the cases which you describe, except to call them influenza of a somewhat peculiar form. I think I have met with cases more or less like them. A—— ——'s disease, which took him down about eight weeks ago, was not very unlike in its general character and course—particularly he had the foul breath, and foul perspiration, The severe symptoms did not, however, yield so soon. Then he had clear physical signs of pneumonitis—but he had little cough and no sputa, so that except for a very careful examination he would never have been suspected to have this disease. The first day of the attack he had a *redness* and *swelling* of the face, which made me apprehend erysipelas, but it vanished soon."

In proceeding to the epidemic of this season, I should premise that erysipelas is endemic here ; particularly in the form of erysipelatous or malignant pustule. In vol. xxxv., page 505, of this Journal, I gave an account of the severest case I have ever witnessed, of erysipelatous or cellular inflammation ; and which occurred in 1842. It originated in a blister on the joint of the fore-finger. From dressing this patient's hand and arm, I contracted pustules and sores, such as I have fully described in the paper alluded to, and again in this Journal vol. xliv., page 169. They have been also fully described by Dr. Peirson in the last volume, page 75, in relation to the case of Mr. Robert Rantoul, whose disease commenced in this form of erysipelas.

These pustules or sores have since been very common here. They are attended with an immense amount of constitutional irritation ; often

13

confining the patient to his bed for a longer or shorter period ; and threatening the loss of the limb, if not of life.

These pustules are so little generally understood, that it is the common practice of physicians, especially when they appear upon the end of the finger, to treat them as felons, and cut down to the bone, or even to *scrape the bone.* This treatment invariably makes them worse.

Dr. Peirson thinks that these pustules are the result of animal poison. I have thought that they might be produced here, by handling rags ; or by something used in the manufacture of paper. But they often appear in subjects not at all exposed to such causes, and who reside at a considerable distance from the paper mills.

They often appear, also, on parts protected by the clothing ; and under such circumstances that they must be attributed to miasm. I have recently had an ample opportunity of observing a fine crop of these pustules upon the epigastrium. They arise in the manner stated by Dr. Peirson, very much resemble the pustules of chicken-pox, and itch and burn, when one pustule will generally take the lead, the others remaining stationary for an indefinite length of time. Sydenham compared the pain of erysipelas to the stinging of bees ; but conceive a bee with a long sting extending from this pustule to the heart and to the stomach, either through the hand and arm, or direct from the epigastric surface ; and also imagine a fine iron wire heated to a red (not a white) heat, boring by the side of this sting ; and you may form a slight conception of the pain of these tubercles. Now if one of these occur in a subject of extreme susceptibility, or previously exhausted by fatigue and mental anxiety, is it wonderful if death ensues ?

Another variety, perhaps also a pustule of this nature, differing only in situation, I will allude to. Some years since, a female domestic, of fleshy and gross habit, came into my family. Shortly after, she complained of violent pain in the ear ; and there appeared diffuse inflammation of the external ear and the meatus externus, attended with excruciating suffering, lasting for several days. It finally was relieved by a discharge from the meatus. Subsequently another member of my family had the same affection, attended with similar suffering.

It may well be imagined that these pustules are exceedingly alarming, both to patient and physician, when met with for the first time. The loss of the hand or arm ; and, in severer cases, that of life, is predicted. Yet I have never known a graver result produced by those which occur in this neighborhood, than stiffness of the finger-joint, which occurred in two cases only ; and a slight deformity of the thumb in one. Cases like that of Mr. Rantoul, and even the more rapid ones which we sometimes hear of, probably require at least three conditions for their development :—a strong constitutional predisposition, a state of the system such as is produced by long-continued anxiety and fatigue, and a constitution of the atmosphere peculiarly favoring the development of the disease.

A simple bread and milk poultice will often allay the irritation, as promptly as opium does a pain in the bowels. Nitrate of silver, thoroughly and promptly applied on the inflamed and sound parts beyond, arrests the inflammation, and quinine hastens the cure.

If sent for in the first instance, I apply the nitrate to the part affected, have it instantly followed by a poultice, and give tr. sulphat. quinin., from eight to sixty drops, according to the age of the patient and the severity of the attack, three times a-day. This has frequently cut short the disease within twenty-four hours. But as they are generally regarded at first as matters of very little consequence, and neglected, the cure is long and protracted. It is a peculiarity of these pustules, that, after being entirely healed, they are always ready to break out upon very slight provocation ; like the wounds inflicted by splinters from the lance of an elfin king, in days of yore.

The first case, I will relate, bears a strong relation to the concluding one in my former communication.

CASE 1.—Somewhere about November, 1852, a patient, Mr. A., who resided about a mile and a half distant, called to see me with his grandson, a boy about 7 years old, whom he wished me to vaccinate. On my informing him that I had no vaccine matter, he said he hoped I could vaccinate him from matter taken from another grandchild two years before. He mentioned, also, that he called to pay his bill ; a trifling one which he had paid about that same time. The lapse of time he seemed entirely to have forgotten.

I called at his house and vaccinated the child Nov. 23d ; and on this, and my subsequent visit, Nov. 30th, Mr. A. was absent on his customary avocations. The vaccination did well, and there was no unusual soreness or inflammation.

Dec. 18th.—I was sent for to visit Mr. A. He came in from his barn, and I was informed that he had been for some time unwell, though he had continued to pursue his usual out-of-door avocations. He appeared dull and heavy, but could give no clear account of his ailments. His digestive functions were deranged ; he was costive, and suffered much from earache. I prescribed laudanum for the ear, and a laxative.

20th.—I visited him again, and he sat down, intending, as I supposed, to give me an account of his symptoms ; but he went off into a detail of a surgical case which happened some years since in Maine. When I came to inquire into his own symptoms, he could give me no clear account of them. His ear was better ; but his throat was now troublesome. On examining the throat, I found very considerable inflammation and swelling of both tonsils. I prescribed a gargle of muriatic acid with confection of roses ; Dover's powders at night, and advised his keeping house.

22d.—Finding that his throat did not improve, I commenced applying the nitrate of silver daily. The left tonsil suppurated, and he extracted the slough or core with forceps. A foul ulcer formed. The application of the nitrate gave temporary relief ; but, on the whole, he continued stationary.

His breath was very foul, and I now learned that his perspiration, which was generally considerable at night, was also very foul, rendering the linen quite offensive. His pulse varied very much. It was small and not generally accelerated, at my morning visit, but I was told he had fever turns during the day.

I always found him sitting up and dressed, but dull and silent, answering questions with great difficulty, as if from mental stupor. He objected to hearty food, at first from fear of its creating fever, and afterwards from the idea that he could not swallow it. When urged, however, he could swallow without difficulty. He made the same objections to the medicines, which, nevertheless, he took, though with great reluctance.

My treatment at first consisted in laxatives, when absolutely required by costiveness, the gargle and nitrate as I have mentioned, and nourishing food. To this I added elixir of vitriol in water, and on yellowness of the skin coming on, one grain of blue pill with half a grain of opium for a night or two. Subsequently I added quinine to the vitriol, and then omitted the vitriol, giving quinine only.

He had at times pain in the head ; wandering pains in the limbs and bowels. There was about as much fulness of the abdomen and tympanitis as in typhoid fever. There was no tenderness on pressure, nor were there spots of any kind. The circulation was torpid, the pulse continued slow and small, and he had coldness of the extremities. There was great restlessness at night ; and he could not sleep well during the latter part of his sickness, even under the influence of opiates. There was at no time any absolute difficulty of getting down food ; and the swelling of the tonsils did not essentially obstruct the breathing, though the liquids were sometimes regurgitated through the nostrils. His diet, through the whole, was nourishing ; and, during the latter part of the time, I rigidly enforced the regular administration of broth, beef-tea and wine.

He very gradually became feebler, and his nights still more restless. The heaviness of mind and failure of memory increased. Still he could answer questions correctly, and was perfectly rational when roused. He died January 16th, retaining his consciousness to the very last moment.

The affection of the ear in the commencement of the disease, and its attacking the throat on leaving the ear, together with many of the symptoms, show its relation to the other cases which I have related, and which I am about to relate. The question might be asked whether the disease of the mind, or at least of the memory, preceded, or whether it was induced by the disease in question ?

Mr. Nunneley, in considering the question whether erysipelas attacks the arachnoid membrane of the brain, describes two kinds of inflammation affecting this membrane. One is violent, attended with full pulse, &c. ; in the other, the mind is rendered dull, and there is a depression of the mental powers ; the pulse is rapid, neither full nor hard, and all the secretions more deranged than in the former case, especially the abdominal. In the former the secretions are often suppressed ; in the latter, perverted. This description, with the exception of the rapid pulse, corresponds very closely with the symptoms above described ; and as we know the long duration of the pustules in many cases, there can be no difficulty in conceiving diffuse inflammation of the arachnoid of a chronic character. Perhaps the most wonderful characteristic of erysipelas, is its great rapidity in some instances, and its extreme sluggishness in others.

CASE II.—Dec. 30th. I was called in the night to the grandchild, above mentioned, of Mr. A. I found him in the same room with the latter. He had been unwell with a cold for several days, and was now violently seized with symptoms of croup. He was a boy about 7 years old—large for his age. I found him in extreme distress ; cough and croupy breathing were very strongly marked. Being a *grandchild*, I could not succeed in examining his throat; but I was enabled once to pass the probang with nitrate of silver. I gave him syrup of ipecac., which vomited him ; and this was repeated several times through the night. I directed warm applications to be made to the throat, and the room to be kept warm and moist.

The next morning I found him greatly relieved. He now took an expectorant mixture of squills, ipecac., &c. ; and in two or three days was perfectly well.

Here was a case, the infectious origin of which was evident, and greatly resembling case No. IX. in my former paper. In that case the patient was much younger, and more delicate both from sex and constitution, and already debilitated by previous disease. The superior vigor of the boy's system saved him.

CASE III.—Dec. 2d. A young married lady, who had a child of about five months old, after walking in the garden in a raw day, was suddenly seized with symptoms of a very violent character. She had severe chills, violent pain in the side, difficult breathing, &c. Her friends administered a purgative, a warm bath, mustard poultices, and subsequently an emetic of ipecac., and such other remedies as they could think of; but finding her not relieved, sent for me about twenty-four hours after her seizure.

Her appearance was unfavorable. Countenance sallow and anxious, forehead contracted as with pain, difficult breathing, and dry cough, with pain in the right side. The bowels were full ; perhaps not more so than is common in typhoid fever. The physical signs indicated considerable difficulty upon the right side. The skin was moist, and the pulse rather rapid, but not full. It was not the pulse of common inflammation ; but this might be accounted for by the course of medication which she had gone through.

I prescribed antimon. tart., gr. iv., in four ounces of water, a teaspoonful every four hours, increasing gradually to two teaspoonsful, if it produced no nausea. A blister to the right side ; morphine at night.

Dec. 4th.—Found her much relieved ; the pain in the side is entirely gone, and her breathing is easier. She has borne the antimony well, and it is now increased to two teaspoonsful.

5th.—Took two doses of the solution after I saw her, and some vomiting ensued ; since which she cannot retain food, and has frequent alvine evacuations. Both nausea and the looseness of the bowels were readily checked by effervescing soda water, and a small dose of morphine. She now expectorates freely, her cough is easy, and she has no pain or tenderness upon the right side ; but complains of pain in her left. Her voice is strong but interrupted, and her muscular strength good. I directed a blister to the left side ; an expectorant mixture ; morphine at night.

6th.—Found her nearly the same.

7th.—Cough continues easy, and expectoration free. Complains of no pain. She lies on her back, with her head low ; and upon attempting to move, contracts her forehead in the manner seen in organic disease. But on being questioned says she has no pain of any consequence. There is no pain upon pressure. She has a mucous rattle in the throat, but temporary. Abdomen very full, and a great deal of flatus.

8th.—Mucous rattle gone. Appears as well. Asks if there is any chance for her. Had some wandering of mind last night, and great restlessness. She now lies with her feet drawn up in bed ; is restless, but complains of no pain. There is still no tenderness upon pressure. Cough and expectoration continue free. She has had free perspirations during her whole sickness.

9th.—Has had a bad night. A good deal of restlessness. This morning is more comfortable. Voice is strong, but somewhat interrupted ; muscular strength good. 10, P.M.—Pulse fluttering, restlessness increased ; mucous rattle in the throat has returned.

10th.—Early part of the night very restless. Had an opiate injection ; and this not relieving her, she had a quarter of a grain of morphine in a pill. After this she slept, and continued to sleep until morning ; readily roused, retaining her senses perfectly, and knowing those around her. In this state I found her on my visit ; and was informed that she had just been roused and had spoken to her husband. She was now, however, pulseless, and on attempting to rouse her, I found it impossible. She died during my visit.

After death, I found the abdomen immensely distended. There was at first much discoloration, but this disappeared and the body resumed a natural color.

In this case, despite of some bad appearances through the whole, the pleuritic symptoms were so much relieved, that I hoped for a favorable issue. The pain in the side had gone, the cough was easy, and expectoration free. There was nothing to call my attention particularly to the abdomen. Diffuse peritonitis, however, must have supervened one or two days before death.

[To be continued]

M. RICORD'S LETTERS UPON SYPHILIS.

Addressed to the Editor of L'Union Medicale—Translated from the French by D. D SLADE, M.D, Boston, and communicated for the Boston Medical and Surgical Journal.

TWENTY-SECOND LETTER.

My Dear Friend,—I had a great desire to say a word to you upon the treatment of chancre, but according to the plan which we have adopted, I cannot in this connection enter into great detail.

Perhaps you will permit me to say to you first something upon the prophylaxis, and upon the medical police, which has gained much ground during a few years, and especially since I instituted, and which has been adopted after me, the examination with the speculum in the special hospitals, and in the dispensary for the public health.

It is very certain that since this mode of investigation has been generally employed, we can observe a great improvement in the health of the public women. Thus, according to Parent-Duchâtelet, in 1800 one diseased woman was met with in nine; now we do not encounter, since 1834, but one in sixty. Consequently, the speculum has played its great part in this amelioration.

But if we wish to do the business well, we must, as I have always professed, visit the women, every three days, without distinction of rank, whether they are in a house or en carte, whether they inhabit Paris or the Barrieres. You remember that from the second day of an artificial inoculation, we may already have inoculable pus. Swediaur admitted that the chancre could be developed in twelve hours; it is necessary then that the visits should be frequent, and the examination always made with the speculum, in order that the inspection of public women should offer a certain guarantee.

I write designedly this word *guarantee*, for there are some who, after their adventurous amours, think that they have a right to reclaim indemnity from the administration. You believe, perhaps, that I am not serious; here is a fact which goes to prove to you my assertion :—A few years ago a merchant of Lyons came to me in a state of very great exasperation against the prefect of the police. He came to get a certificate stating that he had contracted a chancre in a public house that he believed *guaranteed* by the authorities. His intention was to follow it up with damages and interest. He did not know that the *tolerance* is a sort of brevet, which, like all brevets is without guarantee from the government.

I hasten to say that the ameliorations which are introduced every day in the inspection of prostitution, and that the zeal of our colleagues charged with the painful business of the dispensary of health, and of the hospital of Saint Lazare, will give more and more happy results.

That public women are a necessary evil, is generally agreed upon at the present day. I wish neither to combat nor to support this sad proposition ; it is not the place to examine this here; but if the evil is necessary, it should not be extended, so far as the number is concerned, as a learned colleague of Belgium recently appeared to desire, but special attention should be paid to its quality.

In requiring that public women should not communicate disease, it ought to be well arranged so that those who frequent them, should not expose them to it. How shall we do ? Must we institute an examination for the individuals who frequent them, and prevent them if they are diseased ? But in addition to all the difficulties of such an institution, the danger which we might wish to prevent by this institution would be rendered greater, for in place of falling into a sink which the police can clean out, the filth would go elsewhere.

We cannot certainly think, at the present day, of establishing lazarettos, quarantines, of demanding with a certificate of vaccination, a clean bill of health from the verole, as my friend Diday, of Lyons, wrote in a moment of praiseworthy philanthropy, a bill which should be demandable, and as indispensable as the passport, a bill without which one could not be admitted to any public function. Whatever the ingenious author of this proposition has said, the difficulties of its execution appear insurmountable.

There was a time, as you know, when the infected, banished from Paris, were condemned to the cord if they reëntered the city ; an epoch when in the insane asylum of Bicêtre they whipped the patients at their entrance and at their exit. All this did not diminish their number ; on the contrary, the whippers merited in their turn to be whipped : these barbarous measures have fallen into disuse.

It is doubtless necessary to submit to a rigorous inspection all those that we can reach, soldiers for example, to sequester all the patients upon whom we can have any authority ; but a certain tolerance, the pardon of a fault quite often involuntary, and good hospitals with the succor which can be found in them at the present day, and which we can still ameliorate, herein consist the best means for a general prophylaxis, or those at least which shall tend to render the disease less and less grave.

Besides, all those who are acquainted with the sad conditions of the work and remuneration which is made to women in our present condition of society, have for a long time understood and proclaimed that herein was one of the most abundant sources of prostitution, and consequently of the propagation of syphilis. To ameliorate the condition of woman's labor, is then to make at the same time a work of humanity, of morality and of public health.

You remember what I said to you of the manner in which chancres are produced. It is necessary to remember it in order to avoid them. What science possesses most certain as regards the prophylactic treatment, is to avoid chancres. This appears a little *naïf*, but let the debauched remember that it is the truth. I am going to touch here upon a delicate subject, and one filled with dangers. It is still a question of morality and of medical deontology not yet resolved, to know whether the physician can and ought to give advice to preserve from evil those who are exposed to take it from a degraded source. I do not pretend to be more rigorous than the austere Parent-Duchatelet, who commenced this subject with the purity of intention which you are acquainted with in him. On the other hand, am I not re-assured by the nature even of the Journal which gives such liberal hospitality to my letters ? I address myself to the learned, to physicians ; and was it not you, my friend, who said, that science is chaste, even in a state of nudity ? After all, be re-assured, I shall not do more than touch upon this ticklish subject.

There does not exist any sure and absolute preservative from the chancre ; this is my declaration :—

If, in spite of this, one wishes to run the chance of it, some precautions can be taken. One must first bear in mind the precept of Nicolas

Marsa, so forcibly translated by the elder Cullerier—the relations ought not to be voluntarily prolonged; at this time one must be egotistical, as the grave Hunter remarked, but not egotistical after the manner of Madame de Stael, who called love the egotism of two.

Attention to the most minute cleanliness on the part of suspected persons, ought to be exacted in public houses. What we know for a long time past of the deposit of the virulent pus which may be kept in reserve in the genital organs of women, shows the necessity of this. It is a means of always preventing mediate contagion. I have told you that numerous experiments have shown that it sufficed to decompose the virulent pus in order to neutralize it. Alcohol in water, water mixed with a fifth part of Labarraque's disinfecting fluid, all the acids diluted with water so as not to be caustic, wine, the solution of zinc and of the acetate of lead, suffice to prevent the virulent pus from being inoculable; while that if this same pus is not altered, it suffices that the quantity should be excessively small, homœopathic, if you please, in order to act. M. Puche has told us, at the Hospital du Midi, that he had obtained effects from inoculation of a drop of pus mixed with half a glass of water.

The use of fatty substances is very useful, especially for medical men who practise touching upon dangerous parts. Astringent lotions which tan the tissues a little have often served to ward off the contagion.

But if the precautions of neatness are necessary before connection in the person who might infect, they ought to be minute after the act in the individual who is exposed.

There is a method which morality repudiates, and in which debauchees put much confidence, which doubtless often guarantees, but which, as a woman of much *esprit* has remarked, is a cuirass against pleasure, and a cobweb against danger. This mediate agent is often rotten, or has already been made use of; it is frequently displaced; it performs the office of a bad umbrella which the storm may tear, and which under all circumstances, guaranteeing badly from the storm, does not prevent the feet from getting wet. In fact, I have seen quite often ulcerations upon the root of the penis, upon the peno-scrotal angle, upon the scrotum, &c., in persons who had taken these useless precautions.

Many patients believe themselves safe from contagion in not terminating the venereal act. A lady who consulted me about herself, was much astonished in having communicated disease to her lover, inasmuch, said she, *that he did not finish.*

Some medical writers upon syphilis believe that the infection of the urethra particularly, is produced after the emission which made the vacuum, and from the horror which nature has of a vacuum. But numerous facts have taught me the contrary. The emission in fact ought to be considered as a powerful injection from behind forwards, and which thus cleanses the urethra; and if the urethral affections already so common are not more frequent, it is perhaps to this condition that it is to be attributed. Thus an old and excellent precept is that which recommends a speedy micturition after every suspicious connection. At one time, fortunately remote from us, they made use of jugglers.

The circumcision of the prepuce, the excision of the nymphæ which are too long, ought also to constitute an hygienic law as regards the genital organs, for these appendages greatly favor contagion.

I ask your pardon for this digression—but it is necessary that science should seek to take away from charlatanism the dangerous execution of a deceitful prophylaxis. We should be able always to indicate all which can favor the avoidance of contagion, and therefore the propagation of syphilis—not in order to protect or to favor libertinism, but to thereby guarantee virtue and chastity, which become too often the victims of it.

There remains to me now to speak to you upon cauterization as an abortive means, and as curative of chancre. But in order not to divide this subject, I shall make it the topic of my next letter.

Yours,   RICORD.

DR. KING'S ADDRESS ON QUACKERY—ITS CAUSES AND EFFECTS.

[Concluded from page 249.]

THERE are some medical societies in New England whose by-laws declare that it shall be deemed disreputable and unlawful for any fellow of such society to consult, directly or indirectly, with any person who is not a fellow—such offences being punishable with fine or expulsion. In some of the States, no one is allowed to practise medicine or prescribe for the sick until he has a diploma recorded on the books of the town in which he is located. In France, every new scheme that is rejected by the regular faculty is instantly suppressed. All these are salutary provisions, and tend to guard the public against imposition. The importance of medical societies has been too much overlooked. Besides State societies, district and village societies, with their quarterly or monthly meetings, should be everywhere established. These are schools in which every member may learn something, and by comparing himself with others keep regulated and posted up, and become an abler and better practitioner. Here a healthy emulation is encouraged, private animosities are dismissed, jealousies and heart-burnings are cured. Here the passions are hushed, the feelings chastened, and the tongue curbed. Some poet says, " Mountains interposed make enemies of nations, which else, like kindred drops, had mingled into one." Scripture, reason and all experience, assure us that a house divided against itself cannot stand. When any class of men wish to accomplish an object for the good of the whole, they find it necessary to form associations and act in concert. By such means, men who could do nothing as individuals, form powerful associations and accomplish important purposes with perfect ease. Political parties are always wide awake upon this subject; when an election is pending the cry is, organize, organize. Religious and moral associations act upon the same principle, and acquire power by similar means. Mechanics and laborers, without capital, and without influence as individuals, by forming associations and acting in unison acquire immense power. They can almost change the time of the sun's rising ; they have already shortened the day from about fourteen to ten hours.

When they think proper, they raise their wages. 'Nothing is wanted to accomplish anything they wish, but perfect and unflinching concert of action.

But physicians seem to be heedless of all this, and are sometimes alarmed because a few puny, straggling quacks threaten to annihilate the whole profession. Let the physicians of the United States unite and act in concert as they ought to do, and quackery would perish as a viper beneath the foot of the elephant. But the timid, cringing, time-serving course pursued by far too many, tends to counteract the influence of the high-minded and honorable. It is said that a courageous man may look the lion out of countenance ; whilst the braying of some long-eared animal might frighten the timid out of himself. The profession has lost much of its authority and influence by the conduct of men, who, from an excessive desire to please everybody, always endeavor to accommodate themselves to surrounding circumstances ; men who think it safest for them at least to ride two or more hobbies at the same time. Every honorable physician should look upon such obsequious truckling with utter contempt ; he should nail his colors to the mast, and, like Cato of old, disdain everything that his unrighteous enemies have power to offer. And the man who has not courage to do this had better, for the honor of his cause, give himself up at once and go home on parole.

The art of healing, as our profession is sometimes called, has always been too much shrouded in mystery. Its origin is probably nearly coeval with the human race, although very little is known of its early history. More than two thousand years ago we find her in Egypt the bantling of a superstitious priesthood, having darkness for her mantle and mystery for her swaddling clothes ; and from that day to the present, this same evil genius has clung to her skirts and prowled around her temples, polluting her sanctuaries and dishonoring her disciples. Under its shadow quackery reposes. It is the ambrosia and nectar which sustains it, the banner under which its disciples rally, and the tower of refuge to which they fly. Science seeks to banish mystery from the world, and expose to open day every important truth ; to strip medicine of every unhallowed covering, and show, not merely to physicians, but to the public as far as it may be understood, every physiological, pathological and therapeutic process. The patient and his friends should be allowed to know all that they can correctly understand of the nature and treatment of his case. The more genuine knowledge an individual possesses, the less is he liable to be imposed upon by false pretenders ; but a knowledge of one science or art is no sure protection against fraud or imposition connected with some other science. There are men who are learned in everything else but medicine, and who become the unaccountable dupes of new and false medical schemes, and thereby do much mischief ; for the public erroneously suppose that because a man understands the languages, mathematics, &c., he must of course know everything else. In general, the man who has the most plain common sense, who is accustomed to reason at every step he treads, is least liable to be suddenly carried away by new schemes. Those who are sound to the core, whose minds are thoroughly disciplined and trained to correctness of thought, are not easily led astray by phantoms. Such men were Jefferson and Adams, Calhoun and Clay, Story and Webster. Neither of these men ever swallowed a Brandreth's pill, or tasted Swain's Panacea, or drank Townsend's Sarsaparilla, or bathed in Davis's Pain Killer. No irregular practitioner ever entered their doors, or prescribed for their families. Their medical advisers were among the most learned and accomplished of the profession. No Botanic, Thomsonian, Hydropath, Homœopath or Eclectic, was ever summoned to their sick chamber or wanted beside their beds. In their most trying moments they took advice only of regular physicians, and obeyed them implicitly. No others were allowed to moisten their burning lips or wipe the cold damp from their brows. Every one of these men has added his dying seal to the testimony of his whole life, against quackery of every kind, and in favor of regular scientific medicine,. This is testimony of a high order, and it behoves the world to heed it. It stands out in bold relief, which no finesse can hide or sophistry destroy.

From the moment the tyro commences reading medical books, to the last hour of his practice, one continued course of study is required. It is indispensable. Besides standard works, every practitioner should take one or more medical periodicals. And to insure this, I will venture to make a single suggestion. The annual tax of each member is now two dollars ; and as the number of members probably increases faster than the incidental expenses of the society, some part of this amount might be applied towards the payment for a periodical ; and by doubling the tax, making it one dollar per quarter, I think every member of the Massachusetts Medical Society might be constantly supplied with some good weekly or monthly publication, free from further expense. The large number of copies required would enable the publisher to furnish the work at a low price, and at the same time perhaps the society might have some control over its pages. Such a course would carry to every member much useful and seasonable information, and enable him to keep himself always posted up.

Another matter deserves consideration. The public are shockingly imposed upon, and regular physicians disgraced, by scores of ignorant quacks, who, without any qualifications at all, affix M.D. to their signatures. If a man assumes the office of a petty magistrate when he has no such commission, he becomes liable by law to pay a fine or suffer imprisonment, although no harm may be done, to any one, because such conduct would diminish the respect due to the civil magistrate and dishonor all civil authority. But governments are not thus careful to protect from insult the conservators of human life. There is no law that I know of in this State that hinders any one from adding M.D. to his signature, and holding himself out to the public as a graduate in medicine when he has no such credentials. This is a kind of counterfeiting that deserves to be punished in the most summary manner ; and yet it is every day practised with perfect impunity. Ought not application to be made to the Legislature of this State for some act to suppress it ? Is it not as important to protect human life from false pretense, as the goods of a merchant ? In France such villains would soon find it necessary to abbreviate their signatures, or the government would abbreviate their liberties. It ought to be so everywhere. The science of medicine occupies a kind of middle station between the sciences that are fixed and positive, and those that are probable or presumptive; portions of it, only, are susceptible of clear and positive demonstration, while others are only reasonable and presumptive. Its knowledge has been chiefly derived from observation and experience, and is now the aggregate of what has been garnered up throughout all past time. It is necessarily progressive. The improvements in arts and sciences, and the refinements in social and domestic life, constantly increase its necessity and importance, and no imaginary limits can be set to either. Perhaps the science and practice of medicine may forever continue to improve; but from the nature of its office it must forever be in a measure imperfect. There are doubtless many diseases to which these animal machines are liable, which in some stages, at least, will forever defy all therapeutic means. It must fail once, at least, with every human being. But the science is no less necessary or important on account of its imperfections. All other institutions are also imperfect. No code of laws has ever been sufficient wholly to prevent crime. No tribunals have been able always to distinguish between the innocent and the guilty, nor do the councils and admonitions of good men induce all to become virtuous. But this I do say—cultivate and improve our profession, prune it of its cumbersome branches, make it what it ought to be, elevate it to its proper station, give it its just scope and influence; and in everything that is necessary and valuable in society, in all that concerns the happiness, usefulness and honor of men in this life, it will have no superior.

The followers and supporters of new schemes in medicine have always supposed that some mighty revolution was taking place, and that the old practice, as they have always called the only true system, was destined soon to be forgotten. So thought the followers of Serapion, Empiricus, Paracelsus, and a host of other pseudo-reformers of previous times; and so think now the friends and followers of each of the phantom schemes of the present day. But this is a grand mistake. All the baseless visions of ancient times have long since passed away as a dream of the night, and those which have cast their phosphorescent glimmerings upon the present age are fast passing into twilight. In those wild fields no century plants have yet been found; all belong to the cryptogamic class and mushroom genus.

From a review of the past and a contemplation of the future, I see no cause of alarm or discouragement, if the profession will only be faithful to its high vocation. Some of the ancients believed that the art of healing was a direct gift from heaven. This sentiment, although fabulous in its origin, should nevertheless be had in everlasting remembrance. It accords with the just dignity and importance of the office of the art. If physicians will do all their duty, no lasting ills can betide them. An immutable law declares that all that is false must pass away. The empty ravings of fanatic quackery must lash themselves into repose, and everything that is erroneous in our own system should be cast off without regret, whilst all that is true and valuable will stand firm and unimpaired by time. Occasional whirlwinds and hurricanes must be encountered ; but even these help to purify the atmosphere and make it more serene. And if some darker hour shall come, when errors and mistakes, and falsehood and fraud, in one confused mass, threaten society with an universal deluge ; when reason seems to have left her throne to madness and folly ; when impostors have multiplied like clouds of locusts, and the whole horizon becomes filled with the coruscations of strange stars, even then every honest and true man may look around with unconcern, and say with the poet, " Truth, crushed to earth, shall rise again." Volcanoes may demolish mountains and bury cities in their dust and lava ; pyramids may crumble to atoms, ocean waves dissolve the continents, and time place his desolating hand upon all material objects ; but truth is eternal, and can never be overthrown.

REMARKABLE ACCIDENT FROM THE USE OF THE CANULE-DUPUYTREN.

BY JOHN H. DIX, M.D., BOSTON.

[Communicated for the Boston Medical and Surgical Journal.]

A professional friend has just directed my attention to an article in the Courier des Etats Unis, for April 3, 1853, copied from the Courier de la Gironde. The case is intelligently, though not technically detailed, and being not in itself improbable, I see no cause to doubt its truth. Without, however, vouching for its authenticity, I have made a translation of it, very much abridged for your pages, not merely on account of its singularity, but because it adds to various others, one, and a very striking objection to this mode of operation for obstruction of the lachrymal duct.

Notwithstanding its immobility by the wearer, the difficulty and uncertainty of its removal by the surgeon, and the chance of its becoming permanently obstructed by mucous deposits, the tube or canule-Dupuytren is still occasionally inserted in this country. Poisoning by an oxide of copper is not, perhaps, one of the possible results of it among us, the material being here, within my observation at least, invariably gold or silver. But, of whatever material it may be, the liability to swallow an indigestible tube an inch long and from a sixteenth to an eighth of an inch in diameter, is decisive as to the propriety of placing it in the lachrymal duct.

The case is as follows, omitting details and explanations, which to medical readers are unnecessary.

Madame Ch——, residing a short distance from Bordeaux, had for two years suffered from obstruction of the lachrymal duct. By advice of her physician, she went to Paris, where a headless tube, of the sort first proposed and used by Baron Dupuytren, was inserted. This tube was of copper, plated with silver. The result was satisfactory, and Madame Ch—— considered herself cured. Ten months afterwards she began to be again troubled with an overflow of tears, and at about the same time was attacked with pains in the abdomen and vomiting.

These symptoms continued, with increasing violence, and in defiance of medical treatment. She died, and on making the autopsy, in one of the intestines was found the *canule-Dupuytren*, divested of its silver plating, and coated with verdigris.

QUININE IN RHEUMATISM—PRIORITY OF PRACTICE.

To the Editor of the Boston Medical and Surgical Journal.

DEAR SIR,—In your editorial notice, April 6, you say that Briquet used the quinine in rheumatism as early as 1843. By reference to Dr. Reese's Journal, you will see, if my memory is correct, for I am unable to find the copy, that the case I reported occurred in 1844 or 43, and was peculiarly successful ; but in looking over some fugitive cases I have upon record, I find my first use of the article occurred in the spring of 1842, but was not as satisfactory as I anticipated. I do not wish to deprive M. Briquet of a laurel ; far from it. If he was the first on the other side of the water to call attention to it, he is entitled to the honor accruing. From the tenor of your article, I should say there was a wide difference in our doses ; he used only 15 or 20 grains, while I exhibited it in much larger quantities ; and I believe upon therapeutic principles I am correct. But, after all we have said, doctor, rheumatism is a very painful and intractable disease, which often defies all the suggestions ever made, from Hippocrates down to Briquet, or any other of the *quinine gentry.* I recollect Dr. Reese and myself had a spicy little talk about the matter in the Gazette, and he doubtless could give all the facts pertaining to it. How general the use of the remedy has become South, I cannot say, but pretty common, I suspect, from the fact that quinine is given in nearly everything, at least with a great many practitioners. I have seen it used in acute meningitis, and I have stood by the dying bed of a hale man, who was toxicologically quininized ; but it was all done *à la science*, and it passed. *We pray for principles in medicine.* God send them in the 19th century.

In haste, your friend, H. A. RAMSAY.

Thompson, Geo., April 17, 1853.

THE BOSTON MEDICAL AND SURGICAL JOURNAL.

BOSTON, APRIL 27, 1853.

Massachusetts Medical Society.—On the next anniversary, the meeting will be held in Boston. Members generally are anticipating a pleasant reunion. A discourse, the annual business, and a dinner, comprise the ordinary doings. It will be seen by an advertisement in this Journal, that a committee has been appointed to adopt measures to increase the interest of these annual meetings, by means of scientific communications. It is hoped members will co-operate with the committee in bringing about the contemplated improvement. Whether the plan of erecting an edifice for the special accommodation of the society, will be revived, is quite uncertain. Some have supposed that a building for the purpose, located in this city, would centralize the society, and have a good influence on the attendance. It is easier if not more economical to go from any part of the Commonwealth to the capital, than to almost any other town in the State. Very many make it a point to transact various kinds of business on the same trip, and hence they prefer to go to the largest market. In short, from various considerations, it is believed that a majority of the whole prefer to have the annual meetings in Boston, and it is a fact that there are always more together when the anniversaries are in the metropolis. If the project of a hall, a favorite scheme of long standing, is ever to be undertaken, this is a period as favorable as any future day is likely to be. Real estate is dear, but there are no indications of its being cheaper; and besides, a suitable plot of ground cannot be found a few years hence without taking down buildings which are already productive property.

Human Electricity.—At a scientific meeting in this city, week before last, a distinguished clergyman of Boston stated that peculiar electrical phenomena had been observed in his family, which might possibly be produced or influenced by the locality of the house where he resides—a remarkably dry, and somewhat elevated spot. By sliding the feet rapidly across the room, and then immediately holding a finger to the burner, a spark from its extremity would light the gas instantly. On one occasion he blew out the flame and re-lighted the gas a second time with his finger, before leaving the chair on which he was standing. For the amusement of friends, he is frequently in the habit of performing this feat. Even his little children have learned the trick of charging themselves on the floor, for the purpose of giving a shock, by way of surprising those who are proper subjects for sport. The apartment in which these curious acts are accomplished, is carpeted in the ordinary manner, and a piece of bocking covers the centre, which is thought to favor the speedy accumulation of electricity. If the air is clear, dry, and the weather cold, the spark is more certain and the effect strongly marked. Small cork balls are moved about marvellously by a current from the Rev. gentleman's digits.

Colored Physicians for Liberia.—Two colored natives of Boston, distinguished for their good characters and progress in a preparatory course, have been studying medicine a year or two under the patronage of the Massachusetts Colonization Society, with the express object of qualifying them to practise medicine and surgery in Liberia. Not being successful in gaining admission to witness hospital practice here, one of them proceeded to London, where his advantages have been of a superior order. The other is still in Boston, but losing precious time on account of the lack of opportunities for studying disease at the bed-side. They both wish for medical degrees, that they may not be denied the right to practise on their arrival in Africa. In the meanwhile, the society is in a quandary, not knowing what to do next. A purer act of benevolence was never undertaken, than the medical education of these colored beneficiaries. If Africa is to be civilized and Christianized, science and art must be introduced there. Physicians are needed very much in Liberia—a colony that has been sustained by the American Colonization Society, till its independence has been acknowledged by many of the governments of Europe. What can be done for these young men to complete the course so far advanced ? Their ambition is to go where the field of employment would be extensive, and where they can aid in the promotion of human happiness.

Invalid Food.—More interest has been exhibited in the arabica, or, as it is more commonly called, invalid food, than was anticipated when it was first introduced into this country. Many physicians have given in their adhesion, having ascertained that it fully comes up to the representations of its friends. Since Dr. Litchfield opened an agency for it in Boston, we have had occasion to become somewhat acquainted with its properties. An aged lady, very feeble and partially paralytic, bears the strongest testimony in its favor. When no other aliment in the ordinary catalogue of eatables relished, she found the arabica agreeable and particularly nutritious. This, to be sure, is only a single case, within our own immediate sphere of observation ; but it corresponds so satisfactorily with the representations of others, that those who are prostrated by long-continued disease, are confidently recommended to make trial of this much praised dietetic regimen.

Treatment of Diabetes.—In the " Edinburgh Monthly Journal of Medical Science," for October last, it is stated that Dr. Gray, of Glasgow, had been induced to make trial of *rennet* in a case of diabetes, in the hope that, as this body converts sugar out of the body into lactic acid, it might be found to produce a similar change within the stomach, and the lactic acid thus generated might be eliminated from the system, or rather decomposed by the respiratory process. A teaspoonful of rennet was given three times a day. In eight days, the specific gravity of the urine was reduced to 1025, with but a trace of sugar ; in twenty-five days, the quantity was four pints, and the density 1022.5, and no sugar could be detected. At the end of six weeks, the urine remained free from sugar, and the patient had so far improved in health and strength as to return to his work.

Dr. Wood, of Philadelphia, as appears by the last number of the Transactions of the College of Physicians of that city, has made use, with success in one case, of yeast as a remedy in diabetes. A teaspoonful, three times a day, was the prescription employed.

Increase of Smallpox in Glasgow.—The number of deaths by smallpox in Glasgow for the last three years has been as follows:—1850, 456 ; 1851, 618 ; and 1852, 584. During the same period, the number of cases and deaths in the Royal Infirmary of that city were as follows:—In 1850, number of cases, 78; deaths, 18. In 1851, cases, 163 ; deaths, 30. In 1852, cases, 115 ; deaths, 19. During six years between 1836 and 1852, in the same infirmary, the whole number of cases of smallpox admitted was 536. Of this number, 265 had been vaccinated, and 271 were unvaccinated. Of the vaccinated, 19 died ; of the unvaccinated, 86. A very interesting and elaborate article, by Dr. John C. Steele, of the above-named Infirmary, is contained in the Glasgow Medical Journal, the first number of which is just published. From this article the above items have been gleaned, and we may make further extracts from it hereafter.

Leave Taking.—Jefferson Medical College.—Prof. Bache, of the Jefferson Medical College, spoke with energy and feeling to the medical graduates of that celebrated school, on bidding them farewell at the termination of the late course of lectures. ♯He recommended them to peruse medical journals, and to join a medical society. If they follow this advice, the public as well as themselves will reap the advantage. The idea of keeping pace with science, and especially that of medicine, without being familiar with the intelligence which is periodically wafted over the world, is absurd. A merchant might as well neglect consulting the price currents, or shipping lists. The age is one of incessant activity, and those who do not read as they go, will certainly be left in ignorance behind. Dr. Bache holds up empiricism to detestation, while its pretensions are dissected by a skilful hand. " What would the captain of a vessel think of us," asks the speaker, " if we gave him a receipt for sailing from Philadelphia to the West India Islands? Suppose we should lay down, in our directions, the manner in which he should set his sails, and prescribe the position to be given to the rudder. What! he would exclaim, am I not to be influenced in the sailing of my vessel, by its constitution as a frame-work of timbers, by the strength with which these are put together; by its newness, or oldness, by the quantity and quality of its cargo; and, above all, am I not to take into consideration the direction and force of the wind, the nature of the sea I am navigating, the proximity of rocks and shoals, and a thousand other circumstances bearing more or less on the main object of the voyage, that of reaching the desired port in safety?" Dr. B. scarcely leaves a point untouched, which might be of importance in promoting the usefulness, respectability or medical reputation of a young physician. He is a safe adviser, and a judicious counsellor. There is much in the occasions of these farewell addresses, at the termination of years of study, when new relations to society are about being established, that calls into play the warmest feelings of the heart. It is a fitting time for making impressions; and when students are then addressed, by those for whom they entertain a profound respect, the admonitions received have a lasting influence.

Western Lunatic Asylum.—By the recent influx of reports from all sections of the Union, it is pretty conclusively shown that lunacy is not confined to New England. The Western Asylum is a Virginia institution, located at Williamsburg, of which John M. Galt, M.D., is medical superintendent. According to the report, the directors are of opinion that an appropriation from the State of $30,000 for the support of the asylum the ensuing year will be necessary, besides $2,000 to pay the travelling expenses of patients. Dr. Galt's annual report is a clear, well-digested document, creditable to him as a man of benevolence as well as science. He suggests some relief for idiots, who are probably sent to his humane care because people know not where else to send them. They have been culpably neglected throughout the country. New York and Massachusetts are making some atonement for an age of neglect, by creating retreats for their special benefit. Virginia ought to complete the circle of home charities, by at once providing an asylum for these unfortunate beings.

The Virginia Medical and Surgical Journal.—This new periodical has been received. The claims of its conductors on the profession of the Old Dominion are strong, and the new Journal should by no means suffer from neglect, either in subscriptions or original communications. Drs. Otis and Thomas, in this specimen number, show a correct taste in the arrangement of articles, good judgment in selecting, and an ambition to meet the expectations of their many friends. Their messenger will appear monthly, and we have no doubt will abound with information always welcome to a practitioner. The price is five dollars a year. As opportunity occurs, we shall show by extracts how deserving this enterprise is of the hearty assistance and patronage of the brotherhood both in Virginia and the surrounding country.

Homœopathic Agencies.—M. M. Pallen, M.D., of the University of St. Louis, gave a farewell discourse before the medical graduates of the school on the first of March. It is distinguished for its keen and searching analysis of the homœopathic school of medicine. Dr. Allen cuts both ways, without the slightest appearance of respect either for the doctrine, or those who pretend to practise it. Yet he approves of inquiry. To condemn what is not understood, is absurd. He therefore has examined for himself, and decides, on mature investigation of the writings of Hahnemann, just as thousands have done before him, that the whole matter is a humbug. Were this the first article that ever had been published condemnatory of the pellicles, the sugar of milk and the like, it would be serviceable to make extracts from it. But it is not now necessary. If gentlemen commanding the artillery of the homœopathic publications allow him to escape by giving him small doses only in exchange, it will be some evidence that his propositions are unanswerable. We leave the discourse, with the conviction that the author is a racy, pungent commentator, when the full measure of his powers is exerted.

Medical Institution of Yale College.—At the annual examination of candidates for the medical degree, at the New Haven Medical School, in January last, fifteen were recommended and received their degree. The annual address to the candidates was given by Dr. Benj. Welch, of Salisbury. Prof. Benj. Silliman having given notice to the Board of Examiners that he had resigned his professorship, the following resolution was offered and unanimously adopted.

Resolved, That the thanks of the Committee of Examination in the Medical Institution of Yale College are due to Benjamin Silliman, LL.D. for the faithful and very satisfactory manner in which he has for forty years discharged the duties of Professor of Chemistry in this Institution; and we learn with unfeigned regret, that he has retired from the chair, which he has so long filled with such distinguished ability.

To CORRESPONDENTS.—"Justice" on Medical Advertising has been received.

DIED,—In Philadelphia, Dr. E. Cooley, 82.—At Litchfield, Conn, Dr. Ashbel Wessels, 83. —At Bloomfield, Conn, Dr. John Tyer, 88.—At Louisville, Ky., Dr. Richard Ferguson, 76.

Deaths in Boston for the week ending Saturday noon, April 23d, 94. Males, 46—females, 48. Accident, 2—apoplexy, 1—inflammation of the bowels, 1—inflammation of the brain, 4—disease of the brain, 2—consumption, 22—convulsions, 5—croup, 5—cancer, 2—dropsy, 4—dropsy in the head, 2—infantile diseases, 11—erysipelas, 1—gravel, 1—scarlet fever, 6—typhus fever, 1—typhoid do., 1—hooping cough, 1—disease of the heart, 2—inflammation of the lungs, 9—marasmus, 3—mortification, 1—old age, 2—pleurisy, 1—suicide, 1—teething, 3. Under 5 years, 45—between 5 and 20 years, 7—between 20 and 40 years, 25—between 40 and 60 years, 9—over 60 years, 8. Born in the United States, 71 — Ireland, 21—England, 2. The above includes 7 deaths in the city institutions.

Portland Medico-Chirurgical Society.—This Society held its third Annual Meeting March 14, 1853, at the usual time and place. The meeting being called to order, by Dr. Robinson the President, the minutes of the previous meeting were read, and the society proceeded to the election of officers. Dr. James C. Weston was chosen *President ;* Dr. C. S. D. Fessenden, *Vice President*; Dr. W. C. Robinson, *Recording Secretary and Treasurer ;* Dr. H. T. Cummings. *Corresponding Secretary ;* Drs. J. Houghton, S. B. Chase and O. E. Durgin, *Censors.* After the election had been completed, the report of the Secretary was read and accepted, and the Association listened to an interesting address by Dr. Chas. S. D. Fessenden, on the General History of the Science of Medicine, from the earliest age to the present day. The society then adjourned to the next regular semi-monthly meeting.   H T. Cummings, M.D.,
Corresponding Secretary.

Meteorological Phenomenon.—During a storm of wind and rain, on the night of the 25th of March, a yellow, impalpable powder fell in this city and neighborhood, in such quantities as in some places to cover the ground. Being light, it floated upon the water, and formed a thick film along the sides of the gutters. The phenomenon gains interest from the circumstance that a similar precipitate occurred in Tennessee ten years ago (March, 1843), after a cold, backward spring, much like the present. Then, as recently, it was accompanied by a rain which succeeded a day of high southerly winds. The powder had very much the appearance of *flowers of sulphur.* It was combustible, and burnt with the odor of vegetable matter. The explanation generally given of it is, that it is the pollen of flowers wafted into our region by the winds from the South.—*West. (Louisville) Med. Journal.*

Chloroform in Midwifery.—At the late meeting of the New York State Medical Society, the use of chloroform in midwifery was discussed—a majority of those who took part in the discussion being in favor of its use. The subject was introduced by Dr. Burwell, who read a paper upon it. " He had administered chloroform, in one hundred and eighty cases—one hundred and twenty-two of which were greatly relieved, fifty-five partially, and three got'no relief from its use. In seventeen cases, labor was terminated by the use of forceps—in one case by craniotomy—in one by turning. Eighty-eight of these cases were patients in labor for the first time. And in all these cases there had been not a single accident resulting from its use. He considered at length its effects upon the mental faculties, the muscular system, the pulse and respiration. He gave general rules by which to be governed in its use, and particular directions about the manner in which it should be administered, and the quantity to be given."

Death of M. Orfila.—M. Orfila, the celebrated French toxicologist, died at Paris on Saturday the 12th ult. of inflammation of the lungs. He had long filled the chair of Medical Chemistry in the Faculty of Medicine at Paris, and few of our professional friends who have recently visited the French capital, can fail to recall his kindness of manner and anxiety to impart information. M. Orfila has bequeathed a sum of 126,000 francs to various medical institutions, of which sum 60,600 francs are to be appropriated to the magnificent museum which bears his name. His funeral on the 19th ult. was attended by the *elite* of the Medical Faculty of Paris.—*Glasgow Med. Journ.*

THE
BOSTON MEDICAL AND SURGICAL JOURNAL.

Vol. XLVIII.   WEDNESDAY, MAY 4, 1853.   No. 14.

LECTURES OF M. VALLEIX ON DISPLACEMENTS OF THE UTERUS.

TRANSLATED FROM THE FRENCH BY L. PARKS, JR., M.D.

NUMBER III.

GENTLEMEN,—After the historic view, doubtless very incomplete, which I have just presented to you, it remains for me to lay before you the materials which are to serve us in describing displacements of the uterus.

It was in 1849 that Professor Simpson's treatise became known in France, and it was then only that I commenced to occupy myself actively with displacements of the womb. Since then I have been able to bring together 68 cases, for the most part complete, of divers displacements; and it is principally upon what I have myself seen that I shall found my description of these diseases. But, before proceeding to these details, I must endeavor to make you familiar with the exact and methodical exploration of the uterus, without which you would have difficulty in following the descriptions I shall present to you. Before speaking, also, of the uterus in the state of displacement, it is evidently necessary to establish what is its normal state.

EXPLORATION OF THE UTERUS.

The Uterus in the Normal State.—You will easily comprehend, gentlemen, that we need hardly occupy ourselves, here, with any other points than the situation, direction and volume of this organ, together with the normal state of its cavity. As to the intimate structure of its tissue—the presence or absence of a mucous membrane—the origin and mode of distribution of its vessels and nerves—these, relatively to the subject of which we are treating, are but secondary questions, for the elucidation of which your previous anatomical knowledge must suffice.

Situation.—The uterus, situated in the cavity of the pelvis, is, so to speak, suspended between the bladder and the rectum, the two folds of peritoneum known by the name of the *broad ligaments* expanding from its sides. Its cervix forms a projection into the vagina below it, and its fundus or superior surface is situated beneath the intestinal convolutions (which surround it on all sides, and tend to glide in front, between the uterus and bladder, or behind, between the uterus and rectum), in such a manner that the organ is interposed between the intestines and the finger introduced into the vagina.

14

Direction.—Its direction is that of the axis of the brim, whilst the vagina follows that of the outlet. Now, you very well know that the axis of the brim being directed obliquely downward and backward, and that of the outlet being also oblique, but directed upward and backward, there results from the intersection of these two axes an obtuse angle, the sides of which diverge anteriorly. The axes, then, of the uterus and vagina intersect each other at the same angle.

Surrounding Tissues.—The fundus of the uterus is covered by the peritoneum, which spreads out from the sides to form the broad ligaments, and is reflected upon the bladder in front and upon the rectum behind. Between the lower portion of the uterus and the rectum, beneath the fold or *cul-de-sac* formed by the peritoneum, and above the posterior *cul-de-sac* of the vagina, there is a space occupied by cellular tissue of an extremely delicate character, and liable, in consequence of inflammation, to be the seat of the tumors about which I have several times discoursed to you, and which, on a superficial examination, might be mistaken for the body of the uterus felt from behind. This, then, is a point very important to notice.

Dimensions.—Although I have taken the dimensions upon several subjects, my researches have not been made upon a sufficient number, to enable me at present to substitute my mensuration for that given in the books. The uterus is generally described as from 7—8 centimetres in length, and in breadth from 3—4 centimetres in its widest part. In virgins, according to Müller, the total length is from 5—6 centimetres, the breadth 32 millimetres, and the length of the cervix 18 millimetres.

Cavities.—The uterus presents for our consideration two cavities communicating with each other. *That of the body* is in the form of a triangle with its base uppermost, and has a capacity of about 10 millimetres. The sound, as soon as it has cleared the internal os, penetrates this cavity with ease, and is capable of movement to a certain extent.

The oval *cavity of the cervix* is quite well figured as well as that of the body, in a plate given in Dr. Bennet's work, although, in my opinion, the proportions are impeachable, in that the cervix is too large as compared with the dimensions of the body. The cavity of the cervix is narrowed below, where is found the *os externum* which is its channel of communication with the vagina. A still more marked contraction exists at the point where it is continuous with the cavity of the body. This is the *os internum*, which is situated nearly at the point of union of the body with the cervix, and which is about 2 millimetres in breadth. It is always smaller than the external orifice, and may arrest a sound which has passed the latter. The sound may also be temporarily arrested even in the interior of the cervical cavity, by the valvular prominences, which are nothing else than the projecting folds which form what has been named the *arbor vitæ*, and which are ordinarily much more marked in women who have not borne children than in those who have.

Sensibility.—The sensibility of the *os externum* and of the cavity of the cervix is, in the ordinary state, null. But the passage of the uterine sound (by which especially sensibility may be developed) through the *os internum*, is always more or less painful. This orifice once cleared, the cavity of the body appears a little less sensible. But, as soon as the extremity of the sound strikes the fundus of the uterus, females experience a peculiar indefinable sensation, " which goes to their hearts," to employ the expression which they generally use. At the same time the liability of the uterus to contract in a spasmodic manner (for they feel pains resembling those of labor, though infinitely less severe), is a new cause of the difficulty one experiences in passing this orifice.—I hasten to add, that nothing being more variable than this sensibility of the uterus, it will often occur to you to find it morbidly exalted in the points I have just mentioned as points which should be insensible.

EXAMINATION OF THE UTERUS IN STATE OF DISPLACEMENT.

Definition of Displacement.—Previously to laying before you with all the necessary details the state of the organ, the divers means of exploring it, and their utility in uterine displacements, it is necessary first to establish what should be understood by the words *displacements of the uterus.* *There is displacement whenever the axis of the uterus ceases to correspond, wholly or in part, with that of the brim of the pelvis.*

This definition, as you see, comprehends all displacements, in whatever direction they may take place, and to whatever degree they may be carried ; and, as you conceive, may include very limited as well as very extensive derangements. The axis of the uterus may depart more or less from that of the brim, from the slightest divergence to such a degree as even to form a right angle in a direction the inverse of the normal one. We must now, therefore, endeavor to ascertain the point up to which these displacements may be compatible with health, and to what extent they must be carried in order to constitute a disease. This limit is very difficult to fix in an exact manner, as in certain subjects there needs but a slight divergence for the production of symptoms, while in others a more considerable displacement may pass unperceived. Meanwhile, when it has been said that considerable displacements often exercise no influence upon the health, it is my belief that the mistake has been committed of generalizing upon exceptional facts. If the uterus is supple, light, not adherent to the neighboring parts, and if, at the same time, the displacement be inconsiderable, it is possible that no marked trouble may result. Under contrary circumstances, it is very rare that a certain number of symptoms is not developed. These symptoms may not, perhaps, attract the attention of the patient, or, if they do, their cause may be unknown. One sees, for example, women to whom walking is not painful, but who, after a long promenade, are easily fatigued, and then experience a sensation of weight in the lower part of the body, lancinating pains in the loins, and numbness in the thighs. Others are subject to the same symptoms when they go up or down stairs, although walking does not fatigue them at all. Some, all the while experiencing but very slightly-marked symptoms on the side of the uterus, emaciate, become blanched, lose appetite, suffer from indigestion, and yet know of no cause to explain these symptoms. Sometimes, even, there are, in addition, particular nervous troubles and symptoms of all sorts, equally inexplicable. If, then, by an attentive examination, the existence of a displacement is ascertained, we find that by removing this we put an end to all the symptoms, and restore the patient to a perfect state of health.

I cannot abstain from citing to you, in connection with this subject, a case, which is not uncomplicated, it is true, and which presented other symptoms than those produced by the displacement, but which in this latter point of view possesses interesting peculiarities.

CASE 1.—The patient was a lady, 36 years of age, of a robust constitution, who had always observed the rules of hygiene, and had committed no excess of any kind. She has had three children, and at her last confinement, which took place seven years ago, gave birth to twins at the full term. Neither have any of her labors been accompanied or followed by bad symptoms, nor has she since experienced any peculiar troubles, as menstrual derangements—leucorrhœa—pains in the pelvis and loins. Three years ago she commenced to experience attacks of dizziness, returning at long intervals and accompanied by considerable swelling of the stomach, with vomiting and a sense of oppression. These symptoms were followed by a transient diarrhœa, then by general prostration and numbness in the left side of the head. The patient could not move the left eye, nor turn her head to the left side without experiencing nausea and an inclination to vomit. Soon, there supervened attacks of dizziness and painful buzzing in the ears, especially upon the left side. There was no sign of paralysis. In the intervals of these attacks the general health was perfect, all the functions were regularly performed, and walking was not painful. Later, the attacks having become more frequent, the existence of numerous neuralgic points was ascertained in the lumbar region, and in the chest as well on the right side as on the left, and becoming more painful during the attacks. Then, during the effort of vomiting, there was developed on the left side of the neck, invading a little the median line, a tumor, which occupied very evidently the thyroid gland, and which was augmented at each contraction of the stomach.

When, on the 3d of December last, I saw the patient, the attacks recurred every ten or twelve days, and independently of what I have just told you, I learned, on interrogating her more closely, that she was troubled with a sense of oppression and constriction, which taking its departure from the epigastrium ascended, not to the throat but to the middle of the sternum.

She had been treated by diet and emollients with no relief, the disease having rather augmented. Later, narcotics and purgatives had produced a little amelioration.

I prescribed narcotics and antispasmodics, to which I added cold douches, and blisters dressed with morphine upon the painful points. These two last means effected a marked alleviation.

On seeing the patient again, the 17th of December, I interrogated her with still more care, upon the symptoms which might be attributed to an internal affection, and learned that she felt no pain in walking, that she could accomplish quite long distances on foot, without great fatigue, without a feeling of weight in the pelvis or on the perineum, that she was not troubled with very frequent desire to pass the urine, though obliged to empty the bladder twice during each night, and that defecation alone was sometimes but rarely difficult.

Yet, on making a tactile examination I did not find the uterus in its normal position. The finger introduced into the vagina, and following its anterior wall, encountered, immediately behind the pubis, the globular body of the uterus, its anterior surface being easily felt, while it was not easy to explore the cervix, directed, as it was, backward and upward towards the sacrum, its mouth being so elevated that the finger with difficulty attained it. As to the posterior surface, it could not be reached at all. By making the uterus swing over by means of the finger in the vagina, I found that it was easily dislodged, but that it was heavy and quickly fell back into its vicious position. I had a good deal of difficulty in finding the os uteri, in order to introduce the sound, on account of the great elevation and backward direction of the cervix ; but once having reached the opening, I easily passed in the instrument by carrying the handle well downward and backward. The patient felt no pain from this manœuvre, and the uterus was easily brought into its normal position. I inferred, then, the existence of an anteversion with engorgement of the uterus. It was not till this moment that the patient imparted to me the knowledge of an important phenomenon, to which she had not, up to that time, paid much attention. When she rose at night to void the urine, she felt in the abdomen a weight which descended in proportion as the bladder was emptied. Then she was seized with nausea, giddiness, vertigo, in a word with all the symptoms which announced the attacks of which I have spoken to you, and was obliged quickly to resume the horizontal position from the fear that one of them was about to supervene. The knowledge of this phenomenon is interesting, especially as it enables us in some sort to witness the movement which the anteverted uterus must execute in the abdomen. As it presses upon the bladder, it must, if mobile, be raised when the latter is distended with urine, and again in proportion as the bladder is emptied, its point of support failing, it must tend to return to its vicious position. It is this movement which this lady in fact very distinctly felt.

I repeated the introduction of the sound on three consecutive days, without the supervention of pain or of vaginal hæmorrhage. But, at this time, the patient was seized with a general bronchitis of a very violent character, during the course of which, the symptoms above-mentioned were re-produced with renewed intensity, so that I was obliged temporarily to suspend the treatment of the anteversion, not to recommence it till the 24th of January. After four days of preparation, by means of the sound, the stem-pessary was applied, and retained without untoward symptoms till the second of February. The menses here setting in, I removed it, and on the 10th ascertained that the uterus was much less inclined forward than on the first day, but was far from being completely re-placed in the axis of the brim. The intra-uterine pessary applied anew on the 10th, remained till the 17th, on which day I removed it, on account of the supervention of a slight distension of, and pains in, the abdomen, but without vomiting or chills. I was then able to satisfy myself that the uterus had entirely resumed its normal direction, which condition it has maintained ever since, the attacks above described becoming less severe and less frequent. This lady has been able to take a journey of a month's duration, without experiencing any recurrence of her troubles, and since her return to Paris has been menaced with them but once, the attack limiting itself to the first symptoms, which were promptly dissipated. She rises but once at night for the purpose of micturition, and has remarked that she no longer feels the descent of the heavy body during the voiding of the bladder.

If we reflect upon the series of symptoms presented by this patient, we cannot avoid recognizing hysteria (and you know how varied are its phenomena), characterized by the sense of oppression, of distension of the stomach, the vomitings, the painful numbness entirely confined to the left side of the face; the constriction which ascends from the epigastrium to the top of the sternum, in a word, by all those extremely varied nervous phenomena, the combination of which constituted each attack. On the ground of the dizziness, of the pains in the head affecting more especially two organs of sense—the eye and the ear—and accompanied by vomiting, the supposition of a cerebral affection might have been entertained. But, there never was a symptom of paralysis, and in the intervals of the attacks the health was always perfect, and the strength intact. If some cerebral affections, as tubercles, hydatids, or other tumors, offer alternations of remission or renewal, never, in the intervals, is the health as good, nor is the strength regained, and there remains in the affected limbs either paralysis or a sensation of numbness which in our patient was but transient. In these cases, moreover, the attacks, at each renewal, have an epileptic character, which they had not in our case, and the malady is always incurable.

Hysteria, as you know, gentlemen, is so frequent in persons affected with uterine diseases, that very competent authors have regarded it as actually an affection of the uterus betraying itself externally by nervous symptoms. We have then to inquire what influence displacement of the uterus may have exercised in this case on the production of hysteric phenomena. This influence is real, and the more incontestable, that once the displacement cured, we have seen the nervous symptoms diminish rapidly in intensity. If they have persisted to some extent since, it is perhaps because there remains still a certain degree of engorgement of the uterus to which they could be referred. They might also have been re-produced through habit, for we have in this one of the principal characters of hysteria, that it does not completely disappear till quite a long time has elapsed. We cannot as yet say that recovery will take place, and still less that it will be definitive and complete, but we may, after what has already occurred, hope for a great modification in the intensity and frequency of these symptoms.

I could cite to you other facts to prove that it is sufficient to interrogate patients and examine them with care to obtain a report of many symptoms to be attributed to uterine displacements, even when these diseases do not present themselves with the whole train of symptoms which habitually accompany them ; but we will recur to this point in the course of these lectures.

EPIDEMIC OF 1852-53 IN NEWTON AND VICINITY.

BY EDWARD WARREN, M.D., NEWTON, MASS.

[Continued from page 254.]

CASE IV.—The infant child of the patient last mentioned, was taken charge of by Mrs. ———, in whose house she boarded. For about a fortnight it continued in good health. It was fed, I believe, principally upon a solution of seed-cake in water, or milk and water, which seems to be preferred by some mothers or nurses here, to milk or cream.

January 8th.—I was called to visit this child, who seemed to be in great distress. I learned it had been carried into Boston two days before in the cars, but had suffered no exposure. It was now seized apparently with colic pains in the bowels, which subsided and returned, allowing intervals of rest. Thinking it possible that its food had distressed it, I gave an emetic, followed by an enema, and had a sinapism applied to the bowels. This seemed to give some relief; and I followed it by one or two drops of laudanum, once in three hours.

9th.—My attention was called to a birth-mark which I had previously seen, and had found somewhat raised above the surrounding skin. A tumor had now formed, of which this was the surface or covering, and had the appearance of a common circumscribed scrofulous swelling. I directed bread and milk poultices to be applied to it, and these seemed to give great relief. My additional prescription was Dover's powders three times a-day, and a wet nurse.

In a day or two the abscess opened and discharged; and soon after the slough or core came out, leaving a tumor with a hollow centre, precisely like the pustules or tubercles which I have spoken of above. From the time the discharge commenced, it showed no signs of pain. A wet nurse being obtained January 15th, it nursed very heartily and began to thrive.

18th.—She was removed with her nurse to a house about half a mile distant. In the evening I was called to visit her in haste, and found her in spasms. It was particularly noticed that while she kept her right arm in constant motion, the left arm, upon the side of the tumor, seemed to be palsied. She was entirely voiceless. I administered syrup of ipecac., a warm bath and sinapisms. Under this treatment she recovered, and began to move the left arm again; showing that everything like paralysis had disappeared. In the course of the night, however, a similar attack came on, and she died towards morning. There was considerable swelling of the bowels, and a purple appearance of the left side after death. The abscess had nothing malignant in its appearance; the lips were soft, and it was entirely superficial.

CASE V.—Jan. 9th, the day after this child was seized, a lad in the same house, about 12 years of age, was attacked pretty violently in a manner resembling the attacks of the preceding season. He had severe chills, nausea, very red cheeks; but cold hands, pulse slow and languid, and tongue thickly coated. Severe pain in the head. I gave him an emetic of ipecac., followed by Dover's powders.

The next day I found him much better; and in a day or two he was quite well.

Case IV.—Mrs. ———, the mother of the preceding patient, who had encountered a good deal of anxiety and fatigue in her attentions to the mother and child above mentioned, went in to Boston on the 13th of January, in the midst of one of the severest snow-storms of the season, and walked about much of the day in the deep snow, in search of a wet nurse.

On the 14th, I found her quite ill in bed. She complained of pain in the side, nausea, headache, &c. She informed me that she could not take ipecac. in any form, neither as an emetic or in Dover's powder. She proposed to take a cathartic of senna and salts. I recommended compound infus. of senna, as milder in its effects; and also a blister to the side. To the latter she objected, as the pain, she said, was entirely "muscular"—meaning, probably, that it was not pleurisy. She took the compound infus., and one of James's powders with a little opium at bed-time.

On my visit the next morning, she came up from her kitchen, where she had been superintending the cooking, and preparing paste for pies. She continued to go about house until Tuesday, the 18th, when she again sent for me. She had now pain in the right side just below the ribs, tongue coated with a thick white fur, extremities cool, pulse not much accelerated. On a preceding day, she had called my attention to the redness of her cheeks. There was at that time a flush of hectic appearance in one cheek only. It was very transient in its duration. I prescribed a blister to be applied to the seat of the pain, and a febrifuge of paregoric, antimony and nitrous ether. By her own prescription, she took a blue pill at night, followed by a laxative in the morning.

On Wednesday, the 19th, I found her very much the same. Her muscular strength seemed good, and her voice strong and natural. She took notice of everything passing in the house, and laughed when any ludicrous idea was suggested. Her manner, however, was quick, and slightly excited; and she complained that her ideas were not clear.

20th.—Finding that the pain had returned, I prescribed an opiate and warm fomentations to the bowels. She complained of fulness and sinking at the stomach, and some wandering pain in the limbs. The symptoms, with the exception of the white tongue, were now decidedly those of enteritis. She considered herself so unwell that she sent for Dr. Perry, of Boston, who had always been her family physician, to meet me in consultation. He did not arrive at the time expected, and I was sent for to see her alone. I found her, at the time of my visit, much as in the morning. She was at the time composed and quiet, pulse not much accelerated. She complained of an increase of pain and distension in the bowels. I recommended warm applications, and the free and repeated use of laudanum by the mouth or injections, until the pain entirely subsided. I advised her to take no other medicine; no peppermint, spirits of nitre, herb tea, or anything of the kind, but to trust entirely to the laudanum. Her previous uneasiness had led her to take various doses of that character. I advised her to keep the stomach empty.

Dr. Perry arrived in the evening, about three hours after my visit. I was prevented, by my engagements, from meeting him. On his first glance, he probably saw something to alarm him. He found her at his visit restless, tossing in the bed, pulse over 100, tongue dry and dark red. On examining, however, he probably found no very tangible symptoms, answering to his first impression ; his opinion, as related to me in the morning, being that he feared either incipient inflammation or typhoid fever. He simply enforced my prescription of the use of laudanum, and of entire rest. He subsequently informed me that he considered her too much reduced by fatigue and anxiety; to advise any active measures ; and that the inflammatory character of the disease of course prohibited tonics and nourishing diet.

21st.—I found her much better. The laudanum had given relief to the pain, and she had passed a good night. In the afternoon, however, the pain returned, and she sent for me again. I advised a repetition of the laudanum.

22d, Saturday.—I found her alone, and still in pain. Her night had not been so good as the preceding. As in the case of the other lady (Case III.), there was fulness of the abdomen, but no pain on pressure. On endeavoring to show where its seat was, it would shift its place or disappear. She had free perspiration. Tongue covered with a thin brown coat. Although there was no definite change in the symptoms, her general appearance, for the first time, seriously alarmed me. Her voice was strong, and her mind clear. She not only took charge of herself, but even of her family, giving directions, and listening to every sound that was made. During the whole course of her disease, she was cognisant of everything that took place in her house. She was her own nurse, and, in fact, almost her own physician. Whether from necessity, or from the restlessness of disease, she changed her room several times during her illness.

I now wished for a consultation with Dr. Perry ; but unwilling to propose it to her, I concluded to wait for the return of her husband from Boston. As she had now been for some time without alvine evacuation, I prescribed an injection of gruel, to be followed by a gentle opiate ; also hot applications to the abdomen.

In the afternoon I found her not relieved ; the injection had been imperfectly administered, and had possibly worried her ; at least by the necessity of directing and superintending its administration herself. It was considered too late in the day, to send for Dr. Perry ; and as I had proposed the consultation for my own sake rather than the patient's, I did not urge it. It is a pretty old saying that " in the multitude of counsel there is safety—for the physicians."

Sunday morning, Jan. 23d, I found her again in a different chamber. She expressed herself greatly better—almost well ; but her voice was broken and interrupted, pulse almost imperceptible ; her attitude in the bed, and whole appearance, of the most alarming character.

Dr. Perry was sent for, and I met him at 2 o'clock ; but the patient was now *in articulo mortis,* and died within an hour. His view in relation to the treatment I have already given—that as an inflammation, the disease prohibited anything of a stimulating nature or very nourishing food. On the other hand, any lowering measures were equally objectionable, in consequence of her previous exhaustion. The disease commenced with enteritis, and continued to evince every symptom of this disease ; and if the inflammation finally extended from the mucous to the peritoneal coat, it was still an inflammation.

It is possible that could the danger of a fatal termination have been foreseen, the placing her under the care of a nurse, and the enforcement of absolute rest and repose of body and mind, would have been more favorable ; but it is one great peculiarity of the present epidemic, that producing no muscular prostration, there is an uneasiness which keeps the mind active. I do not think that she ever fully complied with my opiate course, although I enforced it at every visit. At all events, keeping her mind always upon the stretch, and retaining charge of a large family, what opiates she took did not have the favorable effect which I hoped. Opiates, if properly used and regularly continued so long as required, are tonics.

Simple enteritis is a formidable and dangerous disease ; more formidable than typhoid fever.

CASE VII.——Jan. 13th. I was requested to be in readiness to attend a young married lady, who had come from Boston to her mother's house in November, expecting to be confined in the course of that month. She had already gone a number of weeks beyond the time calculated, and had felt pains for a day or two ; but this evening the labor seemed to be coming on in earnest. The pains left her, however, towards morning, to return again in the evening ; and pursued this course for four or five days.

On the 17th, the pains showed more signs of continuing, and I was sent for in the morning. I found her sitting up, upon two chairs, with her knees drawn up ; and learnt, to my surprise, that she had kept this posture for nearly a week ; not even lying down at night, on account of the pain produced by a recumbent position. Since her coming from Boston, expecting daily to be confined, she had kept in a close warm room, without exercise, and upon a pretty liberal diet.

The pains were pretty irregular through the day, but increased towards evening. Delivery was accomplished towards morning, without anything remarkable occurring. She had a fine healthy-looking boy, weighing ten pounds.

There was not, however, the appearance of relief which generally attends the instant of delivery. The patient lay in a motionless, passive state, perfectly conscious, and showing no signs of exhaustion or faintness ; but not speaking or moving voluntarily. Her countenance had a mottled, rather bloated look, neither flushed nor pale. From the family constitution, I had expected excessive flowing ; but there was much less than is usual. After the birth of the child, the uterus did not contract, and the size of the abdomen remained nearly the same as before.

On attempting to assist the expulsion of the placenta, I found the cord too feeble to be of any use, and attached so high up, that I could not reach its origin with my finger. After several futile attempts to excite uterine contraction, I judged it better to delay for a short time longer. At the end of an hour I examined again, and finding the womb still dilated and perfectly passive, I introduced my hand and removed the placenta without difficulty, and without more pain than attends its ordinary expulsion.

Finding it still impossible to produce contraction of the uterus by gentle measures, friction, &c., I abandoned the attempt, and left her under the care of a skilful and experienced city nurse. As there had been and was no flowing, and no urgent symptoms, I did not think it advisable to give ergot, or to employ any active measures.   I considered it safer to leave the case to nature, than to take it out of her hands.

19th.—On my morning visit, I was informed that she had passed a bad night. The abdomen had been very much distended. She had severe chills, and had passed a large amount of coagula. The nurse had given her gin for the chills, and applied spirit to the bowels. The tumefaction she informed me was much less than it had been. I found her comparatively comfortable. Her pulse was of sufficient fulness, and not accelerated. The abdomen less full than yesterday, with no greater tenderness than in the most favorable cases. She perspired profusely. Her voice was hoarse, but this was attributed to a cold taken before confinement. She lay on her back, with her head low, knees drawn up ; very restless. I advised warm applications to the bowels, and liquid extract of valerian, a teaspoonful every four hours.

20th.—Has passed a bad night. There has been some wandering of the mind, and extreme restlessness. I found her, however, calm and perfectly rational. The abdomen is still greatly swollen, but by the nurse's report less than it has been in the night. The pulse is not accelerated, and there is no more tenderness of the bowels. She continues to perspire profusely. I directed a dose of castor oil, and the continuance of the valerian and fomentations.

21st.—She had again passed a very restless night. The tumefaction of the bowels, however, was less, and there were no bad symptoms. The oil had operated well. She continued to perspire profusely. I now prescribed laudanum, which I had avoided before for what I considered strong reasons.

Up to this time, there was nothing alarming in the symptoms. Some appearances had occurred of an unfavorable character ; but there was nothing, upon strict examination, of a very threatening aspect. I always found her perfectly rational, the pulse not accelerated, the skin always very moist ; the voice, though hoarse, strong. Upon careful examination of the bowels, there was little tenderness upon pressure. At the time of my visits, she appeared free from pain. In fact, all the symptoms of inflammation which I looked for were absent.

At my evening visit this day, Jan. 21st, I found her worse ; the dyspnœa was considerable, and there was a cadaverous smell. This, though remarkable in fatal cases, is not an infallible prognostic. I have frequently noticed it in patients who recovered. The smell may proceed from the discharge of putrid coagula, or other substance. It by no means necessarily implies general gangrene. At this visit I of course found considerable cause for alarm.

I was called to her again about 11, P.M. The nurse thought her very much worse, and could find no pulse. When I arrived, a re-action had taken place. Her pulse was about 80, steady and regular. The dyspnœa had increased ; but her mind was clear : and on being asked about the difficulty of her breathing, she attributed it to a cold ; and she could even smile in answering my questions. I must confess that I felt very strongly encouraged by her appearance even at this time.

About three hours after, I was again called to her, and now found her really pulseless, and unable to speak. She soon became unconscious, and died within an hour. The surface of the body became purple, and the abdomen was enormously distended.

The day after the death of this patient I was called to her infant, which I had not seen for several days. As the mother had no milk for it, a wet-nurse had been obtained, and it had nursed well. I was informed that it had been apparently ill for two or three days, and the monthly nurse had observed from the first a peculiarity in holding one arm, which was now found to be motionless. The child was dying when I was called to it ; the whole surface of the body purple. It died within an hour.

At the time the death of this lady occurred, there was no epidemic of any kind within my circuit. I had not seen any avowed case of erysipelas for some time, either in the form of tubercle, so prevalent here at most times, or in any other. In the adjoining town of Natick, it was quite prevalent. The patient herself, and one or two others of the family, had frequently suffered severely from inflammation and swelling of the tonsils, but I had never considered it of an erysipelatous character. In this immediate neighborhood, three very severe cases of uteritis had occurred at different times some years since, which I reported for this Journal, all which terminated favorably. No case of diffuse puerperal peritonitis had ever occurred. In Case No. III. the symptoms of pleurisy were the only prominent ones. Some circumstances struck me as anomalous at the time ; especially the rapid and fatal issue of the disease, while those symptoms wore a favorable appearance ; but deaths from pleurisy only, are often as sudden. The subject of Case III. resided at some distance from the patient last mentioned, and died Dec. 10th. This one was confined Jan. 18th, five weeks after. But when another fatal case occurred in the very house where the patient No. III. had died, comparing the peculiar symptoms of the three cases, and also those of the infants, there could be no doubt as to the nature of the disease. The first patient died Dec. 10th ; her infant was attacked Jan. 8th, and died Jan. 19th ; the second one was first attacked Jan. 14th, and died Jan. 23d. The third patient was confined on the 18th, and died on the 21st ; her infant upon the 22d. The subject of the first case reported, died Jan. 16th.

Thus all these deaths, except the first mentioned, took place within eight days of each other. The weather at the time was warm for winter, the ground covered with snow, but melting, and there were frequent rains, a particularly violent rain Jan. 23d. The weather, Dec. 10th, was pretty similar.

It is worthy of notice, also, that the two severe cases of erysipelas which I reported some years since, were sporadic, occurring in different years, and that none others occurred at the same time. So also with the erysipelatous pustule ; it is rare to find more than one case in the same family, though certainly highly communicable by actual contact, if not from the breath and emanations.

[To be continued]

PROSECUTION FOR MAL-PRACTICE.

[Communicated for the Boston Medical and Surgical Journal.]

THE Supreme Court of Massachusetts were occupied, last week, in trying an alleged case of mal-practice, of unusual interest. A summary of the evidence is as follows :—

A healthy boy, by the name of Ashworth, 10 years and 3 months old, had his left hand drawn into the picker of a woollen mill, the consequence of which was several severe wounds of the hand and a simple fracture of the radius, midway of its length, with a lacerated wound over the place of fracture, but probably not communicating with it. Dr. Joseph Kittredge, of Andover, was called to the case, and dressed it, in the usual manner, with sutures and plaster for the external wounds ; and a bandage, secured just above the elbow, compresses and splints for the fracture. This took place in the forenoon of Friday, Nov. 21, 1851. No pain, nor loss of sleep or appetite, occurred till Sunday morning, Nov. 23d, when he complained of a little aching in the shoulder. The prick of a pin in the thumb and back of the hand, gave reason to suppose the sensibility was diminished, but not lost. During the latter part of Sunday night he was restless, and had more pain at the shoulder in the morning. Between 3 and 4 o'clock, Monday afternoon, he was again visited by Dr. Kittredge, who found vesication at the uncovered elbow, and, on cutting off the bandages, the arm, destitute of sensation, mortified from the shoulder downward. The dressing was removed, a consultation called, and a fatal prognosis pronounced. The father continued the opiates, cordials and fomentations ordered by the physicians, but of his own accord, at the suggestion of advising neighbors, kept the shoulder and neighboring part of the trunk and the arm wet with brandy and salt, which he also administered internally. On Tuesday considerable ecchymosis of the shoulder and neck was observed, and some vesications on the trunk. On Thursday, sixth day of the accident, a line of demarcation appeared at the shoulder ; and on the 21st day of the accident, the father removed the arm from the scapula by separating the dead from the living parts with a feather. The boy went into the country, where, on dressing the shoulder, the physician found the head of the bone loose in the glenoid cavity, and removed it. The skin cicatrized over the part, and the boy recovered. The fragment of bone was produced, and was found to be formed of the articulating surface and a portion of the shaft of the humerus.

Several physicians were put on the stand, to give opinions in the case, as to the causes of result, and whether proper care and reasonable skill had been shown in the treatment of the case. On the part of the prosecution, Dr. I. D. Pilsbury, of Lowell, testified to the opinion that all the symptoms were caused by too tight bandaging—that dressings of a fracture should be removed to examine it sooner than the fourth day—that the pulse of the injured limb should always be examined to determine if the artery pulsated—that constitutional remedies should be used to prevent injurious symptoms—that there was no necessity for carrying the bandage above the elbow—that he should expect pain in the shoulder from too tight bandaging of the fore-arm. Drs. Hayward, Townsend, H. J. Bigelow, Ainsworth, of Boston ; Dr. Kimball, of Lowell.; Drs. Loring and Peirson, sen., of Salem, testified to the opinion that proper care and skill in the treatment of the case had been shown by the defendant, and that too tight bandaging would indubitably produce pain, which, in a few hours, would become intolerable, and that it was impossible that the bandaging in this case should have caused the gangrene. They unanimously swore to their belief that the plugging of the artery, which must have taken place at the axilla, caused the gangrene by arresting the flow of arterial blood into the arm. Dr. Peirson alone was of opinion that a fracture of the articulating head of the humerus caused an injury to the artery, in consequence of which plugging followed. His opinion was founded on these considerations :—

1. The appearance of the bone and its place of separation. The bone was separated at its cervix through one half of its diameter, and the rest of the separation was below the line of the epiphysis, through the radial or external tubercle, according to the following outline.

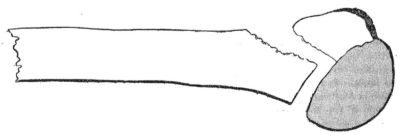

2. The fragment of bone, thus removed with the articulating surface appeared rounded off, as if by absorption, while the shaft of the bone remained as it would have appeared immediately after the fracture.

3. Twenty-one days was probably a shorter time than would have been required for living to have thrown off dead bone, or sooner than it would have been separated by the process of decomposition. The separation of the ulnar, carpal epiphysis, which was exhibited to refute this theory, proved nothing, as it was found to be separated only after the arm had been preserved in spirits for eighteen months.

4. The ecchymosis at the neck and shoulder appeared about the time it was to be expected, as the result of distension of the soft parts which probably occurred after the fracture, which was not suspected, not being

denoted by any pain, the fragments being kept in apposition by the short muscles attached to the shaft of the bone, and by the tendon of the long head of the biceps passing over the upper fragment.

Whether or not this hypothesis explains the cause, the medical testimony, with the exception of that of Dr. Pilsbury, was agreed in assigning interruption of arterial circulation at the axilla as the cause of the gangrene. Notwithstanding this remarkable accordance, the jury gave an award of damages to the amount of $1675. The defendant petitioned for a new trial, on the ground of the verdict being contrary to the evidence.   P.

Salem, April 25, 1853.

TREPHINING IN APOPLEXY AND INFLAMMATION OF THE BRAIN.

To the Editor of the Boston Medical and Surgical Journal.

Sir,—From some experiments upon the gallinaceous tribe, this week, in cerebral hemorrhage and inflammation of the brain, we are inclined to think the trephine worthy of a suggestion in similar diseases in man, and we will give you the reasons for our faith, and leave yourself and readers to your own deductions. In this region of country we have a disease among our fowls, well known to the old matrons of the land, as distemper, but it is really nothing more nor less than a disease of the brain, of an apoplectic or inflammatory character, which is proved by dissection as well as the symptoms. We have had it among our fowls for several years, and as we appreciate our poultry very highly, we tried a variety of means, upon the old woman's plan and our own, for the cure of it, and with passing mortality. This season it attacked our fowls again, and we determined to try a more rational plan. In our slight cases we gave oil, and applied the cold douche with some success; in cases of a worse grade, we gave oil, applied the douche, and introduced a seton in the back of the neck; and in several of our malignant cases, we *trephined the skull*, with decided success. While we write, we have a fine female fowl speedily recovering from a severe and protracted attack, which we attribute to the use of the *trephine.*

Now if the *trephine*, with a simple knife, will relieve the apoplectic condition of the chicken, a very tender animal when compared to man, will it not relieve man of the same affection? All of the great experiments to elucidate the functions of the nervous and other systems, have been performed upon inferior animals, and why should not this be equally legitimate? We performed the operation in several cases, with decided success when we least expected it, for it was a dernier resort with us. Some of the cases operated upon did succumb, and we attribute it to the late hour of the operation. The matter was entirely an accidental occurrence in our hands; but the analogy is so strong, that we cannot resist the inclination to place it before the profession, for further discussion. Some may object to it, on account of its harshness. We reply, nothing is too harsh to protect human life, if no other means will succeed. If arsenic will cure gastritis, and we know it, we will adopt it; and so with everything else. We are an eclectic; and if farther experiments will confirm the position we assume that trephining will relieve or cure apoplexy and inflammation of the brain, we shall be one of the first to adopt it, whenever a proper case presents itself. We extract calculi from the bladder to keep men from dying ; we cut off thighs to protect life ; we excise the maxillary bones to prevent death ; and the operation of *trephining* is not more dangerous than either of them. If tracheotomy will cure epilepsy, as we doubt not it will, we see no good reason why trephining should not cure *apoplexy*. We merely throw out these views to our brethren, as we are no " *wild enthusiast ;*" and we hope every man in the brotherhood will give them a calm and candid reflection ; remembering they are only suggestive upon facts observed in the *chicken* tribe. We shall continue to operate, as cases present themselves to us, and if we find our opinions further corroborated, or not, we will inform the fraternity of it, for we report our cases without regard to success or fatality.

Respectfully, H. A. RAMSAY.

Thompson, Geo., April 18, 1853.

THE BOSTON MEDICAL AND SURGICAL JOURNAL.

BOSTON, MAY 4, 1853.

Drug Inspectors.—Some of our ports of entry are thought to have been poorly guarded against the introduction of worthless drugs and medicines. Many leading members of the profession advocate a grand sweep of the whole body of inspectors, from Eastport in Maine, to New Orleans. A new administration has an undoubted right to place its political friends in the various desirable offices. Many of the present drug inspectors stepped into places from which very respectable incumbents were removed, on account of their politics ; and hence it is reasonable to suppose that the tactics practised by those recently in power, will be copied by each succeeding dominant party. However, on that subject there is not a word to be said here. There have been some poorly qualified individuals put into commission. Originating, as the law of drug inspection did, with the physicians of the United States, represented in the American Medical Association, the inspectors should have been taken from their ranks. Instead of having accomplished, learned men, some of the first set selected by the Secretary of the Treasury were taken from wholesale drug shops, without possessing a single preparation for a post of such importance, beyond knowing the ordinary routine of buying and packing. There were people behind the screen who provided well for their friends and favorites. Wherever an incompetent inspector is found, the sooner he is removed the better. Those best qualified are fairly entitled to the positions. Life and death are somewhat connected with this branch of the revenue service, which demands intelligence, tact and science. Some individuals are also clamorous for a change of medical incumbents in the Marine Hospitals in the various ports of the United States. Rotation in office is the doctrine of the day, and public medical men must therefore take their turn, and retire without complaining.

Throat and Uterine Diseases.—How is it to be accounted for that so many people have ulcerated throats ? Practitioners in former times were rarely consulted upon any difficulty in that region, beyond enlargements of the tonsils in young persons. But now-a-days, throat patients are numerous indeed—so much so, that the treatment of them has become a distinct branch of professional business. . They are perpetually hurrying here and there over the railroads, for the advice of somebody they have heard of who has gained particular distinction on account of his successful treatment of such cases. There must be a direct cause for this wide-spread and increasing malady. Anthracite fires, high-seasoned food, bad water, imperfectly ventilated houses, close sleeping rooms, thin shoes, tobacco, coffee, artificial wines, and numerous other instrumentalities, have been by turns accused, but finally exonerated from having anything to do with the generation of these various conditions of the throat. Therefore the field is open for further investigation.

But another equally perplexing difficulty has arisen in the domain of medical practice, quite as anomalous, viz., variously diseased conditions of the uterus. Has the climate undergone any changes within the last half century to have affected the health of women in this manner ? Either this class of sufferers were entirely overlooked formerly in New England, by the generality of practitioners, or some new cause is operating. From the multiplication of these cases, the treatment of them to some extent has become a specialty. Ladies go great distances for the assistance of those whose names are abroad as successful in restoring unfortunate female sufferers to health. A close study of distinct classes of disease, is fast leading to a subdivision of professional labor. In cities, fifty years hence, the ancient Egyptian system will probably be established—and there will be physicians, as the historian expresses it, for the eye, for the ear, for the mouth, and so on.

A discovery of the cause or causes of the increased prevalence of these two diseases, would lead to happy results. While no satisfactory explanation can be given of their origin, uncertainty in regard to the proper method of medication must characterize the best directed efforts.

Medical Association of Alabama.—There is a massive appearance to the volume just published of the transactions at the sixth annual meeting of this association ; and the contents are eminently worthy of examination. They have the art of persuading the members to contribute liberally, at the south, to the archives of their societies. In medical topography, southern gentlemen have rendered excellent service to the scientific literature of the country. The last gathering of the thrifty State Association of Alabama was at Selma, in December last, commencing on the 13th, and terminating in the evening of the 15th. Instead of hurrying through the secular business, reading papers, choosing officers and dining sumptuously, all in the same day, a rational course is adopted in Alabama, if no where else, of taking ample time for cool deliberation. Dr. A. Denny, of Suggsville, was elected President; Dr. Lopez, of Mobile, Orator ; and Drs. N. Bozeman, of Montgomery, and R. Miller, of Mobile, Recording Secretaries. A diffusive energy is perceivable in the records, that will be felt remotely. Every practitioner can do something towards promoting the respectability and progress of medical science within the jurisdiction of the society ; and a pleasant duty it must be, according to the present published document. Drs. W. H. Anderson and Geo. A. Ketchum's report on the diseases of Mobile, and Dr. Crawford's account of the diseases of Centreville and vicinity, are able, but brief performances. Changeability of disease, by W. Tayler, M.D., of Talladega, and the essay on the summer and autumnal fevers of South Alabama, by I. H. Anderson, M.D., of Sumpterville, are, however, the gems of the publication. Both of them might be greatly enlarged, and sent forth as distinct treatises, for the instruction and guidance of young practitioners. We do not feel at liberty to occupy more space in expressing the gratification derived from the transactions of the Alabama faculty, but cannot refrain from expressing the hope that their organization may long uphold the honor and dignity of the profession in that enterprising State.

Portland Medico-Chirurgical Society.—Till 1850, there appears to have been no medical society in Portland, the principal city of Maine. The constitution and by-laws of the association, which was then formed, bearing the above patronymic, are drawn up with a degree of care that ought to ensure perfect harmony, while the rights and dignities of the brotherhood are protected, and all is done that words can do towards making the members respectable among themselves and respected by the great public. In the organization of these societies, it is very proper to have every regulation clearly explained ; for where there is the least degree of ambiguity, some hair-splitting fault-finder makes his appearance after a while, and delights to harp upon the constitutionality of this thing and that, till the hours appropriated for mutual improvement are frittered away in profitless discussions of no earthly value to any body. A plain, comprehensible instrument may always be understood, and we are happy to perceive that simplicity and fairness characterize the constitution under which the profession of the enterprising city of Portland have united.

Easton Medical Institute.—A private medical institution is working its way into public confidence in the State of Maryland, in the beautiful town of Easton, under the charge of C. C. Cox, M.D., one of the faculty in the Philadelphia College of Medicine. An inducement for a pupil to enter this school, is economy in tuition and board. Charming scenery, refined society, a choice library, good apparatus, thorough instruction and a bland climate, are also among the considerations that might influence a full school of applicants to take up their residence with Dr. Cox.

Transactions of the American Medical Association and of the Kentucky Medical Society.—The Transactions of the American Medical Association, in a large and well-printed volume, and the Transactions of the Kentucky State Medical Society, also got up in a very creditable manner, have been received from the publishers. The former is a document of general interest to the profession throughout the country, and should be extensively circulated. The latter is more local in its character, but every article in it is of practical value, and some of the Reports by the committees are the results of deep research and careful observation. That of Dr. Gross on Surgery, occupying nearly 200 pages, is elaborate and complete. every branch of that department of medical science, especially as connected with Kentucky practice, being taken up and analyzed.

Medical Miscellany.—A woman in Wisconsin became insane from, excess of joy at receiving an unexpected supply of food for her starving family. —A child, not four years old, is insane, and in the Lunatic Hospital at Harrisburg.—No. 5 of Tully's Pharmacology has been received.—The March No. of the New York Dental Recorder is well sustained with original articles.—A new Homœopathic Hospital has been opened at Doncaster, England.—The Philadelphia Journal of Homœopathy says, " we are neither exclusive advocates of high or low potencies."—The population of Lexington, Ky., in a sexual point of view, is singularly divided, there being 2,756 males and 2,755 females.—Dr. Daniel Blair, Surgeon General of British Guiana, has discovered that belladonna has no efficacy as a prophylactic in yellow fever, as he at one time supposed.—By taking Pegu, the British are able to send opium into China without any interruption, by land. —Dr. Robert J. Breckenridge has been appointed Surgeon of the Marine Hospital, New Orleans, in place of Dr. Powell ; and Dr. J. N. Hughes, in place of Dr. M. Pyles.—A man recently died at Clarksville, Georgia, by bleeding at the nose. He expired on the 6th day.—Smallpox is prevailing at New Castle, Henry Co., Indiana.—A female slave, found dead in the bed at Louisville, Ky., was found to have a fatty formation in the heart, between the right auricle and ventricle, that obstructed the circulation.—Dr. Daniel Lee, of the Patent Office. Washington, is to deliver an address before the Agricultural Society, in Franklin Co., Mass., Oct. 7th.—Dr. Boykin has been appointed U. S. Naval Store-keeper at Norfolk, Virg.—A newspaper, under the title of ' The Health Journal," has been commenced at Syracuse, N. Y., which appears to be an emanation from the Eclectic School. —Preparations are making at the various travelling places in the United States for the accommodation of vast multitudes of " well invalids."—The annual meeting of the Mass. Medical Society will be held in this city, Wednesday, May 25th —Dr. Lewis A. Thomas has been appointed Postmaster of New Haven, Conn.—Dr. John G. Dunn has become editor of the Register, Virginia.—A coroner held an inquest over a skeleton, found in a box on its way to Dr. A. Davidson, Huntington, Indiana, in the care of Adams & Co.'s Express.—Dr. Barrett has been elected treasurer of the Savings Bank, Northampton, Mass.—It is stated that eighty American seamen, eighteen captains, ten mates, and as many more foreigners, have died during the past nine months, at Port au Prince, from yellow fever.— Violet Proctor, a female, died in the almshouse, New Bedford, Mass., at the great age of 108 years.—Yellow fever has again broken out frightfully, at Kingston, Jamaica.—Cholera is prevailing near Gaston, N. C.

ERRATUM.—In No. 12, on page 232, 10 lines from the bottom, for " observations," read " reports of cases."

DIED,—Dr. G. W. Baskin, of Mercer, Pa , assassinated. Some one in the dark, as he was returning home and about entering his house, stabbed him with a bowie knife, so that he died as soon as he entered the door.—On the passage to San Francisco, Edward W. Gleason, M.D , of Boston. —At East Hampton, Mass , Dr. Solomon Chapman, 46.—At Bethany, Conn., Dr. Jehiel Castle, 82.

Deaths in Boston for the week ending Saturday noon, April 30th, 75. Males, 38—females, 37. Accident, 1—inflammation of the brain, 2—disease of the brain, 1—congestion of the brain, 2—bronchitis, 2—consumption, 10—convulsions, 1—croup, 3—cancer, 2—diarrhœa, 1—dropsy, 2—dropsy in the head, 4—drowned, 4—debility, 1—infantile diseases, 5—puerperal, 1—erysipelas, 1—fever, 1—typhus fever, 2—scarlet fever, 4—hooping cough, 1—hemorrhage, 1—inflammation of the lungs, 9—congestion of the lungs, 1—marasmus, 1—mania. 1—old age, 4—pleurisy, 1—palsy, 1—peritonitis, 1—inflammation of the stomach, 1—teething, 1—tumor, 2. Under 5 years, 30—between 5 and 20 years. 4—between 20 and 40 years, 20—between 40 and 60 years, 14—over 60 years, 7. Born in the United States, 52 — Ireland, 14—England, 4—Scotland, 2—British Provinces, 2—Germany, 1 The above includes 13 deaths in the city institutions.

University College Hospital.—Death from Chloroform.—On Tuesday last Mr. Wakley held a lengthened inquiry relative to the cause of the death of Caroline Baker, an unmarried woman, aged 28 years, who died in University College Hospital from the effects of chloroform. The inquest-room was crowded by medical gentlemen and others anxious to hear the particulars of the catastrophe. Mr. J. H. Gould, physician's assistant, deposed that on Friday night, the 18th inst., deceased was admitted into the hospital, suffering from sloughing ulceration of the labia and vagina. Mr. Erichsen, one of the surgeons to the hospital, directed Mr. White, the acting house-surgeon, to apply nitric acid to the sores. Accordingly, on Saturday morning, Mr. Gould, the physician's assistant, and Mr. White, proceeded to prepare the patient for the application of the acid; Mr. White, as is the custom on such occasions, first administering chloroform to the patient, Mr. Gould being in readiness to apply the acid. The chloroform, supposed in the first instance to be about a drachm, was poured on lint about five inches square, and folded four or five times over. After a short time the patient became restless, talked loudly, and threw about her arms. Soon afterwards a partial relaxation of the limbs took place, and she became insensible and pulseless. Witness, fearing a fatal result, sent for Mr. Clover, the resident medical officer. Artificial respiration was kept up, galvanism applied, and everything done to resuscitate her, but in vain, as she sank and died.—Mr. Clover corroborated the previous witness, and stated that, although not a qualified practitioner, Mr. White was fully capable of administering chloroform, and that he had only followed the usual practice on such occasions. During four years, chloroform had been applied in 1600 instances in University College Hospital, with but one fatal case occurring. The quantity of chloroform administered was at the option of the operator, and generally averaged from half a drachm to a drachm at the commencement. Professor Erichsen performed the autopsy, and found a fatty degeneration of the heart, and also that the death was produced by a paralysis of the heart from the influence of chloroform. The unfortunate affair was purely an accident, for which no one was to blame.—Dr. R. Quain concurred in Professor Erichsen's opinion, and added that portions of the heart having been handed to him by that gentleman for examination under the microscope, he had found that organ, particularly on the right side, in a state of fatty degeneration. The Coroner summed up, and commented on the great caution that should be used in the administration of chloroform. The jury retired, and, after a brief deliberation, returned a verdict, "that the death was caused by paralysis of the heart, produced by the influence of chloroform, casually, accidentally, and by misfortune." The foreman stated that it was the unanimous opinion of the jury that a medical gentleman of experience should always be present when chloroform was administered; and Mr. Erichsen promised that on all future occasions the recommendation should receive every attention.—*London Lancet,* March 26.

Guano for Mummifying.—From the ship Brandscompt, unloading Peruvian Guano at Leith (Scotland), there were exhumed the remains of three persons, evidently Peruvians, buried in the guano, and which had apparently not been disturbed in the process of loading the ship. It is not known when the bodies were originally interred, but the bones were all found as entire as if they had been preserved in a museum; the hair remained upon the skull, and the clothes were very little decayed.

THE
BOSTON MEDICAL AND SURGICAL JOURNAL.

| Vol. XLVIII. | Wednesday, May 11, 1853. | No. 15. |

EPIDEMIC OF 1852-53 IN NEWTON AND VICINITY.

BY EDWARD WARREN, M.D., NEWTON, MASS.

[Concluded from page 281.]

CASE VIII.—December 2d. I was called to a young married man, about 28 years of age, who was suffering from a very severe attack of inflammation of the tonsils. The pain was intense, and had prevented his sleeping for several nights. I applied nitrate of silver to the tonsils, and gave him a gargle composed of muriatic acid with confect. rosæ and rose water, and a Dover's powder every four hours. This course was continued until the 9th, when his throat was well.

Jan. 31st.—I was sent for to visit him again, and found that he had been suffering for a week with an attack similar to the preceding. I found both the tonsils greatly enlarged, but not filling up the passage of the throat, or causing impediment to the voice or breathing. The pain was more intense than before; the most severe in appearance that I have witnessed from such a cause. As he was unwilling to have the nitrate applied, I prescribed merely opiates, a gargle, and external irritation to the neck. After a day or two, finding he was not essentially relieved, I applied the nitrate of silver again, about the 4th and 5th of February. On the 6th, he informed me that his throat was nearly well; but I found him in bed, complaining of a pain in the right knee. He now told me that he had formerly had rheumatic fever. I advised the application of a blister to the knee, and an opiate at night.

February 7th.—I found the pain in the knee gone; he had pain in the shoulder, and the tongue was covered with a thick white coat. The pulse was small and not rapid.

This afternoon I was called to him suddenly, and found him in great distress from pain in the bowels, especially at the epigastrium. No pain on pressure. On the contrary, he informed me that the pressure of my hand relieved him. I prescribed external irritation and Dover's powders.

8th.—Has passe a bad night. Complains of fulness and distress in the bowels. Coat on tongue brownish. Abdomen and thorax covered with dark-colored circular spots or maculæ. He states that an eruption of this kind came on after his recovery from his last sore throat. Lies on his back, with his head low and his knees drawn up. On moving his

15

body he contracts his forehead with the same expression, as if of organic pain, which I noticed in the other cases ; but says he has no pain. Perspires very freely.

The friends now becoming alarmed, proposed a consultation with a physician who was visiting a patient in the neighborhood. I met him in the afternoon ; and he made a very careful examination of the patient, and decidedly pronounced it a case of typhoid fever. On my calling his attention to the fact, that the maculæ, besides being very different from rose spots, were not confined to the abdomen, but spread over the thorax and a large portion of the body, he thought they resembled the spots of ship fever. He gave a favorable prognosis. Advised a strictly expectant course ; Dover's powder, nitre, &c., and injections when a motion of the bowels was required. I gave my opinion that the disease was of an erysipelatous character, and suggested quinine ; which he thought it too early to give.

My reasons for considering it erysipelatous, were the history of the case, the close resemblance of all the symptoms to those of the cases of peritonitis above described ; the fact that one of the patient's children, during his illness, had an erythematous rash, while another had erysipelatous pustule upon the finger. Their mother had sore throat and incipient pustule, which was cured by nitrate of silver and poulticing. These affections, moreover, were prevailing in all the houses around.

The next morning, Feb. 9th, I found him very much worse. His countenance was quite yellow, tongue dark colored, pulse small, and about 100. Cannot move his left arm. In short, there seemed every probability of his sinking as rapidly as the other three patients. Unwilling to resort to quinine without farther consultation, I prescribed spt. Mindereri as a substitute, and requested a consultation with some one. Dr. Hoyt, of N. Natick, met me about 2 o'clock, P.M. The patient seemed now somewhat better, and the yellowness had greatly disappeared. Dr. H., however, found his pulse over 100. Taking into view the whole history and circumstances of the case, he agreed with me as to its erysipelatous character, and to my great satisfaction advised pretty full doses of quinine. He advised three grains, once in six hours, a conium pill of three grains, and morphine or elixir of opium in doses sufficient to keep him free from pain : also sinapisms to the bowels, and diet of broth and beef-tea. His prognosis was unfavorable.

10th.—Appears better, but says he has passed a bad night. The bowels are easier, but has great pain and soreness in the limbs. Has taken fifty drops of the elixir of opium. Says it is the only thing that has done him any good. Bears quinine well. Pulse a little fuller and less rapid than yesterday.

In brief, he varied greatly from day to day, the disease going from one arm to the other, and to the knees and ankles ; occasionally producing a redness on the joint, and threatening the formation of a tumor or tubercle, but disappearing again, and attended with little if any swelling. The pain was always to be distinguished from rheumatic pain, by being relieved by pressure. The pain or distress which occurred in the bowels early in the disease was very promptly relieved, and did not return.

Pimples or tubercles subsequently made their appearance on his arms, and one large one upon the back. These, however, whether because the disease had exhausted itself, or in consequence of the continued use of quinine, never became very troublesome.

I visited him twice a-day, until the 17th. After continuing the quinine powders for about four days, finding the pulse very full and becoming too rapid, I first omitted one dose in twelve hours, and then substituted a tincture of the sulphate, one drachm to a pound of diluted alcohol, with thirty-five drops of sulphuric acid. As quinine is not perfectly soluble in water or even spirit, it is probable that a much smaller quantity will be effectual when thus prepared. I gave a teaspoonful three times a-day.

I continued my daily visits until about the first of March, at which time he was able to walk out. Two pretty severe cases occurred in another family in the same house ; one in a boy of about 15, the other in a girl of 10 or 12. The symptoms were strikingly similar to those in the preceding case. The boy, however, had great redness of the face, and the girl's attack was preceded by a rash or eruption, which I did not see.

. CASE IX.—I began to visit the above patient Jan. 31st. On the 2d of Feb. I visited a boy of 13 or 14 years of age, in the opposite house, who had an erysipelatous pustule on the end of his thumb. He was the brother of the patient whose case is described in vol. xliv., page 174. The disease had commenced several days before, but was apparently too slight to attract much attention. It was now becoming very painful, and I applied caustic over the sound and diseased parts, and caused it to be poulticed. The inflammation was thus prevented from extending upwards, but the disease continued in the cellular membrane. He had the white-coated tongue, and small, slow pulse, of the others. About Feb. 4th, I commenced the tinct. sulphat. quinine, 15 drops three times a-day. Finding a soft, fluctuating fluid under the skin, I cut through the latter ; but only blood followed the incision, and it became more painful. The tumor continued to increase slowly from day to day. It was much of the time free from pain, and it was advancing on the side opposite to the one I had punctured. In about a week longer, constitutional symptoms developed themselves with great severity ; chills, vomiting, pain across the epigastrium, &c. The pulse, however, when I saw him, was slow, the extremities cool, perspiration very free.

CASE X.—Upon the 14th, when the subject of the preceding case had been two or three days in bed with the severe constitutional symptoms mentioned, his grandmother, a lady of 72 years of age, came towards me in high spirits, exclaiming that the swelling had broken. I found this to be the case, and that it had broken on the side opposite the one on which it had commenced. In the evening I was called to the grandmother, who was said to be dying. She had seemed to me quite well and very active in the morning. She had eaten a hearty supper, which she finished with apple-pie and pickles. After supper, feeling unwell, she went up to her chamber to lie down. The moment her head was upon her pillow, she was violently seized with pain or distress in the back of the head. I saw her within a few minutes. She was sitting in a rocking chair, exclaiming that she was dying, but in a strong and natural voice, and holding her head almost erect. Taking into consideration all the circumstances, I thought expedient to give her a dose of ipecac ; and had mustard applied to the back of the neck. The emetic operated promptly and mildly. She seemed to be somewhat relieved, and I had her placed upon her bed, and directed elixir of opium.

Soon after I left her, she felt an uneasiness in the bowels, which induced her to insist upon getting up. After sitting a moment or two, she dropped backward upon the floor, and became insensible. I found her insensible and stertorous, and she died within an hour. I leave it for others to determine whether her death was or was not the result of epidemic or infectious miasm or virus.

Her grandson soon became able to walk out ; and the thumb has gradually improved, though it is not yet entirely well.

Case XI.—Feb. 2d. I was called to a young man in a house a few steps from the preceding. He had a swelling upon one leg, between the heads of the gastrocnemius muscle, with diffuse inflammation, and severe constitutional symptoms. I had it poulticed, and gave him quinine. In about two days from the time that I saw him, the tumor broke, and he very shortly returned to his business. His mother had at the time a troublesome swelling or puffing up, at the epigastrium, and has since had several attacks of the prevailing epidemic in form ; sudden and severe enough to excite great alarm.

Case XII.—Upon the 12th of February, I was requested to see a young married woman, the mother of two children, who had been out of health all the past summer, apparently with some derangement of the digestive functions. She now had severe cough and palpitation. During the funeral of the puerperal patient, Case VII., she had taken care of the house, and received those who came. She was much exposed to the weather, it being a violent rain ; and also to whatever risk there might be of infection. On examining the cardiac region, the pulsation of the heart was hardly discernible ; but above and upon the left side, near the axilla, was a loud bellows sound. I prescribed a blister over the region of the heart, and an expectorant. The pulse was slow, and, as it were, compressed.

On the 14th of February, the same evening on which the fatal Case No. X. occurred, I was called to her. She stated that she had been suddenly seized with violent throbbing, and her breath was suddenly " sucked in." She had great distress at the epigastrium, and in the head, especially at the back part of it. About an hour after the attack, a fit of trembling or shivering came on. The extremities were cool. Pulse quite slow and small. I directed that she should not be moved from the sofa where I found her. I had sinapisms applied to the bowels ; the head freely bathed with camphor, and gave her spirit ætheris nitrosi, aq. ammoniæ and elixir of opium.

Feb. 15th.—Found her in the same position. She had not raised her head. Pulse as yesterday. Tongue covered with a thick white coat. Great fulness of the bowels, swelling and soreness across the epigastrium ; no spots of any kind. Has perspired freely ; cheeks very red, but the hands cool. I directed a continuance of the mustard poultices, Dover's powders and nitrous ether. Five drops of the ammonia to be given, if any faintness or spasm ensued.

16th.—As yesterday. Lies on her back, with head low. On attempting to raise the head, it brings on great distress. The attempt to raise the left hand to the head brings on throbbing and great difficulty in the chest. Her voice is strong, and her spirits generally good. I prescribed elixir vitriol as a, drink ; spts. Mindereri in place of the nitrous ether. Elixir of opium and ammonia to be used if required.

17th.—As before. Commenced tr. sulphat. quinine, a teaspoonful three times a-day.

18th.—Cannot take the quinine. Reduce the dose to fifteen drops, and increase by five daily. After continuing to improve for about a week, during which her bowels were moved only by injections of gruel, she had a fresh attack, occasioned, it appears, by some slight alarm. I found, however, in the morning, that she was not essentially worse. The circulation had become more free ; the action of the heart was, on the whole, improved. I found that when the quinine was increased to sixty drops, unpleasant symptoms were produced, and it was necessary to go back. Perspiration was always free. Tremblings, throbbings, palpitation, pain in the limbs, particularly in the left arm, frequently returned. For some time, an inadvertent attempt to raise the left hand to the head brought on severe distress in the cardiac region, accompanied with violent throbbing. There were frequent sudden alarms, which occasioned me to be sent for. By the first of April, however, I considered her well enough to discontinue my visits.

This patient had a much better faculty of describing her symptoms than the others. When, towards the end of my attendance, I thought it expedient to prescribe a cathartic, she informed me the next day that she had some pain from the operation. It was real " old-fashioned pain," and the first *pain* she had had since she had been ill. She had suffered a great deal, and had complained of pain, but in the same manner as the others. The truth was, it was a sensation severe and alarming, because different from anything they had ever experienced ; but it was not " old-fashioned pain." On being questioned, the others described it as burning, stinging, or soreness.

During the latter part of her illness, I substituted the application of croton oil for the sinapisms, causing it to be applied alternately to the cardiac region, and to the epigastrium.

In this case I had at first serious reasons to believe that there was severe organic, or, at least, functional derangement of the heart. Nearly all evidence of this kind, however, passed away with her amendment. Most of the symptoms resembled very closely the severe cases which had gone before ; and still more closely the succeeding. The cough and other pneumonic symptoms disappeared entirely when the sudden attack came on. In some of the later cases, the pneumonia has been more severe and the cardiac affection slighter, but palpitation has been very frequent. While, in this case, some of the symptoms were more violent than in any of the others, I never felt any apprehension of immediate danger to life. In Case VIII. I did feel the utmost apprehension of an unfavorable issue.

In the present case, after the first week or two, there was a good appetite; and it was a remarkable feature in this, as in all the other cases, that there was constant craving for solid food; forming a great contrast to the condition in typhoid and typhus fever.

CASE XIII.—The lady who was the subject of Case VI. in my former communication, was attacked in a similar way as before. After keeping about house for nearly a week, she had a fresh access of the complaint, Nov. 14th.

I found her sitting up in bed, as before, with intense distress in the head. Face moderately swollen, and very red. Pulse small, not accelerated. White coat on tongue. Skin cool. In short, the attack was perfectly similar to that of last year; but very much worse. After a few days the distress in the head abated, but severe pain came on in the upper part of one leg, below the ham. On examining, I found diffuse inflammation around a spot between the heads of the gastrocnemius; and the vein in that spot greatly enlarged. The constitutional symptoms had very considerably abated; but the pain in the tumor was very great. I considered it decidedly advisable not to employ depletory measures, but to apply warm poultices at once to the tumor. I gave morphine for the relief of the pain. In about three days, the tumor pointed and began to discharge. A small opening was formed in the vein, from which some blood escaped. After poulticing for a day or two, the inflammation subsided sufficiently to allow me to apply straps and a roller to the limb. About the 18th of November, she began to walk upon it. The wound had healed perfectly, leaving hardly a vestige on the skin, and none upon the vein. An elastic stocking was procured, and has been constantly worn since. There has been no return of disease in the limb.

Here, then, was a case of genuine phlebitis; and its origin could be directly traced, not only to the present and former epidemic attack, but from this, through other members of her family, to the institution, the principal of which died as I have before related. Of course, I cannot say that it was derived by infection from him, or that his disease was the same; but only, that I was informed that a peculiar form of influenza prevailed there among the young ladies; one of whom came home with the symptoms I described.

Feb. 24th.—The subject of this same case had another severe attack, brought on, like the former, from fatigue and anxiety, in attendance upon a sick person. It was attended with more inflammation and swelling about the face, than the preceding ones. I concluded in this case to commence at once with quinine, even before the attack was developed. She took elixir vitriol in water as a drink, which seemed always to benefit her. On the second day of the attack, I gave her, at her own request, an emetic of ipecac.; resuming the quinine as soon as the state of the stomach would allow. On the third day, I found her out of her chamber, and in a day or two she was well. There has been no return of inflammation in the vein.

Whether her rapid recovery was owing to the quinine, or to other causes, I cannot say. The attack was as violent as either of the former, the symptoms were as severe ; and, as in the former case, she had neglected the first warnings, and continued about her usual avocations until absolutely unable to leave her bed.

It is worthy of mention, that the house in which these cases occurred stands in an elevated situation, entirely alone, and about a mile from the village.

CASE XIV.—Feb. 26, I was called in the evening to see a girl of about 12 years of age, who had been suffering for several days from earache. It had now become violent, and was attended with severe constitutional symptoms. I prescribed laudanum for the ear ; and 15 drops of elixir of opium once in four hours. The next morning I found the ear relieved. She had taken three doses of the elixir. The ensuing night I was called up to visit her. The pain had left the ear, and was now in the bowels. She had a white tongue ; had fits of shaking or trembling, and there was great fulness across the epigastrium ; skin cool and moist, pulse slow, cheeks very red. I applied sinapisms to the bowels, and gave her a large dose of elixir of opium. This relieved her, and the pain did not return.

In the morning I found her free from pain, and in high spirits. The coat on the tongue, however, continued. She had good appetite or craving for hearty food. I now put her upon a full dose of the quinine ; a teaspoonful of the tincture I have described. She bore this medicine better than any one to whom I have given it. She was kept in bed for several days, and it was a week or more before the coat left the tongue ; but she improved from day to day, and, in fact, was perfectly comfortable from the time that the night attack was relieved.

CASE XV.—Feb. 24th, a middle-aged married woman, having a family of grown-up children, was taken with severe pain in the right groin, to which she had been subject before, at times. Last night she had chills and palpitation. I found her tongue loaded with a thick white coat, considerable pain in the head, skin cool, pulse very small and feeble, not accelerated. Has had nausea and some vomiting. I gave her an emetic of ipecac., to be followed by Dover's powders ; a blister to the seat of pain in the abdomen.

25th.—About the same. Pain in the groin less. Appetite good.

26th.—Last night had severe chills, which she attributed to sitting up some time. Some nervous excitement or wandering of the mind in the night, and palpitation. Fulness at the epigastrium, and great distress there now. I prescribed tr. sulphat. quinine, a teaspoonful three times a-day, and an opiate at night. The tremblings and a throbbing below the region of the heart came on nightly for some time. Her recovery was retarded by sitting up too much, and by not being free from family cares. I continued to visit her daily until about the 30th of March, when she was well enough for me to leave her ; but she is not yet entirely recovered.

It was my intention to have given other cases, which were exceedingly interesting to me in their peculiar developments ; some of strong robust men, who continued about their usual employments until a fresh and violent access of the disease fairly alarmed and disabled them ; cases coming on with great violence, and disappearing promptly in proportion ; some cases of infants, seized in the most alarming manner either with symptoms of lung fever, or of inflammation of the brain, but disappearing almost as promptly as they came on. But I have already exceeded all reasonable limits.

Latterly the cases have been attended with cough and other symptoms of pneumonia ; sometimes to an alarming degree in infants or young children. Yet I have ventured upon the quinine, although it seemed to be contra-indicated ; and they have rapidly improved. To nursing infants I have given the tincture in doses of five to eight drops three times a-day. Their recovery has been speedy.

I may describe one more attack which I have recently witnessed. As in the other cases, the first stage was passed before I was applied to. On a warm day, on which several new cases occurred, the subject was seized in the evening with headache and fulness or oppression at the stomach, resembling precisely the symptoms of enteritis. This continued through the night and next day ; when towards evening these symptoms disappeared, and a burning sensation was felt from the throat to the stomach, like that of inhaling the burnt air of a close room. Upon going to the outer door, shivering came on, lasting for some minutes. Upon going to bed, the middle of the body, from the thorax to the thigh, including the whole abdomen, was found covered with a scarlet erythema. This remained for about thirty-six hours ; the subject taking quinine, but continuing about his usual avocations. Upon the appearance of the rash, the other symptoms disappeared.

I believe that the disorder generally comes on in this manner. There is a distinct attack, and then twenty-four hours elapse before the chills occur. In this interval, I expect, if an emetic and opiates are given, and entire rest observed, it will be arrested. Perhaps quinine might be given at once, with equal effect.

Quinine, it is well known, is not a new remedy for erysipelatous disease. In its original form of Peruvian bark, it was given and recommended by John Hunter, sixty years ago ; and despite of the authority of Sydenham, Travers, and many other great names, its use has been sustained with much force and clearness by many English writers of the highest eminence.

The description given by Sydenham, applies rather to the sporadic cases, which are often met with in individuals of good constitution when no epidemic is prevalent. He was, perhaps, the closest observer of the epidemic constitutions of different years who has ever written. In erysipelatous diseases attended with debility, he gave tonics. Sir Astley Cooper gave calomel in the first instance, and then resorted to quinine or other tonics. But medical treatment must be adapted, not only to the particular disease, and to the constitution of the patient, but to the locality and the atmospheric constitution of the season.

We have almost given up the use of the lancet. Purgatives are in disrepute among the profession ; though favorites in family practice. Quinine is recommended in rheumatism. The time may come, when it will be considered the sheet anchor in scarlet fever ! Dr. Cain's treatment of scarlet fever, noticed in this Journal in 1851, consisted in inunction by bacon as the base of his treatment, but he employed also tonics and stimulants. This is deserving of consideration. The time may come when opium and bark will form our whole materia medica, relying for everything else upon cracked wheat and molasses, or sometimes a dose of ipecac. !

Mr. Nunnely and other writers describe erysipelas as attended with a quick small pulse. In my cases, at the time of my visit, the pulse was generally slow, but it would vary from hour to hour. The disease was decidedly not one of inflammation, but of irritation, and the, state of the patient at all times was readily affected by mental causes. Hence the appellation of irritative fever seems to be most expressive of the peculiar character of the epidemic, both of this season and the last. It is some years since I examined the work of Dr. Butler, and I do not recollect precisely in what sense he used the term. I would neither attempt to appropriate a name, or to reform nomenclature. I should merely use this name, or *constitutional irritation*, as peculiarly expressive of the present epidemic as I have witnessed it. That it has prevailed and is prevailing to a less or greater degree, not only in other places in the country, but in the city, I am also aware.

In conclusion, I wish to say that I have reported, above, all my fatal cases.

Newton Lower Falls, April 18, 1853.

AN OVER DOSE OF CROTON OIL.

[Communicated for the Boston Medical and Surgical Journal.]

ALL that is important in medicine is made up of facts—and every individual who leaves one fact on record, adds something to the common stock, however trifling the fact, of itself, may be. If you think the following worth a place in your Journal, you are at liberty to insert it ; if not, throw it " under the table."

About the middle of February, S. N., of this town, aged 22, was attacked with acute rheumatism (a disease, by the way, that has been very prevalent in this region the past winter), which continued some six weeks, affecting the heart and diaphragm by metastasis. In the treatment of the case, I relied, mainly, on *copious* bleeding, and calomel combined with Dover's powder. But, to come to the *fact*. The patient so far recovered, as to be out of doors ; and venturing too much, brought on a relapse of the disease, affecting the organs before named, exclusively. I prescribed, among other things, the use of croton oil externally to the epigastrium, and tinct. opil, in doses of ten drops, at intervals. By mistake of the nurse, ten drops of the oil were given, instead of the laudanum. Much alarm was, of course, soon excited ; the patient and his friends having got the impression, which is quite general among *the people,* that this article is given only in cases of "life and death," and then in very small doses. A messenger was sent "for the doctor," in great haste. It happened that I was attending another case at the time, and did not arrive till one hour and twenty minutes had elapsed after the accident. I found that state of mental excitement on the part of the patient and his friends, which naturally results from the apprehension of certain and immediate death. Here was a set of circumstances which, one would think, might give even the uninitiated a faint idea of the responsibilities of a physician. The first thing to be done was to allay the excitement. I said to the patient—"*It won't kill you.*" This produced a calm, which enabled me to sit down for a moment and reflect what was to be done · *physically.* I soon came to the conclusion that it was too late to trust to an emetic ; and determined on giving mucilage to the extent of the stomach's capacity, and wait the result. In *eight hours* there was a *moderate* operation on the bowels. The evacuations which followed, occurred once in thirty minutes, numbering ten in all. The degree of prostration was not great. Not the first symptom of irritation of the stomach appeared. In five days after the accident, the patient was able to walk into another room.

The effect of this occurrence on the public mind, is that "*the oil cured him ;*" which remark has about as much propriety in it, as if we should say of a man recovering from a fit of drunkenness—the "*liquor saved his life.*"   W. B. SMALL, M.D.

E. Livermore, Me., May 2, 1853.

RECUPERATION.

BY GEORGE HOYT, M.D.

[Communicated for the Boston Medical and Surgical Journal.]

THERE is in the animal economy a principle of great value to a physician ; and, if results be considered, of no less importance to the patient, which ought carefully to be studied and apprehended. I refer to the *recuperative* power of the system, by the agency of which an effort is always made to restore a suffering member or diseased body to its original standard of health.

In disease, this principle is always active and more or less obvious. When distinctly seen, it is a valuable and efficient guide ; for a physician is but the handmaid of nature. His province is never to supersede, but to aid her. She has a language of signs, beautiful and distinct, by which her intentions are made manifest, and it is his duty to observe and expound them. In fevers, it is witnessed in the earnest appeals of a patient for water, "cold water," and in his oft inability to slake his thirst. It is not less observable in the delicious sensations arising from the free admission of pure air. It is seen in critical diarrhœas, sometimes in profuse perspiration, often in bleeding at the nose, occasionally in the expectoration of blood, and generally in hemorrhage from the bowels. The following case illustrates the principle.

A young man, of about 18 years of age, in the beautiful town of Hubbardston, where I then resided, was suddenly attacked with pleuro-pneumonitis, apparently investing both surfaces of the serous membrane, and severely affecting the right lung. The disease was fearfully developed before I saw him, and was not arrested till near the end of the second week. After the crisis, his improvement was slight, indeed hardly perceptible, and he continued feeble beyond my expectations. A careful examination by physical signs revealed his true state. An empyema, or, as the sequel proved, a partially-encysted abscess, had formed in his right side; a condition usually fatal, though not necessarily so. At this time it was impossible to determine to what extent the lung was invested.. He was " comfortable," however, and knowing that nothing but an operation could touch the case, I concluded to trust him to the efforts of nature for the present.

From the outset he had been troubled with cough, but with slight expectoration, and did not sensibly change in this respect for quite a length of time. But pus began to appear, gradually increasing in quantity for some months. If he now turned upon his left side, a position he exceedingly disliked, violent paroxysms of coughing ensued, accompanied' by an almost continuous stream of matter—demonstrating, that being unable to make a portal at the side, *nature* had opened a passage to the trachea through the lungs, and furnishing an additional evidence of the general *law.*

. Nearly a year had now elapsed since his attack. He had improved in no particular. Rapid pulse, frequent respiration, night sweats, emaciation and great general debility, were his prominent characteristics. He was evidently incurable, unless it were possible by an operation to relieve him. The objections to this, lay in probable adhesions, the extent of which, it was impossible to determine. In consultation with three eminent physicians, the only one of whom now living, is Dr. Osgood, of Templeton, Mass., it was determined, as a dernier resort, to perform the operation. The consent of all interested being readily obtained, we laid his skeleton body upon a table, and with a scalpel and lancet, I cut to the right lung, betwixt the sixth and seventh ribs. No pus issued ; and the introduction into his side of a curved probe, revealed the reason. Adhesions above the point of incision had taken place, and matter, the abundance of which I could not question, was imprisoned above it. Further dissections were deemed inexpedient, and the case was *again* entrusted to nature. But the wound showed no disposition to unite, and in a few days there burst forth such a quantity of matter, as, in the language of the mother, flooded the bed.

Still the wound did not heal, and within the succeeding ·few days two additional ejections poured from his side, varying in quantity from half a pint to a pint or more, by estimation.

This was the termination of the case. The wound closed, the cough disappeared, expectoration ceased, and his appetite returned. A cheerful mind, with the inspiration of hope, gave him new life, and he ultimately recovered. It is now rising twenty years since that event transpired, the subject is still living, a successful agriculturalist, and the head of a happy family.—There are here *four points* marked by *re-cuperation.*

1st. The empyema, or abscess, the formation of which is *curative.*

2d. The passage for the egress of matter through the trachea.

3d. The *additional* external *impulse* after the operation.

4th. Union of the internal cavities after evacuation of the pus.

FOREIGN BODIES IN THE STOMACH.

FOREIGN substances, of a very singular character, sometimes find their way into the stomach, from which they are frequently extracted with great difficulty. A most remarkable instance of this description, calling forth extraordinary ingenuity on the part of the surgeon, occurred in 1814, in the practice of Dr. Bright, formerly of New Castle, and now of Louisville, Ky. The particulars are too interesting not to be mentioned on this occasion.

" A child near New Castle, in that State, playing with a fish-hook, incautiously swallowed it, while the line to which it was appended hung out of the mouth. The mother instantly seized its hands, and sent for Dr. Bright, who arrived soon after this embarrassing occurrence. Learning that the hook was one of very small size, he made a hole through a rifle-ball, and having passed the line through it, he dropped the ball into the child's throat, which was immediately swallowed. He then, by means of the line, withdrew the hook from the stomach, whilst the bullet prevented its point from injuring the cardia or œsophagus."

My friend, Prof. Gibson, of the University of Pennsylvania, evidently refers to this case in his work on Surgery ; but he attributes it, erroneously, to a New England surgeon. Dr. Bright's case occurred when he was quite a young man ; and while he was a student in Transylvania University, in 1823, he communicated the particulars of it to the late Prof. Brown, of Lexington.

It is known that foreign substances, accidentally introduced into the stomach and other organs, will occasionally migrate to a great distance, and be at length eliminated through the skin. A very remarkable example of this kind occurred, not long ago, in the practice of Dr. N. B. Anderson, of this city. A girl, aged 19 years, on the 20th of April, 1849, in a fit of laughter accidentally swallowed a large brass pin and a medium-sized needle. Nothing of moment occurred for three weeks, when pain and uneasiness began to be felt at the cardiac orifice of the stomach, where it continued for three months, when it gradually changed its position, and fixed itself upon the inferior lobe of the left lung. In this situation it remained for about nine months, without any disturbance of the respiratory function, with the exception of occasional cough and slight hemoptysis. The pain then shifted to the glenoid cavity of the scapula, and then to the axilla, impeding the movements of the superior extremity. The limb continued in this condition until December, 1850, when the pain and uneasy feeling gradually extended down the arm, and at length settled at the elbow, in the belly of the biceps muscle.

Here a dark spot formed, quite sensitive to the touch, which soon terminated in an abscess, filled with bloody matter. and containing the foreign bodies, situated about half an inch apart. The pin was discolored, but the needle retained its polished aspect.

Thus it would seem that these two bodies travelled side by side from the stomach through the diaphragm, and thence through the walls of the chest to the superior extremity, where they finally excited suppuration, leading to their extraction by the knife.—*Prof. Gross's Report on Surgery.*

ON SYRUP OF IODIDE OF IRON AND MANGANESE.

BY WILLIAM PROCTER, JR.

THE attention of the medical profession has recently been awakened to the advantages to be derived from the use of the salts of iron and manganese in combination, when preparations of iron alone have heretofore been indicated. Among the compounds used by M. Petrequin, is a syrup of iodide of iron and manganese, but the method suggested for its preparation from the solid iodides, by M. Burin-Dubuisson is too indefinite to be generally adopted, besides involving the necessity of previously preparing and keeping the solid iodides. The following formula yields a preparation of the strength of the officinal syrupy solution of iodide of iron, and the manner of using it and the doses are the same.

Take of Iodide of Potassium, - - - 1000 grains,
    Proto-sulphate of iron (in crystals) - 630 "
    Proto-sulphate of manganese, " - - 210 "
    Iron filings (free from rust), - - - 100 "
    White sugar (in coarse powder), - - 4800 "
    Distilled or boiled water, a sufficient quantity.

Triturate the sulphates and the iodide separately to powder, mix them with the iron filings, add half a fluid ounce of distilled water, and triturate to a uniform paste. After standing a few minutes, again add half a fluid ounce of distilled water, triturate and allow it to rest fifteen minutes. A third addition of water should now be made and mixed. The sugar should then be introduced into a bottle capable of holding a little more than twelve fluid ounces, and a small funnel, prepared with a moistened filter, inserted into its mouth. The magma of salts should then be carefully removed from the mortar to the filter, and when the dense solution has drained through, distilled or boiled water should be carefully poured on in small portions, until the solution of the iodides is displaced and washed from the magma of crystals of sulphate of potash. Finally, finish the measure of twelve ounces, by adding boiled water, and agitate the bottle until the sugar is dissolved. The solution of the sugar may be facilitated, when desirable, by standing the bottle in warm water for a time, and then agitating.

Each fluid ounce of this syrup contains fifty grains of the mixed anhydrous iodides, in the proportion of three parts of iodide of iron to one part of iodide of manganese, and the dose is from ten drops to half a fluid drachm.

Remarks.—Owing to the slight solubility of the resulting sulphate of potash, and the small quantity of water employed to effect the interchange of elements, but little of that salt is contained in the syrup. The object of the iron filings is to saturate any free iodine that may be eliminated during the exposure consequent on the gradual re-action of the salts. The use of either distilled, or cold recently-boiled water, is necessary to obviate the effect of air on the iodides. It is necessary to allow sufficient time for the complete decomposition of the sulphate of iron, else the syrup will be contaminated with it. The proper moment to lixiviate the sulphate is known by the cessation of the crystallization of the sulphate of potash. The bottle should be shaken from time to time during the filtration to protect the filtered solution, and the washing process should be stopped as soon as the sulphate ceases to have a well-marked taste of the iodides. Practically in this, as in all cases where syrups are made by agitation, and are not to be filtered, it is best to use pure lump sugar, and coarsely powder it for the occasion, as the commercial powdered sugar frequently contains dusty impurities. The preparation when finished has a very pale straw color ; if the salts have not been all decomposed before the washing, the syrup will have a greenish color, and subsequently deposit crystals of sulphate of potash by standing.—*Journal of Pharmacy.*

THE BOSTON MEDICAL AND SURGICAL JOURNAL.

BOSTON, MAY 11, 1853.

Meeting of the American Medical Association.—The sixth Annual Meeting of this Association took place in the city of New York on Tuesday, May 3d. Dr. Jonathan Knight, of New Haven, was chosen President. But little business was transacted on the first day of the session, and in the evening the members, about 500 in number, were entertained at the residences of several of the profession in the city. On Wednesday the reports of the various Standing Committees were called for. Prof. Meigs, of Philadelphia, Chairman of the Committee on Diseases of the Cervix Uteri, desired that his report, which was strictly professional, might not be read to the meeting, as many were present who did not belong to the profession. Dr Condie, of Philadelphia, was unable to present his report on Tubercular Disease, and the committee were continued another year. Dr. Emerson, of Philadelphia, presented his report on the Agency of Refrigeration produced by upward radiation of heat as an exciting cause of disease—the sanatory lesson of which was the great importance of guarding against the refrigerating effects of *nocturnal radiation*, especially in sickly places and during epidemic periods. Dr. Campbell, of Augusta, Geo., reported on Typhoid Fever. Dr. Atlee, of Pennsylvania, reported on the epidemics of New Jersey, Delaware, and Pennsylvania. Dr. Sutton, of Kentucky, reported on the epidemics of that State. Dr. Pitcher, of Detroit, presented a report on Medical Education.—Dr. Smith, of New

York, chairman of the Committee on Voluntary Essays, reported fifteen received, and premiums were awarded to the authors of the two following: " On the Cell, its pathology," &c. by Dr. Waldo J. Burnett, of Boston; " Fibrous Diseases of the Uterus hitherto considered incurable," by Washington L. Atlee, of Philadelphia.—A resolution was proposed by Prof. Palmer, of Chicago, and was adopted—" That this Association earnestly recommends to the local Societies in different portions of our country, to appoint Committees, whose duty it shall be to record the prevalence of epidemic or other diseases, and the general state of health in their respective localities, and transmit the said-reports to the Committee of this body on Epidemics, through the State Societies, where they exist."—Dr. Chas. A. Lee offered a resolution censuring the medical Schools which give two courses of lectures annually—which was laid on the table.—Dr. Buck, of New York, read a paper on morbid growths in the larynx.—The subject of assimilated rank in the navy was discussed, many members taking part in it, and a Committee was appointed to bring the matter before Congress. —Dr. Peaslee, of New Hampshire. offered a resolution that no diplomas should be granted to those who intend to practise irregularly. A warm discussion followed. Dr. Sears thought the faculty who granted diplomas in such cases should have the power of taking them back. The resolution was laid over.

On Thursday, several resolutions were presented by Dr. G. J. Ziegler, of Philadelphia, and referred to the Committee previously appointed on local societies. They recommend the adoption of measures for the formation of State and County Medical Societies throughout the country; and, to secure a more general membership, that instead of the present voluntary application for admission to County Societies by individuals, every unassociated eligible physician be elected to such; and that those thus elected, and neglecting to respond to or unite themselves with the general profession, be considered as not entitled to the usual rights and privileges of professional intercourse and fellowship.—Dr. N. S. Davis, of Illinois, read the report on Medical Literature. The periodical medical literature of the country, it was stated, comprises annually 16.000 pages, 7,100 being devoted to original matter, 2,380 to reviews, and 6.390 to selections and editorials. Complaint is made, that in the original articles. writers are apt to describe particular modes of treatment which they have found serviceable, and to recommend such modes to others without regard to seasons, the topography of the place, or other local influences.—Dr. Winslow Lewis, of Boston, offered a resolution, recommending the passage by Congress of a law compelling importers of medical compounds to state on them their true constituent parts; and that State Legislatures compel venders of the same to do so in the respective States. Dr. Welford, of Va., moved that the statement be made in English, as the spirit of such a law had been evaded in Maine by the Chinese language being used! Drs. Bond of Baltimore, Sears and Cocks of New York, C. T. Jackson of Boston, Cox of Maryland, and Richards of Ohio, opposed the resolution; and Drs. Parker and Bolton of Va., and W. Hooker of Conn., advocated it. It was lost by a large majority.—Dr. Yandell, of Ky., read the report on Malignant Diseases.—A resolution offered by Dr. Gooch, of Va., to secure a more strict adherence to the code of ethics, and proposing that medical degrees be conferred on the condition that they be forfeited if the orthodox system of medicine be deserted, caused much discussion. The subject was disposed of by the passage of a resolution recommending to Medical Colleges and examining boards to require from graduates and licentiates their signature to the code of ethics; and that the formal administration of a pledge faithfully to observe the same, form part of the public exercises at medical commencements.—The Constitution was amended so that four members of the Medical Board of the Army and Navy be admitted to the Convention, and that the American Medical Society in Paris be entitled to a representation.—A Standing Committee was appointed, to report at the next meeting, concerning any cases of death during the year from the use of anæsthetic agents.—The next yearly meeting was appointed to be held at St. Louis.—A banquet was given in the evening, at Metropolitan Hall, about 1,000 being present, which excelled any thing of the kind in New York—as asserted by the Tribune, from which the preceding brief sketch has been condensed—since the reception of Kossuth by the Bar. On Friday, the delegates were invited to visit the city institutions, and those from the North who accepted the invitation, escaped the risk to life and limb which was incurred by many who returned home by the land route on the morning of that fatal day.

Prosecution for Mal-practice.—Our readers were made acquainted last week, by one of the medical witnesses in the case (now, alas! no longer in the land of the living), with the principal points connected with the late trial for mal-practice at Lowell. If a course like this is to be pursued against surgeons, when their professional success falls short of a miracle, some new system of practice must be adopted in self-defence. Not knowing the full bearing of the testimony, it would hardly be warrantable to attempt defending Dr. Kittredge; but it seems very unlikely that a practitioner of general observation and much-experience, should have bound up an arm so tightly as to put a stop to the circulation. Every surgeon in the community is liable to a lawsuit for damages. Juries appear to have been particularly sympathizing with plaintiffs, in these transactions. The case of Dr. Manning, of Lunenburg, is a remarkable instance of a disposition and determination to break down a physician. He had justice at last, at the hands of the judges, but a great injury was inflicted upon his health and property. A Boston surgeon observed, while commenting on the decision at Lowell, that a few years ago he obliged his patients, before acting professionally, to enter into an obligation not to prosecute him. Not unfrequently some rival practitioner has been called to the stand, and his testimony has added fuel to the fire. Such should speak with extreme caution under these circumstances, and be sure that prejudice has no influence over the judgment.

Medical Degrees Claimed by Colored Students.— John P. Barnell, a colored young man, has applied for a mandamus to compel the College of Physicians and Surgeons in the city of New York, to admit him to the profession. This is the statement published. Whether the object is to oblige the College to grant him a degree, or in some other way permit him to have and enjoy the rights and privileges belonging to licensed medical practitioners, is not understood. Some months since, a case very much like this occurred in New England. The parties interested were persuaded to relinquish the project of prosecuting for privileges thought necessary to a respectable entrance into the medical profession. The question came up—has any chartered institution, created expressly for the education of the people, a right to exclude, on account of color, any person of good character and properly qualified, from receiving the benefits of study under instructers thus stationed at the portals of knowledge ? In answer, it was contended that if the admission of a certain student would prove prejudicial to the reputation or harmony of an institution, whether it were an academy or university, the faculty or trustees were bound to exclude the offensive rather than offending individual, and not obliged to declare the cause of their prohibition. So, also, if colored students of medicine demand an examination for a degree, or a license from a medical society, it is competent for the officers to determine whether it is expedient to comply with the wishes of the candidates or not. If by complying, they bring the institution into contempt, and thereby destroy the conservative character it was designed to maintain in providing the community with properly qualified physicians and surgeons, society and even the tribunals would demand a change of policy. But the *law* makes no distinction between men in relation to color here at the North ; and if colored students seek an education, either academical or professional, nothing but public sentiment, operating in favor or against them, can turn the scale. In Boston, a colored attorney was admitted to the bar, and the medical students cannot discover why they have not an equal claim to admission among the Æsculapians. Out of this anomalous condition of things, mixed up with the radicalism of the times, the flow of active christian benevolence, and the strife of political controversy, which brooks no control, it is difficult to foresee how the war of opinion will terminate.

Health of Cities.—A. B. Palmer, M.D., recently addressed a communication to the authorities of the enterprising city of Chicago, relating to the Public Health. It is of a character to command the attention of public functionaries in other places, where the population is dense, and the poor are permitted to make themselves more miserable by tenanting wretched, dilapidated houses, in filthy, out-of-the-way places. We have room for only the following extract.

"Municipal authorities dictate the mode of building for the protection of property from fire, but not for the protection of life, or of property, from disease. We have our limits within which buildings must be so constructed as to resist the ravages of that element—must be made fire-proof—but we have no localities where buildings must be made and kept, typhus, dysentery, scrofula and cholera proof, although the one is about as practicable as the other, if all the other circumstances of the city in reference to the matter be the subjects of regulation. A disease originating and gaining force in a crowded, dense, filthy and illy arranged locality, may spread to other neighborhoods, more insidiously, perhaps (for the pestilence walketh in darkness), but quite as disastrously, as the devouring flames ; and should be equally a subject of municipal regulation.

"The foundation of all hygienic knowledge and sanitary reform, is in accurate and minute statistics, and the undersigned would beg leave to suggest the passage of an ordinance securing the most rigid accuracy and the minutest detail in the registration of deaths, requiring the addition of more particulars than in the present, as to locality, condition, time of residence in the city, &c., of the person—greater minuteness as to the cause of death, continuance of illness, &c., and also a registration of marriages and births."

Blood-letting.—Among the petitions sent to the legislature of New York, a year or two since, was one from Dr. William Turner, praying that physicians may be restrained from drawing blood ! Arguments were produced, conclusive enough to convince a stone, that immense injury had been done by drawing blood from the veins of the citizens of the sovereign State of New York; but either from stupidity, an inability to perceive the force of reasoning, or a recklessness in regard to the value of life among the good people, their constituents, no sumptuary laws were enacted by the law-makers to restrain medical practitioners from acting according to their own individual judgment when at the sick bed. To the petitioners, the criminal neglect of duty in not passing an act to prevent phlebotomy in all cases, and the spilling of blood in operations, was perfectly unaccountable. Notwithstanding the flood of light shed upon the Senate and House of Representatives, even to this day blood-letting is actually practised throughout the Commonwealth of the State of New York. A pamphlet is before us, explanatory of the whole matter.

Death of Physicians by a Railroad Accident.—The late shocking accident at Norwalk, Conn., to a train of cars in which were a large number of delegates on their return from the meeting in New York of the American Medical Association, caused the sudden death of several eminent medical men of New England, who were greatly endeared to the profession and the people. Among them was Dr. A. L. Peirson, of Salem, Mass., a gentleman of the highest respectability, and for many years the leading surgeon in Essex Co. He was the writer of the article on mal-practice in the last number of this Journal, and called at the office to look over a proof of it on his way to New York. Dr. Josiah Bartlett, of Stratham, N. H. (one of a numerous family of physicians, worthy sons of a most estimable medical man); Dr. James M. Smith, of Springfield (a son of the celebrated Dr. Nathan Smith, founder of the Medical School at Dartmouth, and brother to Dr. N. R. Smith, of Baltimore) ; and Dr. J. H. Gray, also of Springfield, were among the victims. On the fatal list we also see the names of Drs. Samuel Beach of Bridgeport, Conn., Alexander Welch of Hartford, and Wm. C. Dwight of Brooklyn, N. Y. Among the physicians who were injured, were Drs. J. W. Bemis of Charlestown, C. H. Browne, of Ipswich, and W. D. Lamb of Lawrence.

Those who were killed were in the two forward passenger cars, which passed over the bridge into the river. In the third car, which did not reach the water, the first half of it being suspended from the bridge and the other half remaining on it, were Dr. J. M. Warren, of this city, with his wife and son, and Dr. Riley with his wife. In the next car, the fourth, which remained uninjured on the bridge, were Drs. Ephraim Buck and George Bartlett of this city, the latter having left one of the forward cars but a few minutes before the accident. Among the list of others who were in the last cars and escaped injury, we notice the names of Drs. Robie of this city, Dickerman of Medford, N. Sanborn of Henniker, N. H., L. Ives and H. G. Wilcox of New Haven, Ct., D. Thompson of Northampton, Benson of Waterville, Me., and Bissell, Bowen, Jones, Nevins, Gloss, Russell, Romer, White and Woodward, whose residences are not stated. It will thus be seen, that of the Boston delegation, which was the largest to the medical convention from any place north, not one was lost or seriously injured ; and this, under Providence, is attributable to the detention of a portion of them in New York for another day, and to the favorable position in which those who returned were placed in the train. The four lamented dead from New Hampshire and Massachusetts were leading members of the profession ; two of them have been known to our readers as contributors to the Journal, and all of them were personally known and respected by us as friends and subscribers.—The whole number of lives lost by this fearful accident was about fifty.

New Medical Rooms.—In consequence of the recent leasing of the first and second stories of the Masonic Temple, in this city, where the archives of the Massachusetts Medical Society have been kept several years, and where the meetings have also been held, new apartments have been procured in Cochituate Hall, Phillips place, Tremont street, opposite King's Chapel, where the business will hereafter be transacted, till more permanent accommodations can be secured. The library, rooms for the Council, together with a fine hall, are all contiguous, and on the whole, convenient and central as could be desired. The annual meeting, however, on the 25th, takes place at the hall of the Lowell Institute, nearly opposite this office.

The Regular Faculty and the Massachusetts Medical Society.—No wonder a correspondent thinks it curious that the Massachusetts Medical Society should be made up of such a singular combination of elements. The following extract from his remarks is not altogether imaginary in its statements. " The members, according to report, represent all shades of medical opinion. Some are allopathic, others homœopathic, while another division have no great amount of good will towards either, because, as they consider, there is a direct violation of the laws of the institution in maintaining a fellowship with persons who ridicule the old school physicians, the original members of the Society. Yet these hostile forces meet together on anniversary days, choose counsellors and committees, dine, and walk away without a word of collision. Which party lacks independence or moral courage to separate this incongruous connection—the oil and water of physic—is one of the problems we cannot solve." We stated in the Journal, recently, that a petition would be presented to the Society, at its next meeting, demanding the expulsion of the homœopaths ; but by the latest intelligence it seems that no one could sufficiently screw his courage up to sign the paper. Being brave behind a high wall, and facing the guns of an enemy, are conditions widely different. At present, therefore, there is no indications of a disruption, although the members represent such different and opposing schools of medicine.

MARRIED,—Wm. J. Morland, M.D , of Boston, to Miss F. S. Dwight.

DIED,—At West Cambridge, Mass., Timothy Wellington, M.D., 70.—At Yale Settlement, Chenango Co. N. Y., Dr. Benjamin Yale, 102 years, 10 months and 3 days old —At Ann Arbor, Michigan, Dr. Ladislaus Gozon, a Hungarian, by shooting himself in a hotel.

Deaths in Boston for the week ending Saturday noon, May 7th, 72. Males, 38—females, 34. Accidental, 1—apoplexy, 2—bronchitis, 1—inflammation of the brain, 1—disease of the brain, 1—congestion of the brain, 1—consumption, 17—convulsions, 1—croup, 3—cancer, 1—dropsy in head, 5—drowned, 2—infantile diseases, 5—puerperal, 5—typhus fever, 1—typhoid fever, 1—scarlet fever, 5—homicide, 1—hooping cough, 1—hæmorrhage, 1—disease of the heart, 2—inflammation of the lungs, 4—congestion of the lungs, 1—disease of the liver, 1—marasmus, 4—mortification, 1—measles, 1—teething, 1—unknown, 1.
Under 5 years, 31—between 5 and 20 years, 5—between 20 and 40 years, 16—between 40 and 60 years, 15—over 60 years, 5. Born in the United States, 53—Ireland, 17—England, 1—Portugal, 1.

Inversion of the Toe-nail.—Dr. E. F. Smith, in a letter from Paris to the editor of the St. Louis Medical and Surgical Journal, thus alludes to a remedy made use of in that city for this troublesome affection :—

"A new operation for the relief of inversion of the toe-nail, or of its growing into the flesh, has been advised and practised by M. Nelaton. This is an extremely painful affection, the irritation produced by the nail producing ulceration and inevitable granulations, which prevents, from the excessive pain, the patient from walking. The ordinary operation, of split-ting the nail, and then with a pair of strong forceps forcibly evulsing a half or the whole nail, has been found unsuccessful, and when after the evulsion of the nail the denuded part is touched with some strong caustic, as caustic potash, it produces a large eschar, which leaves, after its de-tachment, an inevitable and painful sore, which is some time in healing. M. Nelaton's operation consists in removing a portion of the ulcerated and painful flesh adjacent to the nail, and has been several times successfully performed."

New Medical College, Calcutta.—This magnificent structure has just been completed, at a cost of £20,000. It contains 500 beds, and will be incorporated with the old Police Hospital and Eye Infirmary. One wing of the Hospital is for women and children. There are twenty-four wards, each suited to twenty-one patients. The wards are spacious, lofty and ventilated, and each is supplied with water by cast-iron tubes from four large iron cisterns, on the roof, which are filled by a powerful forcing pump communicating with a tank in the vicinity. On the north side is the council-room. and on the south, the operating theatre. The Calcutta Muni-cipal Committee, originated in 1835 by Mr. J. R. Martin, contributed largely towards the erection of the building, the funds for which were ob-tained from the following sources :—Old Fever Hospital subscription, rs. 61 248-7.10 ; New Fever Hospital, rs. 57,771-13-11 ; donation of Pertaub Chund Ling, rs. 50,000.—*London Lancet.*

Hospital for Consumption, Brompton.—The portion of the building completed affords accommodation for 90 in-door patients, and also has every convenience for out-door sick, of whom 100 are daily prescribed for. The new wing, is covered in, and when finished will increase the beds to 230. There are at present no less than 176 patients suffering acutely from pulmonary disease waiting for admission. The Marquis of West-minster has consented to preside at the evening festival in June.—*Ibid.*

Depopulation of the Sandwich Islands.—A Honolulu correspondent of the San Francisco Herald gives statistics respecting the Sandwich Islands. He states the population of eight Islands, according to official documents, to be 80,641 souls. In a given time the number of deaths, compared with the births, among this population, has been more than *six to one ;* e. g., the deaths have been 7,943, and in the same time the births have been only 1,478. According to Capt. Cook's estimate, there were on the islands, when he first discovered them, about 400,000 inhabitants ; and if so, in seventy years there has been the unparalleled mortality of 320,000 out of 400,000 lives. At this ratio another generation will be the last of the Sandwich Islanders.

THE

BOSTON MEDICAL AND SURGICAL JOURNAL.

Vol. XLVIII.   WEDNESDAY, MAY 18, 1853.   No. 16.

SPASMODIC ASTHMA.

BY PROF. EBEN. WATSON, A.M., M.D., GLASGOW, SCOTLAND.

THERE are few cases more distressing to witness, and I might almost add, without fear of contradiction, that there are none more difficult to treat, than those of confirmed spasmodic asthma ; and it is with the hope of contributing something, if only a little, to the resources of the healing art in regard to these obstinate cases, that I venture to submit the following observations to my fellow practitioners. Nor can I better illustrate the importance of this subject, and the call which there is for its renewed and more careful study, than by a reference to the great mortality from that disease occurring annually in our own city.

We find from Dr. Strang's Statistics, that in the year 1851, 212 persons died of asthma in Glasgow ; and in 1852, rather fewer, viz., 202. Now, by the same tables, we also find that the total deaths from all causes, among persons above 15 years of age, amounted in 1851 to 4543, and in 1852 to 4853 ; and seeing that asthma very rarely attacks persons below 15 years of age, it follows that these two numbers afford the means of ascertaining the ratio between the general amount of mortality, and that accruing from asthma. Perhaps the facts will be more tangible if expressed as follows :—

Above 15 Years of Age.	In 1851.	In 1852.
The deaths from all causes were	4543	4853
The deaths from asthma were	212	202
The deaths from all causes except asthma were	4331	4651

Regarding, therefore, the adult population alone, viz., persons above 15 years of age, 1 death was caused by asthma, in 1851, for not more than 20.4 by all other diseases put together ; and in 1852, 1 death was caused by asthma for 23 by all other diseases. Or, to take another view of it, of all deaths happening to persons above 15 years of age, 4.6 per cent. in 1851, and 4.1 per cent. in 1852, arose from asthma. And it still further appears from Dr. Strang's Report, that there were, by the census of 1851, 241,015 persons living in Glasgow above 15 years of age ; so that the proportion of deaths from asthma to those living at the usual age of those liable to that disease, is as 1 to 0.086. If, then, we

16

apply, with the necessary modifications, the formula given by statisti-
cians, viz., that the proportion constantly sick in a population, is double
the annual proportion which the deaths bear to the living, we find that
there are 414·520 persons constantly laboring under asthma in Glasgow alone ; and I believe that this number is rather under than above
reality.

The name of spasmodic asthma was originally founded on the mere
supposition of a spasm in the air-passages, occurring so as to cause the
sudden paroxysms of dyspnœa, to which the patient is liable ; and now
that the structure and functions of the bronchial tubes have been thoroughly investigated and made familiar to every one, we do not *suppose*,
but we *know*, that a spasm really occurs in the air-tubes and causes the
dyspnœa ; so that in this instance modern science has confirmed ancient
hypothesis. But we need not now speak vaguely of a spasm occurring
in the air-tubes, for we know that there are only two portions of those
tubes where spasm can at all take place in such a way as to cause
dyspnœa. These two portions are, in the first place, at the rima glot-
tidis, and in the second, at the extremities of the bronchial tubes, where,
instead of cartilaginous rings, there exist muscular fibres, which were
first discovered by Reisseissen, and which are generally named after
him. In all other parts of the bronchi the rings of cartilage which exist
in their outer wall, prevent anything like complete closure, or even any
considerable constriction of their calibre.

Laennec observed that during the asthmatic paroxysm there was great
diminution, or even complete absence of the respiratory murmur ; a fact
which is at once explained by the pathology of the case, for the small
tubes being contracted, or rather, obliterated, by the spasm, the air cannot pass into and distend the air-vesicles so as to cause the murmur.
When the spasm begins to relax, the patient inspires slowly, and with
difficulty ; a vibratory sound is heard by the by-standers accompanying
the inspiration, and much more loudly through a stethoscope placed over
the thyroid cartilage. In fact, it is caused by the vibration of the glottis, still partially stretched over the entrance to the windpipe. Now, in
my opinion, sufficient importance has not been attached to the spasm
of the glottis in asthmatic cases, and to this I wish to direct special attention ; for it is the glottidean contraction which chiefly hinders the
patient from overcoming that of the much weaker fibres of Reisseissen
in the smaller bronchial tubes. As soon as the muscles of the glottis
relax, and not till then, does the respiratory murmur become re-established ; in other words, it is only then that the patient performs a satisfactory act of respiration.

Observation thus teaches us that the superior constriction, if I may
so call it, is the last to give way, and I believe that in early cases of
asthma it is the first to occur. No doubt, when the disease has become
fully formed, it is difficult to distinguish between the onset of the spasm
in these two places, and I am willing to concede that in such cases it occurs almost simultaneously : but there are two circumstances which prove
satisfactorily to my mind, that the affection does commence at the glottis.
I allude, in the first place, to the fact that many cases of purely laryn-

geal disease end in spasmodic asthma ; and, in the second, that there are cases, though perhaps not very common ones, in which the affection is confined to the glottis—glottidean ásthma, as it might be called.

In my paper on Chronic Laryngitis, published in the Dublin Quarterly Journal of Medical Science, in November, 1850, I stated it as my opinion, that inflammation of the larynx, especially if ulcers have formed, constitutes a not infrequent cause of bronchial asthma, and I supported that opinion by the relation of a case which is so much to my present purpose, that I shall be excused for inserting it here :—

CASE I.—" In the autumn of 1848, a lady, somewhat above middle age, who had for some years been subject to similar attacks, was suddenly seized with a very severe fit of bronchial asthma, the violence of which was subdued in the ordinary way. When she had recovered, I observed that her voice was more than usually weak and husky ; but was informed that such had been its character for many years. She herself complained of a constant pain, of a sharp, lancinating nature, within the thyroid cartilage. On inquiring into the history of her illness, it was found that the patient in early life had been frequently attacked with acute laryngitis, which had ultimately assumed the chronic form, as indicated by the following symptoms which remained, viz., frequent tickling cough, a weak, husky and often hoarse voice, and ere long a constant fixed pain in the region of the glottis, combined with an incessant hawking up of muco-purulent matter, sometimes tinged with blood. On carefully examining this lady's chest after the fit had passed away, the loud sonorous râles, and occasional amphoric breathing, characteristic of partial dilatation of the air-tubes, were at once detected ; the resonance on percussion was deep and full ; the breath-sounds in the larynx were harsh and dry."

This case is peculiarly interesting for the sequence of pathological events which it exhibits. We have first acute laryngitis, producing ulceration, and passing into the chronic state. We then have, not only the usual symptoms of the laryngeal disease, which were persistent, but a new affection excited, viz., spasmodic asthma, and that in a most severe degree. The bronchial tubes ultimately became altered by the violence of the morbid agency that had attacked them. It was not to be expected that at this late stage of the disease any treatment could produce a perfect recovery, but it is satisfactory to be able to state, that after the cure of the laryngeal ulcers by the topical application of solution of caustic, the lady had no such severe asthmatic paroxysms, as those from which she formerly suffered.

The occurrence to which I alluded in the second place, viz., of a kind of asthma confined to the glottis alone, will perhaps be sufficiently illustrated by the following case :—

CASE II.—A young lady consulted me about two years ago for sudden attacks of breathlessness. She had no cough of any consequence, and in the intervals of the attacks she breathed freely enough, but as she seldom enjoyed a night's rest, her general health was somewhat disordered. Her pulse was quiet and natural, and there was no evidence of heart disease, but her complexion was slightly florid and her lips of rather a bluish tinge. When I saw her there was none of the bronchitis which generally attends asthma, and her age forbade the supposition of its being the ordinary kind of that disease. The respiratory sounds in the larynx indicated, by their loudness and harshness, as well as by the exaggerated length of the inspiratory sound, that this portion of the air-tube was in a highly-excited state.

She described the fits of dyspnœa as being always worst at night and in the morning. When the disease was mild she could, by keeping very quiet and still during the evening, avoid the breathlessness for the early part of the night, and thus she got sleep for a time ; but soon after midnight she was sure to awake with frightful dyspnœa, and was obliged either to rise from bed, or at all events to spend in the sitting posture, the rest of the time usually allotted to sleep. Before she came to me, however, on the occasion to which I am now referring, she was always attacked in a similar violent manner in the evening, so that it was only after being completely worn out that she obtained a short repose, from which she was again roused by extreme breathlessness. As I have said, the heart was unaffected by any disease that I could detect, and the lungs were likewise healthy, at all events in the intervals of the paroxysms ; and I believed, from these negative evidences and from the positive signs which could be detected in the larynx, that the chief, nay only, cause of this distressing malady, was spasm of the glottis. I was supported in this diagnosis, also, by the total absence of any approach to hysteria in this case. I frequently asked my patient and found that she had no feeling of globus, either before or during her attack ; and, indeed, her symptoms, as will at once be granted by every candid reader, were essentially different from the chokings of hysterical patients.

No other treatment was used but the regular application of a solution of caustic (℈j. to ℥j.) to the affected part, at first every day and afterwards every second day. About six weeks of this treatment sufficed to remove all the symptoms, and the lady remained quite well until the following winter, when she caught a slight cold and became affected in a similar way, but she applied to me sooner than on the former occasion, and half the time of the same treatment again produced a cure. During the autumn she again had another attack of her disease, but this time it was so slight, and treated so early, that it did not resist the topical application above a week. Since then she has been entirely free of the spasms, notwithstanding the very changeable and trying weather of the past winter.

I think, then, that I am warranted in concluding, 1st, that local causes of irritation in the larynx may produce spasmodic contractions, not only of the glottis, but also of the lesser bronchial tubes ; and 2d, that spasmodic affections of the glottis may occur periodically for a length of time, without involving the small bronchial tubes in any great or important contraction. Now, if these conclusions be correct, they in turn prove what was formerly asserted, viz., that asthma is a disease which commences in the upper and not in the lower parts of the air-tubes ; and it follows, that in the rational treatment of that disease, the remedies which are most likely to benefit the patient, are such as may be applied to the laryngeal lining and to the glottis itself. But it must be remembered that in a large proportion of these cases, universal bronchitis exists, along with the spasmodic affection of the upper and lower tubes : this may arise either from causes operating simultaneously and capable of exciting both diseases, or the bronchitis may have long existed previously to the occurrence of a true asthmatic paroxysm. The former is then .probably the exciting cause of the latter ; and I am free to admit the difficulty, nay, perhaps impossibility, of ascertaining with accuracy, in this class of cases, whether the spasmodic affection was first excited in the small tubes, or at the top of the larynx. It is enough for all practical purposes, however, to know that the latter region is always affected in such cases at the same time as the inferior bronchi, and with even greater intensity ; and, moreover, that it is the spasm of the glottis which chiefly maintains that of the bronchi, by preventing their expansion by the entrant air during the forcible inspirations of the patient.

[To be concluded next week.]

EXTIRPATION OF PHARYNGEAL TUMORS.

BY L. A. DUGAS, M.D., AUGUSTA, GEO.

THERE are no surgical affections more frequently encountered than tumors, and yet there are none in which the surgeon's skill is so often painfully tested both as to diagnosis and treatment. If, as has been oft-times repeated, no surgeon, however experienced, should ever advance a *positive* opinion as to the true nature of a tumor before seeing its internal structure, the difficulty is, in many instances, not diminished when he is called upon to determine upon the propriety of extirpation. And, even after having advised a resort to the knife, he often finds himself surrounded by dangers to the life of the patient, and to his own reputation, sufficient to deter any one not firmly convinced of the propriety of the course to be adopted, and of his ability to do justice to the patient.

Why these difficulties? Do they necessarily attach to the diseases in question—or, in other words, has the profession given to them the careful attention to which they are entitled? It is true, that we have some good monographs upon the subject of tumors, but they are far from being perfect—far from furnishing to the practitioner all the data he may need on entering upon the duties of his profession. The history of tumors to be found in the systematic works upon surgery, is usually so meagre as to be worth comparatively but little, except in cases of the most ordinary simplicity. It becomes us, therefore, to accumulate and to report facts as they present themselves, in order that materials may be at hand for the construction of a work consisting not merely of generalities, but also of such details as may furnish specimens of whatever may be subsequently observed in practice. A volume that would contain nothing more than the history and treatment of individual tumors, so that we might find in it a parallel for any that we may meet, would be invaluable.

Tumors in the pharynx are comparatively rare, according to written authorities as well as our own observation. It may therefore serve the purpose to which we have just alluded, to publish the following history of a formidable case recently treated.

Branch, a negro man about 35 years of age, the property of Mr. J. A. Smith, of Henry County, Ga., was placed under my charge early in February last. He first noticed, about three years before, a small tumor behind the soft palate, which he represented as being very hard and painless. From that time it gradually increased in size, and was never painful, but rather inconvenient. I found the tumor filling the pharynx, extending upward to the posterior nares, downward as far as the larynx, and laterally from one tonsil to the other, forcing down the right one. The soft palate was carried forward and downward, so as to constitute a prominence the size of a large egg, to the posterior surface of which the tumor was attached. Deglutition was so difficult that he could take no solid food—his articulation was very indistinct, and respiration considerably impeded when he would walk briskly, causing him then to breathe loudly and like a horse affected with the " bellows."

Believing the tumor to be fibrous, I proceeded on the 10th of February to its removal, as follows:—

Provided with actual cauteries, a syringe, sulphate of zinc, &c., to control the hemorrhage from the general surface and smaller vessels, I passed a ligature beneath the right carotid artery, and left it there, ready to be tied should this become necessary. The patient was then seated in a chair, and an incision made from the right angle of the mouth to the masseter muscle—which necessitated the ligature of the facial artery. In the third stage of the operation, a longitudinal incision was made from the side of the uvula to the roof of the mouth, through the soft palate, which was then detached from the tumor in the form of flaps. The tumor now presented a white glistening aspect, and was adherent, posteriorly and laterally, to the adjacent parts by strong cellular tissue. Having free access to the parts, the cutting instruments were laid aside, and the mass was seized with strong tumor forceps and drawn forward, whilst my fingers were passed behind and tore asunder the attachments of the lower portion of the tumor. The fingers were then carried successively behind the left, the upper, and a part of the right portions of the mass, which was now removed. The entire mass thus extirpated constituted one distinct tumor ; but there was still another left in the right side, apparently in intimate connection with and pressing down the tonsil with great force. It did not, like the former, present a white glistening surface to the eye, but was covered by a thin stratum of muscular fibres, derived from the pharyngeal muscles. Upon dividing this stratum with the knife, and pressing it aside, the tumor was found to be of the same character as the former—and it was likewise removed by the fingers and forceps, not, however, without much difficulty. It was found to be attached to the ramus of the lower jaw, near the sigmoid notch, to the pterygoid process of the sphenoid bone and to the posterior aperture of the right nostril, and was brought away in separate fragments. Both tumors, when placed together, formed a mass about the size of a turkey's egg.

The patient bore this protracted and painful operation with wonderful fortitude. The amount of hemorrhage was smaller than could have been anticipated, but had to be checked occasionally by cold water thrown into the pharynx with a syringe. After allowing the patient to rest a little, the cheek was stitched and well brought together with adhesive strips. He was then put to bed with the wound of the neck partially closed, and the ligature was permitted to remain beneath the carotid until the following morning as a precautionary, measure.

The patient's recovery was unattended with any circumstance worthy of note. He did remarkably well, and would have been sent home in about a fortnight, had he not taken cold, which affected his bowels and induced considerable fever for eight or ten days more.

Will this disease return? Microscopic examination by Dr. Harriss showed the tumors to be purely fibrous—nothing indicative of malignancy could be detected in them. Time alone will decide the question.

The structure of these tumors was very similar to that of fibrous polypi, but differed from them in not being pediculated. They were, on the contrary, closely attached to all the tissues with which they came in contact. From the history given by the patient, it appears that there was at first only one tumor, and that it was situated behind the velum palati. That in contact with the right tonsil was of subsequent growth. Would the early removal of the first have prevented the development of the second? Some years ago (in 1347) Dr. B., of an adjoining county, sent us a case upon which we operated, and which has thus far not been reproduced.

The subject was a negro woman about 25 years of age, who presented a tumor about the size of a small hen's egg attached to the posterior surface of the velum palati by a broad base about the size of a half-dollar coin. In this instance, instead of slitting up the soft palate, we plunged a hook into the centre of the protuberance and circumscribed it with a circular incision carried through the soft palate, thus leaving entire the lateral half arches and the uvula. The tumor was then readily drawn through the aperture thus made, for it had no posterior attachments. The wound cicatrized completely in a short time, leaving no deformity.—*Southern Med. and Surg. Jour.*

TREATMENT OF HEMORRHAGE AFTER EXTRACTION OF A TOOTH.

BY F. L. CRANE, D.D.S., EASTON, PENN.

MAY 23d, 1851, 10 o'clock, A.M., extracted a tooth, the upper left second molar, for Mr. Stocker, of Mount Bethel (in this county). This gentleman has been under treatment for some time past for a gastro-hepatic derangement, with a tendency to phthisis, and a hemorrhagic diathesis. Informed me that he had had several attempts at extracting teeth, none of which succeeded. In this case the roots of the tooth were of extraordinary length. A small, thin piece of the alveolar plate came away with the tooth. The bleeding ceased, or nearly so, before he left the office, but he said soon commenced and bled throughout the day. In the evening I learned that he was inquiring for me somewhat anxiously. I found the gum bleeding profusely. Tried the usual styptics without much effect. Called Dr. V. M. Swayze, a skilful dentist, of this borough, to assist me. Plugged the cavity tightly with cotton, and placed a piece of cork upon it to shut against, tied a handkerchief over his head to keep his mouth shut, and dismissed him with little or no bleeding. In the night he awoke with his bed flooded with blood ; one of our physicians, Dr. Abernethy, was sent for, who exhausted his skill in attempts to arrest the bleeding, without effect. In the morning I was informed that Mr. Stocker was in danger of bleeding to death, and was requested to do what I could to prevent so dire a calamity. Dr. Abernethy proposed taking up the carotid artery. I told him I had yet one resource left, requesting him to do what he could for the gentleman, while I was making preparations. The patient had already fainted from the loss of blood, and the household were pretty thoroughly frightened, for a large quantity of blood had been lost. I went quickly to my office, and got wherewith to take an impression of the gum and remaining teeth, made a plaster cast, drying it over a spirit lamp ; made metal casts and struck up a silver plate, soldered on clasps to fasten upon the remaining teeth, covered the plate with powdered alum—this last was perhaps of no use—had his mouth cleansed of coagulum, cotton, &c., and put the plate in its place ; found the fit good, and the bleeding instantly ceased. Perhaps one circumstance which rendered my fixture successful was somewhat accidental. I found that one of my silver clasps was so broad that a lower tooth hit upon it when the mouth was closed, and pressed the plate tightly against the gum, rendering it impossible for blood to escape. The plate was worn four days before removing.

Dr. Saltonstall's case, reported in the Journal of Dental Science of October last, differs somewhat from the above. Both methods had the same desirable results, viz., the saving of life.

I was the more prompt in adopting the above plan to arrest hemorrhage in this case, from the fact that a child of a Mr. Randolph, in this place, had a short time previously died in consequence of continued hemorrhage from the gum. The child was teething ; a physician lanced the gum, cutting down, as I understood, upon a lower incisor. The bleeding continued day after day, and the physicians were unable to arrest it. I heard of the case through one of the physicians, and began to cogitate upon what I would do in case I should be called upon, which I was not. I had resolved to strike up a plate, and make a soft pad to put upon it to close against the opposite gum, keeping the mouth closed by a bandage over the head, assisting the formation of coagulum by a styptic under the plate. Would such a proceeding answer, in the absence of so perfect a fixture as the " Alveolar Hemorrhage Compress " of Dr. Reid ? The principal objection, perhaps, would be the necessity of removing it to give the child sustenance, and then replacing it.—*American Journal of Dental Science.*

REGISTRATION OF MARRIAGES, BIRTHS AND DEATHS.

WE understand that the measure proposed to the Virginia Legislature two years ago, by the Medical Society of the State, relative to the registration of marriages, births and deaths, was passed just before the adjournment of the General Assembly, and will therefore be a law of the Commonwealth, after the first of next July. We shall take an early opportunity of publishing the bill at length, for the information of the profession.

The necessity of statistics of the population for the elucidation of truths affecting the welfare of mankind, is universally acknowledged, and we rejoice to see this first step towards the accumulation of materials for future laborers in the field of public hygiene.

It seems a difficult matter to convince our legislators that the lives and physical well being of the community, as well as its pecuniary interests, deserve consideration; and, nevertheless, nothing is more true than that the prosperity of a country is directly proportional to the corporeal vigor and health of its laboring population; and that a wise government will earnestly investigate and remove, when possible, every cause which may exert a deleterious influence upon the health of the masses.

We hear the governments of Europe denounced as remorseless despotisms, regardless of the happiness of the people; still they do something to ameliorate the physical condition of their subjects. London, Paris, and the chief cities of the Continent, abound in public baths and wash-houses, many of which are free, while others are open to the poor at prices varying from three to five cents. In all of the large European cities, model lodging houses are springing up, under the auspices of the governments, to provide well-ventilated and comfortable abodes for the lower classes. The vast pile of buildings in Paris called "cité Napoléon" may be taken as an example of these establishments. This structure encloses a quadrangular court, occupied by a fountain, in an elevated and airy locality. It is already occupied by 250 inmates, and 500 will be accommodated when the remaining buildings are completed. The lodgings are rented at prices varying from twelve to thirty-six dollars per annum; for the larger sum the laborer is entitled to two rooms and a closet for cooking. Baths, laundries and a free dispensary are attached to the establishment. Notwithstanding this moderate rent, the revenue is equal to the interest of the capital invested.

There is no mechanical art, the pursuit of which involves a sacrifice of health, which escapes the vigilance of the public authorities. Men of science are employed to discover means to diminish as much as possible its noxious influence, or to propose harmless materials which may be substituted for the deleterious substances used by the artisan. At this very time a commission of the Council of Health of the department of the Seine, composed of Magendie, Chevreul, Legentil, and others eminent in science or the industrial arts, are engaged in determining the practicability of the substitution of zinc paint for the poisonous white lead now universally employed with such disastrous effects.

The police inspect with care the markets ; the deposits of grain ; the bread assize ; the cleansing of the streets, sewers, &c. ; all noisome establishments, such as breweries, chemical manufactories and cemeteries.   The heaviest penalties are inflicted on those found guilty of adulterating drugs ; the closest restrictions prevent the sale of poisons and deleterious agents.

Vaccination is rendered obligatory in Italy and the South of Europe, and the governments of France and England are now discussing the propriety of a similar law.   The highest medical authorities are paid to furnish advice to the government on questions relating to epidemics, quarantines, and public hygiene in general.   Asylums for the insane, the blind, the deaf and dumb, the aged and the infirm, are everywhere in abundance.   London alone, with its population of three millions, contains thirteen general hospitals, with a collective staff of one hundred and fifty physicians and surgeons, which render relief to three hundred thousand patients annually.   The Royal Hospital of St. Bartholomew alone, succors nearly five thousand in-patients and eighty thousand out-patients every year.   And this vast system of relief, and the immense amount of medical and surgical skill consumed in its bestowal, are almost—the latter entirely—gratuitous.

The subject of medical education is jealously cared for.   The medical schools are generally of the highest order.   Few leave them whose minds have not been refined and elevated by liberal studies ; and yet their graduates undergo a rigid examination by public teachers before they receive a license to practise medicine.

Thus, then, we have briefly stated a few of the means employed by European governments to preserve the health of the population, and to provide proper counsel and relief for those who become sick.   It is painful to inquire what has been done in our country ; still more so to ask what has been done in Virginia.   As regards sanitary police regulations, we have absolutely none.   Diseased meat is daily sold in New York ; cesspools and filthy sewers fill the air of all our large cities with noxious effluvia ; intramural interments are practised ; and every kind of manufacture, injurious to the public health, is freely sanctioned.   In regard to drugs, the falsifications which they undergo are notorious.—*Virginia Medical and Surgical Journal.*

LECTURES OF M. VALLEIX ON DISPLACEMENTS OF THE UTERUS.

TRANSLATED FROM THE FRENCH BY L. PARKS, JR., M.D.

NUMBER IV.

NOMENCLATURE.—Different denominations have been made use of to designate displacements.   Thus, Levret employed the expression *transverse inversion (renversement transversal)* forward or backward, to designate complete displacement in the one or the other of these two directions.   Desgranges first employed the words *anteversion* and *retroversion*.   In 1803, the Germans, among whom Mœller should be mentioned, called retroversion *reclinatio,* and anteversion *pronatio* uteri.

Before these terms came into use, the single word *delapsus* was employed—a term very badly chosen. It was, as I have already told you, M. Ameline who definitively adopted the expressions *anteflexion* and *retroflexion*, which have been admitted into general use, together with the names *anteversion* and *retroversion* proposed by Desgranges. Within a short time the terms *lateroflexion* and *lateroversion* have been with propriety added.

Frequency of Displacements.—As I have already told you, the frequency of these diseases is great. Yet authors are not agreed upon this subject, especially in reference to the question of the relative degree of frequency of each of the different species of displacements. With some, anteversion is the most frequent, while, according to others, it is retroversion which prevails the most. In the opinion of a third class, finally, the various flexions outweigh the other forms.

Among the 68 cases which I have collected, there were 11 simple anteflexions, and 12 simple retroflexions; 24 anteversions with or without flexions, and 21 retroversions with or without flexions. This would make 35 anterior to 33 posterior displacements; or, with a trifling difference, about as many in one direction as in the other. I give these figures, however, merely as data which may be consulted at need, when other facts shall be added to those I have analyzed, since, at present, their number is too inconsiderable to enable us to found upon them a statement of the relative frequency of the different displacements.

Species.—The different species admissible are as follows, viz. :—

(A) In a first group,
    1st. Simple Anteversion.
    2d. Anteflexion.
    3d. Varieties consisting each of an anteversion with one or more inconsiderable flexions.

(B) In a second group,
    1st. Simple Retroversion.
    2d. Retroflexion.
    3d Varieties analogous to the preceding.

(C) In a third group,
    1st. Lateroversions.
    2d. Lateroflexions.

The application of these different denominations should always be made with reference to the position of the body of the uterus, and not, as has been, in our opinon, erroneously done by some authors, to that of the cervix. In order that there should be anteversion, it is necessary that the *body should be inclined forward,* which would cause the cervix to be elevated posteriorly, and to press up against the rectum. In retroversion, on the contrary, the body *leans directly backward upon* the rectum, and carries the cervix upward against the lower portion of the bladder.

As to flexions, they are also designated according to the position of the body—thus, *anteflexion when the fundus lies in front, retroflexion when it is behind.* In a word, *it is in all cases the position of the body which determines the denomination.* It is important that physicians should be agreed upon this point, in order to avoid the misapprehension which but too often occurs.

Perhaps it may be thought the proper course to study together all these different species of displacements, contenting ourselves with indicating, in the course of a general description, whatever is peculiar to each species. And, assuredly, it may be said in favor of this mode of proceeding that the causes are often the same, that there are many common symptoms, and that we have a uniform treatment for all the different species of displacements. But it is not less true that each particular species may present some peculiar symptoms quite important to be known, that the tactile examination, and more especially the sound, furnish differential signs of great value, and that, further, though the treatment be the same, yet its application, in the different cases, presents modifications, the apprehension of which is essential, since it is often upon them alone that all our success depends.

In order to bring out well all these differences, and put you in the way of seizing the characteristics of each particular species, I foresee that a general description would be insufficient, and that it would be better to describe separately each of these species of displacements in the order in which I have enumerated them.

When we shall have given the history of each displacement in particular, we shall close with a general summary, which will permit us to embrace at a glance whatever they may present in common.

EXPLORATION OF THE UTERUS.

But, first of all, I must make you acquainted with the different means of exploration at our disposal—to be employed for all displacements without distinction.

Examination per Vaginam.—In the first rank, comes manual exploration, and especially the *examination per vaginam*—a means, the employment of which in the diagnosis of uterine displacements, cannot be dispensed with, since it furnishes extremely useful information. I practise it, in the first instance while the woman is in the erect posture, because in this position the degree of displacement is better appreciated. Besides the first symptoms being especially manifest when she is erect, it is important to know precisely what is then the direction of the uterus, this direction being, perhaps, no longer the same when the patient is in the horizontal posture. The index finger, with which the examination is performed, should follow the axis of the vagina, in order to arrive at the cervix—and I cannot urge you too much to proceed gently, gradually—without attempting to carry the finger at once upon the cervix—and above all, to avoid pushing back the parts too forcibly, and causing pain.

If it should happen that the index finger could not reach the cervix, it would be well to introduce, at the same time, the middle finger, which being about a centimetre longer, would permit an exploration to a greater depth.

Certain authors have advised attempts to penetrate further by making the hip or the knee a point of support for the elbow. But, in adopting this method, above all, we should proceed very slowly, and with great caution. Especially, should our attention never be exclusively occupied with the purpose of reaching the cervix, but, on the contrary, we should endeavor to take account of everything which presents itself to the finger.

Let us forthwith call to mind what is found by means of the tactile examination—*when the uterus is in the normal state*—in order that we may have a standard of comparison.

If the uterus occupies its normal position, we meet first its anterior lip, and, then, immediately, below, the opening of the cervix, which is quite easy to reach. By carrying the finger in front, we find the anterior surface of the cervix continuous superiorly with the anterior surface of the body, which cannot be completely followed out, and, which is directed obliquely upward and forward, with an inclination toward the anterior abdominal wall, as though passing on to join it.

In front of the body is felt the soft resistance peculiar to the intestine. The bladder distended by urine, sometimes gives a sensation of fluctuation, and may, in some cases, be sufficiently voluminous to obstruct the exploration. It should then be evacuated by the catheter, if the patient cannot pass the urine spontaneously.

Behind the opening of the cervix the finger meets the posterior *cul-de-sac* of the vagina, into which one penetrates in following the posterior surface of the cervix. The finger cannot reach further than the junction of the cervix with the body—directly behind which nothing more is felt than the intestine yielding its peculiar sensation of softness, unless, always provided, there is no accumulation of fæcal matters in the rectum, the resistance of which is felt through the recto-vaginal parietes.

If you are thoroughly possessed of the principles which I have just explained, it will be easy for you to apply them to the exploration of displacements of the uterus. It is evident, in fact, that in displacements of the cervix, the finger, in executing the tactile examination. will no longer find this part in the same position ; or else, if it is the direction of the body which has changed, there may be felt, at different points, salient or retreating angles—but these are differences upon which I shall insist more particularly in speaking of each species of displacement, by itself.

The tactile examination further enables us to ascertain the state of the cervix, its volume, its consistence, its temperature, its exterior conformation. We should satisfy ourselves as to whether or not there are granulations or ulcerations* upon it, and as to whether or not its opening is regular. Finally, the finger should not be withdrawn from the vagina without having impressed on the cervix movements tending to make the uterus swing over, in order that you may know whether or not it moves easily—whether or not the tissues that surround it are supple—whether or not it has contracted abnormal adhesions with the neighbor-

---

This, we have the authority of Bennet for saying, it is difficult to do without the aid of the speculum.—TRANS.

ing parts—bends when its displacement is attempted—is heavier than it ought to be.

It is also very important to endeavor to seize with the other hand the fundus of the organ through the abdominal parietes, whilst the finger in the vagina pushes up the cervix—a manœuvre which aids' our appreciation of the volume of the uterus and also of its direction.

Examination per Rectum.—As to the examination *per rectum*, you will see, at a later period, that in anteversion and anteflexion it teaches but little, and that in retroversion and retroflexion it may also be often neglected without inconvenience. You will take care, then, to practise it only when it shall appear to you indispensable—for, first of all, gentlemen, it becomes us to give heed in practice to the retrenchment of explorations of this sort, when not absolutely necessary to an exact diagnosis.

The finger introduced into the rectum, when the uterus occupies its normal position, feels nothing that it does not meet behind the cervix in the examination *per vaginam ;* only, as it is able to reach higher, it can also follow a little higher the direction of the organ. In case of displacement, the extremity of the cervix is felt if there is an anteversion, or the globular tumor formed by the body of the uterus, if there is a retroversion on a retroflexion. But these are points to which we will return more in detail.

CASE OF CYANOSIS.

[Communicated for the Boston Medical and Surgical Journal.]

THE subject of the following case, a child aged 11 months, suddenly expired on the night of 3d of March ult. At its birth it was small and feeble, but nothing unusual was observed for the first three months. At the end of that time its development almost ceased, and at the age of six months it appeared to have ceased entirely. It was then of a peculiar livid color, and all the functions of animal life were tardily performed.

An autopsy was made 36 hours after death, and the following appearances noted. The chest was small and contracted, abdomen large, and extremities small and shrunken. The lungs were small, the right nearly filled with blood, except at the lower portion, where several miliary tubercles were deposited. The heart was the seat of the primary and most important lesions. The parietes of the right auricle were thinned by absorption, and somewhat softened. The right ventricle was normal ; the left ventricle hypertrophied and hardened, indeed of almost a cartilaginous feel. The left auricle was normal. The foramen ovale was entirely open, freely admitting the blood from one side to the other. The aorta, near its origin, was dilated to about twice its natural size. The liver large, nearly twice its usual size—but no evidence of being further diseased. The gall-bladder was distended with thick, viscid bile, and its inner membrane thickened. No further examination was made.

There was no hereditary tendency whatever to disease in the family.

Carthage, Ill., April 26, 1853. GEO. W. HALL.

THE BOSTON MEDICAL AND SURGICAL JOURNAL.

BOSTON, MAY 18, 1853.

The late Accidental Death of Physicians.—Four of the seven medical gentlemen who were killed on the New Haven railroad, as related last week, were personal acquaintances; but we are not sufficiently familiar with their early history to attempt a memoir of either of them. There must be some among their brethren who could do justice to their memories, and we hereby urge the undertaking upon them. Dr. Peirson, of Salem, was a learned and accomplished practitioner. But that was not all; through the whole course of an active professional life, he was distinguished for energy, uprightness and usefulness in all the relations he bore to society. Dr. P. was President of the Essex South District Medical Society. At a special meeting of the Society, held in consequence of his death, appropriate resolutions were passed, from which we copy the two following.

"*Resolved,* That, in his uniform fidelity in the discharge of all the duties of an arduous profession; in his unremitting diligence; in the kindness and suavity of his manners; in his large benevolence; in his kindly professional charities; and in his zealous and watchful care of the various interests entrusted to him, he leaves to his brethren a worthy example.

"*Resolved,* That, while the Society over which he so ably presided deplore the loss of the wise counsellor and constant friend, the community will mourn the public spirited citizen and the accomplished physician and surgeon, whose active and useful life has been so suddenly terminated."

Drs. Smith and Gray, of Springfield, held a high place in the public estimation. To the city of Springfield, their loss is a melancholy one—to their families, irreparable. Dr. Bartlett's loss, in that portion of New Hampshire in which he resided, will be long felt. A condensed biographical sketch, embodying the prominent points in the character and circumstances of these very useful, talented and exemplary practitioners, would confer a favor on the profession as well as on their personal friends.

The late Meeting of the American Medical Association.—From all accounts, a happier meeting has never been held than the late assemblage at New York. The elegant hospitalities of the profession in that city, are the theme of every medical man whose good fortune it was to be present. Dr. Knight, of New Haven, the president, is a good presiding officer. He was in the chair in Philadelphia, at the organization of the Association. A brief notice of the doings at the meeting was given in last week's Journal. The delegates acquitted themselves, we should judge, to the satisfaction of their constituents. On the whole, this Institution may be regarded with pride by the people. It is not a sectional combination of men for party or individual purposes, but strictly a great representation of the medical practitioners of the United States, who have adopted this plan to collect and diffuse the results of their experience for the benefit of themselves and the community.

The annual volume emanating from the Association is a concentration of the discoveries, researches and inquiries of the preceding year, and will if continued constitute a valuable series for future use.

Medicine in Iowa.—Not many years ago, curiosity prompted us to visit the far-off west, for the purpose of seeing the Indians on their own territories, before they should become enfeebled by intercourse with the whites, and their customs and manners be modified by mingling with the pale-faces from the Atlantic border. Since that period, the fine hunting grounds have passed into other hands, and the Winnebagoes, Chippewas and Sioux tribes have been urged away still further towards the setting sun. In the places where they then pursued their game, towns and villages have sprung into existence, and art, science and civilization are appreciated. All this has taken place in Iowa within the memory of young men. Dubuque was regarded as an extreme settlement on the Upper Mississippi, as recently as in 1844. Now that same Dubuque is a great town, with brick blocks, and an active, industrious, enterprising population. Schools, churches, the hum of business, and the running to and fro of men in eager haste to acquire wealth, are the sights and sounds that surprise the traveller. Among other evidences of a well-regulated community, physicians have established themselves there. On account of a growing demand for their services, or because it is a happy place for a residence, with flattering prospects, they have multiplied to a degree that has warranted the organization of a medical association, under the title of the North Western Medical Society. The constitution and code of by-laws are framed admirably to secure the interests and moral elevation of the members. In the code of medical ethics, a judicious view is taken of the relations of practitioners; their duties, privileges and expectations. More might have been said in regard to the obligations of the public to physicians. It is quite certain that the people have no proper conception of their duty towards those who attend upon the sick and the dying.

Medical Character.—Prof. H. V. Wooten, of the chair of Principles and Practice of Medicine in the Medical College of Memphis, Tenn., delivered a parting address to the graduates of the Institution on the 28th of February, a copy of which has found its way to Boston. After summing up the events belonging to the life of a student, and assuring the gentlemen that with the diploma they have assumed a new position, the accomplished speaker proceeds to discourse on the inestimable value of a good character. " There is the great group of virtues which go to make up what is comprehended in the term *morality.* Among these are the social feelings or sentiments—a refined sense of our relations to those around us—a just regard for our duties to our day and generation—and a fostering care for those gentler and ennobling sentiments and impulses of our nature, which elevate and dignify man, above the passions and practices of mere animal sensuality. A great and cultivated intellect, under control of an immoral will, is as deadly in its influences upon all that is true and pure in man, as the exhalations of the famous Upas." Prudence, firmness, self-reliance and economy are themes upon which Dr. Wooten dwells with enthusiasm. He is a man of soundness, and of elevated moral dignity.

New York Medical Society Transactions.—A volume, of truly respectable dimensions, is every year made up of the papers, journal of proceedings, catalogue of members, &c., of this Society. The present volume, containing the results of the last annual meeting, at Albany, in February, is quite a valuable one, and in the order of its arrangement is a model publication. Among the articles, Dr. Tuthill's on registration, and Dr. Van Buren's case of ligature of the subclavian artery, will be read with profit. Dr. J. S. Sprague is president, and Dr. Armsby secretary.

Polytechnic Journal.—Charles G. Page, M.D., is the leading editor of a recently-commenced Journal with this name, which abounds with information in the mechanic arts and agriculture. Five numbers of the work have been published. Engravings are liberally spread through the pages, explanatory of newly-invented machines, patents, and processes in the cultivation of the earth. An equal amount of information, from elevated and reliable sources, could hardly be purchased elsewhere so economically as in the American Polytechnic Journal, issued at No. 6 Wall street, New York, and opposite the Patent Office in the City of Washington.

Bleeding.—Among the strong cases brought forward by the anti-phlebotomists, is that of the celebrated Madame Malibran, the inimitable queen of song. She was playing upon the stage when last seen in public—entering with all her soul into the character, and giving intense interest to the piece before an immense audience. At the point in which all her powers were taxed to the utmost stretch of a naturally delicate organization, she fainted, from extreme physical exhaustion. A physician, seated in front, leaped instantly to her assistance; and instead of administering a cordial, he bled the already debilitated woman. She never rallied.

Lord Byron, in his last sickness, said to the medical attendants, "do with me what you like, but bleed me you shall not." After much reasoning and repeated entreaties, says the narrative, Mr. Millengen at length succeeded in obtaining from him a promise, that should he feel his fever increase at night, he would allow Dr. Bruno to bleed him. They drew about twenty ounces. On the following morning, April 17th, the bleeding was twice repeated. On the 19th the poet died.

John Hunter proved, continue the opponents of bloodletting, that the blood lives;—every drop, therefore, that is abstracted by artificial or other means, is actually a drop of life irrecoverably lost. The Jews cautiously avoided the loss of this precious fluid; and hence another argument has been drawn against the practice of bleeding.

Notwithstanding the opposing theories on this subject, and the different conclusions drawn from the same premises, it is the province as well as the privilege of every physician to act according to circumstances, and in the use of his best judgment he is justified in prescribing what he verily believes is for the best interest of his patient, without regard to the whims, caprices or theoretical lucubrations of any man or party of men.

A Restless Tongue.—A Boston lady has at this time a somewhat novel disease—a continual motion of the tongue, which no device, effort of the will, or medication, controls. We do not mean that she is a nuisance as a talker or a retailer of street gossip. On the contrary, a worthier woman does not exist. She has expended five hundred dollars among the dentists for artificial teeth, which her unruly member has knocked out so repeatedly, that they are now wholly abandoned; she is therefore a good representative of one of Shakspeare's seven ages—viz., *sans teeth.* Her tongue is moving nimbly and involuntarily within the mouth, against the walls of the cheeks. In conversation, the organ takes on a normal action, but runs instantly into its usual rapidity of motion at the conclusion of a sentence.

Orris Tooth Soap.—Dr. Angell, of Providence, R. I., has been eminently successful in his new composition for the preservation of the teeth. It is assumed by those most familiar with the matter, that charcoal is the best antiseptic employed to keep the teeth in a good condition. By making it impalpable before mixing with the orris and soap, Dr. A. produces an admirable article, which, we understand, meets the approval of the dental profession.

Microscopical Science.—The second number of the Quarterly Journal of Microscopical Science from London, is a beautiful specimen of the patient industry of a few indefatigable laborers in this revived, if not quite new, field for explorations, and also of the art of photography. The articles are quite too technical for the mass of readers. For the library, and as a record of the progress of discovery with the microscope, this London Journal cannot be rivalled.

Officers of the American Medical Association.—We mentioned last week, that Dr. Jonathan Knight, of New Haven, Ct., was chosen President of the Association for the current year. The following are the other officers : *Vice Presidents*—Drs. Usher Parsons, of Rhode Island ; Lewis Condit, of New Jersey ; Henry R Frost, of South Carolina ; R. L. Howard, of Ohio. *Secretaries*—Drs. Edward L. Bedell, of New York ; Edwin L. Lemoine, of Missouri. *Treasurer*—Dr. Francis Condie, of Pennsylvania.

Medical Associations in Cincinnati.—A correspondent of the Journal, a visiter in Cincinnati from the farther West, writes as follows, under date of May 2, 1853 :—

" A few evenings since I had the pleasure of attending a meeting of the Cincinnati Medical Society, which was held at the residence of Prof. A. H. Baker. It is the custom of this Society to meet at the houses of its members, which makes a very respectable circle for the drawing room when all the members are in attendance, as the Society numbers fifty-nine members. A paper was read by Prof. Locke on the analysis of the blood, in which the author presented some cases wherein the value of analysis was made apparent. He also gave the methods as practised by himself.

" An older and more numerous Society is the Medico-Chirurgical Society of Cincinnati. This numbers about 80 members. The objects of the two Societies are nearly identical.   C."

Operation for Inversion of the Toe-nail. Mr. Editor,—An operation for the relief of inversion of the toe-nail, as advised and practised by M. Nelaton, of Paris, is described as new in the Journal of last week. The operation is a good one, but not new. I believe it has been frequently done here. I am sure I heard Dr. Jeffries say, it had been his reliance in bad cases for twenty years ; and I rarely treat this troublesome affection in any other way, having long since considered splitting nails, and strong caustic applications, as contributing materially to the obstinacy of an otherwise simple case. Perhaps some of your readers may inform us who first used the knife in this malady, and thus elevated the method to the dignity of an operation. The principle involved in the incision is as old as the " surgery of ulcers "—the diseased action is singularly suggestive of proper remedial measures. M. Nelaton is of the progressive school ; and as this " operation " has been successful in his hands, undoubtedly it will be repeated in " home cases," by some conservatives who can do nothing in surgery or medicine but copy European models or recipes.

I have no doubt that many of your readers will decide that M. Nelaton is not the first surgeon in the world, if he is the first in Paris, whose operation consists in " removing a portion of the ulcerated and painful flesh adjacent to the nail," for the cure of inversion of the toe-nail.　　　J.

Medical Miscellany.—Dr. James S. Arthur has been appointed Superintendent of the Indiana Lunatic Hospital, vice Dr. Patterson resigned.— Dr. Roberts, of Georgia, was lately sent to the State Prison for fourteen years, for robbery.—Mr. Nourse, of Andover, Mass., weighs 388 lbs. A Dr. Brown, late of Springfield but now of New York. weighs 408 lbs —Dr. J. G. Elliot has received a commission of post master at Littleton Centre, Mass.—Dr. Gibbs, of Stockbridge, Vt., was fined $10 and costs, a day or two since, for selling to a female a mixture of half a pint of alcohol with camphor gum.—Smallpox is prevailing to a fearful extent in western and southwestern Georgia. It rages also at Girard, Ala.—The post-mortem examination of a young lady in Paris disclosed the fact that three of the ribs had encroached upon the liver to such an extent as to produce death. She perished of tight lacing.—Dr. Tuthill's able paper read before the New York State Medical Society, on the registration of births, deaths and marriages. may be had in a pamphlet form.—Monica, a servant woman of Mrs. Eliza Lancaster, of Cobb Neck, Charles Co., Md., died on the 30t ult., aged 120 years.—A German, in a fit of delirium tremens, at New Orleans, amputated his penis close to the pubis. He recovered without tying a vessel.—Edward D. Fenner, M.D., is President of the Medical Society of Louisiana.—Gerlack's General and Special Histology. with additional notes, from the latest French and German authorities, is translating in Boston, by I. O. Noyes, M.D., and will soon be ready for the press.

To CORRESPONDENTS —Dr. Deane's paper on Divided Fingers is on file for publication.—An article on the treatment of insanity has also been received, but is considered inadmissible, as the main treatment is only described under a name indefinite and unknown to the regular faculty.

MARRIED,—Wm. W. Morland, M.D., of Boston, to Miss F. S. Lyman.

DIED,—At Savannah, Geo., J. B Gilbert, M.D., 33.

Deaths in Boston for the week ending Saturday noon, May 14th, 84. Males, 43—females, 41· Inflammation of the bowels, 1—congestion of the brain, 1—bronchitis, 1—consumption, 19—convulsions, 5—croup, 5—dysentery, 1—dropsy, 1—dropsy in head, 6—drowned, 1—infantile diseases, 6—puerperal, 2—erysipelas 1—scarlet fever, 5—hooping cough, 1—disease of heart, 1—intemperance, 2—inflammation of the lungs, 3—disease of liver, 1—marasmus, 5—measles, 3—mortification, 1—old age, 3—pleurisy, 1—palsy, 2—suicide, 1—scrofula, 1—suffocation, 1—teething, 1.
Under 5 years, 47—between 5 and 20 years. 5—between 20 and 40 years, 18—between 40 and 60 years, 8—over 60 years, 6. Born in the United States, 68—Ireland, 2—England, 1—British Provinces, 2—at sea, 1.

Therapeutic Properties of Belladonna—Conclusions arrived at by M. Dubois.—1. That belladonna is not without efficacy in some phlegmasiæ, especially in those of the globe of the eye.

2. That it is the best remedy known in the photophobia which so frequently accompanies inflammations of the eye.

3. That its power as a prophylactic in scarlatina can hardly be contested.

4. That it sometimes cures certain hæmorrhages, such as hæmoptysis, hæmatemesis and metrorrhagia.

5. That it is the remedy *par excellence* for neuralgia, for hooping cough, and most of the neuroses.

6. That it is the remedy *par excellence* to combat pain, especially when external.

7. That it alleviates more than any other remedy the pains of cancer, and cures sometimes, if not cancer, diseases closely resembling it.

8. That it can be advantageously employed in spasmodic contraction and occlusion of the pupil; to reduce procidentia of the iris and to break up adhesions; to prevent the inflammation of the iris so frequent after this operation; to maintain dilatation of the pupil, and to diminish the chances of adhesions after the operation of couching; to prevent secondary cataract; to re-establish vision, temporarily at least, when the lens is opaque in the centre, or when there are opacities of the cornea; to assist the diagnosis in some diseases of the eye.

9, That it is of real efficacy in some cases of strangulated hernia.

10. That its property of facilitating labor in spasmodic constriction of the uterine neck is powerful and incontestible.

11. That it produces advantageous results in some cases of fissure of the anus.

12. That its employment may be more or less useful in spasmodic contraction of the bowels, in constipation, in spasmodic constriction of the rectum, of the anus, and of the vulva; in phimosis and paraphimosis, spasmodic stricture of the urethra, retention of urine, strangury, spasmodic stricture of the larynx and œsophagus; in blepharospasm, incontinence of urine, nephritic colic, hemorrhoids, &c.

13. Finally, that belladonna should be placed in the first rank of medicinal substances.—*Bulletin of the Med. Society of Gand.—(Gaz. Médicale.)*

A Conscientious Patient.—It is stated in the Courier des Etats Unis, that a dentist of high reputation, residing on the Boulevard, at Paris, was surprised by having his door-bell rung with great violence every day for sometime at precisely the same hour. On going to the door each time, his servant found no visiter, but instead thereof, a five-franc piece placed upon the mat. This was repeated for several days in succession, but the manner in which the money was placed there was finally discovered by waiting behind the door for the mysterious ringer, who was no other than an unhappy sufferer who came there every day for the purpose of having an aching tooth extracted. But on arriving at the door, the pain immediately ceased. which he attributed to the sudden approach of the dentist, whom with fastidious honesty he thus repaid. The dentist, who was an equally honest man, had much difficulty in persuading his singular patient to accept money, which the latter thought a very moderate remuneration for the benefit he had derived from approaching his door.— *Amer. Journal of Dental Science.*

THE

THE
BOSTON MEDICAL AND SURGICAL JOURNAL.

| Vol. XLVIII. | Wednesday, May 25, 1853. | No. 17. |

UNION OF DIVIDED FINGERS.

[Communicated for the Boston Medical and Surgical Journal.]

I HAVE sometimes succeeded in establishing the union of divided fingers under circumstances so apparently unpromising, as to induce the belief that the deformity caused by the partial loss of these members may often be prevented. If the cut be clean, oblique, and near the extremity of the finger, and adaptation of the surfaces be timely made and accurately maintained, 1 think, as a general thing, success will follow. In corroboration of this opinion, I offer the following facts.

A young man accidentally divided the fore finger obliquely through the third phalanx. The cut was smooth, and the day being cold there was little bleeding, although the patient walked half a mile. I regretted that he had not brought the separated fragment, whereupon he produced it from his pocket. It had been struck off full thirty minutes, and was cold and bloodless. I immediately adjusted the incised surfaces and applied the necessary dressings. On the fifth day, union by first intention was established, although subsequently the nail separated.

The sequel of this injury was deplorable. The young man returned to his occupation at the expiration of three weeks, and soon after, as he supposed, took cold in the throat, which pretty nearly prevented motion of the lower jaw. He, however, paid no attention to it for several days, until he became much worse, and then I was called to see him, and found him laboring under a seizure of tetanus. He was in great pain in the epigastric region, with violent spasms in the back and neck, and his face presented the expression peculiar to the sustained contraction of its muscles, the sardonic laugh. His mind was anxious but depressed, his respiration at times painful and difficult, and the circulation feeble, rapid and tremulous. In spite of all remedial measures, the spasms became more general and severe, and his sufferings were very great until the seventh day from the attack, when in the act of swallowing he was seized with violent spasms in the throat and suddenly expired.

In another instance, a young man struck off two of his fingers by a straw cutter, and I was sent for to dress the wounds. I inquired for the amputated fragments, and found they had received no attention whatever; but search was made, and they were soon produced. The direction of the incisions was obliquely through the third phalanges. The truncated

17

portions were immersed in warm water and accurately applied, and upon the subsequent dressing it was found that union had taken place in one by first intention, and in the other the integuments were gangrenous.

In this case the period of separation was at least thirty minutes ; but the chance of success will be in proportion to the speedy adaptation of the incised surfaces.

A similar case is reported by A. Graham, Esq. A joiner cut through the index finger of the left hand, between the first and second phalanges. He immediately walked a few yards to a place where Mr. Graham happened to be, when adaptation was made by sutures and adhesive straps, and complete union followed.

A case is related in Johnson's Journal for 1834, of a medical student who accidentally divided the last phalanx of the left fore finger, which was immediately replaced and secured by proper dressings, and union produced. This happened in Italy ; and Dr. Angello della Cella exultingly invites M. Richerand and his followers to cross the Alps and pay him a visit upon the banks of the Entella, and see with their own eyes, and try to believe, they having ridiculed the doctrines of Tagliacozzi as unworthy of credit.

Liston, in his fifth Lecture, makes some observations on the re-union of divided surfaces. He says the native rulers in India inflicted punishment upon a certain caste by cutting off the nose, and that the natives were in the habit after a time of picking up the detached part and clapping it on again, and that it often stuck. After that, they were thrown into hot ovens and baked. Even in colder climes, he says, and in less favorable subjects, adhesions will sometimes take place in parts that are completely separated from the body. In this country many fingers have been cut off and put on again. There is a story told to the following effect by Garingeot, which may be familiar to some of you :—In a quarrel, a man bit off the nose of his antagonist. He picked it up and threw it into an apothecary's shop ; and having beaten his opponent soundly he returned to the apothecary, who put it on and there it grew.

Greenfield, May, 1853. JAMES DEANE.

RAIL ROAD ACCIDENTS.

BY EDW. WARREN, M.D.

[Communicated for the Boston Medical and Surgical Journal.]

THE recent disaster at Norwalk, by which so many valuable members of our profession have been destroyed, and from which so many more have escaped only by the intervention of a benevolent providence, seems to render some remarks upon disasters of this nature justifiable, if not strictly belonging to a medical journal. It is the highest duty of the medical man, to save life, and prevent injury to life and limb, by every means in his power. Indeed, a cool, disinterested observer might form the opinion, that to our profession, alone, it is left to feel for disasters of the character in question. Had we, what we have always boasted of in this country, a free and untrammelled daily press, the remarks I wish to make might more appropriately be expressed in that. But if that is under the iron influence of rail-road companies, I hope at least that the medical press may continue, as it has always been, free.

When an accident happened upon a branch of one of our leading rail roads, a year since, a talented writer—the author of Zenobia and Probus—who with his youngest son had often unsuspiciously incurred the danger, which proved fatal in the case referred to, wrote an article on the subject of this and similar accidents ; and will it be believed, he could find no newspaper that would publish it. At this same time, Dr. M., of Boston, sent to a respectable daily paper a notice of the accident and of the causes that led to it. His bare statement of the accident was published, docked and curtailed of everything that could imply a censure upon the company. Some other writer, I know not who, was fortunate in obtaining admission in the Traveller. He drew down the thunders of the president or superintendent upon his head, for calling the place "a trap." So the trap still remains set. Another terrible accident having occurred within a week after this, I prepared, by permission, an article for a religious periodical, upon the express condition that I should imply no censure against directors. It was not my intention to do so. I regard the directors as servants of the proprietors ; and it is not until proprietors, and every one who owns a share in a rail road, can be properly impressed with their responsibility, that accidents will be prevented.

A distinguished clergyman of Boston, I understand, has, in relation to the late accident, preached from the text—"Thou shalt do no murder." But if murder has been done, who are the murderers? This is a solemn question to put to the community. Who is the principal? *Qui facit per alium facit per se.* The deed of the agent is the deed of the employer. It is unfair in all these cases to place the blame upon fireman, engineman, conductor or directors. It is not until it can be impressed upon the mind of every stockholder in a rail road, that he is actually guilty of murder, if he does not exert his voice, his vote, and, if a writer, his pen, to prevent the destruction of human life, however valueless to the community, that these disasters can be prevented.

If I were to find a drunken man in the road, and knock out his brains, should I, or should I not, be indictable for murder? If a rail-road company find a drunken man upon their track, and run over him, coroner's jury and the daily papers all pronounce that he comes to his death by his own fault. If a heap of ashes or a pile of snow is left in a country road, and a gentleman rides over it and demolishes his gig, a jury will give him heavy damages. I speak seriously, and I have ample proof of what I say.

Rail-road accidents have become so frequent, and so little interest on common occasions is excited, that when we hear that a man is run over on a rail-road track, it attracts as little interest as if it was a kitten. Yet every one who speaks lightly of such accidents ; every editor who slurs them over, or apologizes for them, is an abettor to the deed, at least an accessory after the fact. It is the light manner in which accidents are passed over that affect one or two lives, with their immediate circle of friends, that is the remote cause of such disasters as that at Norwalk. If we could be brought into the palace of truth, and compelled to declare the fact, we must say that it is the shareholders in all rail roads that are the murderers ; and the whole community accessories.

Nothing effectual can or will be done by our legislatures. They will meet and talk ; rail-road directors will meet and talk, and perhaps eat a dinner at the expense of the company, the cost of which might save many lives ; but nothing will be done until it is fully impressed upon the stockholders that each and every one of them is accountable for every death that has occurred or does occur. One has given one hundred dollars, another one thousand, another ten thousand, but each and every one has paid his share towards the murder. Each one is a principal, so long as he does not attend the meetings either in person or by proxy, and do his utmost to prevent these single or wholesale homicides.

A daily paper is rather indignant that a legislator is supposed to have contemplated a law that each company should pay ten thousand dollars for every man they killed by negligence. But let such a measure be carried into effect, with the approbation of the community ; still better, let there be a definite sum to be paid for every man they killed (negligence or no negligence), and rail-road accidents would cease.

Rail roads might be hermetically sealed against trespassers ; a man might always be kept upon the look-out, in front of the train, who should never leave his post, or gossip with passengers or employees. The cost might be somewhat greater to the proprietors ; but perhaps if they attended meetings and examined accounts, they might find means to prevent a diminution of their dividends. Rail-road directors are, like those whom Mark Antony speaks of, " *all honorable men* " ; and I have no idea of disparaging them. But I believe they are rather employed to make money for the stockholders, than to save human life. Would that the associations for the abolition of capital punishment, and the temperance societies, would turn their attention to rail-road reform. Every daily paper teaches us that walking on rail roads is a capital crime.

Under the present system, who, I would solemnly ask, are responsible for rail-way accidents ? The conductor is busied in taking tickets, entertaining the ladies, and attending to the children under his charge. The engineman or driver is employed with his engine, the fireman in keeping up his fire, and the brakemen at their brakes ; each have enough to do. Were a man to be kept upon the watch, and the engineman and conductor compelled to stop the train on the appearance of an obstacle, if it were only a deaf man, or a drunken man, or a private individual of any kind, even at the risk of injuring the engine, many accidents might be prevented.

But recklessness in one point, leads to recklessness in another. Those who abet and apologize for a single homicide, encourage the feeling which leads to a wholesale one.

I had hoped that a paper, in a religious periodical of high standing and influence, might make some impression upon a portion, at least, of those whom I regard as principals—the rail-road stockholders. My paper was rejected, on the ground that *the editors could feel no interest in the subject,* and they thought that their readers would feel none. I presume that they were right, and it is to this indifference in the public that we owe the loss of so many valuable lives.

We boast that increased civilization has taught us to value human life more highly. I doubt whether there prevailed, in Greece or Rome, a recklessness which equals ours. I doubt whether the Goth or Vandal would have tolerated that destruction which with us has become almost a matter of course.

The Norwalk disaster has sufficiently aroused the feelings of the community for the time. Wide numbers, who might have felt indifference had they been themselves exposed, have had their feelings roused to the utmost by the loss or danger of their friends ; and now should be the time for action.

I would repeat it, every stockholder, every rail-road director, every editor, who does not exert himself to prevent the recurrence of such accidents ; every one who slurs over or conceals facts ; every coroner's jury who gives too lenient a verdict ; every one who prefers money to human life, is an accessory to the murder.

Newton Lower Falls, May, 1853.

SOURCES OF VITALITY IN THE TEETH—REMOVAL OF THE DENTAL PULP NOT "IMPRACTICABLE"—RHIZODONTRYPO-NEURHÆMAXIS.

[Communicated for the Boston Medical and Surgical Journal.]

FROM the earliest efforts of the human mind to examine the relations of cause and effect—to investigate the phenomena of nature, or produce practical results from philosophic reasoning, it has ever been active in the pursuit of knowledge. Prone to investigate, it has, not infrequently, indulged in theories and speculations, some of which, although they have not fully realized the expectations created, yet have contributed, in some degree, to that perfection in the arts and sciences which distinguishes the present from the past. It is by degrees, and through difficulties, that our present position in scientific knowledge has been attained ; and, as science progresses, still greater mysteries will be solved—seemingly " conflicting principles " explained—unexplored regions penetrated, and many of its treasures, *now* veiled in obscurity, fully developed.

Every age has produced important discoveries and inventions, and every era has had its sceptics. In astronomy, the Copernican system was violently assailed, at different periods, and denounced as a doctrine contravening the word of God ; the teaching of which brought down the horrors of the inquisition upon Galileo and others who dared promulgate it. The discovery of the circulation of the blood by Harvey met with bitter opposition from some of the most eminent medical men of his time. And the theory of inoculation for the smallpox was attacked by the ablest writers of the day. So great was the hostility to it, that the clergy were called upon to preach against it and pro-

nounced it "a usurpation of the sacred prerogative of God." They
declared the practice "a diabolical operation and anti-providential project that insults our religion and banishes Providence out of the world "
—an operation originated by the *devil* and *first* practised upon *Job.*"
The discovery of vaccination, at a later period, by Jenner, incurred
a similar displeasure, although less violent, perhaps, and of shorter duration, owing to the improved intelligence of the age in which he lived ;
but which arose from the same cause—ignorance and superstition. In
our own time, when it was first announced that the inhalation of the
nitrous oxide, or "laughing gas," or breathing the vapors of ether and
chloroform, would paralyze the intellectual functions and suspend sensation and voluntary motion during a severe and protracted surgical
operation, the *fact* was doubted and denied, by many, for want of knowledge that these agents had the power to produce such effects. And
yet, all these theories and discoveries, with many others that might be
cited, are now well established and matters of record in medical history.

There appeared in Vol. XLVIII., No. 1 (Feb. 2d), of this Journal,
an article on "Impracticable Theories," by M. M. Frisselle, M.D., in
which the writer called in question certain theories, systems of practice,
&c., and among them, the "new operation on the teeth." It is not
my purpose, in connection with this subject, to discuss the comparative
merits of the various systems of medical practice, as each is based upon
a distinct theory, and has its supporters who will look after its special
interests. Nor do I claim that my experiments on the dental nerves,
and the result in which they terminated, detailed in the Journal for October 20, 1852, equal in importance or admit of comparison with the
subjects referred to ; or that they have excited hostility, or particular interest, in the medical profession *generally ;* but my object is to show
that discoveries, theories, &c., by far transcending mine in their results
to mankind, which have been subjects of ridicule and scepticism, and those
who originated or tolerated them, in some instances the victims, not only of
virulent opposition, but of *religious intolerance*, have proved the basis of
many a beautiful and enduring superstructure. Hence it is unwise to call
this or that theory impracticable, simply because it has not gained the
popular voice and been universally acknowledged, without offering sufficient proof to refute it. The folly of such a course has been forcibly
shown by the history of the past, especially in the subjects alluded to.
Not more unwise is that class of experimenters who "first form an
opinion, and then labor to make their experiments prove their opinions
correct." Dr. Frisselle says, "No man, from a limited number of experiments, or cases that may have come under his observation, can sit
down and draw out a theory—ingenious though it may be, and plausible,
but mingled as theories usually are, with conjectures, certainties and suppositions—without being liable to be called upon to enlighten the public

* The subject of the experiments referred to has not met with *universal* favor, either among
physicians or dentists, for want of due consideration. Not long since, in conversation with a medical friend, who is also a dentist of high reputation, notwithstanding he was assured of the success
of the operation, he utterly denied the possibility of performing it, saying—"it cannot be done."
There is, however, a rapidly-increasing opinion in its favor, derived from experience, by those
who have adopted it.

and the profession, relative to what seems to them conflicting principles." This passage being an implied call for an explanation relative to what seems to the doctor " conflicting principles," other extracts will be cited and commented upon by way of illustration.

" A limited number of experiments, or cases," &c. If a physician should treat nearly three hundred cases of fever, or *any* specific disease, involving danger, or perform an equal number of surgical operations, and all for a similar purpose, within the space of two and a half years, and lose but *one* patient, and either *cure* or *greatly benefit* a large majority of the remainder, would he not be apt to come to the " grand conclusion " that the theory, upon which his practice was based, was not " impracticable " ? It would seem so ; and that he might " sit down and draw out a theory based upon and well built up by facts." " In order to judge correctly of any question or practice, the evils as well as the benefits growing out of it should be considered." The comparative success which the treatment has met with in my hands, has been stated in a previous number, and, I may add, several dentists to whom I communicated the results of my experiments, more than two years ago, have adopted it in their practice, and report favorably, without, as yet, having encountered evils sufficient to induce them to abandon it. One of them (Dr. Flagg), whose medical attainments and large experience in dental practice enable him thoroughly to understand the physiology and pathology of the dental organs, and to compare the new treatment with other methods that have preceded it, in a letter to me says—" You spoke with a degree of confidence which induced me to adopt the treatment, and the results encourage me to continue it." And this is the universal testimony of all who have practised it to any considerable extent, within my knowledge.

" The advocates of the new operation, claim, I believe," says Dr. F., " that the surgeon is enabled to plug the carious tooth when the dental pulp is exposed, without pain, and preserve the vitality of the tooth." As one of the " advocates," I have carefully avoided saying that any part of the operation, preparatory to the introduction of the filling, can be done without pain, although it is less painful than is generally supposed ; on the contrary, I have expressly stated that the division of the nerve and removal of the pulp in the few cases in which either or both operations have been done, consumed more time and were *more painful* than when the nerve was merely punctured ; therefore, for *general practice*, these operations were given up within a few weeks after my first experiment.

Again, Dr. F. says—" I do not quite understand how the nerves and bloodvessels can be severed, and, as in some cases stated, the dental pulp removed, without destroying the vitality of the organ. It has always been my impression that when the circulation of the nervous communication is cut off from an organ, it immediately loses its vitality, and nature soon makes effort to remove it. I cannot see why the same rule does not apply to the teeth. So far as my observation goes, it does ; for when the vitality of a tooth is destroyed, nature makes effort to rid herself of it, and will do so, sooner or later, either by ulceration taking place around the fang, or by absorption." From this extract the writer is of opinion, if I rightly understand him, that the principle of vitality in a tooth resides in its central ganglion *only*—that it has no *other* source, and when *that* is cut off, it " *immediately* loses its vitality, and nature soon makes effort to remove it." If such be the case, as a general rule, in common with others, and among them the ablest of the profession, I must confess to having been engaged, for nearly twenty years, in a practice founded on an " impracticable theory," indeed. It is admitted that whenever the circulation of the nervous communication is *wholly* cut off from an organ, it loses its vitality, but the destruction of a dental nerve deprives the tooth of a *portion* of its vitality *only*, as will be shown hereafter. Allowing, for the argument, that nature *does* make effort to remove a tooth after its inner membrane has been destroyed, shall nothing be done to save the organ and prolong its usefulness a few years? Is it the custom, and does it comport with the duties of the physician and the obligations of humanity, to suspend treatment because the patient is to be removed by death, " sooner or later "? If so, why do the promptings of the human heart resort to consultation—to this or that measure, except on the ground that " effort " is often successful?

And not only this, but unremitted exertion is often continued from *hope*, after it has become a " fixed fact " that the patient cannot long survive. The cases are parallel, and to be treated on the same general principles. The structure of the teeth differs, somewhat, from that of other bones; hence, a corresponding difference in their functions, diseases, and the means of cure. Observation teaches that the loss of teeth is often occasioned by the gradual absorption of the gum, alveolus, and periosteum, which deprives them of their external support, notwithstanding the nerve remain alive until the absorbents have nearly finished their work; therefore, nature does not wait for the nerve to be destroyed, or, as Dr. Frisselle would have it, the " circulation of the nervous communication to be cut off," before she commences a removal of the organ. A tissue may have vitality, and yet possess little sensibility. Uninflamed bone, cartilage and tendon, are examples; but when their sensibility becomes exalted, they are highly sensitive. Although the removal of the central ganglion deprives the tooth of its interior source of vitality, and lessens its sensibility to impressions from heat and cold, it does not deprive it of its exterior, or that support which it receives through the medium of its investing membrane; for if it does, the almost universal practice of trying to save such teeth, and the ably written articles on the treatment of the dental pulp, show that the dental profession have labored, for a long time, without reasonable hope of success, and are a stupid set of fellows for not knowing it until Dr. F. made the discovery. Individuals, otherwise well informed, are often to be found, whose notions respecting the vitality of the teeth are based on the idea that it is *entirely* dependent on the nerve and bloodvessels comprising the pulp. To show that such notions are incorrect, Thomas Bell, an eminent English writer on the " Anatomy, Physiology. and Diseases of the Teeth," in speaking of their organization, says—" The fang is covered by a periosteum, and the internal cavity is lined by a highly nervous and vascular membrane ; both of these are intimately connected with the bony structure of the tooth. Now, unless we suppose that these membranes are the media by which vessels and nerves are sent to the bony substance of the tooth, and by which, in fact, its vitality is supported, and its connection with the general system preserved, it will be impossible to assign any purpose which can be answered by their existence. The presence of a nervous and vascular connection between these membranes and the tooth, will appear the more probable, when it is considered that the adhesion between these parts is so strong as to require a slight degree of force to remove them ; which can only be accounted for by the presence of numerous vessels, &c., passing from the one to the other. We are, therefore, justified, I think, in considering this connection as identical with that which exists between the bones and their periosteum."

[To be concluded next week.]

MICROSCOPIC PREPARATIONS,

To the Editor of the Boston Medical and Surgical Journal.

I SEND you a page or two relating to microscopic matters, which some of the students who read your Journal may like to see, if you can find room for so much in any of your coming numbers.

Yours very truly,   O. W. HOLMES.

Many of the readers of this Journal, and especially many of its younger readers, are interested in the microscope in its application to anatomy, physiology and pathology. Most of the young physicians who complete their studies in Europe bring home a " Nachet" or an " Oberhaeuser," and a certain amount of skill in handling it, which they find abundant leisure to improve in the early times of their practice. There are now many good instruments among us in the hands of those who know how to use them, and several of the highest excellence. Our microscopists are beginning to be known somewhat beyond their own immediate circle. Dr. Dalton and Dr. Burnett have been honored by two of the four prizes conferred by the American Medical Association, for essays based in great part or wholly on microscopic investigations. Other observers are at work, who will be heard from in due season.

In the mean time attention has been drawn in this country to the art of making the instruments upon which so many departments of medical science are more or less dependent. Mr. Spencer's labors and triumphs are well known. It is not so generally understood that excellent lenses have been made in this city. Mr. Alvan Clark, distinguished as an artist and as a maker of astronomical instruments, has employed his leisure, occasionally, in making objectives, several of which I have seen and found to compare very favorably with the best of the imported glasses of similar power. There has been little done as yet, however, in the way of providing the microscopist with those numerous accessories which he is constantly requiring, and which in London or Paris he can readily obtain.   To get *very thin* glass, one must hunt up in New York the American agency of Messrs. Chance, of Birmingham, which · is to be found in an obscure warehouse remote from the common markets of scientific commodities.   As for a set of delicate tests, it is doubtful if they can be had without importing them expressly.   Some of Hett's and Topping's injected preparations may be had in New York, but only such as have been left after careful culling by others.

We shall have to find out that we can make many of these things for ourselves, which we are in the habit of importing ; *all* of them, as soon as it will pay to make them.   It would not be surprising to find, in ten years from this time, that there were more microscopists in America than in Europe.   For here everybody must know something of everything ; and as a microscope is *prima facie* evidence that the owner is a microscopist, it will become as necessary a part of the stock in trade as a stethoscope ; which implies that the owner is a stethoscopist —even if he does not know which end to put to his ear, as once happened in a consultation in this region.   Thus there will be growing up among us a market for microscopes and all that belongs to microscopic art, and the skill which has never failed to show itself whenever it has been called for, will find a new channel in providing for this want.

The art of *minute injection* has been until of late very little practised in this country.   Dr. Horner's preparations in the Wistar Museum are among the most successful examples of it.   The application of the achromatic microscope to the study of the tissues has given a fresh impulse to this branch of anatomical art, and many beautiful results have been obtained ; such as we can hardly believe that Ruysch or Lieberkuhn can have approached, by what we know of their performances. Many of the injections of Berres and others are figured in the work of Gerber ; Hassall gives figures of those of several of the English anatomists ; Dr. Neill, of Philadelphia, has given very beautiful representations of some of his own injections of the mucous membrane of the stomach.   From these plates, those who have not access to the original preparations may form some idea of their delicacy and brilliancy.

Preparations of this kind, properly put up in preservative fluid, are of very great importance, especially to the teacher of microscopic art and science.   It is in this capacity that I have had occasion to employ many such preparations, of some of which a few remarks will be here made.

The first I used were some made by or under the direction of Retzius of Stockholm, lent me by Dr. Ware.   One of these, an injection of the lobules of the liver, is a very beautiful exhibition of the two veins and the duct filled with different kinds of injections.   They are put up in a somewhat rough way between two thick plates of glass.

The preparations of Mr. Hett, some of which were selected by Mr. Burnett in London, and others purchased of the importer, are put up with great neatness, and on the whole the most brilliant specimens of minute injection of all those mentioned.   They become infested with air-bubbles in the course of a year or two, which will in time require them to be taken out and the cells re-filled with fluid.

Those of Mr. Topping are injected in many cases with yellow instead of red, which makes them somewhat less showy than the others. They are, however, well filled and neatly mounted.

I have received from Dr. John Neill, of Philadelphia, specimens prepared by himself, the last received very perfect; the colored figures before referred to, which may be found in the American Journal of Medical Sciences for Jan., 1851, show the delicacy of the injection and the use of such preparations in bringing out the nicer points of structure.

We have in this city a microscopist who has devoted himself with great assiduity and success to preparing and mounting specimens, many of which are injected by him with great nicety. Dr. Durkee, the gentleman referred to, has been his own instructor, and has succeeded, after many trials, in acquiring to a great extent the skill which is almost confined to a few persons abroad who make a business of preparing objects for microscopists. I will mention a few of these which I have seen, to give an idea of the points which they illustrate. Several of these which Dr. Durkee had the kindness to give me, I have used with much satisfaction in my demonstrations.

1. Fœtal stomach, near cardiac orifice. A perfect injection, showing ridges, areolæ, but no villi.

2. Skin of the back of the hand, showing vascular net-work.

3. Mucous membrane of gall-bladder, finely injected, showing ridges, running into villi.

4. Membrana tympani injected, showing a non-vascular spot about the attachment of the handle of the malleus.

5. Malpighian corpuscles of the kidney in the human subject and in the ox, beautifully shown.

6. Tongue, showing the filiform papillæ, finely injected.

I have selected these as among the most successful preparations, but there are many others of much interest. Among the rest I should not forget the sections of bone, which Dr. Durkee has the art of making in a very superior way. I have made hundreds of them, and seen a great many made in this country and in Europe, but never saw more than one specimen equal to the best made by Dr. Durkee.

The injected preparations made in this country are apt to be inferior in color to the imported ones. The vermilion is not equal in brilliancy to that used by Mr. Hett. Once in a while it is found to contain specks which take off a little from the beauty of the specimen containing them. But it is evident that we are in the way of learning to do for ourselves what others have done for us, and there can be no doubt that the slight difficulties which stand in the way of absolute perfection will be overcome as the principal ones have already been. It was said at the beginning of this communication, that the young practitioner had *time enough* to improve his knowledge of the microscope in his early years of practice. There are many hours which he must pass in his office, quite undisturbed, in company with his books and his thoughts. Let him add a microscope as a companion to these, and time will be wonderfully lightened for him, while he is acquiring the knowledge he will be very glad of in the busy years that are coming.

The microscope is of all philosophical instruments the most unfailing and untiring companion. The astronomer tells us that hardly more than a dozen nights in the year are adapted to his observations. He must watch all night, exposed to cold and damp, surrounded by costly and cumbrous machinery. The microscopist sits down at his fireside or his window, with a little instrument before him, a mere toy to look at—a giant mightier than the slave of the lamp or the ring in its power of transformation. All that he wishes to observe upon, nature is ready to furnish him. Nothing is too precious or rare for him to covet ; he wishes but a mere speck, a particle, such as the koh-i-noor could spare him. Nothing is repulsive, examined in its infinitesimal shape. The disease which infected the wards of a hospital does not betray itself in the narrow apartment where he studies all its intimate details. He may study and work until *practice* comes and takes him off his feet and floats him away into a world of other cares and duties, and year after year, every day will bring him something new to examine. I will say nothing of the utility, even the necessity of the microscope to the practical physician and the surgeon. As a mere illustrative companion to scientific study, as a mere intelligent plaything, it is the most precious gift to all who love to look at the universe as its inner life is revealed to the senses. To all who have done and are doing anything to render it more available for the purposes of study, we are under obligations which it is a pleasure to express, even if it is done as in this slight notice, which was suggested by the pleasure derived from examining the preparations made by Dr. Durkee.

SPASMODIC ASTHMA.

[Concluded from page 313.]

Case III.—A lady above middle age had for several years been the subject of chronic bronchitis, when suddenly, and without any very apparent cause, she was seized with marked symptoms of asthma, and after a short, but severe paroxysm, she found her former symptoms importantly changed. The expectoration was diminished, the cough came on in fits of greater length, and the succession of coughs was more rapid, while the accompanying dyspnœa was so severe as to oblige her to maintain the sitting posture day and night. I need not add, that her face had a livid color and most anxious expression, and that her extremities were apt to become cold. The physical signs corresponded with the general symptoms. The percussion sound was less clear than natural, the respiratory murmur was feeble, and obscured by loud bronchial râles, and during the paroxysms it was entirely absent for a short time. Its return was ushered in by a long stridulous inspiration, and loud sonorous ronchi throughout the chest.

Here then was a case of chronic bronchitis ending in asthma, and there can be no doubt that the glottis was very much affected by the spasmodic contraction. · If anything is wanted to prove this, it is to be found in the nature of the treatment which was successfully employed in combating the disease. For, with the exception of a few blisters to counteract the bronchial inflammation, and some anodyne draughts to procure ease and gain time, the only remedial means used were topical applications of solution of caustic to the .glottis. In three weeks the patient was free of all asthmatic tendency, the bronchitis remaining little changed from what it had been for years previously ; and it is worthy of remark, though I do not wish to build anything upon it, that no return of the asthma has occurred since the one attack just mentioned, which happened fully two years ago.

Such happy results are by no means always to be looked for, and I am far from wishing to laud the topical applications beyond what they deserve. But I am sure every medical practitioner will bear me out in saying, that the ordinary treatment by bleeding. general or local, by emetics, antispasmodics. opiates, and mercurials internally, with blisters, and various other counter-irritants, externally, has seldom been followed by even a partial success in these cases ; and I am sanguine enough to hope that I have even already in this short paper adduced sufficient reasons, both theoretical and practical, for the trial of a more rational plan of treatment.

That plan does not involve a total overthrow of former practices. It is not meant, in adopting the new, to set aside as useless all older measures, but only to employ them when really indicated. For instance. it is, I think, established both by clinical observation, and by Dr. Williams's experiments. that bleeding carried to any length can never diminish the tendency to spasmodic contraction in the air-tubes ; but during a bad fit of asthma, such a measure may be absolutely necessary to relieve congestions, arising secondarily, either in the brain, or in the lungs themselves. Again, though emetics cannot save the patient from a renewal of the spasm, they may assist in overcoming that which exists, as well as in clearing away the mucus which clogs up the smaller tubes ; and antispasmodics may assist in prolonging their good effects for a short time. In some cases where there is much bronchitis, blisters have a good and more lasting effect, but they do not exercise much influence over the spasmodic asthma. In like manner, a slight mercurialization often benefits the bronchitis of the more sthenic variety, as indicated by the expectoration containing plastic matter, mixed with mucous globules, but it can have no effect on the paroxysmal disease. Opium only lulls for a time—an effect by no means to be lightly esteemed— but when the paroxysm becomes severe it utterly fails.

There is here, therefore, an evident blank in therapeutics. There is no agent hitherto proposed which is capable of removing or greatly diminishing the morbid contractility of the air-tubes. And I think that a solution of caustic applied to the interior of the larynx supplies this defect—fills up the blank. In proof of its having this exhausting effect upon the irritability of the glottis, and ultimately on that of the air-tubes, I can only refer to the results of its use in hooping cough. a disease which is so analogous to spasmodic asthma in its pathology, that it

is almost enough to show the efficacy of a remedy in the treatment of
one of those diseases, to prove its suitableness for the other. Now, in
proof that the topical treatment of hooping cough is most efficacious and
successful, it is enough to state, that, combining the cases treated by me
since I first proposed the plan in 1849, with those treated by M. Joubert,
of Cherion, and published in the *Bulletin de Therapeutique* for January,
1852, we have as follows :—

A speedy cure (in 10 to 14 days) resulted in   - - - 78 cases.
Shortening of disease (3 or 4 weeks' duration), - - - 39 cases.
No change was effected in   - - - - - - -\ - - 8 cases.
                                                            ———
Total number treated   - - . - 125

There was not one death among all the cases treated, and taking their
per centage, we have—

62·4 were cured within a fortnight.
31·2 were cured in 3 or 4 weeks.
6·4 resisted the treatment.
                        ———
100·0

I feel assured that no similar statement could be made regarding the results of any other method of treating hooping cough.

I cannot, as yet, speak of great numbers of cases of spasmodic asthma
treated in this way, but I have been very successful with the topical
method in some cases that had previously been treated without much
benefit in the ordinary manner.   Of these I shall give two examples,
and did time and space permit, I could more than double them.

CASE IV.—Last summer, Dr. Peter Stewart, of this city, sent me a
patient who had come to town to consult him for confirmed bronchial asthma.   He had undergone all the ordinary remedies for that
disease in the country, including, if I recollect right, a somewhat common, and in my opinion, a barbarous species of counter-irritation when
applied to a large surface, viz., croton oil—but all was in vain.   His
dyspnœa was excessively severe, and occurred frequently during the day,
as well as prevented his lying down to rest at night.

I pursued no other treatment but that of a simple tonic to recruit his
shattered energies, and the daily application of solution of caustic to the
larynx.   In about a month's time he was so much better that I advised
him to spend a few weeks at the coast, after which he returned home
much improved in general health, and comparatively free of the dyspnœa.   I recommended him to continue the use of the solution of caustic, applied by himself, as far down his throat as he could reach,
and to wear a respirator ; and as I have not heard from him since, I believe that these means have been sufficient to keep in check, if not altogether to remove, the remnants of his severe complaint.

CASE V.—Another case, at present under my care, and recommended to me by Dr. Smellie, of Buccleuch street, is so similar to the above,
that I need not give any particular account of it here.   Suffice it to
mention, that the paroxysms in this case were very severe, and unmiti-

gated by the kind attention and judicious general treatment of Dr. Smellie ; but that a few days ago, when the patient last called on me, he expressed himself as feeling better than he had done for the two previous years. This was after the topical measures had been used for only two or three weeks, and I have no doubt that the improvement will be increased and perpetuated by the treatment being employed for a more lengthened period.

It is well known that heart disease is a frequent concomitant of asthma, and in such cases it is often supposed that the former is the cause of the latter disease ; but this is by no means the constant relation of the two morbid states, for the disturbance to the pulmonary circulation, occasioned by frequent asthmatic paroxysms, is quite as likely to produce the heart disease as the reverse. It is, however, more important at present to call attention to the fact of the great difference between simple spasmodic asthma, and that which co-exists with heart disease. The pathology of the former has already been explained as an affection wholly confined to the bronchial tubes. But in cardiac asthma, this is, I may venture to say, never the case. In that disease, the substance of the lung is always more or less altered ; generally the air-cells have become much distended, their walls atrophied, and even in some places ruptured ; and it is this vesicular emphysema, not spasmodic contraction of any part of the bronchi, which produces the urgent thirst for air so distressingly experienced by these patients. I need hardly remark, that there could be no good object served by introducing solution of caustic into the larynx in such cases. Indeed, I fear it must be confessed that, in the present state of medicine, little more can be done for such patients than to endeavor as far as possible to palliate their most urgent symptoms, and render more tolerable the short and uncertain period which remains for them to live.

There are, besides the topical application to the larynx, two other remedial measures which I have for some time employed in cases of spasmodic asthma, but regarding which I am not at present able to speak with precision. I may, however, mention them in this place, that others may assist in determining whether or not they have any value in the treatment of that formidable disease. The one is electricity, applied, in a gentle current, as much as possible along the course of the larynx and bronchi. In his experiments on the lower animals, Dr. C. J. B. Williams found that such a current destroyed the contractility of the tubes, and in several instances I have thought that it co-operated with other means, in diminishing the frequency and severity of the asthmatic paroxysms. This, however, might be the effect, not only of its local, but of its general action as a tonic on the nervous system. The other agent referred to is strychnia, which I have used in repeated small doses of 1-20th or 1-16th part of a grain, and I believe with good effect in some cases. Dr. Williams found that when the animals he experimented on had been poisoned by this substance, the air-tubes did not exhibit contractility, and he thought that they were retained in a tonic spasm by the operation of the poison. This very probably was the case, but of course the use of strychnia in medicinal doses produces totally different effects on the human system, and the benefit accruing therefrom must have another explanation. Now, I believe that this medicine, in such doses as I have mentioned above, will be found a powerful equalizer of nervous action in the body, and therefore a good means of diverting that action, if I may so speak, from concentrating in any particular organ, such as the bronchi in spasmodic asthma. It is with this view, chiefly, that I look for benefit from the administration of strychnia in these cases, but I prefer stating this as a mere suggestion, and leaving it to future experience to confirm it or set it aside.

In conclusion, I shall now recapitulate in brief terms the chief propositions sought to be established in the preceding pages.

1st. That very many cases of bronchial asthma have their origin in laryngeal disease; that some remain for a variable period, as a spasmodic affection of the glottidean muscles, and that in all cases of the disease in question, although the bronchi have long been affected, the chief contraction still occurs in the larynx.

2d. That if this contraction at the glottis be in any way overcome, that of the smaller bronchi either simultaneously or speedily relaxes.

3d. That the usual remedies employed in cases of spasmodic asthma, are either such as are directed against the complications of the disease, and not against its proximate cause, or such as have been found in practice incapable of accomplishing its removal. The latter are therefore useless, and the former unfit to fulfil the indication referred to above.

4th. But this indication may be answered more or less perfectly in different cases, by the application of a solution of caustic of moderate strength (gr. xv., or $\ni$ j. to ζ j) to the glottis, which is the organ chiefly affected.

5th. Cardiac asthma, as it is called, does not usually depend proximately on simple spasmodic contraction of the bronchial tubes, but rather on vesicular emphysema. Cases of this kind are therefore unfit for topical treatment.

6th, and lastly. Electricity passed in gentle currents, as much as possible along the bronchial tubes, may be found to diminish their contractility; and repeated small doses of strychnia may likewise co-operate with the other means of treatment, probably by withdrawing the nervous energy to other parts, at a distance from the affected air-tubes.—*Glasgow Medical Journal.*

THE BOSTON MEDICAL AND SURGICAL JOURNAL.

BOSTON, MAY 25, 1853.

" *The Order of Hippocrates.*"—A singular paper, by Albert W. Ely, M.D., of New Orleans, on the subject of the formation of a secret medical association, is a leading article in the May number of the New Orleans Medical and Surgical Journal. The sum and substance of the communication is, that the regular profession is so poorly protected against the designs of unprincipled practitioners, that a secret society is necessary, into which the very worthiest only of the faculty should be initiated. Signs and passes are to be made use of, so that the members may know each other, whenever they meet. Dr. Ely would have the Society "something like the Masonic order, or the order of Odd Fellows." He thus elaborates his scheme:—"We mean to say, that the great interests of the science of medicine require the establishment of a great medical order, having one great head, to which all others shall be subordinate. We have chosen to give this order a name—that of the *Order of Hippocrates;* but some other might perhaps be better. Our idea of the organization of this great order is as follows: it should consist of divisions, called subordinate colleges, deriving their charters from one *grand college* for the whole United States, holding its sessions quarterly, or semi-annually, in some central point of the union. The form and ceremonies of initiation should be of the most solemn and imposing character, accompanied with oaths or obligations binding the initiated to sustain the interests of the order." He goes on to describe it more fully, till a plan is set forth, than which, as a whole, one more ridiculous was never suggested, or one better calculated for utterly destroying the respectability which belongs to the faculty. An institution organized with the avowed object of keeping medical secrets, and aggrandizing individuals, who of course would be "most noble," "right worshipful," or "puissant" physicians, in the lodge of free and accepted M.D.'s, would be the laughing stock of the nation, and a by-word for street idlers. The creation of a central college, on which fifty-five others would be dependent for their existence, would not be in harmony with our republican doctrines, though all of a piece with the signs, grips and passes of the proposed grand "order." A fundamental principle with all medical institutions of this country, is that which disclaims all unnecessary concealment or mystery. Yet, a member of our profession, in full fellowship, acknowledging the code of ethics interwoven with the constitutional frame work of medical associations every where, actually proposes an organization whose members are bound, to secresy, and among whom would soon grow up, unchecked, abuses more flagrant than any characterizing the various phases of quackery throughout the land. Another consideration may be alluded to. In Massachusetts, extra-judicial oaths are forbidden by law, and are therefore closely looked after by the grand jury. How these affairs are conducted in other States, we do not know. That they are untramelled by legislative action, in that respect, is possible; but that would not prevent the unpopularity of a secret conclave of medical men whose meetings were expressly for the benevolent purpose of raising themselves on the ruin of others! Democratic principles are too thoroughly inculcated in our ranks and throughout the community to tolerate the "Order of Hippocrates;" and we think therefore that Dr. Ely will never live to witness in actual operation his proposed remedy for the evils that threaten the respectability of the ancient and honorable profession of medicine.

Medical Testimony.—Mortifying results have followed, in several courts of law in Massachusetts of late, in regard to the influence of medical testimony. Gentlemen of the best professional attainments have stated facts, as well as given their opinions, on the stand, neither of which have had any more weight with a jury than the prattling of a child. There is an evident disposition to underrate the experience of practitioners, and when it is brought forward, as in the famous arm trial at Lowell, a few weeks since, science, in its highest sense, relating as it did, on that occasion, to the laws of life, is lighter than a feather in the scales of justice. Perhaps this low es imate of medical learning has grown out of an impression that there is no essential difference between the flood of quacks who flourish throughout the land, and the thoroughly trained medical student. Something has weakened the public confidence-in the profession, and no other cause more probable than this can be suggested. It is ridiculous to pretend, as a reason, that physicians are monopolists, or that they have interests to protect, oppressive or injurious to the people. They only ask not to have their acts misrepresented or their motives impugned.

Massachusetts Medical Society.—To-day the anniversary meeting is held in this city. Some of the prominent transactions of the meeting will be noticed hereafter. The counsellors for the year are to be chosen, a discourse delivered, and the fellows will then dine together in Faneuil Hall. To-morrow the new board of counsellors elect the president and other executive officers. Medical strangers in the city will be cordially received. The business affairs of the Society will be attended to at the Hall of the Lowell Institute, instead of Cochituate Hall.

Vision Restorator.—A novel instrument has been patented, and is on sale, for elongating the axis of vision. It consists of a beautifully wrought wooden cup, that fits over the eye, attached to which is a small hollow India rubber ball, communicating by a tube with the cup. By pressing the ball, the air is excluded, and then adjusting the cup, and letting go of the ball, the air in the former is exhausted. The fluids in the chambers consequently expanding, the cornea is made more convex by the outward pressure from within towards the vacuum. Thus the convexity of the eye, in an aged person, for example, is instantly restored to the condition of youth, and objects can be seen without the assistance of convex glasses, and at a convenient distance. Large sums of money have been made within a year or two in producing this same result by manipulating the eyes, the operator compressing them with his fingers, and gradually producing a little increase of convexity. Immediately after, the individual is conscious of being able to read without further artificial assistance, and in the enthusiasm of the moment conceives himself permanently benefited. This, however, is a fallacy, for the vessels, made turgid by friction and the compression of the recti muscles, soon return to their normal condition, and vision is precisely what it was before. The vision restorator accomplishes this temporary distinctness of sight more readily and elegantly than by the means mentioned, and far more economically. Now comes the question, is this instrument useful or injurious? Accompanying it, besides several recommendatory certificates from persons entirely unqualified to give an opinion, are directions for guiding the purchaser. We strongly urge upon our medical friends to be cautious in applying these cups, since there is, in our opinion, more probability of injuring than benefiting those who may seek relief by their means.

Medical Coroner.—At the suggestion of eminent medical gentlemen, Charles H. Stedman, M.D., of Boston, has been appointed a coroner. A more suitable person could not have been found. It is very complimentary to Dr. S. to have been selected, without solicitation, by his professional brethren. Repeated efforts have been made, heretofore, to persuade the Governor of the State to place physicians in that office, as is customary in Europe, but unsuccessfully. No class of citizens can be so thoroughly qualified for researches into the causes of death, as they are, and this is a sufficient reason for giving them the preference. An impression exists that the Attorney General will issue an order requiring that bodies brought before inquests shall be examined, and that Dr. Stedman will hereafter exclusively attend to that essential service in this county. We congratulate both Dr. Stedman and the public on this excellent appointment.

Norfolk District Medical Society.—This Society held its annual meeting at Dedham, on Wednesday, the 18th inst., and elected the following officers :—

Dr. Ebenezer Alden, of Randolph, *President.* Dr. Appleton Howe, of Weymouth, *Vice President.* Dr. Edward Jarvis, of Dorchester, *Secretary.* Dr. Danforth P. Wight, of Dedham, *Treasurer.* Dr. Lemuel Dickerman, of Medfield, *Librarian.* Drs. Erasmus D. Miller, of Dorchester. Theophilus E. Wood, of East Randolph, *Committee of Supervision.* Drs. Ebenezer Stone, of Walpole ; Henry Bartlett, of Roxbury ; Benjamin Mann, of Roxbury ; Simeon Tucker, of Stoughton ; Stephen Salisbury, of Brookline, *Censors.* Drs. Simeon Tucker, of Stoughton ; Henry Bartlett, of Roxbury ; Ebenezer Woodward. of Quincy ; Jonathan Ware, of Milton ; Erasmus D. Miller, of Dorchester ; Benjamin Mann, of Roxbury ; Benjamin E. Cotting, of Roxbury ; Danforth P. Wight, of Dedham ; Edward Jarvis, of Dorchester, *Counsellors.*

The President, Dr. Alden, read a very learned and elaborate discourse, giving the history or notice of all the former and deceased physicians of the county. The Society voted to print this address for the use of the members and for distribution. It will form a very valuable addition to our medical history.

The Society voted to have a general discussion of the prevailing diseases of the autumn at the next semi-annual meeting in November. They have had similar discussions at the previous meetings in the autumn, and these have elicited much that was profitable and satisfactory to the members of the association.

To CORRESPONDENTS —Dr. North's account of the late meeting in New York ; Dr. Stradley on Boring the Cranium ; and a notice of the meeting in Baltimore, of the Superintendents of Lunatic Asylums, have been received.

MARRIED,—J. F. Dyer, M.D., of Annisquam, Mass., to Miss M. T. French.

DIED,—In North Adams, Mass., Dr. Thomas Taylor, 46 —Dr. Wm. Beaumont, a distinguished physician, of St. Louis, who was a surgeon in the army during the war of 1812, died a few days ago.

Deaths in Boston for the week ending Saturday noon, May 21st, 74. Males, 40—females, 34. Accidents, 2—asthma, 1—inflammation of the bowels, 1—disease of the bladder, 1—inflammation of the brain, 2—disease of the brain, 1—consumption, 9—convulsions, 6—croup, 2—dysentery, 1 —dropsy, 1—dropsy in head, 3—drowned, 2—debility, 1—infantile diseases, 7—scarlet fever, 7 —hooping cough, 2—disease of heart, 1—intemperance, 1—inflammation of the lungs, 7—marasmus, 1—measles, 3—old age. 1—palsy, 1—rheumatism, 1—sun stroke, 1—teething, 2—unknown, 2— worms. 2—disease of the bowels, 2.

Under 5 years, 37—between 5 and 20 years, 8—between 20 and 40 years, 11—between 40 and 60 years, 14—over 60 years, 4. Born in the United States, 54 —Ireland, 13—England, 4.—British Provinces, 3. The above includes 10 deaths in the city institutions.

Tetanic Symptoms from the Use of Iodide of Potassium. By D. P. PHILLIPS, M.D., Passed Assistant Surgeon, U. S. N.—A case of some singularity having occurred under my own observation, and thinking that it might not be devoid of interest to you, I have concluded briefly to give its history.

Whilst Acting Surgeon of the U. S. Ship Massachusetts, a fireman, named J. White, was admitted upon my sick list with rheumatism. I ordered the administration of iodide of potassium, grs. viii. ter in die, to be taken before meals in a spoonful of water. Soon after commencing with the remedy (probably the second day) he complained of some uneasiness and stiffness in the jaws; but supposing it to be some trivial affair, I paid but little attention to it. On the next day the difficulty had increased, and I directed frictions with some stimulating liniment; but when I saw him the day after, the jaws were immoveable. Upon careful inquiry, I ascertained that ever since he had been using the iodide he had experienced a burning and uneasy sensation in the œsophagus and stomach. Upon learning this, I discontinued the medicine, and ordered counter-irritation over the stomach. In a few days the tetanic symptoms entirely disappeared, and the iodide of potassium was renewed, but diluted in a tumbler half full of water, and given *after* each meal. The patient entirely recovered from rheumatism, and had no return of the trismus. I attributed the unusual symptoms entirely to the use of iodide of potassium in too concentrated a form.—*Philad. Medical Examiner.*

Medical Students on the Sabbath.—"An exchange paper states that sixty students in the medical department of the University of Louisville, Ky., are to be seen every Sabbath morning in the Sabbath School of the Chesnut street Presbyterian Church, diligently engaged in the study of the Holy Scriptures, under the instruction of Drs. Yandell and Silliman, two of the University Professors.".

To our mind, the above simple announcement speaks volumes in favor of the young gentlemen referred to. We shall fear nothing for the science of medicine when it is in the hands of competent men, of established Christian principles. As a rule, it is not they who are "carried about by every wind" of medical doctrine.—*New Jersey Med. Reporter.*

Buffalo Hospital of the Sisters of Charity.—This hospital has been enlarged by the addition of a wing, which will increase its capacity by nearly one-third. The new wards are now ready for occupancy. Vacant lots in front and rear have been purchased, securing for the institution grounds sufficiently ample for quiet, pure air, and any future additions which may be required. The bounty of the State has enabled the trustees to make these important improvements, placing the institution on a firmer basis, and augmenting its charitable resources.—*Buffalo Med. Journal.*

Aneurism.—Dr. Pravas of Lyons, has been experimenting with a concentrated solution of the per-chloride of iron, by injecting a few drops into isolated portions of the arteries, with the effect of coagulating the blood. He proposes thus to cure aneurisms. He employs a very finely pointed trocar, introduced into the vessel by a sort of rotary motion, and a syringe the piston of which is worked by a screw. His experiments on inferior animals have been successful.—*New York Med. Gaz.*

THE

BOSTON MEDICAL AND SURGICAL JOURNAL.

| Vol. XLVIII. | Wednesday, June 1, 1853. | No. 18. |

THE ANNUAL MEDICAL FESTIVAL OF 1853.

T) the Editor of the Boston Medical and Surgical Journal.

Dear Sir,—Having received, at the last anniversary of the American Medical Association at New York, some friendly reproofs for having of late suspended my contributions to your Journal, I send to your disposal a few discursive thoughts on the character and doings of that body, without the least pretence of rendering a full report of their proceedings.

Having been for years excused from the bustle and attrition of routine practice, and limited mostly to office business, I had considered the meetings of this national high court of medicine to be enjoyed rather through the columns of our medical periodicals and newspapers, than by seeing and hearing. But, on the morning of May 3d, I repaired to the Bleecker Street Church, and, being ineligible to membership, I complied with the suggestion of several friends and took and maintained a position where I could both see and hear. And I must say, my dear editor, those were delightful days! I had no responsibilities nor labors. Hence I could look on. And, such happy reunions! So many dear old friends and acquaintances, men who had extended the most marked courtesy and kindness to myself in my past lonely wanderings in quest of health; and from many quarters, Georgia, Louisiana, St. Louis, Philadelphia, Boston, &c. And there, too, the very men with whom I toiled twenty—thirty years ago, in New England. Aye, and dear, departed Dr. Welch, too, of Hartford, with whom I slept the last night but one of his pilgrimage! I allow you to say that he led us in family prayer only twenty-six hours before his Father called for him.

Here, too, I saw, for the first time, many of the princes of our profession. It was most cheering. Cordial, amicable was their greeting. Many saw their friends mingled among the mass of six or seven hundred, without the power of exchanging salutations. It seemed as if the whole day *should* be devoted to social enjoyments exclusively; but it was one continued scene of hard labor, earnest discussion, pithy, pointed addresses and reports, very free from gas or egotistical inflation, and pointing exclusively to the advancement of medical science.

And there appeared to be great soundness of views on the varied and multiplied topics of the meeting. There was certainly great harmony of opinion and action. I am not going to be so simple as to particularize, where wisdom seemed to abound on every side. But I will say that some of the gentlemen from Maryland and Virginia stirred up an unwonted tide of complacency and satisfaction in my heart. I wanted to say to them, what I *will* say through your types, good doctor, if your sheet should ever chance to meet their eyes, that I was particularly gratified with the treatment which quacks and outsiders received at the hands of these gentlemen and others.

Some thirteen years ago, next November, I was listening to Dr. Meigs's introductory lecture to the many hundred young men who had just assembled in Philadelphia in attendance on the then three medical schools of that city. " Young gentlemen," said he, " make it your care and effort to become *necessary*, by your superior skill and assiduity, and you will not be supplanted." This comprehensive maxim embraces the whole scheme of medical success. If not much mistaken, I saw evidence, during those three days, that our profession are mainly satisfied that all our talk about quacks, interlopers, and *our* rights and privileges, is worse than useless. How instantly does the common citizen set all this *denunciation* down to self-interest. It *did* seem, the other day, as if the medical faculty of this country had decided that the very best way of meeting the "*pathies*" is to qualify our young men and laborers in medicine, by rapidly pushing them into the secrets of successfully combating and removing disease, to " make themselves more necessary " to the community in the hour of pain and peril, than all or any pretenders. And, can't it be done? Let every lecture, every recitation, every clinique, discussion or public movement, be based upon this great and benevolent idea, and the thing is done. Why not? Are not the opposition lines manned mostly from abortions in our regular, medical schools—men who have failed in fair competition? Men, who, in a majority of instances, truckle to some popular whim, and who employ that whim to ride into employment, as men use a balloon? I may be deceived. But it is my immovable conviction that our profession is going right—north and south, east and west; and it was this conviction that made those days, just before that awful sunset, so bright and sunny to me. Why, Sir, for fifteen years, it has seemed to me that the world were delighted in persecuting and mangling our faculty, caressing novices, listening to wild plans of therapeutics, encouraging pretenders, and treating with significant buts—buts—the very men who are bound by public opinion to leave their beds at midnight to administer relief to muttering, thankless beings! And this is not all. The world, nay, editors, have begun to acknowledge that there *is some* merit due our profession for their readiness to risk all among immigrants from smallpox, scarlet fever, &c., from which so many of our numbers have been sacrificed.

But I must close. I want to name many in that assembly. I want to particularize the specimens of eloquence and business sagacity I witnessed. I want to speak of three or four men who toiled like blacksmiths, and on whose efficient arrangements such despatch attended. I will not name my old friend, Dr. Knight, nor his predecessor, Dr. Welford, of Virginia. No! But I *must* name Dr. Condie, of Philadelphia, and Dr. Joseph M. Smith, of New York. There were probably others whose agencies were equally employed in keeping the machinery moving without creaking or entanglement; but the labors of these men seemed to me so important that I *cannot* withhold this feeble tribute of my admiration and applause.

But, farewell the happy days, and delightful, hospitable evenings, and the excursions of this great and splendid medical festival of our nation. I expect never to see another. But, during the brief remainder of my medical journey I shall not cease to be grateful and animated at the prospects of my own profession. I am quite sure our men are making such solid improvements in physic and surgery—such concentrated efforts to become skilful in removing disease and suffering, that their persecutions and wrongs are already on the wane; and the younger men will yet see *their* fraternity *the only* body of respectable practitioners; not doubting, however, that there will evermore be a certain portion of men and women who will prefer to be gulled and peeled and robbed and poisoned by unprincipled quacks and nostrum venders.

Saratoga Springs, May 20th, 1853.   M. L. NORTH.

LECTURES OF M. VALLEIX ON DISPLACEMENTS OF THE UTERUS.

TRANSLATED FROM THE FRENCH BY L. PARKS, JR., M.D.

NUMBER V.

EXAMINATION BY MEANS OF THE SPECULUM.—We do not, as I have already told you, neglect the use of the speculum, as a means of diagnosis in cases of displacement of the uterus. We prefer the full speculum, or a valvular one with three or four valves, which, when open, corresponds to the full speculum. The bivalve speculum, in my opinion, cannot be usefully employed in those cases where it is specially important to know how the cervix uteri is placed relatively to the field of the instrument. These two valves, in fact, describe, in separating, an arc of a circle, the centre of which is near the vulva, and at their point of articulation—the movement which results being sufficient, if the uterus is mobile, to alter its existing direction.

The speculum should be introduced slowly, with precaution, and in the direction of the axis of the vagina. Still less than in the tactile examination should you attempt to fall directly and at once upon the cervix, or to seize it always at will; but, if you do not find it in its habitual situation, you should direct your speculum toward another point. The necessity of executing this manœuvre, which, as I have already told you, had attracted attention without its whole import having been appreciated, is always due to a displacement.

Now, if, in such a case, you seize the neck of the uterus, it is only by having caused the organ to swing over, and it is then no longer possible for you to appreciate its real situation. You may, however, obtain a perfect appreciation of its position by proceeding in the following manner; viz., as soon as your speculum has passed the orifice of the vagina, the obturator must be withdrawn. The walls of the vagina, then, being constantly applied to each other, you will see them unfold

before the extremity of the instrument, forming, as it were, an architectural rose (rosace), the centre of which is necessarily situated in the
axis of the vagina.   This appearance will seem to retreat as the speculum advances, and, if you take good care constantly to maintain the
centre of convergence of the vaginal walls in correspondence with the field
of the instrument, you will, of necessity, keep in the axis of the vagina.
By proceeding thus you will arrive at the cervix, which, in the normal
position of the uterus, will not present itself directly to you ; as you must
recollect that the axis of the uterus is not continuous with that of the
vagina, but forms with this last an obtuse angle open in front.   It follows, then, that the cervix must present itself rather by its anterior than
by its posterior surface, and, in fact, one sees a larger portion of the anterior than of the posterior lip.   As to the external orifice, it is situated
somewhat posteriorly.

Such is the normal presentation of the cervix of the uterus.   When
you do not find it in this position, be sure that there is a displacement.
If, for example, the external orifice shows itself at the very centre of the
portion of the cervix in view, the latter is displaced forward, as is the
fact in certain cases of retroversion.   This displacement will be more
marked still if the orifice approaches near the anterior wall of the
speculum.   .

In this last case, one sees at the outset a great extent of the posterior
surface of the cervix.   But if, on the contrary, you perceive a great
extent of its anterior surface, and if the os externum tends to conceal
itself deeply toward the posterior wall of the instrument, it is probable that you have to deal with an anteversion.   I say it is probable,
because in flexions the cervix no longer follows the axis of the body,
and perceiving only the cervix, you cannot yet decide whether there is
a version or a flexion.   You see, then, that the speculum informs you
of the existence of a displacement—a point of some importance—but that
by itself alone it cannot enable you to distinguish exactly the species.

In the lateral displacements, the external orifice, which normally is
situated in the median line, is inclined toward the side opposite to that
of the displacement, and a greater or less extent of one of the lateral
surfaces of the cervix can be very well seen in the field of the speculum.   While examining the situation of the cervix by means of the
speculum one should not neglect to note its volume and its color ; also,
the state of its opening, together with the existence or absence of the
different alterations which it may present.   As Dr. Bennet advises, the
bivalve speculum is to be employed for the purpose of separating the
lips of the cervix, and of examining its cavity to a certain depth.   But,
as you will apprehend, this can be done only in cases in which the
cervix is large, and sufficiently open either in consequence of inflammation or after numerous labors.

Examination by means of the Sound.—We come, gentlemen, to a
means of exploration of very different importance.   I allude to the
employment of the uterine sound.   In a word, although by the " toucher " and the speculum we can collect many and useful indications, we
may always with the aid of the sound arrive at a precise, rigorous,

and I had almost said mathematically exact diagnosis. Prof. Simpson, who was the first to use the instrument in a methodical manner, employed a metallic rod with a great curvature. This I have already shown you. I have also called your attention to the divisions upon it marked by alternate prominences and depressions which can be felt by the finger.

For some time past, M. Huguier has made use of a sound much less curved, which is divided into centimetres on its concave surface, and has a movable slide governed by means of a rod passing through the handle. This slide is destined to indicate the point to which the sound has penetrated into the uterus. M. Huguier has given to this instrument the name of *hysterometer.* The sound which I use is very similar, although I have not retained the slide, the finger answering to mark the depth to which the instrument has penetrated. M. Charrière has rendered this instrument more portable, and consequently more convenient, by dividing it into two pieces which are screwed to each other. A screw entering the handle upon the side corresponding to the concave surface, serves to maintain the two portions more firmly united, and, at the same time, indicates the side on which the concave surface is, without the necessity of ascertaining it with the finger. If made of a flexible metal, its curvature can be increased or diminished at need, a property which is sometimes of use, when the uterus is in a state of retroflexion. It is owing to his having attended particularly to this species of displacement that Prof. Simpson has thought proper to give so great a curvature to his sound. Experience, nevertheless, has demonstrated to me that this exaggerated curvature is not necessary, and that a straighter sound penetrates quite as well, because, in proportion as it advances, the uterus being raised by it, accommodates itself to the direction given to it, and, so to speak, is unplaited. But, if it was too firmly united to the neighboring parts, or not sufficiently flexible to permit of replacement by this means, the instrument would be arrested at the level of the displacement, and a sound more curved than ours would enter no better, for, however extreme might be the curvature of the instrument, it would never be as great as that of the uterus itself when bent. Thus much having been said to justify our choice of the sound we prefer, let us see how it should be employed. Some make use of the speculum in introducing the sound—a means perhaps serviceable in aiding those not experienced in this little operation to penetrate the external orifice. In this case, the speculum should be withdrawn as soon as it has reached the cavity of the cervix, as, after this, it would impede the different movements which it is necessary for the sound to execute. For this reason, I prefer not to employ the speculum, and content myself with passing along the extremity of the sound upon the index finger of the left hand, previously introduced into the vagina, and having its pulp placed upon the opening of the cervix. Here, at the outset, a primary difficulty may present itself, independently of that which you might experience, if not practised in distinguishing the opening of the cervix in women who have not yet borne children. This opening may happen to be extremely small, and so contracted that the sound cannot be made to enter. Three times I have met with this insurmountable resistance

—once, in the case of a woman who had borne children but who had been frequently cauterized. Here the internal orifice was not contracted like the external os. The two other cases were of women who had not borne children, and in whom the contraction existed also at the internal orifice. In fact for one of them, who is still in our wards, it has been necessary to have a pessary made expressly, with an extremely slender stem, the ordinary stems not being capable of introduction. In such cases it is sufficient, after having introduced the speculum, to make a few scarifications with a bistoury around the opening of the cervix, when penetration is effected with facility. As to the internal orifice, we are sometimes able to pass it only after often-repeated trials.

Once within the cavity of the cervix, the sound should then be passed in the direction of the axis of the brim, provided the uterus be in its normal position ; and though some resistance be encountered from the valvular folds of the mucous membrane, we must not endeavor to clear them by pushing roughly and with force, but, on the contrary, proceed gently, giving a slight motion to the sound which will enable it to pass these obstacles and to arrive at the os internum. Then, at first, quite a considerable degree of resistance may present itself in consequence of the contraction of which I have just spoken to you. After passing this point, a peculiar sensation—more or less intense, according to the idiosyncrasy of the patient, is always aroused, so that if the sound is small, and the os internum sufficiently large, the instrument may pass from the cavity of the cervix into that of the body without your experiencing the feeling of resistance which informs you of the moment when this passage takes place. You will always, however, be warned of the moment of passing the internal os by the sensibility of that sphincter, since the cervix being in all cases nearly insensible, and its internal orifice being endowed with very great sensibility, there is produced, even in those who suffer least from the introduction of the sound, a disagreeable sensation which the patient will ordinarily mention, and the knowledge of which will never escape you, provided you give sufficient attention to the matter. In some patients there is quite severe pain with slight griping sensations, similar to those produced by contractions of the uterus, since the woman complains of suffering as from the slight pains which announce the approach of labor. Once in the cavity of the body, the sensibility ceases, to re-appear the moment the sound touches the fundus of the uterus, and gives rise to that peculiar pain which, according to the expression of the patients, " goes to their hearts." It is easy also to assure ourselves that the walls of the cavity of the body are everywhere sensible by touching them with the end of the sound ; and, if, after having cleared the internal orifice, this sensibility appears to cease, it is because the sound glides gently between these walls. When the sound penetrates more easily into the body of the uterus, it is felt to be more free and to be moved about more easily.

If you should experience a more considerable resistance from the walls themselves of the uterus, before arriving at the fundus of the organ, it is because there is a displacement, and then, in place of pushing on in the normal direction, you should incline the end of the sound in the direction toward which a tactile examination may lead you to suppose that this displacement exists. If there was a retroflexion, for example, the concavity should be directed backward instead of forward, and the sound should be made to describe a circle passing through the handle, and having its centre in the ' extremity, which, consequently, would revolve upon itself alone. If the handle were made to rotate upon itself, the. extremity would have to describe a large arc of a circle —a movement which could not be effected without pain, nor without injury, as the walls of the uterus would be in consequence necessarily contused.

The sound having thus taken the direction of the canal into which it is to penetrate, the uterus becomes righted as the instrument is introduced, in such a manner that the retroflexion, which I have taken for an example, is transformed into a retroversion, on the arrival of the sound at the fundus.

The sound once introduced, the displaced organ should be brought into its normal position. In order to do this, we should always act with gentleness, giving to the sound a movement the reverse of that by which it is introduced. In order to judge approximatively as to whether the sound has reached the fundus of the uterus, I have placed at the distance of six and a quarter centimetres (a length which represents the normal depth of this organ) from the extremity of the instrument, a depression which can be felt by the finger, without the necessity of withdrawing it. So long as the sound has not penetrated to this point, there is reason to think, if an obstacle presents itself, that it is not the fundus of the uterus, and, accordingly, we may endeavor to overcome it, whilst if the point in question has been passed, it is not prudent to attempt any further progress.

I ascertain the depth of the uterus, by retaining, while I withdraw the sound, the index finger of the left hand upon the point which corresponds to the external orifice, and thus supply the place of the slide of M. Huguier. It is important, indeed, to know the exact depth of the uterus, if it is wished to apply the intra-uterine pessary, in order to make the stem of a length a little less than this depth.

As to the length of the cervix, this may be recognized by noting the peculiar sensation which patients experience, and the resistance which exists at the internal orifice. We have only to withdraw the instrument when it reaches this point.

I must repeat an injunction which I have already given you, but which is important in practice, never to persist in efforts to introduce the sound, if you meet with too great resistance. It is better to desist, and then to renew your attempts, two, three, or even four times, than to seek to penetrate by main force; for you may, by taking the latter course, cause injury, or at least pain sufficiently severe to disgust patients at the outset with a mode of treatment which must necessarily be quite protracted.

I would secure your attention further to the importance of *combining the tactile examination* of the uterus, *with the exploration by means of the sound.* The finger introduced into the vagina to guide the instrument, explores the cervix, estimates the thickness of its walls, recognizes certain sinuosities in its course, which would otherwise remain unknown (the sound meanwhile retaining the organ fixed), and judges as to whether any tumors exist in the neighborhood, and especially whether or not these remain stationary, when the uterus is moved. Prof. Simpson thinks, that in cases of retroflexion, we should endeavor to feel the end of the sound at the moment when it reaches the tumor formed by the uterus behind the cervix. For my part, I have never been able to feel it, even when employing sounds curved as much as those of Prof. Simpson, the inability to do so being explained by the righting of the uterus by the sound itself, in the manner I have explained to you. In these cases, in fact, the uterus is no longer felt in the same place, the introduction of the sound having had the effect to raise it, even before we have given to the instrument the movement intended to bring the organ into its normal situation.

The movements given to the uterus by means of the sound, will permit you to appreciate the rigidity or the suppleness of the surrounding tissues, and any adhesions the organ may have contracted with them. As soon as you have brought the body of the womb into its normal position, relatively to the cervix, you will proceed slowly, and without violence, as by attempting to replace it roughly, you would expose yourself to the danger of causing ruptures or strains which would be followed by formidable inflammations.

While withdrawing the sound, it is well to push back the cervix with the finger, in order to maintain it, as long as possible, in the direction which has been given to it.

Now, gentlemen, the different means of exploration of which we are in the habit of making use being known, we proceed to consider the information to be obtained by them in each particular species of displacement. This we shall do, while giving the description of each by itself—a task which we shall undertake at once, commencing with anteversion.

BORING THE CRANIUM.

To the Editor of the Boston Medical and Surgical Journal.

Sir,—In support of the conclusions arrived at, from experiments upon the "gallinaceous tribe," by your correspondent, Dr. H. A. Ramsay, with reference to the operation of trephining in apoplexy and inflammation of the brain, I offer the following remarks upon the subject, from an ancient and forgotten work. After bringing forward, in long and formidable array, the remedies of the time—as issues, ligatures, frictions, suppositories, and scarifications—the author continues, " 'Tis not amiss to bore the skull and let out the fuliginous vapours, because this humour hardly yields to other physic, and the head bored in two or three places avails much to the exhalation of the vapours. I saw a man with brain disease at Rome, that by no remedies could be healed, but when by chance he was wounded in the head and his skull broken, he was excellently cured. Another, breaking his head with a fall from on high, was instantly recovered of his disease."

The matter is at least worthy of the serious consideration of the brotherhood, which I trust it will receive. Yours, J. STRADLEY.

Frederica, Del., May, 1853.

OBITUARY OF DR. A. WELCH.

[Communicated for the Boston Medical and Surgical Journal.]

AMONG the many physicians whose lives were so suddenly terminated by the distressing railway disaster at Norwalk, Conn., the death of none can be more deeply lamented than that of the late Dr. Archibald Welch, of Hartford. Dr. W. was son of the Rev. Móses C. Welch, one of the most distinguished divines in New England, and was born in Mansfield, Conn. He practised medicine for many years in his native town, then removed to Wethersfield, and afterwards to Hartford. He was elected a member of the State Legislature in the two former towns, was for many years President of the State Medical Society, was one of the Medical Examiners at Yale College, and held many other important offices of trust. As a friend, he was constant and sincere, noble in his aims, clear in his views, and held a high rank in his profession. He was greatly endeared to his patients by his kind and tender sympathies —and a large circle of warm friends now greatly mourn his departure from earth. When we consider his noble qualities, we feel that his place cannot be easily filled. But now his usefulness, his toils and hardships, are ended. No more can he stand around the beds of the sick and administer to their many wants. No more can he soothe or cheer the dying sufferer, or comfort the afflicted ; for in that world where we trust he has entered, there are no sorrows to assuage, no sufferings to alleviate.

Mansfield, Ct., May, 1853. W. H. RICHARDSON.

DR. MILLER ON THE REMOVAL OF THE DENTAL PULP.

[Concluded from page 337.]

THIS being the current physiological doctrine of the day, it will be seen that the vitality of the teeth is sustained, and their connection with the general system preserved, by means of nerves and bloodvessels which enter their bony substance through the agency of both their inner and outer membranes ; and when, from any cause, the inner membrane is destroyed, their vitality and functions are dependent on the nervous and vascular communications kept up through the medium of the periosteum *alone.* Suppose the case reversed, and the tooth correspondingly denuded of its periosteum, how firm and how long would it be retained in its socket ? It would become an isolated organ—a foreign body at once, having no sympathy or connection with the general system. It is evident, then, that a tooth is *more* dependent for its connection with the animal economy on its *periosteum*, than on the highly nervous and vascular membrane which lines its internal cavity.

In support of this theory, is the long-established practice, well known to the profession and the public, of *mechanically* destroying the nerve previous to setting a tooth upon the root, and of *chemically* destroying it prior to filling teeth. Although failures have been frequent, yet a sufficient degree of success has attended cases of this sort to warrant a continuance of the practice by the dental profession generally, to a considerable extent.* The same principle is applicable to any other branch of medicine, and to diseases in general. In selecting the following cases for illustration, it is proper to state that they were more successful than the average—that the success of an operation, however well executed, is greatly owing to the general health and habits of the patient—in these cases more so than to the skill of the operator.

Nearly two years ago I removed the roots of the superior incisor and canine teeth, with a view to a full denture, upon each of which I had engrafted an artificial crown about fourteen years previous. Each root sustained its respective crown during the *whole* of that time, and was tolerably firm in the jaw at the time of extraction, although nearly *all* of the other teeth in *both* jaws had been removed by absorption. Two, out of the six, remained during the whole period without being re-set. In February last, a case came under my observation, in which one of the older dentists of Boston inserted an artificial crown, made from a human tooth, more than nineteen years ago. The crown was considerably decayed, but the root was in a condition to last several years longer, being nearly or quite sound. . It was supplied with another (mineral) crown. Now, if the destruction of the dental pulp causes an *immediate* loss of life, by what means, in the cases referred to, were the teeth retained in a healthy condition so long after the operation, except through the medium of their investing membrane?

March 2, 1839, I removed the superior left second molar tooth for S—— E——, aged 26 years. After the removal, the enamel not being marred, I remarked that it seemed too good to be lost, which induced him to ask if it could not be filled and re-placed. I replied it could, and mentioned the experiments of John Hunter, in transplanting teeth; saying, at the same time, it was not good practice. At his request, I filled the tooth (with tin foil) on its posterior approximal surface, taking care to cover the roots with a silk handkerchief to prevent contact with perspiration from the fingers, and returned it to its socket. In two or three months after the operation, the soreness passed off. On the 14th ult. (April, 1853) I had occasion to fill the same tooth in another place. It was firm in the jaw, and the parts about it in a healthy state, having remained so without interruption. The filling is still good. This patient's teeth have been examined frequently, during the interim, and operated on somewhat extensively, thus affording ample opportunities for critical observations.

* The loss of teeth from the use of chemical agents has been greatly diminished by Dr Flagg, of Boston, who in 1847 published an article on a course of practice which he had been pursuing for two years previous, differing from the one *now* exciting attention, in *principle* mainly—the modus operandi being similar.

A few years after, I tried a similar experiment on one of my own teeth—an inferior incisor—which became firm, shortly after the operation, and proved a useful member several years. Having a constitutional tendency to absorption of the gum and alveoli, it eventually loosened, in common with others *not* affected by caries, was extracted a second time, and required as much force to remove it as the other teeth.

These experiments are not referred to for the purpose of recommending them, but to illustrate the theory under consideration.

There is one *other* physiological fact in confirmation of this doctrine. The dental nerves of elderly people frequently become absorbed, and their canals filled with a bony deposit. The same thing occurs in the teeth of middle-aged persons, in which the action of the absorbents and exhalants is increased by irritation produced by the close proximity of the nerves to the abraded surfaces—also in the teeth of cattle. Now, in cases of this sort, where there has been no surgical operation whatever—no destruction of the central ganglion, either by mechanical means, chemical agents or ulceration, but by *absorption,* and the teeth remain firm and healthy years afterwards—do they *immediately* lose their vitality, and nature soon make effort to remove them? As the dental nerves diminish in size, as age advances, there is good reason to believe that they are *entirely* absorbed oftener than we are aware of. Is a theory in medicine or surgery to be discarded because the practice founded upon it may not always be successful? If so, what theory would not fall under condemnation? What treatment, for whatever disease, has not sometimes failed? The *causes* of failure are oftener owing to circumstances not under the control of the physician or surgeon, than theory.

Enough has been said to show that the removal of the dental pulp is not based on a new or impracticable theory ; the method of doing it is all that is novel. Nor is it a new discovery that a tooth, from which it has been removed, is not sensible to impressions from heat and cold. Although I do not recommend for general practice, to sever the nerve, and remove the pulp, or to amputate and allow it to remain, for reasons previously given, yet the practicability of these operations has been established by successful experiments on the single and bicuspid teeth, and, I should have no doubt of an equally good effect on the molar teeth, but for their being more difficult of access and having a greater number of roots, with corresponding nerves, which always embarrass, more or less, any means of cure for this class of teeth. Amputation of the fore-arm and shoulder are both practicable, yet one is vastly more complicated and hazardous than the other. And so it may be said of many other operations, that are not abandoned because of an occasional failure.

From the tenor of Dr. Frisselle's article, he appears to be under a wrong impression, in that he makes no distinction between my early experiments and the operation to which they were the stepping stone. They were successful beyond expectation ; but, for general use, gave way to improvements. Those experiments eventuated in *rhizodontrypo-neurhæmaxis*—the operation of drilling the root of a tooth, either *through* the

gum or *under* its margin, to the nerve, " wounding it as little as possible,"*
so as not to impair its vitality or function, but to open its vessels and relieve
them from the increased pressure of blood consequent upon irritation excited by operating on the diseased organ. " Ubi irritatio ibi fluxus." This
operation, with few exceptions, I had practised more than two years before the subject was introduced to the profession through the pages
of this Journal. Owing to the smallness of the nerve, occasionally, it
is nearly impossible to puncture, without cutting it off; therefore great
caution should be used.

In reply to the doctor's criticism on the anatomy of the teeth, I have
to say, the " exceptions," which he admits, were what I wished to provide for in commencing a new series of experiments. I have a large
number of bicuspids with two nerves, and several with three—two recently extracted from the under jaw. The nerves of the bicuspid
teeth are somewhat flattened, usually more so in the superior than inferior ; and in those that *have* two nerves, the bifurcations commence at
different distances from their necks. Knowing such to be the fact, and
not feeling certain as to results, in my third and fourth operations, which
were on the bicuspids, the drill was introduced further from the margin of the gum than when operating on the single teeth, in order to accomplish what I *then* considered necessary, viz., amputation of the nerve.
The reasons, both physiologic and pathologic, which induced me to
consider the subject, were occasional failures in the employment of
other modes of practice, in common use, as stated in a former number.
Nor did I expect *entire* success in this. The *theory* was founded on
well-known principles in surgery. When the edges of a wound are
placed in apposition and properly dressed, inflammation follows, causing
an effusion of fibrin which forms the bond of union. Within a few
days after the parts become united, the new structure is organized with
bloodvessels, nerves and absorbents, which restore the circulation and
nervous communication. In *tenotomy*, for club foot, &c. after the tendon is cut, the parts are separated and retained in position until new tendinous matter is deposited sufficient to re-establish the communication.
The *farrier* is familiar with this fact, and adapts his treatment to the
end to be accomplished. Relying on the recuperative power of the
animal economy, it occurred that the principle was applicable as well
to nerves as tendons, and that a dental nerve might be divided and re-
unite, and the nervous and vascular communications be re-established
as in other wounds. Knowing that punctured wounds are considered
among the more dangerous, being liable to produce tetanus, I did not
venture to ´puncture the nerve, merely, until it occurred that amputation could not be applied to the molar teeth having three or more roots,
and as many nerves, and that the dental nerves had not only been
punctured through the carious cavity, often, but crushed for the purpose
of setting teeth, without serious consequences; also that they are not
nerves of motion, but of sensation, being derived from the sensitive portion of the fifth pair ; therefore, a puncture might not be attended with

---

* From the original manuscript containing a description of the operation, dated Oct. 12th, 1850.

the same consequences as in a motor nerve.* 1 am ·not aware that tetanus has ever occurred from wounds inflicted on the dental nerves, although they have been subjected to severe treatment, oftener, perhaps, than any other class. Whether, if it has not,' it be owing to their being sensitive instead of motor nerves, is mere. conjecture. These speculations induced me to try the puncture, which I found a safe substitute for amputation. They are not mentioned, however, as having foundation in philosophy, but as being incidental upon entering a new field of investigation. S. P. MILLER.

Worcester, Mass., May 12th, 1853.

RAIL-ROAD MURDERS.

[Communicated for the Boston Medical and Surgical Journal.]

THE late most shocking disaster at Norwalk, has excited in the public mind a degree of indignation that is somewhat proportionate to the criminality that should attach to those who were the immediate agents in producing it. For several years, accidents, or rather, acts ⌐of this kind, have been becoming more and more frequent ; the public have felt keenly, have sympathized sincerely, and have given strong expressions of the deep indignation entertained against those who were the cause— but, after all, no change for the better has been brought about. At this juncture, is it enough for us to say, " something must be done," and then let the subject go to a speedy oblivion ? Have we no more sense of the value of human life than to say, by such a course, we do not regard it as a sacred thing ? If an individual is found guilty of a *single* murder, he is pursued by the community till a full expiation of his crime to the law of the land is obtained. But if a wretch, in the employ of a great and rich corporation, through the improper use of intoxicating liquor, a stupid indifference, or spirit of recklessness which characterizes too many of our rail-road employees, consigns to the grave scores of the most valuable lives in the community, *he may be turned out of employment,* receive a few epithets from the newspaper vocabulary, which have about as much effect upon him as the pattering of so many drops of rain on the back of a *goose,* and then be re-instated in business. It is clear that more stringent laws are called for in relation to the management of rail roads, as well as for the speedy punishment of those persons who are culpably negligent in carrying out the regulations which are, and may be, established by rail-road corporations. These things being so, it is necessary for somebody to move in the business ; and who can more appropriately make the move, than the medical profession ? As conservators of the physical well-being of the public, it seems fit that they should lead off in a work, the accomplishment of which is so loudly called for, by the frequent and awful accounts of the destruction of human life and health which are brought to our notice. And, above all inducements for action on the part of our profession in

* The fifth is the only pair of encephalic nerves having two roots ; it is, therefore, a nerve both of sensation and motion, on which account Sir Charles Bell classed it with the spinal nerves.

relation to this subject, is the one arising from the fact that some ten of its most valuable members have been sacrificed by the late disaster at Norwalk.

It appears to me that the " sons of thunder," as well as the " sons of consolation," in the medical ranks, should pour a " living stream of elo-quence, argument and fact " into the public ear, and also through the me-dium of the press, that powerful engine in its sphere, clearly present some of the more startling truths and fearful facts which have become *fixed* in regard to this subject, till a rational public sentiment is established, and the servants of the people, whose duty it is to make laws for the good of the community, shall be forced to an action more consonant with the acknowledged principles of humanity. When railroading was in its in-fancy in this country, managers were restrained by the general appre-hension and fear that existed in the public mind in regard to them. But long familiarity with them has blunted the sense of danger with which they are always attended. We are hurried on, from one fearful disaster to another, without being benefited by the awful lessons which they should teach us. It is undoubtedly true, that instead of being more cautious, managers are more careless by experience. Instead of a diminution of the loss of life, it is fearfully on the increase. In the State of New York alone, the annual deaths by rail roads amount to more than three hundred.

But I did not intend, when I commenced this communication, to do much more than express the opinion that physicians should take hold of this subject and pursue it till the object is accomplished, hoping that some of your *able* correspondents will show it up in the light of all the facts that exist in relation to it.   Medicus.

E. Livermore, Me., May 23d, 1853.

MEMOIR OF THE LATE DR. SAVARY.

(Communicated for the Boston Medical and Surgical Journal.

Phineas Savary, the subject of this brief memoir, was born at Ware-ham, Mass., A.D. 1800. After being graduated at Brown University, and pursuing the usual studies, he took the degree of Doctor of Medi-cine, and commenced practising as a physician in Attleborough, twenty-six years ago. Dr. Savary's sound professional acquirements, suavity of manner, and real kindness of heart, soon gained for him an extensive circle of practice and a warmth of friendship which remained unimpaired to the time of his death. A long continuance in the same community, extending over more than a quarter of a century ; his self-denying faith-fulness in the discharge of every duty ; and his high moral worth, gave him a place in the general estimation, which few men ever attain. To be in need was a sufficient claim upon his services, irrespective of con-dition ; and his attendance upon the sick was uninfluenced by motives of personal interest or emolument. Prodigal in the expenditure of time and ease for the benefit of his patients, no effort was too much, and no sacri-fice of personal convenience too great, to enable him to minister to their wants or relieve distress.   Benevolence was ever a prominent trait. Multitudes can bear witness to the consolation of his presence.   A cheerful temperament enabled him to inspire hope and encouragement, and induce that frame of mind most favorable for the restoration of health.

Dr. Savary had never taken a part in the discussion of the prominent topics of the day, nor in the field of politics.   Yet his intellectual capacity, and practical good sense, united with a bearing dignified and conciliatory, eminently fitted him for the active duties of public life. The especial sphere of his labor was clinical practice.   In the sick-room he was unrivalled.   His fine tact and sympathy admirably fitted him for the duties of the obstetrician, in which department his services and skill were widely sought and appreciated.

As a citizen, no man was more esteemed.   The cause of education and the interest of the common schools were objects of his sedulous care.   He maintained his character as a student, and kept himself informed of the modern advances in medical science.   The Latin classics were his delight, and with them he preserved a constant familiarity.

He was emphatically a man who exemplified the religion which he professed.   Prompt and conscientious in the performance of every duty, his influence was ever on the side of virtue and charity.   His moral character colored his whole life and intercourse.   No temporizing policy of self-interest ever tempted him to resort to questionable expedients. His unvarying rectitude never subjected him to distrust, and no one ever doubted the integrity of his opinion.   He was a shining illustration of the language of Lamartine—" Un médecin doit être bon ; c'est plus de la moitié de son genie."   And again, the words of the same writer are appropriate—" La science de médecine n'a que des axioms ; son cœur a des divinations.   La volonté de soulager est par elle-meme un puissance qui soulage."   It may be said of him he had not an enemy ; and no man in private life has left a larger circle of sincere mourners.   The memory of the " beloved physician " will long be preserved.

Dr. Savary died on the 19th inst. from apoplexy.   Many months since be suffered a light attack, attended by slight muscular paralysis. This was apparently recovered from, and at the expiration of a few weeks his ordinary business was resumed.   Ten days before his death there was a recurrence of the apoplectic symptoms, accompanied by complete hemiplegia.   He had retired for the night in usual health, after spending a cheerful evening at home ; and within an hour or two fell into the apoplectic condition from which he never recovered.   The loss of power on the left side was sudden and complete, consciousness was impaired, and speech difficult and incoherent.   The power of deglutition likewise suffered ; respiration was stertorous and involuntary.   Complete anæsthesia prevailed over one half the body.

Under one order of classification, cases commencing in this manner are termed paralytic, rather than apoplectic.   Yet as serous effusion or cerebral hemorrhage is always found, and more commonly sanguineous extravasation prevails, there seems to be no inaccuracy in including the affection under the generic name of apoplexy.   The facial muscles of the left side, to which the ramuli of the portio dura of the 7th pair of nerves are distributed, lost their tonicity and became relaxed, thereby permitting the symmetrical muscles of the other side to draw the centre of the face across the median line. The condition of the temporal and masseter muscles was not observed, but the entire anæsthesia of the left side of the face, renders it probable that as the lesion was within the cranium and farther back than the origin of the 5th pair, the muscles to which the anterior root of the 5th is distributed, partook of the loss of function.

Breathing became more and more difficult, and the lungs were clogged with mucus. The countenance was turgid and discolored by the imperfectly arterialized blood. During the last days there was excessive vascular action, and death resulted finally from the combined effects of coma and asthenia.

The involuntary muscles which appertain to the function of organic life, and never acknowledge the direction of the will, are not necessarily dependent upon any influence derived from the nervous centres ; and though they might continue to act if a due supply of arterial blood were kept up, even in the absence of a brain, still experiment has shown that the readiest way to affect the heart and other involuntary muscles through the nervous system, is to act upon a large portion of that system at once. The marked affection of the involuntary muscles in this case seems to imply that the cerebral lesion was extensive and severe. The intensity of the other symptoms likewise indicates the probability of a considerable cranial hemorrhage and laceration of the structure of the brain.

Treatment *secundum artem* was adopted, under the direction of experienced advisers. " *Nil prosunt artes ; erat immedicabile vulnus.*"

Paracentesis capitis has lately been proposed as an *ultimum remedium* in apoplexy. Autopsies have revealed, that there is almost always a communication formed between the original cavity and the ventricles, or with the surface of the brain. When the effused blood lies beneath the membranes, the trephine may give it issue ; or even if the clot is in or near the corpora striata or optic thalami, where it not infrequently is found, removal of a portion of the cranial parietes may abate the pressure from within and afford a chance for restoration.   E. S.

Attleborough, May 24th, 1853.

THE BOSTON MEDICAL AND SURGICAL JOURNAL.

BOSTON, JUNE 1, 1853.

Massachusetts Medical Society Anniversary.—On Wednesday last there was a grand gathering of the members of the Society, in the forenoon at the Lowell Institute Hall, and in the afternoon at Faneuil Hall. At the meeting in the forenoon, the subject of homœopathy was referred to the Council, to report next year. It may be considered, therefore, as consigned to the tomb of the Capulets. Dr. Jackson's discourse on Morbid Anatomy, was a good one, and was listened to with much attention. The dinner at Faneuil Hall passed off with much satisfaction. The Chairman exhibited a happy tact at drawing out speakers, and some excellent sentiments were offered. A general expression of satisfaction was observed in regard to the speech of the Rev. Dr. Blagden. Dr. Hayward, who the day before was re-elected President, made some able and appropriate observations, which will soon appear in the Journal. On Thursday there was an adjourned session. But little business was transacted, however, besides voting the publication of a catalogue of the fellows, to accompany the transactions of the Society, soon to appear. In 1854, the anniversary meeting is to be held at Fitchburg—an enterprising, beautiful town, about forty miles from Boston, and which probably is to be the next city chartered in Massachusetts.

Association of Medical Superintendents of Hospitals and other Establishments for the Insane.—This Society held its annual meeting in Baltimore, on Tuesday, the 10th ult., and continued its sessions through the three succeeding days. It was a large meeting. There were twenty members present, having the care of nineteen Lunatic Hospitals, and one in similar private practice, in eleven different States. They were—Dr. Luther V. Bell (President), Somerville; Dr. Clement A. Walker, Boston; and Dr. Edward Jarvis, Dorchester, Massachusetts. Dr. John W. Tyler, Concord, N. H. Dr. Isaac Ray, Providence, R. I. Dr. N. D. Benedict, Utica; Dr. D. T. Brown, Bloomingdale; and Dr. Francis Bulloch, Flushing, New York. Dr. Horace A. Buttolph, Trenton, N. J. Dr. Stewart, and Dr. Thomas S. Kirkbride, of Philadelphia; Dr. Joshua Worthington, Frankford; and Dr. John Curwen, Harrisburgh, Pa. Dr. John Fonerden, and Dr. William Stokes, Baltimore, Md. Dr. Charles Nichols, Washington, D. C. Dr. Francis Stribling, Staunton, Va. Dr. Elijah Kendrick, Columbus, Ohio. Dr. Richard J. Patterson, Indianapolis, Ia. Dr. Turner R. H. Smith, Fulton, Mo.

This is truly a working Association. Their meetings have been held for several years in various parts of the country, and always well attended. The members prepare dissertations upon subjects previously designated by the president, or selected by themselves. These are read at the meetings, and followed by full and free discussions upon their several subjects in all their bearings.

At the last meeting, Dr. Kirkbride read a paper on the employment and duties of night watchers, and the best management of hospitals, for their security, during the hours of sleeping. Dr. K. read another paper upon the appointment of trustees, superintendents, and all other officers and assistants in hospitals, and their mutual relations and several duties. This article has a general as well as a special interest, and should, and probably will, be so published, that the world may see it. Its great object was to so arrange the government in all its branches, from the highest to the lowest, that each should perform its duty for the best good of the patients, and each should discharge its responsibility without conflicting with others. Dr. Bell read a very able article upon the position, duties and responsibilities of medical witnesses, in regard to cases of lunacy, real or supposed, which are brought before the courts of law. Dr. Stokes read a paper upon the propriety of establishing boards of experts in lunacy, who should examine into, and testify concerning, doubtful cases, subject to the adjudication of courts. A paper was presented from Dr. John M. Galt, of Williamsburgh (Virginia), Eastern Asylum, on the social relation of the patients in hospitals in regard to their friends and the world. Dr. Ray read a dissertation describing some anomalous forms of mental disease. Dr. Jarvis read a paper on the effect of excessive and perverse or wrong uses of the brain in producing insanity. He showed the connection of the mind with its physical organ in health and in disease, and then the analogy of the effects of over action, wrong action, or the misapplication of the powers of the brain upon the mind, with the effect of excessive or perverted use of the stomach upon digestion. In both, the functions are disturbed or impaired; and in the one case dyspepsia, and in the other insanity or imbecility, is the result.

Several other papers were read, all of great value and interest to those who are especially engaged in the care of the insane, and all were discussed with careful attention to their merits and their bearings. Most of these will probably be printed in the Journal of Insanity.

While the Association was at Baltimore, they received much hospitality from the citizens of the town who are engaged in the management of the Lunatic Hospitals. They visited and minutely examined the Maryland Hospital, the St. Vincent's Asylum, and the site for the new hospital which is to be built about five miles out of the city. They also went to Washington, and visited the site selected for the new national hospital for the army and navy and the District of Columbia.—After a very laborious and agreeable session of four days, and a happy visit at the South, they adjourned on Friday, to meet next year at Washington. It is to be hoped, that, at the next meeting, more of our Southern brethren will be present.

Besides the nineteen physicians present at the last meeting, there are others who are engaged in the same pursuits, and who are considered as members of the association; viz., Dr. John M. Galt, of the Eastern Asylum, Williamsburgh, Va.; Dr. James Parker, Columbia, S. C.; Dr. Thomas F. Green, Milledgeville, Geo.; Dr. Preston Pond, Jackson, La.; Dr. Boyd M'Nairy, Nashville, Tenn.; Dr. John R. Allen, Lexington, Ky.; Dr. James Higgins, Jacksonville, Ill.; Dr. M. H. Ranney, New York, N. Y.; Dr. John S. Butler, Hartford, Ct.; Dr. George Chandler, Worcester, Mass.; Dr. Wm. H. Rockwell, Brattleboro', Vt.; Dr. Henry M. Harlow, Augusta, Me. All of these have charge of public hospitals. Dr. Edward Mead, of Cincinnati, O.; Dr. Nehemiah Cutter, of Pepperell, Mass.; Dr. H. T. Buel, Flushing, N. Y.; have the care of private asylums. Drs. Fremont and Mauran have the charge of Beaufort Asylum, near Quebec, Canada; and Dr. Douglas of the Provincial Asylum, St. John, N. B. All of these establishments, except that of Louisiana, have been represented at some of the meetings of the Association, which may be said thus to include all those engaged in the care of the insane in the United States.

American Medical Association.—Our thanks are due to the Editor of the New Yrok Medical Times for a full report of the proceedings of the Association at the late meeting in New York. It makes a pamphlet of 18 pages, and appears to have been prepared with much care. We shall copy from it a list of the chairmen of the various Special Committees, as soon as we can find space. We also notice a full report in the New Jersey Medical Reporter, comprising about twenty pages of the last number of that monthly journal.

Anatomical Depot.—Not unfrequently the inquiry is made, where skeletons and anatomical preparations can be purchased. Dr. Codman, in Tremont Row, Boston, has commenced importing disarticulated crania, skeletons, and some of almost everything a medical student or minute demonstrator might require. This will be a great convenience to the profession generally. In addition to these articles, instruments without number, of the most approved patterns, from celebrated manufacturers, are on sale, and will prove a convenience to medical strangers. Dr. Codman was educated a physician, and therefore understands precisely the proper shape and quality of surgical cutlery, dental apparatus, &c.

Action of Medicines.—A diversity of opinion exists in regard to the manner in which the system is acted upon by medicines introduced into the stomach. Nothing short of positive demonstration, therefore, is entitled to much consideration. There seems to be no end to theoretical suggestions on this point, but something certain is wanted, and when a fact has been positively established, it should be made known as a guide in future efforts at medication. The London Medical Society awarded the Fothergillian prize, in 1852, to Frederick William Headland, B.A., for an able work on this subject, which bears the title of " The Action of Medicines in the System." It has been re-printed in this country, and is fresh from the press of Messrs. Lindsay & Blakiston, Philadelphia, comprising 56 pages octavo, is well printed, and reasonable in price. The chapters in the book relate to the more important classifications of medicines ; the general modes of their action ; and some of the more important medicines in particular. A succession of propositions are ably discussed, illustrated by reference to various sources of information of the highest scientific worth.

Medical Miscellany.—Dr. Marshall Hall, in his tour westward, spent a week in Cincinnati. The Western Lancet thinks he is inclined to make the United States his future home.—Drs. Warren of Boston, and Mott of New York, have been elected members of the French Academy of Medicine.—Dr. Wm. B. Rogers has resigned the chair of Natural Philosophy, and Dr. Lawrence Smith that of Materia Mdica and Chemistry, in the University of Virginia.—M. Dubois has been appointed accoucheur to the Empress of the French.

To Correspondents.—Papers on the Treatment of Hemorrhage after Extraction of a Tooth, and on the Treatment of Scarlet and Typhoid Fevers, have been received.

Married,—At Quebec, Dr. Wm. A. Sassamille to Miss Kate Boxer.

Died,—At Brooklyn, N. Y , Charles D. Rossiter, M.D , 27 —In Albany, N. Y , Lewis C. Beck. M.D.— At Dubuque, Iowa, Dr. George W. Richards —At Lempster, N. H., Dr. Truman Abell, 74; for many years author of the New England Farmer's Almanac, and the writer of various articles in former volumes of this Journal.

Deaths in Boston for the week ending Saturday noon, May 28th, 79. Males, 38—females, 41. Accidental, 1—apoplexy, 1—disease of the bowels, 1—inflammation of the brain, 2—consumption, 17—croup, 2—dysentery, 2—dropsy, 1—dropsy in head, 4—infantile, 4—puerperal, 1—erysipelas, 1—fever, 3—typhus fever, 1—typhoid fever, 3—scarlet fever, 4—gravel, 1—hooping cough, 2—disease of heart, 3—intemperance, 1—laryngitis, 1—inflammation of the lungs, 7—marasmus, 3 —measles, 3—old age, 3—palsy, 1—pleurisy, 2—scrofula, 2—teething, 2—thrush, 1.
  Under 5 years, 34—between 5 and 20 years, 8—between 20 and 40 years, 20—between 40 and 60 years, 7—over 60 years, 10. Born in the United States, 53 —Ireland, 19—England, 2—British Provinces, 5. The above includes 12 deaths in the city institutions.

The Memory of the Deceased Physicians.—At the annual meeting of the Massachusetts Medical Society, held in this city May 25, 1853, the following Resolutions, presented by Dr. John Ware, of Boston, were unanimously adopted.

Whereas, It has happened, as one of the results of the late appalling calamity, which has cast a gloom over the whole community, and plunged many families into the deepest affliction, that several members of our profession, some of them our own honored associates, and some, of distinguished character from our sister states, have perished by a sudden and dreadful death, whilst others have barely escaped the same untimely fate, we, the Fellows of the Massachusetts Medical Society, assembled in annual meeting, in order to give expression to the sentiments which this occasion has excited, do unanimously resolve—

That, while, in common with all our fellow citizens, we have been deeply affected by this recent dispensation of Divine Providence, our attention is at this time especially called to the loss which this Society and the profession of medicine have sustained in the death of men not only eminent as physicians, but personally honored and beloved in the communities to which they belonged.

That we cannot but feel that this event has cast a shade of sadness and solemnity over this usually cheerful and happy anniversary.

That to those communities, which have been thus deprived of the medical advisers on whose skill and humanity they have been accustomed to rely in times of suffering and danger, we tender the expression of our profound regret.

That we offer to the families and friends of our deceased associates the assurance of our heartfelt sympathy in their affliction, and of the high respect in which we hold the character, and shall cherish the memory, of those who have been thus suddenly taken from them.

GEORGE HAYWARD, *President.*

CHARLES E. WARE, *Rec. Sec'ry.*

On motion of Dr. W. J. Dale, it was voted that these Resolutions be entered on the records of the Society, that a copy of them be transmitted to the families of the deceased, and that they be published in the Boston Medical and Surgical Journal.

Recuperative Powers of the Burmese.—Dr. Palmer, of the East India Company's service, recently arrived in Boston from Calcutta. He was surgeon in the Burmese war still raging, and was at the taking of the great city of Prome by the British, last autumn. Dr. P. stated a curious fact, the other day, illustrative of the recuperative powers of those people. Like the Chinese, they seem to recover from wounds that would be fatal to almost any other race of men. A married woman with one child, being upon her hands and knees while crawling under the awning of a boat, was shot with a ball which entered her body about an inch from the right side of the anus. In about half an hour after, the ball was discovered on the right side of the navel, imbedded in the loose structure, and after some difficulty was extracted. In its course it had penetrated both the bladder and uterus. A bloody discharge, mixed with urine, flowed freely from the wound for three or four days, when it ceased altogether. Little or no inflammation ensued, no antiphlogistic measures were adopted, and although the unfortunate patient suffered violent pains the two first days, Dr. Palmer kept her quiet with chloroform, and in three weeks she was restored to perfect health.

THE

BOSTON MEDICAL·AND SURGICAL JOURNAL.

Vol. XLVIII.   Wednesday, June 8, 1853.   No. 19.

TYPHUS AND TYPHOID FEVER—CALOMEL AND THE LANCET.

To the Editor of the Boston Medical and Surgical Journal.

Sir,—Should you consider the following remarks worthy of publication, they are at your disposal. They are the result of thirty-four years' experience in an extensive country practice. During my apprenticeship I had some experience in what is called now the old-fashioned typhus fever. I was taught by Prof. Nathan Smith, then professor in Yale College, that it was a disease *sui generis*, having a regular course; that its symptoms might be mitigated, but its progress could not be arrested until its termination by death or by a natural crisis; that it was contagious to a certain extent, and its subjects were exempted from its recurrence; that its character was modified by unknown causes—so much so, that he had never known it presenting the same symptoms at different seasons, and that he had always found too much interference on the part of the physician detrimental.

In 1818, the first year of my practice, I saw much of this form of fever; but having been influenced by the prevalent practice of that day, I gave powders of calomel to the extent of affecting the glands of the mouth, and of promoting a greater or less degree of ptyalism. Those acquainted with this form of fever, are aware that diarrhœa is not a very frequent attendant. This treatment, on the whole, appeared tolerably successful, and but few died. I saw, however, the sad effects of mercury in one case, in the exfoliation of portions of the lower jaw, unquestionably the result of too severe ptyalism. Convalescence was in general very slow.

In the year 1819, typhus (or what is now misnamed typhoid) prevailed very extensively in this section, particularly in the township of Newport, on the west side of Lake Memphremagog. In that season I had a large number of cases; and in one family thirteen were sick with it, several at the same time. This fever assumed all the characteristic symptoms of what has been called of late ship fever. The late Dr. Arnoldi, who saw cases of it in the township that year, pronounced the ship fever recently prevalent in Montreal as identical with that, and my own observation has been confirmatory of his opinion. I think every nurse exposed to this fever took it, with the exception of those who had had the typhus under the old form about five years previous, at which time it had

19

prevailed extensively in the same place. All such escaped this fever, without exception, which fact confirms my opinion of the identity of typhus and typhoid. This fever was ushered in by great prostration of strength, followed by diarrhœa, which proved troublesome through the whole course, connected with much heat and more or less bloating of the abdomen. The latter was so great, in some cases, that I was obliged to use the swathe. The lancet could not be borne in any case; even the most robust patient would swoon from the effects of the loss of four ounces of blood from the arm. In the treatment of these cases I soon found that calomel, either alone or combined with opium, was decidedly injurious.

Having premised thus much, I will briefly give an outline of my practice in typhus fever during the last twenty years. I am aware that individual success is not always a criterion of correct practice in fevers, because experience teaches that their malignity and danger is greater in some seasons than it is in others. During this period, the most cases I have treated in any one year was 35; the most in one family that year, was 5. Of all that I have treated for typhus or typhoid within this period, no case proved fatal. 'It is true that I have seen cases within this time in consultation which proved so; but none under my charge. Having observed the bad effects of calomel in the cases of 1819, I was induced to observe carefully the phenomena presenting themselves in typhus, as well during the different seasons as during the several stages of the disease, noting at the same time the peculiarity of treatment required in consequence of the concentration of the disease, in the development of increased irritation, or of inflammation in particular organs. The result was, that I soon discovered that when the mucous coat of the stomach and intestines became the seat of concentration (which constitutes the typhoid), there was an excessive flow of very yellow bile—so much, that at the first visit the patient had vomited or had in the stomach large quantities of it. This I attributed to the effect of heated blood passing directly from the irritated viscera to the liver, and thus by direct stimulus, with the aid of direct sympathy, exciting that organ to over action, and thus causing it to throw out an excessive quantity of bile (vitiated, of course, by the over excitement of the organ) into the intestines, and often into the stomach from inverted action consequent upon the nausea—such being the condition of the patient in the early stages of the so-called typhoid fever. In such cases I have given at once four or five grains of calomel, to be followed in thirty minutes with a solution of tartrate of antimony, and this to be repeated every half hour until free vomiting was induced.

The question may be asked why I gave calomel in cases where the liver was already over excited? My answer is, that I found it the most effectual means of disengorging the congested vessels of the mucous coat of the stomach and intestines; and, besides, the prostrating effect of the antimony so quickly following prevents any direct stimulating effect of the calomel on the liver. I will observe here, that in cases where diarrhœa was present, I gave an opiate to check the discharge previous to giving the calomel. This course invariably produced free alvine discharges, and left the bowels free of irritating fecal matter. The vomiting is generally less distressing after taking calomel as above.

After this I gave no more calomel in the course of the fever, unless its use was indicated by slate or clay-colored discharges indicating a torpid or inactive state of the liver, from causes which I will soon point out. My next step was to apply a single cotton or linen cloth, sufficiently large to cover the whole abdomen, wet in cold water, or, what I generally used, an infusion of hops with vinegar added, beginning with a temperature which could be borne without causing chills, and this to be so frequently changed as to keep the abdomen at a temperature a little below the natural heat, at the same time directing the spine to be frequently washed with the same. As the object of this was to lessen inflammatory irritation, and particularly to diminish the heat of the blood by which the liver had been kept in a state of over excitement, it will be seen that, unless strictly attended to, the object in view would be lost. In such cases, I consider the reduction of abdominal heat of so great importance, that were I confined to one single remedy in fever, I should prefer this. By its proper use the danger of ulceration in Peyer's glands is obviated, as well as all the ill effects resulting from the irritation of vitiated bile on the sensitive mucous surfaces. If this be neglected, the system becomes prostrated by the abdominal irritation, the glands become ulcerated, and sympathetic irritation is increased in every part of the system. The diarrhœa is also increased by the irritation of an excess of bile, and the fountain of healthy nutriment is cut off.

In order to comprehend, fully, the effect of heated blood on the liver, it must be borne in mind that it is a secreting organ ; that it is a vast reservoir of blood, which it receives directly from the abdominal viscera ; that its secretion is thrown directly into the intestines, and that when vitiated it becomes an exceedingly noxious irritant, adding irritation to the too greatly-excited mucous surfaces. In fever, the blood is ever in a heated state ; but when inflammation occurs in parts not supplying the portal system, the increased heat from this local cause is thrown into the general circulation ; but on the contrary, the heat from inflamed abdominal viscera passes into the portal circulation, and the injury is compound—first, the exhaustion from increased secretion of bile, and second from the irritation on the gastro-enteric mucous surfaces, thus increasing inflammation and diarrhœa, and interrupting wholly the digestive process. It may be said that cold affusion has long been practised in fevers. It is true, and I have tried it ; but the object is not attained by it which is effected by its local use as I have pointed out.

My next object has been (I may as well say *is*, not having wholly left practice), to watch the development of local inflammation in either of the great cavities, which almost invariably supervenes during the progress of this fever. This, if in the chest, I meet with blistering, cupping and leeching, and under certain circumstances with the lancet. If in the head, the same treatment with the addition of cold applications to the scalp.

In regard to the use of the lancet, I have found it of use in all cases where local inflammation has become developed, unless contra-indicated by the location of the febrile irritation on the mucous coat of the intestines, with an attendant diarrhœa. General bloodletting is not borne well in such cases, even in the first stages. This is no doubt in consequence of the destruction, by this irritated action, of that preparatory digestive process which is essential in order to fit the nutriment to go through the change of sanguification. Therefore, in all such cases, the blood that is in the system at the time of attack is all that can sustain the vital powers during the progress of the fever, as no other blood can be formed until the intestinal irritation is subdued or transferred to the chest or head.

I have frequently found, after the irritation of the intestines with the diarrhœa has abated, and inflammatory symptoms become developed in other parts, that the patient has been benefited by the lancet even as late as the eighth or tenth day. Bleeding, however, in typhus, should ever be moderate, not exceeding eight or ten ounces, and this it is not often necessary to repeat unless the disorganization of some organ is feared. If the cold applications be kept too long on the abdomen, and the heat too much reduced, the liver falls into a state of inaction, the alvine discharges become too light, and calomel should be given in doses of two or three grains at night until the secretions are restored. In typhus unattended with diarrhœa, calomel can be given more frequently with advantage. In these cases, especially if attended with thoracic irritation, the liver is very liable to fall into inaction from the diversion of irritation to other parts. I cannot express myself too strongly against the too free repetition of doses of calomel, with ipecacuanha and other irritating substances, during the whole course of typhus fever, as practised by some physicians. The constant use of a solution of tartarized antimony is equally objectionable. Such practice causes continued irritation, which aggravates and prolongs the disease. It has not been my intention to enter any farther into this subject than was necessary in order to give my own views relative to the use of calomel and the lancet in fevers.

In conclusion, I cannot but express my opinion that the effect of heated blood, in the portal circulation, on the liver, has been too much overlooked in other cases besides fever, particularly in the inflammatory complaints of the bowels of children, and also in peritoneal inflammation in adults. Every careful observer will notice, in all cases where there is preternatural heat of the abdomen, that there is invariably an excessive flow of bile. How inconsistent, how injurious, then, must be the effect of continued doses of calomel, adding as it does increased stimulus to an over-excited organ!

I am fully convinced that ulceration of the glands of Peyer and Brunner will hardly ever occur in cases where the abdominal heat has been kept down during the progress of fever.

One other remark I wish to make, in relation to a recent modification of typhus fever—and that is, the tendency to congestion and subsequent inflammation of the serous envelope of the brain and spinal marrow. All practising physicians must have witnessed or read of cases of cerebro-spinal meningitis. These cases are not essentially connected with, typhus fever, as they occur evidently as idiopathic disease. The first change appears as a simply congestive state of the bloodvessels of the serous membrane, frequently preceded or attended for a few days with stiffness in the neck or back. This state, if neglected, runs into inflammation, producing all the characteristic symptoms of cerebro-spinal meningitis. In severe cases there is often developed some degree of paralysis of the nerves going to the vital organs; but as it is not my intention to speak of this disease particularly, I will only observe, that since its prevalence I have observed in typhus fever a modification, dependent, no doubt, on the same endemic influence. This peculiarity has not occurred in all cases which I have seen of late; but as it does occur, I wish to call attention to it. This modification appears dependent on a greater degree of congestion of the neurilema in the first stages of fever than is usual. As far as my observation has extended, its manifestations are a less frequency of the pulse in the onset of fever, together with a want of action in the capillary vessels of the skin, as appears by a purple appearance in the face and extremities. There is also less heat of the extremities and abdomen, and less diarrhœa, than in the common typhoid, but there is a slight tendency to paralysis (often severe) of the nerves going to the viscera. I have noticed this more particularly in the want of contractile power in the bladder. These cases require the use of quinine; but my object in mentioning this peculiarity is that this modification of the fever often requires the use of more calomel, as the excessive secretion of bile usually attendant upon typhoid does not often occur in this; which may be partly owing to the less degree of abdominal heat, and partly to the paralytic tendency of the nerves. Consequently in these cases the cold cloth should at times be omitted, and calomel given often enough to ensure a sufficient secretion of bile.

The conclusion of the whole matter is, that I consider typhoid fever to be essentially typhus, the concentration of febrile irritation being more confined to the gastro-enteric mucous surfaces; that the ulceration of Peyer's glands and the excessive flow of bile are the results of the inflammation or increased irritation of the abdominal viscera, and that calomel and the lancet are not indicated, for the reasons specified; that when the febrile irritation is more general or more concentrated about the chest or head, with less heat of the abdomen, and little or no diarrhœa, we have the old-fashioned typhus, and cases which are more benefited by the use of the lancet and calomel. It is possible that the luxurious living of modern times has increased typhoid-fever by its debilitating effect on the digestive organs. **M. F. Colby, M.D.**

Stanstead, Can. East, May, 1853.

HYGIENICS OF TEMPERANCE.

BY SAMUEL A. CARTWRIGHT, M.D., NEW ORLEANS, LATE OF NATCHEZ.

[Communicated for the Boston Medical and Surgical Journal.]

WHETHER water or alcohol be the better health-preserving agent, is a question to be determined by observation. Some account of the effects of each on a number of the Æsculapii themselves, is herewith respectfully presented to that profession whose office it is to keep in tune the curious harp of man's body, and to take cognizance of everything which preserves or disturbs its harmony. Nothing tends more to preserve or disturb its harmony than water and alcohol. Hence the members of the medical profession, who may take sides in the temperance controversy, now agitating the people of every State in the Union, are not to be regarded as out of their province, but in a field properly belonging to them, where instead of being viewed as intruders or intermeddlers, they are, by virtue of their calling, entitled to rank as chiefs.

The writer is one of three physicians, who located in Natchez thirty years ago. The new comers found only *one* practitioner in the city belonging to the same temperance school with themselves. The country and villages within fifteen miles around afforded only *three* more. All the rest believed in the hygienic virtues of alcoholic drinks, and taught that doctrine by precept and example. Besides the practising physicians, there were ten others in the city and adjacent country who had retired from the profession. They were all temperate. Thus, including the new comers, the total number of temperance physicians, in and near Natchez, thirty years ago, consisted of seventeen. Of these, five have died :—Dr. Henry Tooley, aged about 75 years ; Dr. Andrew M'Creary, aged 70 ; Dr. J. Ker, 60 ; Dr. Wm. Dunbar, 60 ; Dr. James A. Mc Pheeters, 49. In 1823, the average ages of the seventeen was about 34 years. According to the Carlisle tables of mortality, and those of the Equitable Insurance Company of London, seven instead of five would have been the ratio of mortality in England. Those at present living are Drs. D. Lattimore, W. Wren, Stephen Duncan, James Metcalf, W. N. Mercer, G. W. Grant, J. Sanderson, Benj. F. Young, T. G. Elliott, ——— Phœnix, Prof. A. P. Merrill, and the writer.

On the other hand, every physician of Natchez and its vicinity thirty years ago, whether practising or retired, who was in the habit of *tippling*, as the practice of drinking alcoholic beverages is called, has long since been numbered with the dead ! Only two of them, who were comparatively temperate, lived to be gray. Their average term of life did not exceed 35 years, and the average term of life of those who were in the habit of taking alcoholic drinks frequently between meals, on an empty stomach, did not reach thirty years. In less than ten years after they commenced practice, the most of them died, and the whole of them have subsequently fallen, leaving not one behind in the city, country or village, within twenty miles around.

To fill the places of those who died or retired from the profession, sixty-two medical men settled in Natchez and its vicinity between the years 1824 and 1835, embracing a period of ten years ; not counting those of 1823 already mentioned. Of the sixty-two new comers, thirty-seven were temperate, and twenty-five used alcoholic beverages between meals, though not often to the extent of producing intoxication. Of the thirty-seven who trusted to the hygienic virtues of nature's beverage— plain unadulterated water—nine have died, and twenty-eight are living. Of the twenty-five who trusted to the supposed hygienic virtues of ardent spirits, all are dead, except three ! and they have removed to distant parts of the country. Peace be to their ashes ! though mostly noble fellows, misled by the deceitful syren, singing the praises of alcoholic drinks, to live too fast and to be cut off in the outset of useful manhood, it is to be hoped they have not lived in vain ; as by their sacrifice science has gained additional and important proof of the fallacy of the theory, which attributes health-preserving properties, in a southern climate, to alcoholic beverages in any shape or form.

While referred to in the mass, to correct a popular delusion, it would be unnecessary and improper to drag their names before the public. Not so, however, with those who owe life, fortune and reputation to avoiding the shoals on which their brethren were wrecked. The public have a right to know who they are, and the cause of temperance is justly entitled to all the influence attached to their names. According to the Carlisle tables, and those of the Equitable Insurance Company of London, thirty-seven individuals, at the average age of 25 years (which was about the average age of the new comers who settled in Natchez), would, in a quarter of a century, lose nine of their number ; whereas, of the thirty-seven temperance doctors, only nine have died in twenty-eight years. Of these, Drs. Wm. P. Foster, Cornell and Ferguson fell by the yellow fever of 1825 ; Dr. John Bell came to the South, with phthisis pulmonalis, from New Hampshire, and was the son of the Governor ; Dr. H. Perrine, of quinine notoriety, was killed by the Indians in the Florida War ; Dr. E. Johnson returned to Kentucky and died ; Dr. Ogden fell a victim to some chronic ailment ; Dr. J. W. Monette, always a dyspeptic, died after he had finished his history of the Valley of the Mississippi, and had made a handsome fortune by his practice ; and Dr. Thomas Davis was cut off by the yellow fever of 1839—making nine in all. The remaining twenty-eight are still living, or were when last heard from. Dr. Campbell removed to London, where he was practising medicine at last advices. Dr. J. Thistle, a year ago, removed to Davenport, Iowa. Dr. Wm. M. Guin is at present a United States Senator from California. Drs. Stewart, Walker, Pollard. French, Hubbard, Page, Sydney Smith and E. C. Hyde, removed to Louisiana, and are all engaged in the planting business, except the three last. Drs. Freiott and Weston returned to New York, Dr. Holt to Kentucky, Dr. James Young removed to Memphis, and Dr. Woodworth to Illinois. The remainder are still in Natchez and its neighborhood. They are Drs. F. A. W. Davis, Harpour, the two Leggetts, Asa Metcalf, J. Foster, Atchison, Wood, Chamberlain, Ward, Colhoun and Abercrombie.

If the property of all the temperate doctors of Natchez and its vicinity, dead and living, including those who have moved away, and including those who have retired from the profession, embracing those of 1823, and all who came in up to 1835—fifty-four in number—were equally divided, each would have upwards of a hundred thousand dollars for his share. Temperance, in that portion of the South at least, is not only hygienic, but auriferous. They all began life poor, with nothing but their profession for a livelihood. Some of them are in the possession of millions, and have long since retired from the duties of their profession. They nevertheless belong to the medical public, and have no right to object to their names being brought before that public for the scientific purpose of proving to the physicians, at the North, the hygienic virtues of temperance in the South. Many northern temperance men are so weak in the faith, as to be led to believe, on their coming South, that rain and river water (the only kind to be' had in Natchez, New Orleans, and some other parts of the South) actually requires the addition of some stimulating liquid to make it healthful. This weakness or distrust of temperance principles is owing to the want of well-authenticated facts from the South bearing on the question. Facts are better than theory to enable, not only physicians, but the people generally, to form rules of conduct on a subject of such importance. To have their proper weight, they should be authenticated, and the important truth made known, that of the whole number of temperance doctors of 1823 (thirty years ago), in Natchez and its vicinity, more than two thirds are still living in the year 1853, at ages varying from 55 to 85 years; that of the whole number of the intemperate, of the same period, not one remains, in town or country; that of thirty-seven temperate and 25 intemperate physicians, who came in afterwards, between the years 1824 and 1835, all of the former are living except nine, and all of the latter are dead except three. Hence it was necessary to mention the names of the temperance physicians, many of whom are known abroad as well as at home, as living proofs of the important truth, that a temperate and upright life is the surest, safest and best road to health, wealth, longevity and respectability.

Many young medical men, as well as others, on coming South, mistake the noise of bar-rooms and grog-shops for the public sentiment of the country. Hence they are too apt to plunge into dissipation, under the delusion, that water is unwholesome unless mixed with stimulants; and that it is, moreover, essential to popularity and a good introduction to business, "*when in Rome to do as Rome does.*" The error lies in mistaking the purlieus for the true Rome of the South, and in the erroneous theory which attributes to alcoholic beverages the hygienic properties that pure, unadulterated water alone possesses. It was not by dram-drinking that the above-named medical men preserved their health. Their names being known, they can be interrogated and answer for themselves. It was not by grog-shops or the influence or agency of the inmates of such places, that they succeeded in business, and came into the inheritance of the fat of the land.

It is to be deplored that there should be any discrepancy of council among medical men in regard to the use of alcoholic drinks. While physicians, in perfect health, make use of such beverages and attribute to them hygienic virtues, the public will be slow to regard them as poisonous to the blood of a healthy man. Much of the evil lies in the inattention bestowed on the subject in our systems of medical education, since the voice of the American Hippocrates, Benj. Rush, ceased to echo in the lecture-room. "Man, who is the servant and interpreter of nature, can act and understand no further than he has, either in operation or contemplation, observed of the method and order of nature.", Those, who can master this first principle of the Novum Organum, found in its first sentence, will at once perceive why physicians, even the most skilful and experienced, are as liable as other men to fall into error and to be unsafe guides on any subject they have not studied or only superficially examined. They have studied arsenic thoroughly, and they know what effects it produces in large doses and small, in sickness and in health, and can even detect the minutest portion of it in the tissues; but very few of them have thus studied alcohol, and become aware of the truth, that if it be a little slower, it is nevertheless as sure a poison.

Canal St., New Orleans, May 23, 1853.

TRE \TMENT FOR HEMORRHAGE FOLLOWING THE EXTRACTION OF A TOOTH.

[Communicated for the Boston Medical and Surgical Journal.]

On page 315, of vol. xlviii., of this Journal, bearing date May 18, 1853, commences the description of a plan for arresting hemorrhage from the socket of a tooth after extraction; but I have for many years used other means which have always been effectual in my hands. I first clear the socket of all the clotted blood; then with the thumb and finger, press the parts firmly together, and have the mouth well rinsed with cold water. When this is done, I wind a small lock of cotton on a wire or probe, saturate it with a drop or two of creosote, and press it down to the bottom of the socket; then with another small probe, or wire, press on the cotton and withdraw the probe, leaving the cotton in its place. On this I press firmly a larger roll, filling the socket; on this still another firm roll, so that the opposing teeth or jaw will press on it; and if the first application should fail, I clear the socket and repeat the operation directly, and it will not fail to stop the bleeding. Among several which I have had to do with, I will mention two cases only.

CASE I.—In 1842, a young woman had a tooth extracted in the morning. The bleeding continued through the day, when she had caught more than a quart, and I was sent for. I took with me the creosote, and by following the plan above described, the bleeding ceased instantly, and never more returned.

CASE II.—A young man, from Boston, had a tooth extracted in this city in the morning, and bled fearfully till 11 o'clock, A.M., when he sent for me. In his case I used the same means, and the bleeding ceased at once, and he returned to Boston in the noon train of cars.

A good dentist of this city became alarmed by profuse bleeding from the socket, and called on me for aid, when I informed him of my method, which he followed fully, and stopped the bleeding at once. He afterwards informed me that he had no more trouble in similar cases, though he had met with many.   DANIEL MOWE.

Lowell, May 21, 1853.

CASE OF DOUBLE MONSTER—MORBID STATES OF THE PLACENTA.

BY WM. F. MONTGOMERY, A.M., M.D., ETC., DUBLIN.

MARCH 6th, 1851, Mr. O'Donovan was called to Mrs. L., aged 35, mother of three children, and seven months pregnant of her fourth, in very delicate health ; her abdomen enormously enlarged, having the appearance of a twin pregnancy in the ninth month ; lower extremities œdematous ; and she was exceedingly weak and dispirited ; former pregnancies favorable.

11 o'clock, P.M., labor set in rapidly. Mr. O'Donovan found the membranes ruptured and the room deluged with the waters ; the feet and legs of a child were protruded, cold and livid ; at the orifice of the vagina appeared what at first seemed a hand, but being pushed down it was found to be a third leg, then a fourth leg was discovered and brought down.

By passing the finger round the fœtus, Mr. O'Donovan found that the body was single at the umbilicus, the cord lying in the cleft, and a portion of intestine protruding. He assisted the pains, which were few and weak, gradually drew down the body, and, having hooked down the arms, delivered the woman of a full-grown monster fœtus, with two heads and two sets of extremities ; the placenta soon descended and was removed ; the heads passed one after the other, moving, as it were, on a central point, the junction at the neck. There was imperfect contraction of the womb, and a tendency to hemorrhage, which, however, Mr. O'Donovan was enabled to prevent by the usual means, and the mother ultimately did well.

"No description," says M. O'Donovan, " can convey an idea of the horrible appearance of this monster : the heads taken together were much larger than the head of a full-grown healthy child, and were fully developed ; the faces fronting and applied to each other, the mouth of the one being received into that of the other, which was a large chasm, the line of junction commencing at the lower lip and continuing perfect to the umbilicus ; the thorax of each was well formed and distinct except for the juncture ; at the dorsal vertebræ, and opposite the umbilicus, the bodies were drawn towards each other as if compressed by a cord. The gross bulk of the double monster was equal to that of a single child of nine months ; each head was as fully ossified as a natural fœtus of the same age, that is, seven months. The abdominal parietes were deficient at the junction of the funis, where there existed only a thin diaphanous membrane, as if an expansion of the sheath of the cord itself ; the arms of the children embraced each other in the form of a figure of 8. The placenta was about the natural size, part apparently healthy, but nearly a third *presented a vast collection of hydatids*. No examination would be permitted."

Mr. O'Donovan has lately informed me that the lady was again confined last month (February), under his care, of a healthy, full-grown, female child, and had a most favorable labor.

I may observe, in reference to this case, how often anomalous or morbid states of the cord or placenta are, as indeed we might anticipate, found in connection with malformations or monstrosities of the fœtus ; hydatid degeneration of the placenta is often met with, not only accompanied by extreme atrophy of the fœtus, but frequently no trace of it is left remaining.

One of the ugliest and most disgusting-looking monsters I ever saw was connected with an enormous placenta, whose substance was quite unravelled, and the separate branches of capillaries hung down like minute stalactites, at least two inches long, while the twin brother of this monster was a comely child, attached to a healthy placenta and cord.

Such a relation between morbid anomalies of the placenta and malformations or monstrosities in the fœtus must cease to surprise us when we consider that the placenta is, in fact, the organ or apparatus by which the whole *pabulum vitæ* is supplied for the development and support of the child during its intra-uterine life, and if this supply is tainted at its source, or interrupted by morbid changes therein, we can readily understand to what a degree the evolution of the embryo is likely to be thereby affected.

Hence it is, that in those perplexing cases so frequently met with, in which women are, in several successive pregnancies, delivered of dead children, without any discoverable constitutional disease or infirmity in the mother, an examination of the placenta so frequently discloses to us morbid alterations quite sufficient to explain the distressing result. Of these I may just allude to what has been called tubercular disease of the placenta, apoplexy of its substance, hydatid degeneration, inflammation of the placenta or envelopes of the ovum, and especially if producing their adhesion to the surface of the child.

In another instance under my observation, the cord was excessively dropsical, so as to be in some parts two inches in diameter, and in that case 'the child was unequally developed, one side of the body being very much larger than the other ; this inequality, however, gradually disappeared, and the young lady is now of unexceptionable symmetry. " In one of the recorded cases," says Vrolik, " the superior extremities were wanting, and the anus was closed."

Serres considers the absence of one of the umbilical arteries as the efficient cause of that form of monstrosity in which there is *ectopia viscerum abdominalium*, but such a consequence does not always follow such a defect. I have in my museum a specimen of a placenta and umbilical cord with only one artery, and it was connected with a remarkably fine, healthy, and well-formed child.

This want of one umbilical artery was also observed in Sir A. Cooper's imperfect and heartless fœtus, but, with the exception of an umbilical hernia, there was no other *ectopia viscerum abdominalium.*

I have for many years endeavored to impress on my pupils the great advantages to be gained not only in the way of general pathological inquiry, but in the acquisition of a particular species of knowledge of the utmost practical value, by carefully examining the fœtus and its envelopes in every case, but especially in those cases of blight or arrested development, where the size of the fœtus is so entirely at variance with the real date of the pregnancy, a mistake on which point may lead, and has often

led, to giving an opinion which may irreparably injure a really unblemished reputation.

The following case, which was recently brought under my observation,
is a striking illustration of the above remark. Five months after her
husband's departure for a foreign country, a lady miscarried of an ovum
and fœtus, presenting the characters and development of the third month.
For more than two months and a half after the separation of the parties
she had no menstruation, and had other indications of pregnancy ; but
she then had sanguineous discharges from the vagina, which were regarded as a return of her catamenia, and she was no longer considered
pregnant. These, however, ceased, and there was again a suppression for
two months and a half, at the end of which time the lady miscarried of an
ovum and fœtus, presenting conditions corresponding to such a period ;
the result of which was a conviction, on the part of some members of her
husband's family, that she must have been unfaithful to him, and it was
at once decided to inform him of his misfortune. Before doing so, however, the ovum was shown to a medical friend, who, wishing to have his
own judgment in so delicate a matter fortified by the opinion of another,
submitted the ovum to me for careful examination, when the true nature
of the case appeared at once manifest : the envelopes were in a morbid
state, thickened and tuberculated, and had evidently been long separated from their vascular connection with the uterus ; the umbilical cord
also was diseased at its placental end, where it was expanded into a
lotus-shaped sac, filled with a brownish serum. Of the true history of
the case there seemed, then, no doubt ; the lady had conceived just at the
time of her husband's departure, her pregnancy had proceeded undisturbed
until the third month, when she had symptoms of miscarriage, but did not
miscarry ; but the ovum was blighted, and, having lost its vitality, ceased
to grow ; it was, however, retained in the uterus until the expiration of
five months from the date of conception, when it was expelled in the
morbid state already described. This explanation at once set at rest all
the unworthy and undeserved suspicions entertained against this innocent
lady, who would otherwise have been made the subject of a most painful proceeding. Facts of this kind have been heretofore insisted on by
the writer in his work on the Signs of Pregnancy, and some cases related
in illustration.

[The above is taken from an elaborate and carefully-prepared article
in the last number of the Dublin Quarterly Medical Journal. The writer gives descriptions of nine remarkable cases of double monstrosity,
some of them of recent occurrence and never before published. The
interest in each of them is greatly increased by accompanying well-exe-
cuted plates, representing the strange connections which sometimes—
but fortunately so rarely—take place in twin births. The subject is of
interest in this country, while the celebrated Siamese twins are again
exhibiting themselves to the public, and we may, therefore, copy hereafter Dr. Montgomery's account of other cases.—ED.]

OPERATION FOR CANCER IN AGED PERSONS.

Mr. Weedon Cooke stated, at a late meeting of the Medical Society of London, the following case :—W. M———, aged 68, a tall, well-built, bony man, an agricultural laborer from Essex, had suffered for two years from an epithelial cancer of the hand, which commenced as a warty scale upon the thumb. This had progressed in spite of all treatment, until when he came under my care at the Cancer Hospital, Dec. 3, 1852 ; I found the thumb and forefinger separating by ulceration, and the disease extending across the whole of the back of the hand. After a few days' ineffectual attempts to stay the immense purulent discharge, I, on the 22d of December, removed the forearm three inches below the elbow-joint without pain or consciousness, the chloroform having acted very kindly. The only circumstance worth remarking in the course of the operation was the tying a large patulous vein. The patient at this time was weak, had a very red, glazed tongue, with a disposition to diarrhœa. For the first week he did well, slept by means of a grain of opium at night, and took milk, wine, and fish. At this time the stump became inflamed, the stitches sloughed out, and the flaps separated. Generous diet, with porter, bark, and acid, soon set up a healthy action, and granulations began to spring up; but it was a month after the operation before the stump had quite healed. I may state as a small point of detail that I found in this case, as in others, that the ceratum saponis spread on lint was most serviceable in keeping the parts cool and in nice apposition. At the same time that the stump became inflamed, the right leg and foot began to swell, accompanied with considerable tenderness of the calf and along the inner side of the thigh. By means of constantly applied warmth the inflammation was kept down, and entirely subsided in a fortnight, leaving still some œdema of the foot. During the continuance of the phlebitis the tongue retained its glazed, raw-beef appearance, but began to become moist and less red on the twenty-first day after operation. All things after this progressed favorably, and he was sent home with the stump quite healed and general health greatly improved on the 14th of February, being seven weeks after the operation. On the 22d of March he came to town to see me, and exhibited a ruddy, agricultural aspect, quite refreshing to look at. Stump free from pain and quite healthy looking ; no swelling, but some slight weakness of the right leg. The microscopic examination of the cancerous matter exhibited cells having two or three nuclei with a variety of shape, some oblong, some caudate.

The salient points of this case are the age of the patient, showing how tolerant of operations aged people are, the occurrence of phlebitis in a distant part of the body, attributable to the tying a large vein during the operation, and the propriety or otherwise of going beyond a joint in all amputations of this nature. In private practice it is very common to find the friends of patients objecting to operations, when the proposed subjects of them are in advanced age, without considering that some persons have more resilient stamina at 70 than others have at 40. There are many reasons why we should not allow an old person to die of the exhausting effects of a local disease, which may be removed by the knife. First and foremost, the dread and suffering of an operation are removed by chloroform, and old people bear this agent very well, all the accidents that have been recorded being in young persons. Does not the introduction of anæsthesia call upon us to reverse, or at any rate carefully to revise, many of our old opinions with respect to operations—opinions which were perfectly good before the discovery of this great alleviator? Secondly, the offensive discharges of an ulcerated or sloughing sore make life burthensome to the patient and grievous to his friends. Thirdly, the fœtor which is inhaled, and the decaying matter which is absorbed into the blood, poison the system, producing irritative or perhaps hectic fever, so hastening the melancholy termination. Fourthly, the pain, which is excruciating, wastes body and mind, " making both diy and night hideous ;" and lastly, recorded cases and general experience show that after the source of all these evils is taken away there is such a rebound given to the system that the healing process goes on, under the influence of generous diet, satisfactorily and to a happy conclusion—namely, restoration for years to comfort and society. Of course cases are presented to the surgeon, where the powers of life are so low that he would fear either death from the immediate effects of the operation, or from the exhaustive discharges subsequently ; but these cases are as often remarked in the young and middle-aged as in the old, and would in either case be a bar to operative procedure. There is one great distinguishing circumstance between the young and old with respect to operations, and that is in the after-treatment ; for it may be taken as a rule, although having exceptions, that aged persons must be well supported and carefully watched from the very commencement; whilst in the young the inflammatory fever will require to be controlled by antiphlogistics. In the foregoing case the patient had attained to nearly the threescore years and ten, and did well, notwithstanding the ugly complication which retarded restoration—namely, the phlebitis, which was attributable to the tying a large vein in the course of the operation The practice, now so common, but amongst our fathers so feared and reprobated, of tying veins, either when they bleed obstinately in the course of an operation, or for the purpose of obliterating them when in a varicose condition, requires the serious reconsideration of the profession ; for although it would not be wise to inculcate the horror with which any interference with the veins was formerly contemplated, the many serious results which have accrued from the present practice bids us be chary of our ligatures on veins, recollecting that there is the greatest safety in a middle course ; for what man could contemplate with complacency the death of a fellow-creature from the effects of the little operation of tying a saphena. In future I shall certainly prefer cold effusion, or even the actual cautery, to ligatures for obstinate venous hæmorrhage.

One other consideration remains in connection with this case, and that is the propriety of amputation above or below the joint. It was a question I had to decide wholly for myself, since, on the one hand, the professional friends who kindly assisted me counselled removal above the joint, whilst the patient made me promise to leave him as much of his arm as possible. Perhaps this strongly-expressed desire biassed me, but I am inclined to think that there were grounds for my preference of amputation on this side the joint. The disease had commenced in the skin, and although ulceration had extended so far as to destroy some of the cartilages of the metacarpus and phalanges, I did not discover any disease of the bones, and the result will, I think, show that there was none. The advantages of the small piece of forearm left over a straight stump are numerous and patent—to lean, to carry, to push, and even to hold. The only fear, that of recurrence of the disease in the end of the bone soon after the operation, has passed away ; and should the stump again take on the disease, there will be no reason to suppose that the soft parts were not the peccant portions. With respect to the question of operation, there could be no doubt in this case, since the man was sinking from the drain upon his system, and the irritative fever produced by purulent absorption. By removing the diseased hand, life has not only been prolonged but rendered enjoyable.—*London Lancet.*

THE BOSTON MEDICAL AND SURGICAL JOURNAL.

BOSTON, JUNE 8, 1853.

Dr. Hayward's Remarks at the Festival of the Massachusetts Medical Society.—At the dinner of the fellows of the Massachusetts Medical Society, at Faneuil Hall, on Wednesday, May 25th, Dr. Reynolds, the anniversary chairman, presented the following sentiment :—

" The Massachusetts Medical Society—instituted by our Fathers in the Profession for the promotion of sound learning, thorough education, and an honorable character and intercourse among physicians ; may it ever have, as at present, a wise head to direct its counsels, and zealous members to maintain its usefulness, its interests and its honor."

As a matter of course, this brought up the president of the Society, George Hayward, M.D., whose observations were cordially received. Faneuil Hall rang with cheerful voices. We are gratified in being able to present the following report of his remarks, which are of peculiar interest to the members of the ancient institution over which he presides with equal honor to himself and the Society.

"Mr. Chairman,—The place I occupy in this Society requires me, no doubt, to respond to the sentiment that you have just given. And while I regret that I cannot do this in such a way as I could wish, I should be unjust to my own feelings if I were to remain silent ; if I were not to make my grateful acknowledgments, as I now do, for the manner in which I have been noticed by you, and for the kindness with which that notice has been received.

"This too is the first time that I have had an opportunity of meeting the Fellows of this Society since I have been made their presiding officer ; and I avail myself of the occasion to tender them my most sincere thanks. When I consider the number and respectability of the gentlemen who compose the Society, the purposes for which it was instituted and the character of the individuals who have preceded me in this office, I cannot but regard my election as the highest honor of my life, as it is the one that is most grateful to my feelings.

"Those, Mr. Chairman, who know the Society now for the first time, in the full vigor of its manhood, are not aware how feeble and inefficient it was at the outset. It began with less than seventy members; widely separated from each other; without the facilities of intercourse between the different parts of the Commonwealth that now exist, and at one of the darkest periods in the annals of our country. It was incorporated before the close of the revolutionary struggle, when the state of public affairs was the paramount object in the minds of men. Its meetings were consequently thinly attended; they were frequently adjourned for the want of a quorum, and so little interest was felt in its concerns, that for a time it had a very feeble and precarious existence.

"But since its re-organization in 1803, its course has been onward and prosperous. It now numbers more than twelve hundred members, and embraces within its ranks nearly all the medical talent, skill and science of this Commonwealth.

"It is indeed an honor to be the presiding officer of an institution founded for noble and disinterested purposes. You have said truly in the sentiment that you have just given, 'that it was instituted for the promotion of sound learning, thorough education, and an honorable character and intercourse among physicians.' And though adverse circumstances may in its early history have prevented to some extent, for a time, the full accomplishment of the design of its founders, yet for the last fifty years it has steadily advanced in prosperity and usefulness, exerting a most salutary influence upon the public and upon the profession.

"I will not, however, trespass on your time, which can be so much more agreeably occupied by others, in speaking at any length of what it has accomplished; I will merely say, that it gave its early and efficient aid to the cause of temperance; that it induced the authorities of our State to legalize the study of anatomy; that it has labored steadily to raise the standard of medical education; to guard the community from ignorant and designing empiricism; to enlighten the public and the profession in relation to the various epidemics that have appeared in our country from time to time during the last fifty years; and to give a more elevated social position to its Fellows, by promoting among them a love of science, and a dignified, courteous and honorable course of conduct.

"How much good it has effected in all this, I will not pretend to say; but I will say, that it has been actuated by no sinister or selfish motives, in the efforts it has made, and still continues to make, to furnish the community with high-minded, skilful and accomplished physicians.

"When I reflect too, Mr. Chairman, on the character of those who have preceded me in this office, I feel still more deeply the honor that has been conferred upon me. No one can be more fully aware than I am of their great superiority to the present incumbent; but I will not yield to them in ardent attachment to the objects of the institution and a sincere desire to promote them.

Of my sixteen predecessors, eleven are dead, and I am old enough to remember all but two. It would be a most grateful duty, if there were time, to say something of each of them. Of the venerable Holyoke, the first President; of the courteous and dignified Danforth; the learned Rand; the eloquent and sagacious Warren; of Fisher, the modest, amiable and profound student; and of the high-souled and chivalrous Brooks. But this task I leave to abler hands and a fitter occasion.

"The five surviving ex-Presidents have our earnest wishes, that they may long continue to enlighten their brethren by their experience; cheer them by their example; and instruct them by their wisdom.

"Of this number there is one, with whom I was associated in a subordinate capacity, while he was President of the Society; from whom, during forty years, I have received numerous acts of personal kindness, and to whose professional skill I am deeply indebted.

"But these alone would not make it proper that I should speak of him at this time and in this place. There are other considerations, however, that seem to me not only to justify such a notice, but to demand it. For at least fifty years, he has been a most active and efficient member of our Society, and during that long period, has done more than any other individual to promote its interests and elevate its character.

"Nor is this all. His whole life has been a practical illustration of the noble principles by which he has been guided. Every member of our profession, to whom he is known, has entire confidence in his skill, probity and judgment, and feels that he may rely upon him in any emergency as a safe counsellor and a kind friend.

"But I forbear saying more. No one who hears me can doubt to whom I refer. I will therefore with your leave, Sir, propose the health of James Jackson: all who know him, respect him as a physician, revere him as a man, and love him as a friend."

Henlé's General Pathology.—Treatises on this department of medicine are multiplying. This is not an evil, however, but a boon, for which proper expressions of thankfulness should be offered to those who are conferring the benefit of their researches on that great body of practitioners whose devotion to the endless details of business interferes with deliberate, systematic study. Henry C. Preston, M.D., of Providence, R. I., is the translator of a "Treatise on General Pathology, by Dr. J. Henlé, Prof. of Anatomy and Physiology in Heidelberg." The book is from the press of Messrs. Lindsay & Blakiston, Philadelphia. There is no striking feature in it, which gives it entire superiority over preceding works; still, it is excellent, and is calculated to secure the patronage of medical men. Dr. Preston informs us, in his prefatory introduction to American readers, that Dr. Henlé is a distinguished medical teacher, and the best German pathologist, perhaps, now living. He was prosector for Dr. John Müller, at Berlin. Two editions of his treatise have appeared in that country, which shows in what estimation it is held by learned men there. Besides an introduction, embracing the consideration of medical systems, and ending with an elaborate historical view of various periods recognized in the literature of medicine, the body of the volume, a handsome octavo of 391 pages, is divided into four sections. Under the first, the nature of disease and morbid processes is presented; II., general etiology; III., disease in its relation of extent; IV., relations of disease with regard to time. There is some fine writing in reserve for the student who takes this good book in hand. "The whole created world," says Dr. H., "as far as human reason extends, shows such a conformity of the means to the end, that we, on the one hand, consider that which is customary where it appears non-conformable to the design, as abnormal; and that which is conformable to the design, even where we cannot perceive its signification, we consider as normal. So, therefore, upon the way to the ideal, the development changes itself again into an anomaly, if it ceases to accommodate itself to the given relations." The following is a practical paragraph, to be kept in remembrance in certain cases, in determining whether a person is actually dead. "The rigidity of the dead body seems to be a never-failing sign of death ; and in those cases where it is not observed, it only seems to have occurred so early and passed away so quickly, that it has been over-looked. The cause of this remarkable phenomenon has been and is still unknown. Cold accelerates its appearance, but keeping the body warm does not stop it. With the termination of the rigor mortis, coincides the beginning of the infallible signs of decay, the cadaverous smell, and the development of gas, which, in summer, often causes, in a very short time, a complete loss of identity, swelling up the corpse so that it cannot be re-cognized, and often occasioning, after death, evacuations of the contents of the bowels, bladder, and even the uterus, and finally a green color of the abdominal walls. At this time the microscope demonstrates the pre-sence of infusoria, to become whose food is the final destiny of the soul-less organism."

Unity of Disease.—In the recently-published "Transactions of the Ala-bama State Medical Society," is an essay on the Unity of Disease, by H. Backus, M.D., of Selma in that State, which the author says " is so ob-scured by errors, partly original, partly typographical, as to be scarcely in-telligible." That he may not be misunderstood, and go down to posterity with the reputation of being an incomprehensible writer, he has issued a pamphlet, with a corrected text, which very materially alters the sense, be-sides bettering certain expressions that were difficult of comprehension.

Medicine in Burmah.—The phongees or priests, a numerous and pri-vileged body in Burmah, from immemorial time have been writers. They reside in monastic establishments of vast extent, and besides attending to the duties enjoined by the faith of Budhism, they devote much time to the reading of medical books. Their wooden books, says Dr. Palmer, are piled up in immense masses, and those expressly relating to medicine are very numerous. So few missionaries have learned the language of that country, that it is hardly probable any of their works will ever be trans-lated ; and if they were, they would be of no service to science or hu-manity. As curiosities, it might be a gratification to know what they think of diseases, and how they treat them.

Life Insurance.—In the case of the late sudden death of Dr. Peirson of Salem, and Dr. Gray of Springfield, the family of the latter have se-cured to them a sum of money necessary to their comfort; while the other, by neglecting to make the last annual payment, lost all that had been paid for some years, nothing coming back to his bereaved family. A gen-tleman from Connecticut remarked, some three years since, that he took out a policy on his life a long time ago, in Philadelphia, for $5000, and had made punctual payments, till the sum paid in exceeded the amount his family would have were he dead; yet if he stopped paying the annual assessment, the whole would be sacrificed to the company. And he fur-ther observed, that no bargain could be made to allow a hold on the money paid in. "The directors think," he said, "my bones may be good picking ten years longer!" When the insured lives till the annual payments exceed the amount of the policy, life insurance is a poor investment. Had the same sums been placed even in a savings bank at four per cent., the inheritors would have been vastly better served. But here is the rub, in negotiating with a life insurance company—the applicant cannot ascertain whether the chances for life or death preponderate within a specific period. Were he to die immediately, the survivors would be gainers, if money were of more value to them than the industry of the insured. If, on the contrary, an annual drainage upon a small purse absorbs all the property of the family or individual, and life is still prolonged, nothing is gained by the operation. Before proposing for insurance, it is all important to ascertain the character and resources of the company. An immense amount of iniquity is practised by rotten concerns, whose runners are perpetually on the go into counting-rooms, work-shops, factories, &c., persuading people to provide by life insurance for those dependent upon them. All companies, even the soundest, must be receiving large sums, through the neglect or inability of the insured to pay the annual premium stipulated in the contract. As corporations are without souls, a forfeit is good luck—and money never refunded, should the unfortunate owner of the policy be reduced to beggary. An office that would return one half, under either aspect of misfortune, would soon be well patronized.

Medical Miscellany.—Dr. Leigh's well-written thesis, entitled Respiration Subservient to Nutrition," has been published in a pamphlet, and is deserving of an extensive sale.—The East Tennessee Record of Medicine and Surgery, having reached its fourth quarterly number, has been discontinued. Dr. F. A. Ramsey, the editor, a man of learning and enterprise, is hereafter to be connected with the medical journal published at Nashville, Tenn.—One hundred and fifty gentlemen regularly qualified doctores medicinæ, are registered in the Homœopathic Medical Society of the State of New York.—Dr. C. P. Gage, of Concord, N. H., has been appointed Coroner for the County of Merrimack.

To CORRESPONDENTS.—A paper by Dr. Ramsay on the Pulse, Cranial Dimensions, &c. of the Southern Negro Child, has been received.

MARRIED,—At Aroostook, Me., on the 25th ult E. G. Decker, M D, to Miss Jessie A. Howard.—At Rahway, N. J., E. M. Hunt, M.D., to Miss E. L. Ayres.—In New York, Richard S. Seaman, M D., to Miss Mary G. Byrne.

DIED,—On the 18th ult. at his residence in Springfield, N. H., of pulmonary consumption, Dr. Joseph Nichols, in the 57th year of his age. A brief sketch of the distinguished merits of the deceased as a moral, intellectual and medical man, will be furnished for publication in the Journal.—At Cayuga, N. Y., Dr. John Lawrence Milledoler, son of the late Rev. Philip Milledoler.—At Waterford, Vt, Dr. Abner Miles, 74.—At Cambridge, Vt.. Dr. B. S. Minor, 55.—At Theresa, N. Y., Dr. Oliver Brewster, 50—a lineal descendant of Elder Brewster, who came over in the Mayflower.

Deaths in Boston for the week ending Saturday noon, June 4th, 66. Males, 33—females, 33. Abscess, 1—accidental, 1—inflammation of the bowels, 1—inflammation of the brain, 2—disease of the bladder, 1—consumption, 13—convulsions, 4—croup, 2—diarrhœa, 1—dropsy in head, 5—infantile diseases, 3—typhoid fever, 1—scarlet fever, 6—homicide, 1—disease of heart, 1—inflammation of the lungs, 3—marasmus 3—measles, 2—old age, 1—poison, 1—palsy, 1—rheumatism, 1—smallpox, 1—suicide, 1—disease of the spine, 1—teething, 1—throat disease, 2—thrush, 1—unknown, 2—worms, 2.
Under 5 years, 32—between 5 and 20 years, 5—between 20 and 40 years, 21—between 40 and 60 years, 3—over 60 years, 5. Born in the United States, 46—Ireland, 16—England, 2—British Provinces, 1—Scotland, 1. The above includes 8 deaths in the city institutions.

Special Committees of the American Medical Association.—The following is a list of Chairmen of the Special Committees chosen at the last meeting of the American Medical Association, with the subjects to them committed.

1. Dr. D. F. Condie, of Philadelphia, Penn., "On the Causes of Tubercular Disease."
2. Dr James Jones, of New Orleans, La., "On the Mutual Relations of Yellow and Bilious Remittent Fever."
3. Dr. R. S. Holmes, of St. Louis, Mo., "On Epidemic Erysipelas."
4. Dr. George B. Wood, of Philadelphia, Penn., "On Diseases of Parasitic Origin."
5 Dr. R. D. Arnold, of Savannah, Geo., "On the Physiological Peculiarities and Diseases of Negroes."
6. Dr. James R Wood, of New York, "On Statistics of the Operation for the removal of Stone in the Bladder."
7. Dr. F. Peyre Porcher, of Charleston, S. C., "On the Toxicological and Medicinal Properties of our Cryptogamic Plants."
8. Dr. Goodrich A. Wilson, of Virginia, "On Cholera, and its Relation to Congestive Fever—their Ahalogy or Identity."
9. Dr. Worthington Hooker, of Connecticut, "On Epidemics of New England and New York.'
10. Dr. John L. Atlee, of Lancaster, Penn., "On Epidemics of New Jersey, Pennsylvania' Delaware and Maryland."
11. Dr. D. J. Cain, of Charleston, S. C., "On Epidemics of South Carolina, Florida, Georgia and Alabama."
12. Dr. W. L. Sutton, of Georgetown, Ky., "On Epidemics of Tennessee and Kentucky."
13. Dr. Thomas Reyburn, of St. Louis, Mo., "On Epidemics of Missouri, Illinois, Iowa and Wisconsin."
14. Dr. George Mendenhall, of Cincinnati, Ohio, "On Epidemics of Ohio, Indiana and Michigan."
15. Dr. E. D. Fenner, of New Orleans, La., "On Epidemics of Mississippi, Louisiana, Texas and Arkansas."
16. Dr. Charles A. Lee, of New York, "On Domestic Hygiene."
17. Dr. Daniel Brainard, of Chicago, Ill., "On the Constitutional and Local Treatment of Carcinoma ".
18. Dr. N. S. Davis, of Chicago, Ill., "On the Influence of Local Circumstances on the Origin and Prevalence of Typhoid Fever."
19. Dr. George Engelman, of St. Louis, Mo, "On the Influence of Geological Formation on the Character of Disease"
20. Dr. Henry M. Bullitt, of Louisville, Ky., "On the Use and Effect of Applications of Nitrate of Silver to the Throat, either in Local or General Disease."
21. Dr. Robert F. Campbell, of Augusta, Geo, "On the Pathogenic Influence of Feather Beds."
22. Dr. James Bolton, of Richmond, Va., "On the Administration of Anæsthetic Agents during Parturition."
23. Dr. Henry Taylor, of Mount Clemens, Mich, "On Dysentery."
24. Dr. F. Donaldson, of Baltimore, Md., "On the Present and Prospective Value of the Microscope in Disease."
25. Dr. R L. Howard, of Columbus, Ohio, "On the Pathology and Treatment of Scrofula."

Committee on Plans of Organization for State and County Societies.—Isaac Hays, M D, of Pennsylvania, Chairman; Worthington Hooker, M.D., of Connecticut; Josiah Andrews, M.D., of Michigan; B. R. Wellford, M D., of Virginia; A L. Peirson, M.D., of Massachusetts.

Committee on Medical Literature—T. S. Bell, M D, of Kentucky, Chairman; Samuel H. Pennington, M.D., of New Jersey; Edward H. Parker, M D, of New Hampshire; William K. Bowling, M.D, of Tennessee; Zina Pitcher, M D., of Michigan.

Committee on Medical Education.—B R. Wellford, M D., of Virginia, Chairman; Resign Lowe, M D., of Iowa; Lyndon A. Smith, M.D., of New Jersey; Jacob Bigelow, M.D., of Massachusetts; L. A. Dugas, M.D., of Georgia.

Committee on Volunteer Communications—Drs. C. A. Pope, Thomas Reyburn, John S. Moore, J. B. Johnson and A. Linton, of St. Louis, Mo.

Committee of Arrangements.—Drs. J. R. Washington, J. S. Moore, S. Pollok, Thos. Reyburn, L O'Farrar, W. M McPheeters, C. W. Hempstead and E. S. Lemoine, of St. Louis, Mo.

Committee on Publications.—Dr. D. F. Condie, Pennsylvania, Chairman; Dr. E. L. Beadle, of New York; Dr. A. Stillé, of Pennsylvania; Dr. I. Hays, Pennsylvania; Dr. E. S. Lemoine, of Missouri; Dr. G. Emerson and Dr. G. W. Norris, Pennsylvania.

On motion of Dr. Watson, of New York, the name of the Committee on Volunteer Communications was changed to that of Committee on Prize Essays.

Dr. Beaumont, whose death was mentioned in the Journal of May 25, was a native of Lebanon, Conn., where he was born in 1785. In 1812, after studying medicine at St. Albans, Vt., for two years, he joined the Sixth Infantry as an Assistant Surgeon. For more than twenty years he was a member of the medical staff of the Army, being stationed at various points on the Northern frontier. In 1830, he was stationed at Jefferson Barracks, and subsequently at St. Louis. About this time he resigned his commission, and resided in St. Louis, where he enjoyed an extensive private practice. A severe fall, producing severe contusions upon the back part of his head, is supposed to have caused his death. His experiments on digestion, in the person of Alexis St. Martin, the Canadian, some years since, have caused him to be well known.

THE

BOSTON MEDICAL AND SURGICAL JOURNAL.

| Vol. XLVIII. | Wednesday, June 15, 1853. | No. 20. |

SCARLET FEVER.

To the Editor of the Boston Medical and Surgical Journal.

SIR,—Having just perused, in your Journal of the 16th of February, Dr. Wood's treatment of scarlet fever, I have taken the liberty of sending you my own views and practice in this disease. We country physicians not being so much guarded as others by rules of professional etiquette, are perhaps too apt to adopt independent rules of practice, and to adhere to them whether right or wrong. Those who look with contempt on the practice and experience of country physicians, do so without reflection. Our opportunities for observation are far greater than such persons anticipate; and not being able to visit our patients so often, we are led to anticipate more closely changes which may occur in our absence. We cannot at all times call in a fellow practitioner, to return us a compliment which we may have made him, by strengthening our position with the friends, by the declaration that all is right; but we have to make good our position and abide its consequences—and I can assure you that we are very strictly watched. You see, therefore, that we are often thrown on our own resources, in cases where a city physician could readily call in some one to divide his responsibility.

I have had formerly much experience in scarlet fever. In the year 1832 I had nearly 800 cases, which assumed all shades and all degrees of malignity, from the mildness of the flea-bite to the virulence of the plague. What puzzled me much, was the great diversity in the character of the disease, and the great discrepancy among authors as to its nature and treatment. I found it breaking out here and there without exposure. In some cases several were sick in a family, and in others one or two; and besides, in some cases the rash would appear without the sore throat, in others the affection of the throat without the rash, in others both combined. In some cases in the same family it would manifest itself in enlargement of the parotid gland; but this usually occurred in infants at the breast. In others, the patient would be found in a state of collapse, with mottled, checked or purple appearance beneath or in the skin, without eruption or elevation of the surface. Now, thought I, can this be a contagious disease, exhibiting itself in such a diversity of forms? If so, why does it appear here and there without exposure ?   And besides, contagious diseases have something specific in their progress ; but in this, all appeared chaotic, not only in its protean character, but also in the treatment as laid down by different authors.   Now can order be brought out of confusion ?   With such reflections I carefully observed the different forms of the disease. At the same time I examined the throats of hundreds within its endemic influence, but who were not sick.   In all these cases I found congestion and engorgement of the papillæ of the tongue, with elongation of the soft palate, and some degree of purple appearance about the fauces. The cases of collapse resembled the appearances which I had observed in those exposed to fixed air from burning charcoal, and I had also observed in the latter an eruption somewhat analogous to that of scarlatina.

From these facts I came to the conclusion that the cause producing scarlatina was atmospheric ; that the first abnormal change was congestion or passive engorgement, or apoplexy of the mucous membrane, extending from the mouth through all its ramifications in the stomach and intestines, the bronchiæ and air-cells of the lungs, as well as in the nostrils and Eustachian tubes to the internal ear.   Now what is the first and immediate effect of this congested state of the mucous membrane ?   An impaired function of the lungs ; the blood is imperfectly decarbonized, and so great is the suspension of the function of aeration, that in severe cases the patient falls into a state of collapse, and dies as he would from the respiration of fixed air, without re-action— the dark-mottled appearance of the skin, in these cases, furnishing the only characteristic symptom as pointing out the nature of the disease. In slighter cases this first stage is not observed, and there appears no indication of illness till the eruption appears in the skin.   In other more severe cases, the soft palate and fauces become dark and ulcerated, or the retained carbon and perhaps some other noxious principle which induced the disease is spent by irritation of the parotid glands.   This engorgement of the capillary vessels, which constitutes essentially the disease (all the other morbid states being the result), produces as stated an impaired state of the function of respiration, or suspension of it.   In the latter case the patient falls into a state of collapse, and dies ; but when the function is impaired, the carbon is retained and its deleterious effect is manifested by the peculiar eruption which gives the name to this disease.   In the congestive stage the vessels of the throat are so over-distended as to lose their vitality, and the parts fall into ulceration or gangrene.   If this congestion be removed before the contractile power of the vessels is lost, they fall into a state of collapse ; but the function of the mucous surface is not immediately restored—the membrane assuming a shining and glazed appearance.   This state of the tongue is without doubt an index to that of the lining membrane of the stomach. By this condition of its mucous coat its function is impaired, and it is from this cause that so many fatal cases of relapse occur from improper food, even after slight cases of scarlatina.   I believe that in the mildest cases of this disease, this red and glazed appearance of the tongue is ever an attendant, so much so that an experienced observer can tell by this the character of the disease.

Having taken this view of cause and effect, as constituting this disease in all its protean characteristics, I was led to the adoption of the following practice, and twenty-five years' experience has confirmed my opinion of its correctness. In the early stage, while there is still congestion in the mucous membrane, I give an infusion of Cayenne pepper, repeating every ten or fifteen minutes till some effect is observed in the lessening of the purple appearance in the throat—giving it, perhaps, six or eight times. I then give ipecac. to produce free vomiting; and in case the throat is dark and somewhat ulcerated, I add sulphate of copper. In this case the pepper excites the vessels to action, and the concussion produced by the emetic is generally sufficient to relieve the oppressed membrane, and to restore the function of the lungs. If, however, there remain any purple appearance about the fauces and soft palate, I continue the pepper every hour till it is removed. I then treat the disease as mildly inflammatory. As this disease is one of extreme irritability, and the mucous coat of the stomach is in a glazed state, with its function impaired, I give but very little medicine. I usually give mucilages, and occasionally a little warm sage tea, and put the patient under the influence of belladonna. I use the German solution of the extract (three grains to the ounce). This I continue during the whole progress of the disease; and I am confident that no physician who has not given it a thorough trial is aware of its good effect. It lessens the violence of the disease, keeps out the eruption, and effectually equalizes the circulation in the capillary vessels. Since 1832 I have given it as a preventive, with invariable success whenever the directions were complied with. In fact, as I view the disease, no one can take it if brought under the influence of belladonna, for it effectually, by its action on the capillary vessels, prevents the congestion which primarily constitutes the disease. The tincture of colchicum and that of the Phytolacca Decandra, would unquestionably exert the same preventive powers. The relapse in scarlatina depends, no doubt, on the retention of too much carbon in the blood, with perhaps some of the deleterious miasm which first induced the disease, and as free action of the skin tends to eliminate this, Dr. Wood's practice would probably prove beneficial. If exposure to cold be avoided, and a careful regimen prescribed for a few days, there will be no danger of relapse. I think no solid food should be taken until the tongue has lost its glazed appearance. Cayenne pepper should never be used after the congestion in the mucous membrane is removed. I must, however, say, that, as far as I have observed the practice of others in this disease, the indiscriminate use of pepper, as practised by Thomsonians, has been far more successful than that of some physicians who treat it as inflammatory from its commencement (without reference to that passive state of engorgement which ushers in the disease), with their calomel, antimony, and cathartics. The one unnecessarily keeps up irritation, but his practice has removed the first morbid condition; while the other permits this congestion to continue, until fatal results ensue, which are often accelerated by calomel and other irritating medicines.

The question may be asked—Do you consider this disease contagious? I answer—Certainly not. In 1832 it prevailed for 50 miles around me, ever occurring in isolated families. Why, then, do those who are exposed take it ? They do not take it from the sick, but from the same endemic influence, and you will find its effects in examining all in the same locality. But why do several in the same family have it, while others escape ? Because there is similarity of constitution, and the same susceptibility to receive morbid impressions. Such members would have had it if kept a mile apart in the same locality. Such cases I have known. Contagious diseases cannot be prevented by medicine, but belladonna will prevent the access of this disease (if the extract is good) ; and besides, contagious diseases do not expose to relapse, while exposure to cold or over-eating disposes to it in this, during any period within two weeks.   M. F. COLBY, M.D.

Stanstead, Can. East, May 19, 1853.

LECTURES OF M. VALLEIX ON DISPLACEMENTS OF THE UTERUS.

TRANSLATED FROM THE FRENCH BY L. PARKS, JR., M.D.

NUMBER VI.

IT would be easy to unite in the same description simple anteversion, anteflexion, and anteversion with flexion, since these forms of displacement have extremely numerous points of resemblance ; but, as there are also certain differences, I think we shall be able to give a more exact and more complete view, by first describing simple anteversion, and then indicating wherein the two other forms differ from or resemble it.

In respect to anteversion, I shall enter into somewhat extended details, which will enable us to proceed more rapidly in the description of the other displacements, because then we shall have a type—a point of departure necessary to the understanding of the subject.

Definition.—There is simple anteversion *(pronatio-uteri)*— when, there being no flexion of the organ, the body of the uterus is inclined forward.

As the movement of inclination takes place about an imaginary point, situated not at the inferior portion of the neck of the womb, but near the junction of the body with the cervix, it occurs, as a natural result, that the cervix is borne upward and backward, when the body is inclined downward and forward.

Among the cases of anteversion which have come under our observation, 21 have been observed in a manner sufficiently exact to be of service in the study of this disease. The thesis of M. Ameline contains 18 cases, but since he did not observe them all himself, since he was not possessed of all the information relative to them which could be desired, and since he was not able in any way to verify those which were communicated to him, I shall avail myself only of the 21 cases collected by myself, having recourse to those of the above-mentioned writer, or to those recorded by other authors, merely for the purpose of comparison.

Causes.—We would mention first among the causes of anteversion, as well as of all other displacements, the *form* and the *anatomical posi-*

tion of the uterus. This organ possesses a considerable degree of mobility in the pelvis. It is supported by lax ligaments, susceptible of elongation, or of contraction, and may be consequently pushed forward, backward, or laterally, by changes in surrounding organs, by tumors, &c. Furthermore, the large extremity of the uterus being situated superiorly, allows the centre of gravity to be shifted, and the organ to swing over more easily than these changes could take place under opposite conditions.

It has been thought, further, that the *periodical congestions* to which the uterus is subjected during menstruation must favor the operation of these causes. But, to this it may be objected that if the length of the womb augments, at the catamenial period, all its other diameters increase in the same proportion, and thus the centre of gravity is not shifted.

The other physiological causes to which great importance has been attached are, first, the *changes in volume to which the organs surrounding the uterus are subjected,* and which, as I have just said, may push this organ in different directions ; and, secondly, the *relaxation of the ligaments,* in consequence of the traction undergone by them during pregnancy, in such a manner that they lose the power of effectually resisting the action of the causes just enumerated.

I must tell you, gentlemen, that several of these so-called causes have been alleged to be such from physiological considerations, and, that the study of cases has not as yet established their existence. It would be necessary, in order to remove all uncertainty on this head, that we should be able to consult the results of quite a considerable number of autopsies. But, at present, science possesses only a few records of post-mortem examinations, the greater part of which have been made upon subjects in which the disease had not been observed during life. Thus, when the state of the uterus and its appendages or of the organs in its neighborhood, is spoken of, reference is almost uniformly made to inferences drawn from the examination of these parts in the living subject, and not to strict demonstrations derived from necroscopic researches. But, I dwell no longer upon these causes, which, I repeat, are common to all displacements, and to which, consequently, I shall not have to recur.

Age.—M. Ameline says he has never seen anteversion before puberty. M. Huguier, however, has seen a case of congenital anteversion, and I myself met with the following probable case :—A young girl who had been directed to me, at the " Hôpital Beaujon," by M. Gillette, died of a typhoid fever, without having complained of the slightest symptom on the part of the uterus. There was no occasion, in such an affection, for examining this organ during life. But, at the autopsy, we found it lying transversely, and so situated that the body of the organ actually rested upon the bladder. It was light and not bulky, and had contracted no abnormal adhesions to the neighboring tissues.

This case tends to prove that displacement can exist without symptoms, up to a certain age. But, would not this condition of the parts be a sufficient reason for us to fear the appearance of symptoms, at a later period, when the organ should have attained its entire develop-

ment ? As to the patients who presented themselves to us with symptoms sufficiently grave to induce them to ask our interference, they were
from 20 to 38 years of age, at the time we first saw them—the average age of the whole being 30 years.   But it should be recollected,
that in all these cases, the disease had been in existence a certain length
of time.   In 17 cases only, we were able to ascertain, in an exact
manner, the precise epoch of the commencement of the complaint.
We found that its first appearance was between the ages of 19 and
33 years, with a mean age of 25 years and a very small fraction.   This
difference, which amounts to five years between the average age of
the patients at the commencement of the affection, and the average age
attained at the time of coming under our observation, is sufficient to
show us how great is the tendency of this disease to prolongation when
left to itself.

Constitution.*—The constitution was originally robust in 10 cases ;
in 9, moderately vigorous, and in 2, feeble.   But, generally, if the disease had been of any considerable duration, it was very rare that the
constitution was not more or less affected.

Temperament.—The difficulty which results in the appreciation of
temperaments from the numerous combinations of the elements of each,
in different individuals, led us to give special attention to this predisposing cause.   Eighteen of our patients, only, have appeared to offer
sufficiently predominant signs of this or that temperament to enable us to
note it.   In 6 the elements of the lymphatic temperament predominated,
especially in one, in which the muscles were flaccid, the surface exsan-
guine, and the submaxillary ganglions engorged.   In 6 others we found
the elements of the lymphatic united to those of the nervous temperament.   Five had a sanguine, and one a bilious temperament.

Leucorrhœa.—Leucorrhœa has been considered one of the causes of
anteversion.   Although, in order to elucidate this point, we have inquired
as to its existence before the appearance of the other symptoms, information on this head has most often either failed us, or been extremely
vague.   Four patients very positively assured us that they were free from
the discharge in question previously to their other troubles.   Three only
recollected having had it for a long time.   A fourth told us that she
had had it at a former period, as a sequence of a fall, and that it had
disappeared a long time before the commencement of the anteversion.
The rest gave us but very imperfect information on the subject.

Menstruation.—In relation to menstruation, we found it to have
been generally well established at the outset, with the exception of
those slight irregularities which almost always occur, and of which we
shall make no account.   One patient had been chlorotic for a year before the appearance of her menses, and three others had experienced
during the first months, irregularities—delays sufficient to lead us to attach a certain degree of importance to them.   Of those in whom menstruation had been once well established, four were affected with *dys-
menorrhœa* occurring before the other symptoms, while in one alone there

* " The General Health " of Marshall Hall ?—TRANS.

was a complete suppression of the menses during quite a long period of time. In this latter case, however, they had returned a very great while before the manifestation of the anteversion. We do not find, then, a single case in which suppression of the menses can be really regarded as a cause of this disease ; and, I ask myself the question, if the authors who have mentioned this disorder in this light, have not taken the effect for the cause.

Parturition.—The influence of parturition is more interesting to study than that of the causes above enumerated. Of the 20 cases which can be of service to us in this investigation, 18 women had had one or more labors at the full term. Of this number, 12 had borne a single child, and had then gone 2, 3, and 5 years without having any. One among them had had two miscarriages after child-bearing.

Of the 6 others who had borne children, 1 had had two, 2 had had three, 1 had had four, one other five, and the last had borne six. In two cases the labor had been severe ; in another it had been followed by hemorrhage ; and in a fourth by inflammation. Saving these few exceptions, the labors had presented nothing peculiar.

One only of our patients *had risen too soon* (four days) after delivery. All the others had kept the bed at least nine days.

Such, gentlemen, are the facts I have been able to collect upon this subject. I give them to you not as an exact representation of that which is, or of that which must be, in the majority of cases (of which last I have not a sufficient number on which to found such a representation), but as a document which may be usefully consulted at need.

Miscarriage.—Three only of our patients had miscarried. In two of these the miscarriages had been followed by delivery at the full term, and, by consequence, had not been concerned in bringing about the displacements supervening at a later period. In the third, on the contrary, two successive miscarriages took place, after a first labor at the full term. The history of this case is so interesting that I feel compelled to lay it before you.

Case II.*—A. C. entered the " Hôpital Beaujon," Sept. 27th, 1851 —pale, thin, of a moderately good constitution. From the age of 12 to that of 16 years she had leucorrhœa, ceasing after the commencement of menstruation, which was laborious, and furnished but a scanty discharge. At 17, she underwent delivery at the full term, the labor lasting twenty-four hours, and there being no unfavorable symptom. She avoided undue exertion for several weeks, and the menses re-appeared regularly after the second month. At 26 years of age, after nine years of perfect health, she had a miscarriage at the second month, followed by attacks of hemorrhage, in consequence of which anemia set in, was treated by iron, and was succeeded by the re-establishment of health. But two years later a new pregnancy took place, at the commencement of which the patient was troubled with lumbar pains. Hemorrhage oc-

---

* All the cases cited having been explained at length, at the clinical visits, and remaining still in the hands of M. Valleix, to be, in all probability, re-produced at a future time, I shall give here only as succinct a summary as possible, and shall abstain especially from detailing the examination of the patients, when it presents nothing extraordinary —T. GALLARD.

curred at the third month, and was followed by a new abortion. According to the statement of her physician, a portion of the placenta remained in the uterus,' and was not expelled till several days had elapsed, and after the administration of ergot. A. C. was then obliged to keep the bed for six months, the menses not re-appearing till the third month. From that time she constantly experienced weakness in the limbs, feelings of weight and dragging sensations *(tiraillemens)* in the pelvis, in the loins, and in the groins. The appetite was irregular and the digestion impaired. There was no trouble either in defecation or in micturition. The pain occasioned by walking was so severe that latterly she had not left her chamber.

The 27th of December I examined her with M. Danyau, when we ascertained that there was an anteversion of the uterus. We made in conjunction with each other a sketch to recall the position in which we found the organ. This and the few following days the sound was passed. The operation was not painful, and was followed only by the flow of a few drops of blood. On the 30th, application—slightly fatiguing for the patient—of a pessary with an immovable stem *(redresseur à flexion fixe)*, which was taken away, at the end of twenty-four hours, in consequence of the appearance of the menses ten or twelve days before their usual period. They were more abundant than was their wont.

The 10th of October, on examining the patient again with M. Danyau, I found the cervix still directed backward, but presenting its opening in such a manner as to be more easy of attainment. The body was inclined forward in its normal position. To the anteversion there had succeeded a slight flexion with a displacement of the cervix backward. The patient felt better, and at her request was allowed to leave the Hospital.

From the 16th to the 21st, she had quite a severe enteritis.

The 21st, I re-applied the pessary. It remained three days, at the end of which it was thrown out of place by a movement of the patient. Re-placed the 20th, it was well borne for thirteen days. It was taken away the 9th of December, in consequence of the appearance of the menses, which lasted twelve days. Those of January were also very abundant. After the pessary was removed, the uterus was found in its normal position, and has thus remained, as I had an opportunity of ascertaining scarcely a month since. Walking has become easy, and the symptoms which existed in connection with the digestive functions have disappeared. A. C. is in a state of health such as she did not enjoy from the commencement of her symptoms, up to the present time.

THE PULSE, CRANIAL DIMENSIONS, &c., OF THE SOUTHERN NE-
GRO CHILD, WITH SOME REMARKS UPON INFANTILE
THERAPEUTICS.

To the Editor of the Boston Medical and Surgical Journal.

Sir,—As there is much discrepancy existing in the accounts given of the physical characteristics of our negro race, I send you a few of the physico-vital mensurations of the negro child, which I have carefully taken with a neat graduated tape, in the presence of reputable persons. I have thrown them together in tabular form, from which you can deduce your own analogical conclusions. I wish the tables were more extensive; but they were secured amid my daily peregrinations, and as the field is comparatively an unexplored one, I hope you and your readers will not ask too much at once, or hurriedly censure any slight inaccuracies which may occur, and which I shall be pleased to correct.

A Diagram of the Pulse, Cranial Dimensions, &c. of Southern Negro Children at different Ages and of both Sexes.

No.	Age.	Pulse.	Inter-Palpebral Occipito.	Cranial Circumference.	Sex.	Color.
1	3 yrs.	81	$14\frac{1}{2}$	$19\frac{1}{2}$	male.	dark.
2	7 "	82	$15\frac{5}{8}$	21	"	"
3	4 "	83	$15\frac{1}{2}$	$20\frac{1}{4}$	"	"
4	4 "	85	15	$20\frac{1}{2}$	"	"
5	3 "	87	$13\frac{1}{4}$	$19\frac{1}{4}$	"	"
6	4 "	84	$14\frac{5}{8}$	20	"	"
7	6 "	84	$14\frac{1}{4}$	$20\frac{1}{4}$	female.	"
8	2 "	88	$13\frac{3}{4}$	19	male.	"
9	2 "	88	$13\frac{7}{8}$	$19\frac{1}{4}$	"	light.
10	1 "	100	$12\frac{1}{4}$	$16\frac{7}{8}$	"	dark.
11	7 "	92	$14\frac{5}{8}$	$19\frac{1}{2}$	"	"
12	2 "	100	$13\frac{3}{8}$	$19\frac{7}{8}$	"	"
13	5 "	96	$14\frac{1}{2}$	20	"	light.
14	5 "	96	$14\frac{1}{2}$	$19\frac{3}{4}$	"	"
15	7 "	98	$14\frac{3}{8}$	$20\frac{3}{8}$	female.	dark.
16	7 "	81	$14\frac{1}{8}$	$19\frac{7}{8}$	"	light.
17	7 "	81	$14\frac{1}{2}$	$19\frac{3}{4}$	"	"
18	6 "	88	14	$19\frac{3}{4}$	"	dark.
19	5 "	86	14	$19\frac{3}{8}$	male.	"
20	3 "	98	$13\frac{1}{2}$	$20\frac{1}{8}$	"	"
21	1 "	108	$12\frac{1}{4}$	$17\frac{5}{8}$	female.	light.
22	5 "	91	14	$19\frac{7}{8}$	"	dark.
23	5 "	94	$14\frac{1}{2}$	$20\frac{1}{4}$	male.	"
24	3 "	100	$13\frac{1}{2}$	$18\frac{1}{2}$	"	light.
25	5 "	100	$13\frac{5}{8}$	19	female.	"
26	6 "	100	$14\frac{1}{2}$	$19\frac{3}{4}$	"	"
27	7 "	85	$14\frac{1}{2}$	$20\frac{3}{8}$	"	dark.
28	3 "	102	13	19	male.	light.
29	2 "	107	$13\frac{1}{4}$	$18\frac{1}{4}$	"	"
30	6 ms.	116	$10\frac{1}{4}$	$15\frac{1}{4}$	female.	"
31	7 yrs.	92	$14\frac{1}{4}$	$20\frac{7}{8}$	male.	"
32	1 "	108	$13\frac{1}{4}$	$18\frac{1}{4}$	"	dark.

I do not claim for these data that they settle, beyond cavil, any question to which they relate; but as they are the only effort I have seen in this direction, I claim for them just what they *indicate of the subjects to which they refer*, and *no more*, while every one can draw his own conclusions, upon inferential grounds. In the admeasurements I was very careful that they were all taken with a corrected measure; and the arterial beats were noted by a watch, and committed to paper at the moment. In casting up the tables, and making the comparative averages, I may have made some errors, for I did it under pressing professional circumstances; yet I beg the reader to point out all such inaccuracies, for I assure him I want nothing incorrect, as *truth* and *science* are too sacred to be prostituted to erroneous calculations upon statistical data which may be of paramount importance. In connection with these tables it was my design to furnish you with a series of similar ones upon the pulse, &c., of the white child; but circumstances have operated to prevent this, though I hope, at a future time, to fill the vacuum.

The Monthly and Annual Averages of the Negro Child's Pulse, upon Sexual and Non-sexual Principles.

The average rate of the male per min.		93·28
" " female	"	93 80
At the age of 4 to 6 months	"	116·
" of 1 year	"	105.
" of 2 years	"	95.
" of 3 years	"	93·
" of 4 years	"	84·
The male from 1 to 4 years averages		95·
The female from 1 to 4 years averages		108

The Comparative Averages, and Annual Developments of the Negro Child's Head, upon Sexual Principles.

From the inter-palpebral space to basilar part of the occiput, in all sexes and ages tabularized	14	inches
The average circumference in all, &c.	17	"
At 6 months, the inter-palpebral and basilar occip. space, female	$10\frac{1}{4}$	"
1 year " " " "	$12\frac{1}{4}$	"
5 years " " " "	14	"
6 years	$14\frac{1}{4}$	'
7 years " " " "	$14\frac{1}{2}$	'
Average circumference of the female head in all cases,	19	'
At 4 to 6 months " " " "	$15\frac{1}{8}$	"
1 year " " " "	$17\frac{5}{8}$	'
5 years " "	19	".
6 years " " ..	$19\frac{3}{8}$	"
7 years " " " "	$20\frac{1}{8}$	"
The average inter-palpebral and occipital space of male	14·15	"
At 1 year " " " "	12·75	"
2 years " " " "	13·75	"
3 to 4 years " "	16·	"
3 to 7 years " "	16·62	"
The average circumference, male	19·55	"
At 1 year " "	11	"
2 years " "	19	..
3 years ..	19	"
4 to 5 years " ..	19	"
6 years "	20·85	"

. An examination of the above tables will exhibit, that the pulse of the male child is a shade faster than that of the female. This I have no doubt all subsequent investigations will verify. And I am farther inclined to think the pulse of the white child is faster than that of the negro. This is a mere opinion, however, subject to confirmation or disproval hereafter. That climate, temperament, health, &c., control the pulse to some degree in all colors, sexes and ages, every man will admit; hence, it is a very difficult matter, if not impossible, to settle the pulse at any definite beat.

In the cranial developments of the sexes, it will be seen that the growth of the skull advances faster from six months to three years than at any other period. How far further tables may confirm this, I am not prepared to say, but will abide the only correct means of determining it, viz., *the mensuration of more subjects.*

I have thought, for a series of years, and yet think, that southern children weigh more at birth than those of New England, and I would be happy to exchange protocols with some gentleman upon this point. That southern children grow off faster, and develope sooner, than yours of New England, I think scarcely susceptible of controversy.

The southern negro child is a fat, healthy subject. You of Massachusetts would be astonished to see how the southerners raise them in the rural districts. They are the companions and playmates of the planter's own children; they mess together, and it is really amusing to see four or five little white urchins, and as many blacks, get around a dish of "*pot-liquor*" or a pan of molasses, each with a piece of corn bread, and every one master of "*all he surveys.*" I have thought, if there was happiness in the world, this social exhibition and fraternity of feeling among the black and white children of the South, afforded it. If you dare intrude upon the white one of the gang, the black will resent it; if you infringe on the reserved privileges of *Davy*, the white child will repel it. I have not unfrequently seen my little son Johnny fight for his little negro playmates, and *vice versa.* This is a fair picture of the way they are raised in the country South. There may be some few and particular exceptions to it, but what I say is the common plan. The consequence is, when they grow up, under such influences, there is a mutual tie of reciprocal attachment, between the white and black, which nothing can sever. I have no kind of doubt but there are hundreds and thousands of southern blacks so ardently attached to the masters of their childhood, that in no event would they become free, if opportunity offered. But this is a digression, and I will pass on to a more practical and useful theme.

Infantile Therapeutics of the South.—I do not attempt to indite an essay of erudite learning upon this question, but merely to make a few suggestive details, of a practical character, that our brethren North may see how we far-off Georgians do things at home.

Diarrhœa.—Probably the most common of all diseases South, among our children, is *bowel disease.* It originates in the spring and summer months, from the uncontrolled use of fruit, and other causes. The negro and white child South, are the finest specimens of rude democracy and republicanism you ever saw; they eat *plums, apples, peaches, melons, vegetables,* &c., *ad satisfaciendum,* and no man dare interfere at "*that fig tree.*" They eat comparatively little meat. The result is, bowel affections of a lienteric and other characters. Sometimes the affection grows obstinate, inducing fever, intestinal pain, &c. ; and unless a prudent prescription is made, it now and then proves fatal. Indeed, I may say that at least half of our infantile mortality arises from this affection. The most common plan of treating the disease, when febrile symptoms supervene, is the mercurial practice. I have found it very successful, in combination with soda and the cretaceous mixture. I have long since repudiated the idea of a mercurial in everything. I admire its virtues when properly and legitimately administered, but I have no doubt that many a child has been sent to an untimely grave by its injudicious use in this disease. It is perfectly preposterous to suppose that the liver is at fault in every case of infantile diarrhœa, and that a mercurial is therefore the remedy. I am confident many children are sacrificed to this isolated abstraction, which has its origin in error, and its end too often in death. The purgative plan is fallacious. To me it appears unphilosophical to be dosing a child with purgatives, to remedy a disease, the prominent feature of which is *too much purgation.* I usually give a mercurial or other laxative, as may suggest, to clear the track of the intestines of any effete matter. I then use astringent, cretaceous or other mixtures, with poultices, and leeches if necessary, to the abdomen. In obstinate cases of long continuance, 1 have used the persesquin. iron very successfully, in connection with opium. Enemas of tannin, and other astringents, go admirably, but I have never derived much good from nit. argenti.

Trismus Nascentium.—I have heard much of trismus, but have seen little of it, and I am loth to think it is as common as has been suspected. I have seen many children die in convulsions, some of which cases would doubtless be called trismus, but I cannot permit myself to apply a desperate name to every loss I have, merely to cover my bill of mortality in an excusable way. I am fearful that the diagnosis of our brethren is at fault about this trismus question ; or at least that it does not occur as often in country practice as in city. What cases I have seen have been fatal, none recovering. I regard it as a disease of great havoc ; but for the comfort of mothers, I am happy to say, that, so far as my information and observation extends—*it is of very rare occurrence.* I make no therapeutic suggestion, as I have none worthy of confidence.

Remittent and Intermittent Fever.—The diarrhœa of southern children occasionally degenerates into remittent or intermittent fever, or sometimes I have seen an intermittent diarrhœa, with pure febrile signs ; but I imagine pure and uncomplicated remittent and intermittent fever is not so common now as formerly. It sometimes occurs, and it is more difficult to manage than in the adult. I usually, for the first form, adopt the mercurial practice gently, and if I can find a remission sufficiently obvious, I use quinine. If the bowels pass off too much, with tormina, I use poultices, opium, and leeches if necessary. This plan will generally succeed, unless the case is malignant, and then the judgment must determine the general curriculum of management. The intermittent form of the disease yields readily to quinine, arsenic, and other antiperiodics.

Convulsions.—From a variety of causes, such as over-eating, using crude food, &c., southern children often have convulsions. I see a great number of such cases. The best plan of treatment is to clear the bowels rapidly with an enema or brisk purgative. But if the fit depend upon a looseness of bowels, as is sometimes the case, I give invariably an opiate ; leech and poultice the bowels, use the warm bath, with the cold douche, and while in bed keep the temples leeched, and head covered with cold linen, made so by cold water or ice. I have never had any cause to regret this general practice—always cutting the gums if necessary.

Aphtha.—Southern children at the breast frequently have thrush, which I think is caused by an accumulation of milk in the mouth ; and I usually prescribe a prophylactic with marked benefit—that is, *to wash the child's mouth with cold water and a soft linen after nursing, and also the nipple.* Adopting this simple plan, I have never had a case of aphtha in my own family, and I hear the same success follows the adoption of it by others. When, however, I meet a case, I usually prescribe a solution of sulph. zinc, or the chloride soda, for the cure, and I prefer them to all other agents. When the aphtha is complicated with intestinal or bronchial disorder, the treatment must be modified to suit the demand.

Hooping Cough.—This affection sometimes occurs in country practice, and I have seen it occasionally. In this clime it requires a mild expectorant treatment, and is rarely fatal in its simple form. A decoction of peach leaf is a fine domestic remedy for it, assisted with syrup scillæ and paregoric.

Measles and Scarlatina.—Both affections prevail in our rural districts, in an epidemic form sometimes. The former requires but little management to insure safety. Keep warm, drink warm teas, and avoid atmospheric exposure, and the cases usually convalesce. Children here suffer but little from it, unless it is a very malignant variety.

Scarlet fever, in former years, has killed a great many children ; but I am inclined to think it has partly resulted from a therapeutic error. The disease requires the mildest treatment ; gentle emetics, poultices to the throat, gargles, scarifications, and mild laxatives or injections, constitute the rational plan, while harsh medication is deleterious. The learned and complicated plans of treating it put forth by Armstrong, Condie and others, have not only obscured rational thought upon its pathology, but have prevented the use of proper remedies. The treatment laid down by them may do in a frigid clime, but it is death here.

I might extend this paper to a much greater length, but my time and engagements will not permit. I hope the few fugitive thoughts which I have carelessly thrown together, may meet with the attention if not edify the medical practitioners of the North. I am sure, in my own mind, that the difference in our latitudinal positions makes a material one in our therapeutics. I think, also, the southern child is unable to stand the infliction of general venesection, while it bears leeching pretty fairly.

Nor will the child in this region bear drastic medication of any kind, in any considerable degree.

If in any of these opinions I err, I stand ready for correction. I am not forgetful of the old maxim—" To err is human ;" and while I grant its truth in regard to others, in all the charity imaginable, I ask an extension of its kindly influence to myself.   In great haste, &c.,

Thompson, Geo., May 28, 1853.   H. A. RAMSAY.

PERMANENT CURE OF REDUCIBLE HERNIA.

[GEORGE HEATON, M.D., of Boston, whose success in the treatment of hernia is extensively acknowledged, has issued in a pamphlet form a review of the Report of the Committee on Hernia appointed last year by the American Medical Association. Of course we shall not undertake to comment particularly on the matter in dispute between Dr. H. and the Committee, but shall copy a portion of his pamphlet, as we did of theirs, to show our readers what he has published concerning his mode of operating by injection. The question in which the profession are interested, is simply this—Can reducible hernia be cured ? The large number of successful cases cited by Dr. Heaton in his appendix, shows that his method operates well in practice, and would seem to answer the question in the affirmative. Those who have read the report of the Committee alluded to, will be interested in the perusal of the review of it, and they will then be enabled to appreciate the labors of each party in the literature as well as the practice of hernial surgery. The following brief extracts from it are all that it is necessary for us to copy.—ED.]

As the Committee have much to say of the operation by injection, the value of which, in my opinion, they exaggerate entirely, and the origin of which, whether accidentally or intentionally, they attribute to the wrong source, I will give the true account of the origin and value of this operation ; from which, I will premise, two conclusions will be obvious, at variance with those to which the Committee seem to have come. First, that Dr. Pancoast is not the originator of the operation by injection ; that I performed it, and described it to my friend Dr. Mott, of New York ; and, moreover, that Dr. Jayne, of Illinois, had invented an instrument for performing said operation, and secured letters patent on the same two years before Dr. Pancoast, according to his own account, made any experiments with it. Secondly, that the sub-cutaneous operation by injection of the hernial sac, is neither a simple nor advisable operation ; that, although successful in many cases, if rightly performed, the difficulty of performing it without bad consequences ought to condemn it entirely.

My attention, with that of Dr. Hart, of Alton, Illinois, was first directed more particularly to the operation by injection of the sac, for the radical cure of hernia, by Dr. Jayne, who had invented an instrument for performing such an operation, and before coming to us, had, in the year 1840, secured a patent on the same.

Having at that time under our care several cases of reducible hernia, among the convicts in the Penitentiary at Alton, we immediately set about testing the value of the operation on the persons of these, and also on some of the blacks at St. Louis. The operation consisted in injection of the sac subcutaneously with an irritating fluid, by means of the instrument before mentioned. In the selection of a fluid for the purpose, Dr. Jayne gave the preference to some one of the essential oils, using now and then tincture of cantharides. In my first operations I used, also, the essential oils, but soon abandoned them for the tincture of iodine. I believe, therefore, that I performed the operation of injection with iodine, of which so much has been said, before any other man.

Before our experiments, the operation of injection by the subcutaneous method had never been performed in this country or in Europe. At least no report had been made of any such operation, and there is no reason to suppose that it had ever been undertaken.

With the success of these experiments we were much elated, and felt that the desideratum for the radical cure of hernia had at length been discovered. Subsequently, in November, 1841, I communicated the result of the operation to Dr. Valentine Mott, of New York. He expressed himself highly pleased with it, and made a complimentary allusion to it in his lectures before the University. * * * * * *

The operation by injection, in many cases so satisfactory and apparently so permanent, in others was not so. Frequently it required to be repeated several times on the same individual, and in all cases the utmost care was required in its performance to avoid troublesome consequences, as, I understood, those of the Committee who undertook it found out.

Becoming dissatisfied with this operation, and having already, in the course of my investigations, tested every principle of any degree of plausibility which had been suggested or relied upon by operators in times past, for the cure of hernia, with no satisfactory results, I felt that the only hope of permanent cure in all or in a majority of cases of hernia, lay in some *modus operandi*, the effect of which should be an approximation of the pillars of the abdominal ring, or a closure of the tendinous openings. For a long time, therefore, I conducted all my researches with a view of getting at some principle which would enable me to accomplish this.

These researches, in which of necessity I was obliged to rely almost entirely on theory alone, did conduct me, I am happy to say, to precisely such a principle; a principle on which I have based a mode of treatment and operation which closes effectually and permanently the various openings through which hernial protrusions take place. Not only, indeed, does it do this, but in those cases where, from a general weakness resulting from the extreme delicacy of the textures connected with hernia, or a thinness, as it were, of the *parietes abdominales*, there is a positive predisposition to the complaint, I have found that it rendered the part firmer and better able to resist pressure than its original condition.

In such cases, where there has been a recurrence of hernia, I have almost invariably found it occurring at some other opening. Thus, when I have cured a person of oblique inguinal hernia, and he has afterwards, from a fall or violent strain, brought it on anew, it has proved, almost without exception, to be direct inguinal hernia.

THE BOSTON MEDICAL AND SURGICAL JOURNAL.

BOSTON, JUNE 15, 1853.

Galvanism.—C. H. Cleaveland, M.D., formerly of Waterbury, Vt., is the author of a pamphlet, heralding the great remedial powers of galvanism. Almost every disease is represented in it as vanishing before the influence of this extraordinary agent, and on this account it has the appearance of being nothing more nor less than a special advertisement. Towards the close, there are comments on Seymour's Galvanic Supporters, which rather confirms the reader in the opinion that the immense good to the public to be accomplished by the circulation of the pamphlet is to be accompanied by a special benefit to the proprietors. Men are rarely so purely benevolent as to collect and arrange the number of alleged facts brought together in this instance, for no other purpose than the good of those who may read them. Perhaps it may be discovered hereafter, that Dr. Cleaveland, who is well known as a writer in our medical periodicals, has had extensive experience in the administration of this most potent of nature's instrumentalities, and that the instruments he recommends are of great value. No one holds in higher estimation than ourselves, the appropriate use of medical electricity ; but there is an absurdity on the face of the proposition, that because it has proved an efficient remedy in one case, or half a dozen cases, it is therefore a panacea for all others.

Fusel Oil.—A correspondent in Connecticut is desirous to have something more in the Journal about fusel oil. Whether in pulmonary affections any decided benefit has been derived by the use of it, is not precisely settled. Some expectations were raised, at one time, that important results would follow its use. It was even almost believed that the development of tubercles in the lungs might be arrested by the new medical agent. Of late, very little is said upon the subject. Dr. Charles T. Jackson's paper, which was given in this Journal some months since, embraced the whole ground in regard to its chemical origin. Those who have had practical experience in its administration, and are therefore familiar with its therapeutic properties, should make them known to the medical public.

" *Duties, Discouragements and Hopes of the Medical Profession,*" is the title of a discourse before the State Medical Society of Louisiana, by J. M. W. Picton, M.D., late President of the Institution. Here at the North Dr. P. is principally known as a surgeon. A great operation performed by him at New Orleans, some years ago—the life of a negro being saved by the excision of an enormous scrotal enlargement—is still distinctly remembered. We discover by the address that the hopes, duties and discouragements of medical gentlemen at the South, are pretty much like our own in this forty-second degree of north latitude. At the beginning of the address reference is made to the ceaseless activity of the age. The mental energies are necessarily taxed severely, if any additions are intended to be made to the present storehouse of knowledge left us by our predecessors. Those who have the elements of progression in their composition, have a busy time of it. Dr. Picton has an orderly mode of reasoning, and a vigor and cogency in presenting truth, united with an active temperament, a disciplined mind, and a thorough insight into the mysteries of medical life. His cultivated taste is indicated by poetical extracts liberally interspersed through the text. They express sentiments in elegant forms, and by their terseness impress the mind more forcibly than the same thoughts in a different arrangement of language, and are therefore pleasant additions to the author's train of remarks. While Dr. Picton discusses the gratifications and grievances incident to a professional career, he refers to weaknesses belonging to the unrewarded servants of the community. "Even the village surgeon," he says, "now acts according to the newest fashion of some great transatlantic operator; and when two country physicians meet for consultation in the log cabin of a back-woodsman, they discuss the propriety of a practice, which, but thirty days before, had been proposed by a professor in one of the ancient Universities of Europe." A gentleman who can write with so much strength, should either tax himself or be stimulated by his friends to contribute largely to the archives of medical literature.

Suffolk District Medical Society—Dr. Williams's Address.—On the 30th of April, the fourth anniversary meeting of the Suffolk District Medical Society was held in Boston, and Henry W. Williams, M.D., one of the members, delivered an address which has since been published. After a proper allusion to the obligations imposed on the practitioner of medicine, the main subject of the speaker was diseases of the eye. He did not particularize symptoms, or fatigue his audience by tedious descriptions of morbid appearances. In the following sentence he expressed precisely what every one who heard him acknowledged to be true. "It is natural that, sooner or later, almost every physician should acquire a reputation for his knowledge or management of some particular diseases." In this section of the country, and especially in the large cities, individual practitioners are beginning to conduct a single branch of practice. The public believe that a disease can be more securely given in charge to a man whose entire thoughts are bestowed upon one malady, than to one whose mind is distracted with general practice. No matter how many fulminating edicts may be circulated against this tendency of the day, it cannot be arrested. The divisions of practice will be established, and special practitioners are becoming more skilful, while the benefit to the community as well as their own receipts are greater. Dr. Williams is an oculist of whom we hear an excellent account, and he is destined for eminence as such. His remarks in this address are practical and judicious, and may be read with profit by every practitioner. It is complimentary to him that the First Medical District Society in the State should have published his address at their own expense.

Reasoning from Effects.—A reverend gentleman, Dr. Noyes, of Providence, R. I., towards the completion of a series of lectures on the "Truth of the Bible," addressed a note to his friend, Abner Phelps. M.D., of Boston, for the purpose of obtaining his views, as a physiologist, respecting the flow of water from the wound made by the centurion in our Saviour's side, while he was upon the cross. A common opinion seems to be prevalent among theologians, that the pericardium was punctured, and that

the fluid was from that source.   Dr. Phelps returned an answer to Dr.
Noyes's request, which appears at the close of the volume of lectures,
and is of unusual interest.   It presents a critical analysis of the whole
transaction, to its melancholy termination.   Dr. P. shows, that had water
existed in the pericardium, in sufficient quantity to have been called a
flow, it would have indicated disease.   But the Redeemer was without
spot or blemish, and in perfect health, as a man, at the eventful period of
the crucifixion.   After a variety of ingenious and elaborate arguments,
Dr. Phelps presents a new theory, explanatory of the apparent difficulty
of accounting for the water.   He has, with commendable zeal, collected
facts enough to show that at death, the serum is separated, but not before,
and hence the Saviour must have been dead when the wound was made.
Here is the pith of the matter—" The veins generally contain about two
thirds of the whole mass of the blood, without any oxygen in it; while
the arteries contain about one third part, with oxygen.   Consequently, if
the whole mass of blood in the body, contained fifteen pints of water, the
arteries would contain five pints, when the blood therein had coagulated
—or, in other words, had concreted, which is merely the separation of the
serum from the crassamentum."   Dr. Phelps supposes that a cut artery
would permit the escape of serum—and thus the water is accounted for
on plain anatomical principles.

Another question has also been investigated by the same indefatigable
student of the Bible.   Some have imagined that it would be quite impossible to drive a heavy iron spike through the hands or feet, without breaking a bone.   Dr. Phelps went to the medical college, where facilities were
presented for conducting a sufficient number of experiments to satisfy the
most incredulous, and found that the act may be performed many times
in succession, without disturbing essentially the relations of the bony
parts.   Dr. Phelps has secured to himself the reputation of being a bold
inquirer.   He pursues his investigations with an ardor that is never satisfied with anything short of an actual demonstration, where such is
possible.

Nothing New in Medicine.—This is a common observation, and from
being in every body's mouth is presumed to be true.   But, after all, there
must be some advances making in practical medicine, as well as in everything else.   An examination of the past proves, beyond contradiction, that
up to this time, there has been constant progress in the science.   Yet
there are conservatives in the medical ranks, as well as among politicians,
who are perpetually saying, in effect—" pray, gentlemen, let well enough
alone."   Thousands of physicians neither think nor explore beyond the
chart placed before them in the books.   They have a distaste for innovations, and would much prefer to live out their three score and ten years
in the happy conviction that Cullen's Practice and Motherby's folio Dictionary embody all that is worth knowing in the divine art of healing.
They neither purchase new books nor give their sanction to modern pathological investigations.   They firmly set their faces against vaunted discoveries in the materia medica and in surgery ; and, above all, the use of
ether or chloroform, to obliterate sensation under any circumstances,
strikes them with a kind of holy horror.   Could we dwell upon the subject, it might be shown that through the efforts of medical men, sanitary
measures have been put in force ; uninhabited districts changed into delightful residences ; the public health of European and American cities greatly

improved, and the longevity of the world thereby promoted. Who, then, can proclaim, with a show of truth, that there are no advances in medical science ? Each revolving year brings something to delight or astonish the conscientious physician, as each discovery arms him with new powers for contending against prejudice, conservative idleness and the inroads of disease.

Poisonous Dropsical Inoculation.—An accident of a singular and dangerous nature recently befel the celebrated surgeon Prof. Langenbeck, in Berlin. Having been called in to attend a lady of high rank, in a most advanced and perilous stage of dropsy, Dr. L. deemed it necessary to proceed without delay, to puncturation, and this without waiting for other assistance. The operation was, therefore, instantly and successfully performed, and the patient, previously at death's door, relieved and saved. During the operation, however, some of the acrid discharge fell upon his hand, and was of course washed off when the work was completed ; but ere long the hand, arm, throat and neighboring regions began to swell, and all the febrile and inflammatory symptoms of animal poison ensued, Vigorous remedies were forthwith employed, and the danger averted, but the Professor is not yet so entirely recovered as to enjoy the full use of the side affected, whilst the venom has shown its lurking agency by causing eruptions on other parts of the body.

Medical Miscellany.—Dr. Jos. Leidy, of Philadelphia, has been appointed Professor of Anatomy in the University of Pennsylvania, in place of Dr. Horner, deceased ; and Dr. Wm. B. Page has been appointed one of the surgons of St. Joseph's Hospital, Philadelphia, also in place of Dr. Horner. —The American Medical Society of Paris has issued a circular, making known several additions to its constitution, whereby its usefulness will be likely to be increased. All communications and books for the Society are received and forwarded by Mr. Edw. Bossange, 134 Pearl street, New York.—Dr. W. G. Edwards, Professor of Clinical Medicine, &c., in the Medical Department of St. Louis University, has resigned his chair.—A letter from Dr. H. A. Ramsay, of Georgia, to Dr. Bryan, of Philadelphia, on the southern negro, has been issued in a pamphlet. Dr. R. has an article on the same subject in the Journal of to-day.—Dr. J. L. Smith's essay on the sudden coma of typhus and typhoid Fevers, and typhoid pneumonia, has been re-published in a pamphlet from the New York Journal of Medicine.—Drs. Wood and Bache are on a visit from this country to Paris.

MARRIED,—At Bridgewater, Dr. Luther W. Clarke, of Lake Superior, to Miss Mary G. Thacher.

DIED,—At New York, Ralph E. Elliot, M.D., of South Carolina, 55, a graduate of Harvard College in the class of 1818.

Deaths in Boston for the week ending Saturday noon, June 11th, 69. Males, 37—females, 32. Accidents, 2—apoplexy, 1—inflammation of the bowels, 2—disease of the brain, 5—burns and scalds, 1—consumption, 15—convulsions, 1—croup, 2—cancer, 1—dropsy, 1—dropsy in head, 3 —drowned, 1—infantile diseases, 2—puerperal, 4—scarlet fever, 5—disease of heart, 3—disease of hip, 1—intemperance, 1—inflammation, 1—inflammation of the lungs, 6—congestion of the lungs, 1½—marasmus, 3—mortification, 1—sun stroke, 1—teething, 1—pleurisy, 1—thrush, 1—unknown, 2.
Under 5 years, 30—between 5 and 20 years, 11—between 20 and 40 years, 15—between 40 and 60 years, 11—over 60 years, 2. Born in the United States, 49—Ireland, 15—England, 2—Scotland, 1—Wales, 1—Germany, 1. The above includes 7 deaths in the city institutions.

Statistics of Paris for 1853.—The Parisian correspondent of the Virginia Medical and Surgical Journal gives the following minute particulars respecting the mortality and other matters of the city of Paris for the first month in the present year.

"There died, in January 3070 persons; 1569 males, 1501 females, being 539 more than in December. Of these, 272 males and 214 females were less than three months old; between 3 months and 1 year, 91 males, 79 females; between 1 and 6 years 221 males, 230 females; between 6 and 8 years, 23 males, 18 females; between 8 and 15 years, 37 males, 39 females; between 15 and 20 years, 80 males, 75 females; between 20 and 30 years, 177 males, 172 females; between 30 and 40 years 128 males, 140 females; between 40 and 50 years, 144 males, 113 females; between 50 and 60 years, 138 males, 122 females; between 60 and 70 years 112 males, 116 females; between 70 and 80 years, 98 males, 119 females; between 80 and 100 years, 48 males, 67 females. January includes 160 deaths of children under 6 years, and 334 deaths of persons upwards of 15 years, more than occurred in December. 196 males, 205 females, died of pulmonary phthisis; 109 males, 139 females, of pneumonia; 98 males, 125 females, of pulmonary catarrh; 140 males, 143 females. of enteritis; 180 males, 105 females, of typhoid fever; 72 males, 40 females, of brain fever; 55 males, 50 females, of apoplexy. 116 males, 95 females, were stillborn. 21 boys, 27 girls, of croup; 28 boys, 25 girls, of convulsions; 2 adult males, and 6 adult females; 19 boys, 16 girls, and 1 female between 20 and 30 years, of measles; 5 boys, 6 girls under 8 years, 13 males, 10 females, and 1 female of 50, of smallpox; 473 males, 500 females, of divers and unenumerated diseases. 22 males, 7 females between 20—60 years, 1 male and 1 female between 15—20 years, and 2 men above 60 years, committed suicide. 162 lunatics were sent to the asylums, 67 lunatics were liberated, 43 died. The Prefecture of Police placed in the *hospices* 19 children between 2—13 years; 21 temporarily; 119 below 2 years, abandoned; the *hospices* received directly 7 children between 2 —12 years, 48 below 2 years. 16 lost children have been returned to their parents. Of the 119 children below 2 years, 6 have been ascertained to be legitimate, 107 natural, the rest uncertain; 30 were born in the *Maisons Hospitalieres*, 39 in the midwives' houses. Information was obtained about 101 mothers, 14 are Parisians, 87 from the country, 33 have their parents, 37 are orphans, 12 are motherless, 20 fatherless, 36 have previously had children, 96 declare the fathers of their children have abandoned them, 5 receive aid from them. Among the mothers 14 are linen-seamstresses, 10 seamstresses, 8 day-workers, 3 embroiderers, 39 maids, 1 shop book-keeper.

Pulmonary Calcareous Concretions.—We are indebted to Dr. Jas. M. Scaife, of Claiborn Parish, Louisiana, for several very handsome specimens of calcareous concretions expectorated by a patient affected with consumption. The doctor states that quite a large number of them were coughed up with purulent matter.

Such concretions. however, are not confined to phthisical subjects, but have been observed in the lungs of persons who have died without any serious lesion of these organs. They usually consist principally of phosphate of lime—and sometimes exist in very great numbers in the pulmonary tissue.—*Southern Medical and Surgical Journal.*

THE

BOSTON MEDICAL AND SURGICAL JOURNAL.

VOL. XLVIII.   WEDNESDAY, JUNE 22, 1853.   No. 21.

WOUNDS OF THE HEART.

FROM LECTURES BY G. J. GUTHRIE, ESQ., F.R.S.

WOUNDS OF THE HEART are for the most part immediately fatal. Many persons have, however, been known to live for hours, nay days, and even weeks, with wounds which could scarcely be otherwise than destructive ; and several cases are recorded in which the cicatrices discovered after death, in persons known to have been wounded in the vicinity of the heart, have shown that even severe wounds of that most important organ are not necessarily fatal. As our knowledge of the nature of the injury inflicted can never be distinct, it follows that every wound should be considered as curable until it is unfortunately proved to be the contrary.

Auscultatiom and *percussion*, and principally auscultation of the whole præcordial region, have afforded means of judging of injuries of the heart which were not formerly known. A vertical line, coinciding with the left margin of the sternum, has about one third of the heart, consisting of the upper portion of the right ventricle, and the whole of the left, on the left. The apex of the heart beats between the cartilages of the fifth and sixth left ribs, at a point about two inches below the nipple, and an inch on its external side ; or, if one leg of a compass be fixed at a point midway between the junction of the cartilage of the fifth rib on the left side, with the rib and the sternum, and a circle of two inches in diameter be drawn around, it will define as nearly as possible the space of the præcordial region occupied by the heart—whilst uncovered, except by the pericardium and some loose cellular texture. In the rest of the præcordial region it is covered and separated from the walls of the chest by the intervening lung.

If the chest of the dead subject be transfixed with long needles, it will be found that the centre of the first bone of the sternum corresponds with the lower edge of the left subclavian vein, and to the arch of the aorta crossing the trachea ; the centre of the second bone to the upper edge of the appendix of the right ventricle ; and the centre of the third bone corresponds to the right side of the right auricle ; the right ventricle being lower down. A needle penetrating the chest at the costal extremity of the fifth rib, close to the upper edge of its cartilage, will touch the septum of the ventricle. The apex of the heart is an inch and a half below this, and inclined to the left side.

The semilunar valves of the pulmonary artery correspond to a spot a little below the centre of the third bone of the sternum. The aortic valves are a few lines below and behind the pulmonary. The mitral valves are a little lower, and still more deeply seated. The pulmonary artery, after touching the sternum, inclines to the left, and is found close to the sternum, between the second and third ribs. The aorta ascends to the first bone, and crosses it to form the arch.

One third of the heart, consisting of the upper part of the right ventricle and of the whole of the right auricle, is beneath the sternum; the remainder of the right, with the left ventricle and auricle, are to the left side of that bone.

On applying the ear to the præcordial region, the patient being in the erect position, two sounds are distinguishable in a healthy heart—one duller and more prolonged, the other clearer and shorter; between these there is scarcely an appreciable interval. The period of repose is sufficiently marked before the first or duller sound returns. Of the time thus occupied, one half is filled up by the first or dull sound; one quarter by the second or sharp sound; one quarter by the pause or period of repose.

Twenty-nine theories have been proposed, each accounting for the sounds of the heart. The theory of Dr. Billing appears to prevail at present, which supposes that the sounds thus heard " are caused by the valves, which, being membranous, each time they resist the reflux of the blood, are thrown into a state of sudden tension, which produces sound."

The impulse of the heart, so far as it can be felt by the touch, depends much on the position in which the body is placed. In the erect position it is heard between the fifth and sixth ribs. In the recumbent posture the impulse is almost imperceptible. It is, perhaps, more observable when the body is turned on the right side, but decidedly more so when it is turned on the left. A clearer sound proceeds from a thin, and a duller sound from a thick heart; a sound of greater extent from a large heart, and a sound of less extent from a small one. A more forcible impulse is given by a thick heart, and one more feeble by a thin one; the impulse is conveyed to a longer distance from a small heart.

From a clearer sound we believe in the probability of an attenuated heart, but we argue its certainty from a clearer sound joined with a weaker impulse. A stronger impulse denotes the probability of an hypertrophied heart, but we argue its certainty from a stronger impulse with a diminished sound.

The terms endocardial and exocardial are used to designate the alterations which take place in the sounds of the heart under disease; endocardial when they occur within the heart, and exocardial when they take place upon its surface. The endocardial murmur of disease, or bellows-sound, takes place of, and is substituted in certain cases for, the first or second, or even for both the healthy or normal sounds. The exocardial murmur of disease is heard with the normal sounds, but confusing and overpowering, sometimes overwhelming them by its rubbing or crumpling noise. The natural sounds exist, although rendered imperceptible by the greater distinctness and nearer approach of the unnatural or unhealthy ones.

The heart apart from the pericardium never moves without a sound ; the pericardium apart from the heart never gives out one. Under disease the heart gives out the natural sound, diminished, exaggerated, or modified, or, it may be, totally altered. The sounds given out by a diseased pericardium must always be new (there being no old ones), and are described as rubbing, or to-and-fro sounds. The pleura when diseased, being a serous structure, like the inner membrane of the pericardium, gives out less marked, but somewhat similar sounds (the "*frottement*" of the French), in particular stages of the disease.

The alterations in the ordinary sounds constituting the endocardial murmurs of the heart heard under disease, depend principally on the altered state of the endocardium, or membrane lining its cavities ; the sounds given off, and called exocardial, on an altered state of the serous membrane of the pericardium, are reflected over the outer surface of the heart. The endocardial or bellows sound, when it accompanies the normal sounds of the heart, may result from any kind of derangement affecting the internal membrane of that organ, particularly rheumatic inflammation, or from any force which may compress its cavities ; it may depend on the altered quality of the blood, from anæmia. It should be present after excessive hæmorrhages have greatly reduced the powers of the sufferer. When this murmur or sound occurs after injury in the vicinity of the heart, and is accompanied by fever, it indicates inflammation of the lining membrane, although no local pain, no palpitations, nor irregular movements of the heart should be present.

When a murmur or sound is heard of a different kind, possessing the character of friction, or of surfaces moving backward and forward on each other, or to and fro—this sound is the sign of inflammation of the membrane covering the heart, as well as of that lining the fibrous external tissue of the pericardium. The signs of both external and internal inflammation may be present at the same time, and they frequently are in cases of acute rheumatism.

When the heart is supposed to be wounded, even without much loss of blood, there is fainting, palpitation, irregular movement or total cessation of its action ; coldness of the extremities ; ghastliness of countenance, succeeded by great anxiety ; a sense of anguish ; an intermission or cessation of pulse, followed, if the patient should survive, by re-action, which renders it very frequent, and sometimes increases its impulse, whilst the anxiety is increased by pain, sometimes intolerable, referred to the part. These symptoms imply a serious injury, although they may not all be present, and many of them differ in intensity. If the patient should survive, the ordinary sounds of the heart will return, with more or less irregularity, accompanied after a few hours by the endocardial murmur, although something like it may perhaps be observed from the first period of injury. The friction, or attrition sound, indicating the presence of inflammation of the pericardium, may be absent, and will not be discernible, if a layer of blood is effused into the cavity of that membrane, whilst the natural sounds of the heart are rendered more indistinct as the heart is separated from the walls of the chest by the effusion, which distends the pericardium, and impedes the regular action of, but cannot compress the heart, as an empyema does the lung. If inflammation take place without an effusion of blood, the friction sound will be heard, and will usually continue even after some effusion of serum and of lymph have occurred, as the quantity of serum is rarely sufficient to prevent the effused and attached portions of lymph from rolling against each other.

The presence of a larger quantity of fluid may be more distinctly known by percussion ; if it can be borne in cases of injury, the degree and extent of the dulness being the measure of its existence and accumulation. It may extend over a part or the whole of the præcordial region, reaching as high as the second, or even the first rib, beneath the sternum, and even under the cartilage of the ribs of the right side.

That the heart when wounded is capable of recovery by the permanent closure of the wound, in a few rare instances, is indisputable ; and it would seem, from a consideration of the different cases which have been recorded, that such recovery takes place in consequence of there being little blood discharged through the wound, or into the cavity of the pericardium, or into that of the pleura. The absence, or the cessation of hæmorrhage, by the contraction of the wound, or the formation of a coagulum, is the first step towards a cure, and it was to one or other of these circumstances that most of those who survived the injury for several days or weeks owed their existence for the time, although they usually died from the effects of inflammation, more of the inner lining and outer covering, than of the substance of the heart itself.

If the wound be inflicted by a musket or pistol-ball, it cannot be closed, although pressure may be made upon it for a time, so as to suppress the external flow of blood. If this should succeed, it is more than probable that the hæmorrhage will continue internally, and that the patient may die after much suffering, principally from oppression, caused by the escape of blood into the cavity of the chest.

If the wound be a stab, the external opening may be accurately closed, and the escape of blood prevented ; but as the pressure of the blood in the pericardium is unequal to restrain the action of the heart, blood forced out through the opening fills the cavity of the pleura, and causes suffocation, unless from some accidental circumstance the opening in the heart becomes obstructed and the bleeding ceases.

If all the circumstances be considered, there can be no doubt of the propriety of closing the wound in the first instance, if the flow of blood is excessive and appears likely to endanger life. It seems to be as little doubtful that the wound should be re-opened after a time, if the danger from suffocation be imminent. The relief obtained by the escape of a little blood may be efficacious, whilst it does not necessarily follow, although it is more than probable it will be so, that its place will be occupied by a further extravasation of blood, which will prove fatal. It is a choice of difficulties, and death from hæmorrhage is easier than death from suffocation.

In the case of the Duke de Berri, whose right ventricle was wounded, and who died from loss of blood, Steifensand reprehends Dupuytren for having opened the external wound every two hours to prevent suffocation ; but if death were actually impending from the filling of the cavity of the chest being about to cause suffocation, there was nothing to be done but to give relief at all hazards.

When the sufferer has recovered from the imminent danger attendant on the infliction of the injury, and the pericardium is believed to be so full of blood or of serum as to prevent in a great measure the movements of the heart, it has been proposed by the Baron Larrey to open the pericardium by the following operation—equally, as he thinks, applicable in an ordinary case of hydrops pericardii :—

" An oblique incision is to be made from over the edge of the ensiform cartilage, to the united extremities of the cartilages of the seventh and eighth ribs. The cellular tissue being divided with some fibres of the rectus and external oblique muscles, there remain only a portion of the peritonæum, called its false layer, above the pericardium, which can be seen after the division of all intervening cellular tissue, projecting between the first and second digitations of the diaphragm. Into this the bistoury is to be entered, with the precaution of doing it with the edge turned upward, and directed a little from right to left, to avoid the peritonæum. The smallest portion possible of the anterior border of the diaphragm is next to be divided, where it is attached to the inner part of the cartilage of the seventh rib. The internal mammary artery is to the outside. The patient should be placed perpendicularly, and supported on his bed, which inclines the anterior part and base of the pericardium to the fore part of the chest."

Skielderup recommends this operation to be done by trepanning first the sternum, a little below the spot where the cartilage of the fifth rib is united to that bone, at which part the periosteum lining it offers considerable resistance, and should not be divided by the trephine. Below this there is a triangular space formed by the separation of the layers of the mediastinum, free from cellular tissue, and tending a little more to the left than to the right. The apex of this triangle is opposite the fifth rib ; its base touches the diaphragm. The bone having been removed, the patient is made to lean forward, when the projection of the pericardium will enable the operator to feel that a quantity of fluid is within, and to open it with safety.

J. Dierking, a stout, muscular man, of the third regiment of German Hussars, was wounded at the battle of Waterloo by a lance, which penetrated the chest between the fifth and sixth ribs, and was withdrawn. He fell from his horse, lost a good deal of blood by the mouth, and some by the wound, and was carried to Brussels without any particular attention being drawn to the injury. His strength not being restored, whilst he suffered from palpitations of the heart, and other uneasy sensations in the chest, he was sent to England to be invalided, and in November, 1815, to York Hospital, Chelsea, in consequence of an attack of pneumonia, of which he died in two days, without attention being particularly drawn to the cicatrix of the wound.

On examining the body I found that the lance, having injured the edge of the cartilage of the rib, passed through the inferior lobe of the left lung, the track being marked by a depressed narrow cicatrix. It then perforated the pericardium under the heart, and sliced a piece of the outer edge of the right ventricle, which being attached below turned over and hung down from the heart to the extent of two inches, when in the fresh state, the part of the ventricle from which it had been sliced being puckered and covered by a serous membrane like the heart itself. The lance then penetrated the central tendon of the diaphragm, making an oval opening, easily admitting the finger, the edges being smooth and well defined. It then entered the liver, on the surface of which there was a small irregular mark or cicatrix. The heart in front was attached to the pericardium by some strong bands, the result of adhesive inflammation, but the general appearance of the serous membrane showed that this had not been either great or extensive. The pericardium was not thickened.

If this man had lived long enough, he might have furnished an instance of hernia of the stomach or intestine into the pericardium.

That the heart when exposed is insensible, or nearly so, to the touch, was known to Galen and to Harvey. Galen is said to have removed a part of the sternum and pericardium, and to have laid his finger on the heart. Harvey did the same on the son of Lord Montgomery, who was wounded in the chest. Prof. J. K. Jung not only introduced needles into the hearts of animals, but also galvanized them without disadvantage, although Admiral Villeneuve is supposed to have died suddenly from running a pin into his heart with a suicidal intention.

That a person may die from the shock of a blow on the heart, need not be doubted, and that they do die when little blood is lost, is admitted. History preserves the fact, that Latour d'Auvergne, who had obtained the honorable title of " Premier Grenadier de France, and Captain of the 46th demi-brigade," fell and died immediately after receiving a wound from a lance at Neustadt, in the month of July, of the sixth year of the Republic, which struck the left ventricle of the heart, near its apex, but did not penetrate its cavity. He was, however, 68 years of age.

In wounds of the heart, all extraneous matters should be removed, if possible, and all inflammatory symptoms should be subdued by general bleeding, by leeches, by calomel, antimony, opium, &c. The chest should be examined daily by auscultation. If the cavity of the pleura should fill with blood, it ought to be evacuated to give a chance for life, and if the pericardium should become permanently distended by fluid, it should be evacuated.

Lacerations and ruptures of the heart have frequently taken place from blows or other serious contusions.

Ollivier, who devoted much time to reading and collecting the observations made by different writers on the injuries of the heart, says, " that of 49 cases of spontaneous rupture of the heart, 34 were of the left ventricle, 8 only of the right, 2 of the left auricle, 3 of the right, and that in 2 cases both ventricles were torn in several places ; and that these results were in an inverse proportion to those which occurred after blows or contusions ; the right ventricle being ruptured in 8 out of 11 cases, the left ventricle 3 times ; the auricles being also torn in 6 out of these 11 cases ; the ruptures not being confined to one spot, but taking place occasionally in several different parts, or even in the same ventricle." In 8 of the cases he had noticed, the heart was ruptured in several places. That a spontaneous rupture may be cured as well as a wound, seems likely from a case reported by Rostan, of a woman who died after fourteen years' suffering with pain about the heart, and was found to have the ventricle ruptured. A cicatrix was observed to the left side of the recent rupture, half an inch in extent in every direction, and in which the new matter was evidently different from the natural structure of the heart.—*London Lancet.*

SOURCE OF VITALITY IN THE TEETH.

RHIZODONTRYPO-NEURHÆMAXIS, AND THE REMOVAL OF THE DENTAL PULP, NOT FOUNDED ON PHYSIOLOGICAL PRINCIPLES, AND THEREFORE IMPRACTICABLE.

[Communicated for the Boston Medical and Surgical Journal.]

In this progressive, practical, and prolific age, it is not surprising, when we consider the long and diligent cultivation which the various arts and sciences have received from so many hands, that by a careful observation, there should be discovered, here and there, an abnormal growth, or parasite, which needs the amputating knife of the " dresser" to more fully insure the perfect and rapid growth of the true scions. It is the duty of every professional man, and of every man in society, whatever his calling or circumstances may be, to do something to add to the knowledge and interest of that department in which he labors ; and to examine and investigate such projects and theories as may come before him, before fully subscribing to them. It is not expected that all are to make discoveries or inventions ; but all may do something towards *proving* them. From the days of the persecuted " Copernicus, Jenner and Galileo," down through the hosts of false and true, practical and impractical, theorists, even to the days of Perkins with his " tractors," Hahnemann with his working motto, *similia similibus curantur,* Paine with his " light," and Willard and Ericcson with their motive powers, there has been, and there always will be, not a few, who will make it their business to examine and investigate, to see whether the things stated " are so." The world usually attributes merit only to those who succeed ; but every one who makes effort, in a good cause, should receive credit, alike with those who are more successful, as *motive* gives character to action.

The microscope has opened, and is still opening, a wide and interesting field of discovery to the anatomist and pathologist ; and few are the diseases in which the physician has not been made wiser through its use, thereby better understanding the condition of the diseased subject ; and been thus enabled to more accurately apply his therapeutical agencies to the patient's pathological wants. It therefore becomes every membe of the healing art to keep well " posted up," or he·will be exposed to the charge of supporting, both by precept and practice, some theory that *was*.

The remarks recently made through this Journal, on the subject of microscopic observation by the profession generally, have much·force ; and I hope the time is near, when the profession, in the United States, shall take the lead in this department of scientific research.

In the matter of the " new operation " on the teeth, which has already elicited some discussion ; I do not wish to be considered as setting myself up as a teacher (as intimated by my friend Dr. Miller), but as an humble learner, seeking for the true light of science as developed by study, and careful and well-tried experiment and observation.

I am happy in stating that Dr. Miller rightly understood me, when he inferred, from a former article, that it was my opinion " that the principle of vitality in a tooth, resides in its central ganglion *only*—that it has no *other* source, and when *that* is cut off it *immediately* loses its vitality, and nature soon makes an effort to remove it." This position I think I am able to sustain by incontrovertible evidence, drawn from the recent investigations of physiologists ; though, in so doing, I should be sorry, in my efforts to do science and dental patients justice, to necessarily convince·any member of the art, " and among them the ablest of the profession," " of having been engaged·for·nearly·*twenty* years in a practice, founded on an impracticable theory."

In the fifth American edition of " Principles of Human Physiology," by Dr. Wm. B. Carpenter, 1852, from·page 282 to 297, are to be found some very interesting *facts* relative to the structure, development, source of vitality, and death of·the teeth ; and to those who are fond of scientific instruction in·a very entertaining form, I would recommend a perusal of this valuable work. From it I shall make such quotations, in the exact language or sentiment, as shall serve my present purpose.

" The human teeth consist of three distinct substances ; dentine, enamel and cementum." The dentine, which composes the larger part of the tooth, " consists·of a firm substance; in which mineral matter largely·predominates. It is traversed by a vast number of very fine branching, cylindrical, wavy tubuli, which commence at the pulp-cavity (on whose walls their openings may be seen), and radiate towards·the surface. In their course·outward, the tubuli occasionally divide dichotomously ; and they frequently give off minute branches, which again send off smaller ones. These·dentinal tubuli, on their arrival at the line of junction between the enamel and dentine, sometimes recurve and anastomose with contiguous tubes ; sometimes pass for a short distance into the enamel ; others pass into the interspaces that exist among the large granules that form the *outer surface* of the dentine ; and some of them *may* even extend into the cementum and communicate with its radiating cells." Through these tubuli the proper nutriment of the tooth is carried, being absorbed from the pulp-cavity.

Thus we see that the proper vessels·of the tooth commence at the pulp-cavity, and extend to the surface of the dentine ; though M. Tomes has given us, as exceptions, cases where *some* of the tubuli have been seen to extend into the cementum. Dr. Carpenter, in speaking of the vascularity of the cementum as found in some animals, says, "In man, however, in whose teeth the cementum is very thin, such vascular canals do not usually exist, though M. Tomes states that he has occasionally met with them." And he further says that "its presence (the cementum) in the simple teeth of man and the carnivora can be shown only by the application of the microscope." Thus we are shown that the cementum petrosa (or "periosteum") of the tooth possesses usually no vascularity, and consequently cannot be a *source* or even a *medium* of *vitality* to the tooth.

[To be concluded next week.]

MEDICAL TESTIMONY—DR. HEATON'S PAMPHLET ON THE HERNIA REPORT CONSIDERED IN THIS CONNECTION.

To the Editor of the Boston Medical and Surgical Journal.

SIR,—A recent number of the Journal contained an article upon medical testimony, with allusions to the slight importance attached to the opinions of eminent physicians by juries, in cases in which disagreements occurred as to cause and effect, between physicians of the highest reputation and their less known and therefore less appreciated brethren.

Whatever has been said against juries, selected in the usual form for the trial of legal cases, as judges of medical facts, conclusions and inferences, will be said again by individuals who may have a theory disturbed by a particular verdict. Juries are usually composed of men possessing an average share of intelligence and "common sense"—and in scientific issues, are to rely upon the testimony of a class of expositors known to the law as experts. In medical science there is one step requisite to render pathological inquiry as satisfactory as the more demonstrable propositions of chemistry, mechanics, or engineering. The essential element in the process of analysis necessary to understand the merits of a disputed question, is separation of opinion from facts—in medical questions, a result sometimes with difficulty accomplished.

The appearance of a pamphlet, "Review of a Report of a Committee of the American Medical Association on the Permanent Cure of Reducible Hernia or Rupture, by George Heaton, M.D.," suggested to the writer a reference to the article alluded to in the beginning of this communication, at this time. It is not proposed either to consider the "Report of the Committee" or the "Review of the Report" in a critical sense, but only as the two may illustrate the question of medical testimony. A discussion upon the merits of the "hernia" question may be left to the parties interested more directly in the conflict of opinion and fact.

There have been cases tried in our State Courts lately, in which "medical opinion" has been divided, and the verdicts of the juries, so far as they may be considered as decisive upon the medical questions involved, have been given against the weight of authority, or "generally-received opinion"; and physicians have condemned the verdicts of these juries.

Now suppose an action is brought for mal-practice, in a case of operation for the cure of hernia. A medical witness is asked " whether or not there is any surgical operation at present known which can be relied on, with confidence, to produce in all instances, or even in a large proportion of cases, a radical cure of reducible hernia."

Many surgeons in Boston and elsewhere, would probably testify that there is not any such operation known. Three among the most distinguished of them would certainly so testify ; for according to Dr. Heaton's pamphlet they have certified to this opinion, in " a report upon the subject of hernia to the American Medical Association."

We have, however, a contrary " opinion," certified by Dr. George Heaton, who, if he was upon the witness's stand in the case supposed, would testify—" that there is a surgical operation which can be relied on with confidence to produce a radical cure of hernia, not only in a large proportion of cases, but in all cases which one could reasonably expect to be cured." If questioned for reasons for his " opinion," he would reply by reference to " five hundred cases, or more, upon which he had performed this surgical operation, successfully," as he has stated in his pamphlet Review. Now if these five hundred " cases " are " cures," they are affirmative " FACTS "—demonstrating the proposition that there " is known " an operation for the cure of reducible hernia.

A medical writer observes, that " lists of cases, however certified, rather deceive than enlighten." When applied to hernia, however, the objection to " lists of cases " loses its force. The difference between an opinion and a fact is well defined by the same writer, in his objection to " lists of cases." He says, " when a man asserts that he has been cured of a particular disease by a certain drug, he is apt to think he is declaring a fact which he knows to be true ; whereas this assertion includes two opinions, in both of which he may be completely mistaken." But a man generally knows if he have a hernia, and if cured by drug or operation can testify to the cure as a fact.

Now in the case supposed, would a jury subject themselves to just reproof, if in their verdict they should record the fact, that " there is known a surgical operation for the cure of reducible hernia," upon the evidence of the three surgeons on the one part, who certify that they do not know of any such operation, and Dr. Heaton on the other, who has performed the operation " five hundred times or more." Dr. Heaton has not described his operation. Perhaps its theory is against all surgical rule. This opinion is of no weight, certainly, against the published facts of his practice. The writer has never witnessed Dr. Heaton's manipulation for the cure of hernia ; nor has he had opportunities for operating himself for the radical cure, as he could not promise " a cure " upon any self-relying basis, when applied to for that purpose.

The new principle, upon which is based " a mode of treatment and operation which closes effectually and permanently the various openings through which hernial protrusions take place," may yet be discovered by some surgeon, who to a knowledge of the disease and its anatomical relations, with opportunity for experiment, will add perseverance against difficulties, constant application, and liberal appreciation of scientific truth.

Dr. Heaton states his operation to be a simple one. He does not en-lighten us upon it a step beyond the subcutaneous incision. We have, therefore, no means of inferring what is expected, as curative action at the objective point. The direction of the " delicate instrument adapted for the purpose," after it had penetrated the skin, would serve as a key to the destination and action of its point. If I am correctly informed, Dr. Heaton has no objection to operating in the presence of physicians who place patients under his care. I should be pleased to witness an operation, if invited to do so by him, and I frankly state the reason for the desire to do so.

I have an untried theory for a simple operation designed to " approxi-mate the pillars of the abdominal ring," perhaps identical or similar to Dr. Heaton's plan. It was suggested by a case of accidental wound, in which case was a hernia ; the healing of the wound and the cure of the hernia occurring at the same time, under my care, some years ago. No particular importance was attached to the case at the time, other than that the cure seemed against the rule. The divided parts were noticed, and a tardy union expected. The reverse was the fact ; per-fect union by adhesion was accomplished in about ten days, and no de-scent of bowel perceived afterwards. It may be superfluous to add, that I had no idea of a cure of the hernia from this wound. During the process of cure there were present none of the usual signs of inflammation.

Hitherto all the operations performed for the radical cure of hernia have been based upon inflammation or morbid action for producing ad-hesion and closure of the inguinal canal, in inguinal hernia. The means have been varied, but the end proposed has been the same. The fail-ures are counted in large majorities, even when the cure has been at-tempted by the most skilful hands. Dr. Heaton's plan is not included in the list usually described in surgical works, as his *modus operandi* and theory are in company with the concealed " desideratum " ; and whether adhesion in his cases is produced by inflammation or otherwise, can only be inferred by cures in the usual ways attempted in the expe-rience of those conversant with surgical disease.

The structures divided by the accidental incision in the case referred to, under my observation, seem to have much to do with the closure of the dilated canal in hernia, and are to me suggestive of a theory of cure—particularly if these structures are operated upon by subcutaneous incision. Improving upon the hints contained in Dr. Heaton's history of his discovery, I shall make a trial of my conceived method upon the first case of reducible hernia that comes under my care, the patient being willing to take the chance of an untried operation ; and I sincerely hope those surgeons in the midst of a large hospital practice, will, with the opportunities constantly occurring, endeavor to discover what the " sim-ple operation " may be that has enabled Dr. Heaton to treat hernia so successfully.

The tendency to cure is proved by the frequent successful termina-tions under many modes of operation ; although the principle in the in-dividual cases does not appear to have been comprehended, and there-fore fails upon general application.   Your ob't serv't,   **J. S. Jones.**

NECROSIS.

[Communicated for the Boston Medical and Surgical Journal.]

FEW diseases entail more annoyance upon a country practitioner than disease and death of the osseous tissues. The apparently trifling nature of the lesion, at first a small granulating ulcer, seems hardly to justify the medical interference, which obstinacy alone in resisting all simple curative means, has summoned ; and far from anticipating the serious prognosis, which one familiar with its aspect will unhesitatingly deliver, it is only expected that errors perhaps in its previous treatment will be alluded to, and some particular specific applied which will speedily terminate the trouble. Its nature truly defined, and an indefinite but protracted duration announced, incredulity questions the accuracy of your statement, and possibly looks for assistance from other quarters, where the views are more in consonance with the wishes and opinions of the interested party. I have generally found that the class of patients most subject to necrosis, are children who are predisposed, either by inheritance, or exposure to unfavorable influences, to scrofulous affections. The bones in such cases have been slow to take on the process of ossification, and a deficiency of the phosphate of lime has to a greater or less extent been present throughout the entire osseous system. This is usually attributable to an insufficient energy of the circulation, but seems to depend rather on a want of that nutritive principle in the blood, which evinces itself in the pale and wan complexions observable in children who are scantily clothed or subjected to the impure atmosphere of ill-ventilated apartments.

Jan. 12th, 1849.—A boy, about 14 years of age, with hereditary tendency to phthisis, had a slight pain and tumefaction over one of the metatarso-phalangeal joints, followed by ulceration. The probe detected the caries by that peculiar petrous feel which results from contact with dead bone. An incision through the cellular tissue gave exit to a few thin shells of bone, and the ulcer closed. The same occurred with one of the metatarsal bones of the same foot. While this last ulceration was in progress, a depression was noticed over the tibia midway between the epiphyses, which resulted in an extensive ulcer. It then became a question whether the caries could not be arrested at once by excision—whether, by a forcible separation of the sound from the unsound, the integrity of the bone could not be preserved; but I found, on consulting various authorities, that although a few cases had proved fortunate, yet in general, a repetition of the operation had been finally resorted to. Mr. Lawrie, of Glasgow, mentions two cases in which he was successful in thus anticipating the *sequestrum* ; but his success does not seem to have been frequent enough to warrant a pursual of the practice. I concluded, therefore, to wait until the sequestrated portion was entirely enucleated ; and although larger than the *cloaca* through which egress was to be obtained, determined to operate without an enlargement. Having procured a strong pair of curved forceps, with jaws notched for the purpose, they were introduced through the aperture ; and seizing upon the detached bone, I succeeded in crushing it

in several fragments ; and when thus completely disintegrated, a mucilaginous injection was thrown in, which upon flowing out, brought with
it the bruised and minute portions of the sequestrum. By a succession
of injections, the entire cavity was thus emptied. The aperture closed
with but little delay, and the limb became as sound as its fellow.

Hanover, Mass., June, 1853.   B. WHITWELL.

REMARKABLE CASE OF CATALEPSY.

[THE following case is related by Dr. L. C. Dolley, of Rochester, N.
Y., in the Daily Democrat of that city. Although thus sent out in a
daily newspaper, it has the appearance of being authentic, and on account of its remarkable character we copy it into the Journal—ED.]

Cornelius Vroomer, now aged about 37 years, a country laborer, and
resident of Clarkson, Monroe Co., N. Y., of robust and vigorous frame,
middle size, and 165 lbs. weight, about five years since (in June, 1848)
made complaint of an obtuse pain in his head and epigastrium. This
was sufficient to induce him to stop work, and ask medical advice. Dr.
C., of Clarkson, saw him and prescribed little more than guaiacum and
rhubarb, supposing the case one that would prove amenable to mild measures. The pain in the head and stomach continued for about two
weeks, when consciousness, sensorial powers and volition became suspended. His respiration and circulation continued natural, while, without
coma or spasm, muscular rigidity retained the body and limbs in the precise position they were when the attack came on. No apparent change
occurred from this condition for several days, and with the exception of
waking periods of from one to sixteen hours taking place at intervals of
from one week to four months, he has remained in the same condition to
this date.

His conscious periods for the first few months occurred at intervals
seldom exceeding two weeks—latterly seldom less than four, and sometimes not less than eight or ten weeks. His most lengthy period of unconsciousness has been four months ; longest waking interval sixteen
hours. In the great length of the periods of unconsciousness and motionless rigidity, the case is unique and particularly interesting. During
the whole of these periods there has been the most complete anæsthesia.
Powerful excitants have been applied to the surface at various times,
such as blisters over the head and spine, and at one time, accidentally,
sufficient heat to his limbs to vesicate extensively, without causing any
manifestation of pain. The nervous system, it would appear, is but
slightly influenced by all external impressions. None but the slightest
motion of the limbs are induced by currents of magnetic electricity, and
under repeated applications of cold water, including a plunge into Lake
Ontario, he seemed to experience no impression, excepting at one time
under a long-continued douche from a height, he moved himself from
his position, but did not manifest a full return of sense.

The involuntary functions of his system are performed with much
regularity, but with less force and activity than in health. Pulse and

respiration regular but faint.   Evacuation from his bowels occurs once in
from six to nine days—passes his urine more frequently.   These calls
of nature are made manifest to his attendants by a slight uneasiness of his
body, and are kept in abeyance until necessary preparations are made.
From this feature of the case, and the fact that when conscious he has
once or twice evinced a knowledge of events which transpired during
his cataleptic state, and that he possesses the power of balancing himself
when placed erect upon his feet, it is apparent to the physiologist that
everything but the spinal and ganglionic system is not asleep, that the
senses are partly awake, and of a somnambulic character.   I am informed
by his attendants that there are times when his system seems more
completely under the influence of natural sleep than at others ; this so-
porose state is indicated by snoring, and is not attended with the least
relaxation of the muscular rigidity.   Food is usually administered to
him twice a-day, and only by prying the jaws asunder and forcibly introducing it into his mouth and fauces.

His conscious periods return suddenly and at irregular intervals.   During these short waking periods he walks erect, shows no very manifest diminution of strength or natural mobility, greets his old acquaintances, con-
verses freely, and supplies liberally the demands of his stomach.   On
one occasion, not many weeks since, it is said he walked to the beach of
the Lake, a distance of half a mile, and treated himself and friends to a
supply of such grocery luxuries as dried herring and crackers.

Nothing is known of his habits previous to the invasion of this disease, to which it can be referred.   It is known that he " imbibed " only
occasionally, and was a tobacco-chewer, and it is worthy of note that
the last-named habit is completely reformed, as he has not expressed a
desire for the weed for four years.   During the colder months the temperature of his surface is considerably diminished, and at times his extremities are quite cold.   When the surrounding atmosphere is comfort- •
ably warm, the temperature varies but little, if any, from the healthy
standard.

As seen at this time his cast of features is calm and complacent, and
presents nothing particularly unpleasing, except the protrusion of his lips.
The firm pressure of his jaws has forced the incisor teeth to a very acute
angle in front, and almost forced them from their sockets.   The projection of the teeth and the approximation of the maxillæ have forced his
teeth to a prominence quite equal to his nose.   The external surface of
the upper lip lies in close proximity with the nostrils.

Tonic spasm, of not the greatest rigidity, exists throughout his muscular system: His head is brought downward and forward towards the
sternum ; the body is curved foward, the spine forming the arc of a circle, as in emprosthotonos.   The forearms cross the abdomen ; the wrist
joints and those of the fingers are the most firmly fixed.   The thighs and
knees are but slightly flexed, and are firmly fixed at obtuse angles.
When placed upon his feet or seated in a chair, he has the power of sustaining himself in an erect posture as rigid as a statue, from which position he has to be removed mechanically by his attendants.   At one time

he was placed upright upon his feet, and suffered to remain in his motionless position for three days and nights.

' It is unnecessary to specify the various measures which have been adopted by a number of the sons of Æsculapius for his restoration. Their "science and skill," thus far, have seemed to avail nothing in this case. His friends say they have restored consciousness on one or two occasions by administering very copious draughts of whiskey. Nitrous oxide, long-continued cold to the head and spine, and chloroform, are measures which have not been tested.

THE BOSTON MEDICAL AND SURGICAL JOURNAL.

BOSTON, JUNE 22, 1853.

More Alligator Experiments.—We perceive, by the New Orleans Delta, that Drs. Cartwright and Dowler have been engaged in additional experiments on the American crocodile. Three of these animals were secured in the court-yard of Dr. Cartwright; one was operated on by Dr. Dowler, and the other two by Dr. Cartwright. The experiments on the former go to show the possession of a *diffused* sensibility—a local capacity to recognize pain, after the division of the spinal marrow and also of the nerves emerging from it. Dr. Cartwright's experiments, as our readers will surmise, were connected with the motive power of the circulation—and the results were similar to those of former experiments already recorded in this Journal. In addition to the tying of the windpipe in both animals, one of them had the chest opened, and the heart, lungs and stomach exposed; yet after two hours time, both being proved to be dead by exposure over flames of fire, resuscitation was brought about by artificial respiration. In Dr. Dowler's subject, which was bloodless, the inflation failed.

Eccentricities of Medical Men—The Pentateuch in Rhyme.—No profession or trade is without its anomalous characters. Indeed, it is impossible that all minds should be alike. The intellectual world would be dull and monotonous were there no varieties of mental tastes and capacities. Hunkers in thought are as objectionable as those in politics. Neither would allow any progress, if they could prevent it. Contented in their own circumscribed sphere of action, so long as they can hold the first position, and keep others down—a whisper, a suggestion, and, above all, the act of teaching any thing new, calls forth the strongest energies of their nature in opposition. Some of the abnormal sentiments, and especially the whims and eccentricities, of physicians, constitute agreeable episodes in professional life, when they do not interfere with the rights, privileges or happiness of others. Oddity is often connected, too, with great genius. Queer trains of thought, and a disposition always dominant to do and say things differently from other people, make a marked man. In the course of an extensive editorial intercourse with members of the medical profession, in this and other countries, we have been in contact with some very extraordinary persons. Without particularizing, it is sufficient to state the fact that propositions for a multitude of schemes have, over and over again, been submitted to us for consideration, many of which, were they made known, would create a universal shout of laughter; while half of the remainder would seem to show that their authors were stark mad! Some of these are remotely related to medicine, and some not at all. Still, their publication is not unfrequently urged with a pertinacity hardly to be resisted, as the author of each sees clearly—more so than any one else—the vast revolution it is calculated to produce, and always for the best interest of mankind! But were such writers often indulged, spectators would have exclaimed, long ago, in the words of a commentator in the Salmagundi,

"For physic and farces,
Their equal there scarce is;—
Their farces are physic,
Their physic a farce is."

These reflections have grown out of the circumstance of a novelty in literature having recently come under our notice. One of the medical brotherhood has left with us a written paraphrase of the whole Pentateuch, and also other portions of the Bible, actually turned into verse! Simply considered as a labor—to have written so much with one's own hand, indicates immense industry; but when to this is superadded the mental activity necessary to put the books of Genesis, Exodus, Leviticus, Numbers, Deuteronomy, &c., into rhyme, and preserve harmony of measure, the work may be considered as no every-day effort. On the whole, it is the rarest specimen of medico-literary eccentricity within the compass of our recollection. Here is a specimen of the versification.

"A woman having borne a son,
Observ'd seven days separation;
On the eighth after 'twas born,
The boy was of his foreskin shorn."

See how the author relates what happened to Pharaoh for his obstinacy—

"Now came a judgment dire, of frogs,
From rivers, meadows, pools and bogs,
And every house, from oven to the bed,
Was filled with croakers, live or dead."

Naturalists have never determined what kind of marine monster swallowed Jonah; but our author has settled the question without hesitation—

"Oppressed with fear, the prophet roar'd,
'Throw me over—overboard.'—
The foam concealed him from the sail,
As came along a mighty whale,
That swallowed all within his reach
Just as we should suck a peach,
And down went Jonah, neck and haunch,
Into the monster's awful paunch."

But we have not room, even if this were the place, for more extracts from this unique performance.

Stricture of the Urethra—Treatment.—In April last, Paul F. Eve, M.D., of the chair of surgery at the University of Nashville, Tenn., read a paper upon stricture of the urethra, and the rapid and free dilatation of the urethral canal. Dr. Eve's reputation commands confidence, and we are of the opinion that his teachings on this subject are entitled to high consideration. A pamphlet is abroad, which might be ordered by mail from the publisher, J. T. S. Hall, Nashville, that furnishes more reasons for the course of treatment he recommends, than could be transferred to our pages without trespassing on a copy right. Besides furnishing the most recent practice of eminent French surgeons, he gives his own sound views, accompanied by illustrative cases. At the conclusion, there are some propositions that may safely be regarded as rules of practice, two of which are as follows :—" To cure stricture, the orifice of the urethra must be so enlarged that the *canal beyond* it may be dilated *to its original size,* which we ought to recollect is about twice that of the opening leading to it. Instead, therefore, of being satisfied with introducing bougies, of two lines in diameter, through a restricted portion, they should measure four or five lines in thickness." " There is no necessity to confine a patient in bed, in treating stricture ; when an instrument has been once introduced, it has done all it can to expand the passage, and should be withdrawn," says Dr. Eve, that others, larger in size, may be immediately substituted. " While this process ought to be cautiously and very gradually conducted, the more rapidly and freely it can be applied, provided no pain is excited, the sooner the disease will be removed."

Busts of Medical Men.—Within a few weeks, a very beautifully-exe-cuted marble bust of the venerable John Green, M.D., of the city of Wor-cester, Mass., has been placed temporarily in the Boston Athenæum. The expression of the man has been so accurately transferred to the marble, as to create an interest in the artist, Mr. B. H. Kinny, who is destined to a permanent place among the native geniuses of the United States. The power of thus giving vitality to stone is a divine gift : it cannot be taught, or learned ; and whenever and wherever it is manifested, such a rare en-dowment should be liberally encouraged by the community. Civilization is as much advanced by the cultivation of the fine arts, as by the multi-plication of elementary schools of learning. Where there is no public taste leading to the patronage of painting and sculpture, the higher senti-ments are imperfectly developed, and the beautiful in nature is not ap-preciated. If some half a dozen New England fathers in medicine would leave to the scientific institutions of the State, a similar memorial of their existence, they would not only be gladly received, but the fine arts would be encouraged, and the community benefited.

The late Dr. Truman Abell.—Among the necrological notices in the Journal a few weeks since, was that of Truman Abell, M.D., late of Lempster, N. H. Dr. A. was an eminent practitioner, and his industrious, well-spent life, secured for him the respect of a large circle of friends. Besides fulfilling all the duties of an active country physician, he cultivat-ed the highest departments of science, and especially that of astronomy. He saw in the firmament a vast field for contemplation, and an inexhausti-ble source of instruction. The more he studied the exhibitions of divine agency in the heavens, the greater was the moral influence he exerted in the community. For thirty-nine successive years, Dr. Abell conducted the New England Farmer's Almanac. The calendar pages of that use-ful, extensively-circulated, but unobtrusive work, bear unfading evidence of his capacity, accuracy and powers of expression in a difficult branch of knowledge. He was accurate in whatever he undertook, mastering every subject, with equal facility, to which he gave the full force of his ever active mind. In botany he had few if any competitors at the North. At the advanced age of 74 his labors upon earth were completed, and the good man entered upon another and higher state of existence. An interesting account of a very remarkable state of illusive vision, experienced in his own person, was communicated by Dr. A. for this Journal, and may be found in Nos. 21 of vol. xxxiii., and 3 of vol. xxxiv.

Concentrated Medical Agents.—Messrs. Keith & Hendrickson, of New York, have embarked largely in the manufacture of medicinal preparations in a concentrated form. To obtain the active medicinal properties of indigenous and foreign plants is the object contemplated by these gentlemen. There is not an article received into the materia medica, belonging to the vegetable kingdom, from which they cannot extract its essential virtues. Their laboratory is known as the American Chemical Institute. It is not our province to determine whether medicines should be precisely as nature prepared them, either in bark or roots. An immense amount of useless, if not injurious, material may be, and in fact is, absolutely taken into the stomach as the supposed necessary accompaniment of the particular thing which the physician prescribes. The separation of whatever is foreign to the purpose, and simply taking the unmixed, detached medicinal agent, would seem to be an improvement. There are those, however, who object to this process. But they might, it appears to us, with an equal show of reason insist upon eating the shells with the oyster. Certainly there is room for inquiry on this point. Leaving others to decide who is right and who is wrong, it is quite certain that very delicate doses of some of the offensive but excellent remedies are prepared at the establishment alluded to. For example, two grains of jalapine answers all the purposes of a dose of ten or fifteen grains of the pulverized root. An apothecary shop is thus put up in miniature, so that a country practitioner may carry, in one pocket, all the principal medicines used in a mixed business. A full case, as thus prepared for the profession, strongly resembles a homœopathic pocket-book of petit phials. But there is an obvious difference between a trillionth part of a grain of a cathartic drug, in a hogshead of water, a teaspoonful of which is taken once in forty-eight hours, and two grains of an extract, containing the active properties of fifty or a hundred grains. It would be both gratifying and useful to have this matter debated, and the facts brought forward for and against the concentrated drugs. In the mean while, it is represented that the demand upon the manufacturers indicates a preference among the profession for much in a little space. A concise description of each medicine, and the precise dose, in this new form, should go with every package. Some terrible mistakes will assuredly follow, and bring the system into disrepute, if care is not taken, seasonably, to instruct those who have necessarily to learn how to prescribe them.

Taylor's Medical Jurisprudence.—Having examined a copy of the third American, from the fourth London, edition of this book, just from the press of Messrs. Blanchard & Lea, Philadelphia, we feel called upon unhesitatingly to express our confidence in it, as a work of the highest order, and quite indispensable to gentlemen who desire to keep up with the progress that is every day being made in medical jurisprudence. No member of the bar, who pretends to be qualified for conducting an intricate trial, in which the principles of medical science are involved, could very well dispense with it, without depriving himself of an important legal assistant. Edward Hartshorne, M.D., of Philadelphia, has appended to the original a synopsis of some of the State laws, which gives additional value to the volume as a book of reference in criminal law in this country. On a former occasion, the peculiar claims of Dr. Taylor's labors were stated; by simply apprising medical readers, therefore, that in this edition nothing has been taken away from it, but that much that is excellent has been added, further comment is not needed. The book is a large octavo of 621 pages, closely printed, with a fair type, and on good paper.

Registration Laws.—An able paper, by Franklin Tuthill, M.D., which originally appeared in the Transactions of the Medical Society of the State of New York, is published in a separate pamphlet for circulation. It seems that repeated efforts have been made in the Legislature of that State to repeal the act providing for the registry of births, deaths, and marriages, which induced Dr. Tuthill to review the objections brought against it. As a historical document, it is eminently worthy of preservation, because it furnishes a good account of the origin of registration laws in ancient times; and in the next place, it sets forth, both eloquently and cogently, the true reasons why there should be a carefully kept record of three important events in civil life, viz., the birth, marriage and death of every individual. From the skilful manner in which Dr. Tuthill has conducted the argument, and the energy displayed on every page of the discourse, we trust that those who have the honor of the Empire State in their keeping, as legislators, will peruse it carefully, and never lose sight of the great benefits to be derived from a strict system of registration.

School of Practical Pharmacy.—In the autumn of 1849, a school of pharmacy had its origin in Philadelphia, that is still conducted vigorously and advantageously for students. Lectures commence for an autumnal course, in September. A published list of each class for years indicates the prosperity of the institution. The present catalogue gives the names of 154 attending the last course. Whether it is an enterprise of only one man, or of an association of physicians and druggists, is not stated. On the cover we read—" Announcement of Edward Parrish's School of Medical Pharmacy for Medical Students."

Dr. M. R. Woodbury, of Concord, N. H., has been appointed surgeon of the U. S. Marine Hospital at Eastport, Me.

To CORRESPONDENTS.—Dr. Cartwright's account of the Experiments in New Orleans, alluded to on another page, has been received, and will appear next week.

MARRIED,—James Stewart, M D., of Malden, Mass., to Miss S. J. French.—Dr. A. H. Flanders, of Newburyport, Mass., to Miss B. Fields.

DIED,—At South Royalton, Vt., Dr. Byron A Manchester, 24.—At Edgecomb, Me, Dr. John Boutelle, 79.—At New Haven, Ct., James M. Thacher, M.D., of Philadelphia, 30.—In New York, Dr. Peter G. Douglass, late of Boston, 71.

Deaths in Boston for the week ending Saturday noon, June 18th, 55. Males, 30—females, 25. Accidents, 2—congestion of brain, 3—consumption, 12—convulsions, 1—croup, 3—cancer, 1— dysentery, 1—dropsy in head, 2—infantile diseases, 3—erysipelas, 2—scarlet fever, 4—typhoid fever, 1—fracture of skull, 1—hemorrhage, 1—disease of heart. 1—inflammation of the lungs, 3 —disease of the liver, 1—marasmus, 3—measles, 2—palsy, 2—disease of the spine, 1—suicide, 1 —teething, 2—unknown, 2.
Under 5 years, 19—between 5 and 20 years, 8—between 20 and 40 years, 8—between 40 and 60 years, 14—over 60 years, 6. Born in the United States, 38—Ireland, 13—England, 1—Scotland, 1—Germany, 2. The above includes 3 deaths in the city institutions.

Hydropathy in California.—By the following report of a Committee of the House of Representatives in California, it will be perceived that the Chairman was a sensible man, and also that hydropathy is bold in its pretensions there as well as here. There is a vein of wit running through it, which gives it a zest, and the whole tone of it very clearly shows that old birds are not to be caught with chaff. It is taken from the Alta Californian.

"The Committee on State Hospitals, to whom was referred a remonstrance by G. M. Bourne, hydriatic physician of San Francisco, would beg leave respectfully to report,

"That they have carefully weighed the propositions contained in said remonstrance, and found them wanting, as follows:

"1st, Because it assumes that a man has a right to place himself before the public as a practitioner of a science, of the principles of which he is entirely ignorant. He says he is in possession of no other warrant for practising the healing art than that conferred upon him by the great source of his being, or in other words, he was born with a sheep's skin, *ergo* he has, without preparation, the natural right to practise medicine and surgery. Your Committee believe in no such logic.

"2d, In the opinion of your Committee, it is not inimical to the spirit of our free institutions that the flights of erratic genius should be restrained within proper limits. The laws of every State protect its citizens from frauds practised upon them by false pretenders. If, then, the protection of property is deemed so essential, how much more carefully should health and life be protected from the impositions of ignorant pretenders and charlatans.

"3d, That the medical profession has not realized the world's expectation, is lamentably true; but that it has approached any nearer so desirable a consummation since the advent of Priessnitz and hydropathy, your Committee has not been advised.

"The order of Pretender, with whom your remonstrant fraternizes, has no legal existence, and, as your Committee believe, should have none.

"The assertion of your remonstrant, that an immense number of astonishing and miraculous cures have been effected by means of cold water, requires confirmation; and your Committee, all of whom are medical practitioners, cannot conceive in what manner it has been made subservient to the successful management of difficult cases of parturition, and require the testimony of more than one interested witness to establish the fact. Your Committee have searched all the records within their reach, and can find no such statistics, but if, as your remonstrant asserts, a man totally ignorant of medicine and surgery did accomplish so much good, another man equally ignorant might accomplish as much evil.

"Your Committee believe that no system of medicine should receive the protection of the laws of the State, to the exclusion of others. At the same they believe that every practitioner, whether of allopathy, homœopathy, hydropathy, eclectic, botanic, uriscopic, root, herb, Indian or corn doctor, should possess some evidence of his proficiency in such science, other than the ear-marks with which he was born. Your Committee are not aware that any legislative enactments are in contemplation which will have the effect of retarding the progress of medical knowledge, as your remonstrant asserts.

"Those fathers of medicine whom your remonstrant has had the temerity to press into the service of hydropathy, never dreamed of the employment of water as a curative agent, to the exclusion of all other remedies, the advent of Priessnitz having been many centuries subsequent to this time.

"'Literary celebrities' are not, in the opinion of your Committee, the proper persons to decide upon the merits of any system of medicine.

"Sir John Ross and other navigators have recorded their opinion of water, no doubt verifying it as absolutely necessary to the success of navigation.

"*Lie-bigs* experiment of the chemical effects of cold water upon the animal economy, your Committee have not seen; but they can readily conceive, as your remonstrant asserts, that great changes (if not entire dissolution) of the human body would occur under six weeks of active water treatment.

"Notwithstanding 'the great fiscal embarrassment of the State,' your Committee believe it would be more than folly to substitute simple cold water for medicines of known and of proven utility, and discharge from our State Hospitals men of tried ability, and substitute a natural-born doctor on account of cheapness. Your Committee have heard of men who were born kings, and of others who were born fools, but no well attested case of a *born* doctor.

"Your Committee would recognize the right of a female to practise medicine and surgery, if her education qualified her to perform its arduous duties. Her nature peculiarly fits her for ministering to the wants of the sick and afflicted.

"In conclusion, your Committee would recommend that a copy of this report, together with a copy of your remonstrant's manifest, be transmitted to that 'bourne' from whose 'home for the sick' no patient will be likely ever to return, and ask to be discharged from a further consideration of the subject. **J. H. ESTEP,** *Chairman.*"

Abortive Treatment of Typhoid Fever.—Dr. Fenner, of New Orleans, at a late meeting of the Physico-Medical Society of that city, referred to several cases of Typhoid fever, which he had lately under his care in the Charity Hospital; and in which, he had employed the abortive treatment of quinine, given in large doses along with a portion of opium, and with the same advantageous results, as in the cases which he had previously reported to the Society, where the same mode of treatment had been followed. The abortive treatment, in all the cases which were submitted to it three days after the attack, did well. Others again, that came in in all stages of the disease, and on whom the same treatment was tried, did not do so well.

THE

BOSTON MEDICAL AND SURGICAL JOURNAL.

Vol. XLVIII. Wednesday, June 29, 1853. No. 22.

TYPHOID FEVER IN PARIS.

[The following is an extract from the editorial correspondence of the Charleston Medical Journal and Review, under date of Paris, March 5, 1853.—Ed.]

An epidemic of typhoid fever is very prevalent in Paris at present, and it is seen in all the hospitals. In these it is quite interesting to witness the variety of treatment adopted by each physician of note, as his medical tendencies incline ; that pursued respectively by MM. Bouillaud, Briquet and Louis, whom I have followed, presents many points of difference, and it has been difficult to determine on which side the scale of success leans. We hope, however, to be able to send a paper by a medical friend who has watched closely the service of the former, and who can furnish some testimony with respect to his mode of employing the lancet in this disease. M. Louis very generally administers seltzer water, vinous lemonade, and adopts, to a certain extent, the expectant system. M. Briquet at La Charité pursues what appears to me rather a middle course. He abstracts blood in the early stage of some cases which seem peculiarly fitted for it. I may observe here that I have also heard M. Trousseau say, that even as late as during the second and third septenary period, he was in the habit of bleeding to prevent the increase, or destroy the congestion of the lungs which so often exhibits itself, its approach and presence being of course easily discoverable by the physical signs. M. Briquet relies with much confidence (and my own observation in his wards can sustain him) upon the application of cups and scarification to the mastoid region during delirium and coma of typhoid. It completely checks the increase of these dangerous symptoms, as I have repeatedly witnessed. He does not give mercury internally, but applies plasters of mercurial ointment over the entire abdomen until the secretions become active, or the tongue and skin exhibits the desired moisture. This method of using the remedy might more easily reconcile itself to those who so much doubt respecting the advantages of its internal administration. He gives ordinary Bordeaux wine, during the period of convalescence. These means, thus generally expressed, are often associated in his practice with the use of ice, administered in every possible way, and through every channel—bladders filled with it are applied to the scalp, it is dissolved in the mouth, and given with enemata. One

22

of his internes mentioned to me this morning, that he had lost but one case within three weeks. There are between twenty and fifty sick of the disease in each service of the hospitals, and few of these fail to present gargouillement, the characteristic rose mark and sudamina.

As the subject of typhoid fever has been much discussed of late at the South, and in the pages of this Journal, it may not be thought useless to consider the following autopsy which I witnessed at La Charité a few days since. It is instructive as indicating the characteristic march of the disease in an individual in whose system it was not modified by medicines. The subject, a man about 33 years of age, of good conformation when he entered the Hospital, presented a very favorable condition save the existence of the endemic ; this had seized upon him as it had upon most of those who had within the last year or two moved from the country to Paris, and who did not live under favorable bygienic conditions. He had been bled, but absolutely no medicines were taken with the exception of *tisans* and mucilaginous drinks. Notwithstanding, the entire lining membrane of his *stomach* was intensely red and exhibited all the traces of severe inflammation : there was some exudation of plastic lymph, and the particles of coloring matter seemed infiltrated beneath the mucous coat; when scraped off with a sharp bistoury, the surface beneath was white. Thirty of Peyer's glands were enlarged and inflamed, decreasing in size from the commencement of the colon until they disappeared in the small intestines. The largest were about a quarter of an inch in diameter, with elevated edges, presenting, as M. Briquet remarked, precisely the appearance of carcinoma ; the surface of those situated most inferiorly exhibited the yellow summit, indicating the commencement of gangrene. No other portion of the intestinal canal was diseased, if we exclude the above enlarged mesenteric glands. The *spleen* was four times the ordinary size, though it did not appear that the deceased had suffered from intermittent fever. The cavities of the *heart* contained some fibrinous deposits, and its muscular tissues were soft. The *lungs* showed previous inflammation of the bronchia, and the lower lobes were still engorged ; these did not compromise the life of the individual, as quite a large portion was spongy and elastic. The consistence of the *brain* was firm, no fluid was found in the ventricles, but there was venous engorgement on its surface. The *liver* and other organs remained quite natural.

THERAPEUTIC VALUE OF VERATRUM VIRIDE.

BY   W. C. NORWOOD, M.D., OF ABBEVILLE, S. C.

WE know of no agent so peculiarly adapted and so universally applicable to the treatment of febrile and inflammatory affections, as the American Hellebore. With limited exceptions it fulfils the therapeutical indications in these diseases unaided and alone ; and, withal, its results are so invariable that we may expect to realize its effects, when properly administered, with the same certainty with which the husbandman anticipates an abundant harvest from the proper culture of his field.

However numerous or diversified may be the causes of febrile and inflammatory diseases, certain uniform effects or events are sure to follow them, and to correct or modify these effects is the grand aim of the practitioner. To do this successfully, a practical and experimental knowledge of the therapeutical properties of the agents calculated to modify the actions excited by these causes, is necessary ; and this is the reason of my pressing so earnestly on every one, the importance of thoroughly testing, and closely watching for himself, the therapeutical effects of veratrum viride ; for I believe that he who fully understands its powers and applications, is in possession of the key which opens the door to triumphant success in the treatment of many diseases hitherto considered the opprobria of medicine.

I have been charged with enthusiasm, extravagance and fancy, in estimating the value of this remedy, and in urging its claims upon the profession ; but years of close observation and experience have convinced me that, far from exaggerating, I have failed to do justice to the subject. Who can overrate the value of an agent capable of controlling the actions of the heart with demonstrative certainty ? When it was announced, by the Italian physicians, that digitalis possessed the property of subduing and controlling morbid vascular action, medical men ardently anticipated the benefits that were about to be realized. But it proved not to possess the powers ascribed to it, and the field was again open for research and inquiry. After long observation and repeated experiment we are able to affirm, in the most positive manner, that *veratrum viride* entirely fulfils this indication. In less than twenty-four hours it will reduce a pulse of 100 or 160, to between 35 and 85 beats in the minute.

But this drug possesses other important remedial powers. It is a certain and efficacious emetic ; it possesses expectorant and diaphoretic properties in an eminent degree ; its adanagic power is considerable, and it acts as a nervine in allaying morbid irritability.

We trust that these statements, based upon careful clinical observation and mature reflection, will induce the profession to use this remedy, and we believe that the benefits resulting to the sick from its judicious employment will be incalculable.*—*Virginia Med. and Surg. Jour.*

CASE OF DOUBLE MONSTER—RITTA-CRISTINA.

BY WM. F. MONTGOMERY, A.M., M.D., ETC., DUBLIN.

THIS remarkable double monster (possessing two heads and bodies, and two sets of upper extremities, but only one pair of legs and feet) was born at Sassari in Sardinia, 12th March, 1829. The mother was well formed and had previously borne seven perfect children ; in the birth of Ritta-Cristina the labor was not attended with difficulty ; the heads present-

---

* Dr. Norwood publishes (Charleston Medical Journal. November, 1852), his formula for preparing a saturated tincture of the root of veratrum viride :—R. Of the dried root of veratrum viride, viij. oz. ; of alcohol of the shops, xvj. oz. Digest for a fortnight. The dose for an adult is eight drops to be given every three hours.—ED.

ed, and each head was separately baptized and named. They were brought to Paris, and there publicly exhibited, which is said to have hastened their death. It is rather amusing to know that the public authorities interdicted their exhibition except under most stringent restrictions, for fear that it would open a door for psychological speculations and discussions.

On examination after death, the two vertebral columns were found separate in their whole length, and a rudimentary pelvis, formed of a single bone, separated them inferiorly. Another fully developed pelvis was situated in its natural position, and supported two well-formed abdominal limbs; the ossa innominata were widely separated posteriorly, so as to include between them the two sacra and the rudimentary pelvis : there were only eleven ribs at each side; the lower limbs were remarkably meagre and ill nourished.

There existed a single bladder, uterus and rectum, which were common to the two subjects, but behind these organs were found rudimentary traces of others.

There were two distinct hearts in one pericardium, which touched at their apices; all the other thoracic and most of the abdominal viscera were double; examination by the stethoscope indicated only a single heart.

Many interesting observations were made on this monster during life; the nervous systems seemed to have but little communication, except in those parts which were in the line of union, as the anus and sexual organs; for if the right limb was pinched, or the sole of the foot tickled, Ritta only felt it; and if the left, only Cristina; so that of the common pair of limbs, the right seemed to belong to the one individual, and the left to the other. And this was verified on dissection; for the spinal cords were found to be quite separate, and there was no communication between the nerves forming the nervous trunks going to the two abdominal limbs; the only union between the nerves of the two beings was found in the parts in the line of junction. One would sleep while the other remained awake sucking; or smile while the other cried or was quite tranquil.

The two creatures experienced the sensation of hunger at different times, but felt the desire to expel the fæces at the same time. This might be expected from the structure of their alimentary canal, which was double as far as the commencement of the ilium, and single in the rest of its course. There was an anastomosis of the iliac arteries belonging to each.

There was a remarkable difference in the expression of their countenances : Cristina being of a gay and happy look, while Ritta looked sad and melancholy, as if suffering, which was the fact.

They died at Paris, 23d November of the same year, having lived eight months and eleven days; and I believe their survival for such a length of time constitutes an exception to the history of double monsters with two hearts in one pericardium. The account of their last moments is deserving of mention. Ritta, who had always been feeble and ailing, at last became very ill for some days before her death, but during those days Cristina continued in perfect health, was gay and merry, and was playing in her mother's arms when Ritta breathed her last, but on the moment Cristina screamed out and instantly expired. It was remarked also that she became cold and rigid in a few minutes ; but that Ritta became so only at the end of eight hours.

The same authority which objected to their exhibition·while living, wished to prevent their examination after death, and ordered their burial within twenty-four hours ; and it was only at the urgent solicitation of M. Geoffrey St. Hilaire and others, that permission could be obtained for delay, in order to investigate their organization.—*Dublin Quarterly Journal of Medical Science.*

MOTIVE POWER OF THE BLOOD PROVED BY EXPERIMENTS ON FOUR CROCODILES—ONE BROUGHT TO LIFE.

BY SAMUEL A. CARTWRIGHT, M.D., NEW ORLEANS, LATE OF NATCHEZ.

[Communicated for the Boston Medical and Surgical Journal.]

FOUR crocodiles were subjected to vivisection in the court-yard of my office, on the 1st and 6th of the present month. One was nearly ten feet long, another about six and a half feet, and the other two of smaller size.

June 1st, at half past 9 o'clock, I tied the trachea of one of the smaller sized saurians, and turned it loose. At twelve minutes before 10 o'clock, I tied the trachea of another one, and proceeded at once to open the thorax and abdomen, exposing the viscera, even the heart, to view, by opening the pericardium. It was then taken from the table and placed on the floor. The largest crocodile was surrendered to Dr. Dowler, to perform any experiments he might see proper. By this time a number of medical gentlemen had assembled to witness the experiments ; viz., Drs. Copes, Nutt, Hale, Wharton, Weatherly, Chaillie, Chappellier, Greenleaf, Prof. Riddell and his brother, and also Messrs. Brenan and Gordon. While the large crocodile was being secured and made fast to the table, the two others, whose tracheæ had been ligated, were moving about as actively as before the operation. Some doubted whether the ligation would kill them at all ; and others were of the opinion that the exposure of the viscera and serous membranes of one of them, to·the action of the air, would prevent the ligation from proving fatal, as oxygen would be absorbed and carbonic acid expelled by·the tissues thus exposed. The experiment reported at page 394 of the 46th volume of this Journal, June 16, 1852, where an alligator, nearly dead, revived under the scalpel of the dissector, while the ligature was still around the trachea, had given rise to that opinion ; although it was subsequently demonstrated, by attempts at insufflation, that the lungs had been cut by the operator, thus giving egress to the poisonous carbonic acid and ingress to the vivifying oxygen—still the erroneous impression was left on the minds of Dr. Dowler and others, that it was the exposure of the membranes to the air by the dissection· which revived the animal. In the present case the viscera and membranes were as extensively exposed to the air as in that instance. I particularly guarded against cutting the lungs or any branches of the bronchial tubes. Both animals, in less than an hour after the ligation of the trachea, were dead. The one, whose viscera had been exposed, died as soon as the other. When pinching, burning and piercing the most sensitive parts of the body ceased to cause motion or to produce sensation, the first one operated on was re-placed on the table, and the viscera of the thorax and abdomen exposed by dissection. An artery was accidentally cut, and a profuse hemorrhage was the consequence. The temperature of the room was 83°. The inflating process was then commenced, and some faint evidences of returning vitality manifested themselves ; but as the reptile had lost the greater portion of the blood in its body, the very substance I wished to vivify and set in motion by the introduction of fresh air into the lungs, I abandoned the experiment and removed the subject from the table, without regret, intending to make it answer the purposes of another experiment to prove the error of certain reviewers, who had taken the position, " that alligators were curious animals, and might come to life of themselves if let alone." Hence the determination to let this one alone, to prove to sceptics that nothing short of the admission of fresh air into the lungs can restore life in cases of asphyxia or suspended animation. It never came to, or responded to the irritants applied to its nerves, but quickly lost every remaining vestige of life after the insufflation was suspended. Even the irritability of the muscles was destroyed ; thus confirming the experiment reported at page 79 of the 47th volume of this Journal, Aug. 26, 1852, where simple ligation of the trachea not only destroyed life, but muscular irritability, by poisoning the blood by the retention of carbonic acid.

The other crocodile, above mentioned, whose trachea had been tied at a quarter before 10 o'clock, and the viscera immediately exposed, was found to be dead, and at 25 minutes before 11 o'clock was replaced upon the table. Various means were used, as pinching, piercing and burning the most sensitive parts of the body, to extort symptoms of life ; and when they failed to have any effect, the inflating process was commenced. After continuing the insufflation of the lungs for some fifteen or twenty minutes, the animal came to life, snapped its jaws, opened its eyes, moved its limbs, and twisted and worked itself when pinched or cut. In the language of a by-stander—" *it lived again.*" It continued to live for several hours afterwards. It was brought to life at 11 o'clock. At 3 o'clock, when the company left for dinner, it was still alive, and would dodge the finger when thrust at its eyes, although not touched. Several gentlemen, before leaving, convinced themselves by that and other measures, that the reptile was not only alive, but had its sight, hearing, intelligence and the power of motion restored to it. When the company left, it was the only live crocodile in the room. Both the others had been dead for some time. The first one operated on had been dead more than four hours—and the one which Dr. Dowler had been experimenting on was also dead, although it was the last one brought on the table.

On the 6th of June I tied the trachea of a female crocodile, about six and a half feet long, and as large around as a common-sized man—Drs. Dowler, Copes, Wharton, Chappellier, Reynolds, Greenleaf and Backee being present. When animation became nearly suspended, the viscera were exposed by dissection. On opening the pericardium, the auricle of the heart happened to be pierced. The hemorrhage was profuse. A ligature was put around the slit in the auricle, but before the hemorrhage could be arrested the most of the blood in the body had escaped. Insufflation was tried, but it had very little ostensive effect. It excited the heart into action, and restored some degree of motion and sensibility ; but it restored and preserved an amount of vitality sufficient to enable Dr. Dowler, to whom I resigned the half-dead female saurian, to re-produce those astonishing phenomena of the nervous system, which he has heretofore made known to the scientific world. They are of a nature to make a Nilotic ruin, a perfect chaos, of the main foundation of physiology and psychology since the days of Moses. In the report of the experiment on the battle-ground crocodile, published August 25, 1852, in the 47th volume of this Journal, it is stated that after tying the trachea the animal died, and that Dr. Dowler, with fire, hooks and forceps, failed to produce a single nervous phenomenon he had been accustomed to show. But in this instance, a sufficient quantum of vitality remained and was kept up by the inflation, to enable him to verify to the by-standers nearly the whole of those remarkable facts he has heretofore reported in his " Contributions to Physiology." He proved with the half-dead reptile, as also with the ten-foot crocodile on the 1st of June, what he had frequently proved before, viz., that sensibility, motion, the will and intelligence, continue to be manifested in the body after it has been cut off from the brain and spinal marrow ; that pinching the distal portion of any divided nerve will cause motion and sensation in the part to which it is distributed, and that the same phenomena will continue to occur as the nerve is followed downward toward the part to which it is distributed. These experiments with the crocodile prove the fallacy of those dogmas, which have so long made physiology and psychology the most hypothetical, changeable and non-progressive of all the sciences. Until cut loose from the unsound learning of the dark ages, those noble sciences cannot be made to perform their proper part on the arena of practical utility. The hypotheses to which they are chained, make the cerebral system the *subjective or the me*, and the blood the *objective or the not me.* To reach the brain, the supposed seat of the subjectivity, recourse has been had to the supposition, that impressions from without are conveyed by a subtle fluid, oscillations or other means, through the nerves to the brain—the supposed exclusive residence of the mind. The latter is supposed to give its commands, which are conveyed by the same or another set of nerves to the muscles and to the different organs of the body, ordering muscular motions to be performed and pain or pleasure to be felt. Another hypothesis pre-supposes that the chief motive power of the blood is derived from the mechanical propulsion effected by the contraction of a muscle, called the heart. There are more than three millions of species of animals destitute of such an organ, and even in mammals the heart and arteries are of subsequent formation to some other structures of the body abundantly furnished with nutritive fluids. While such unsound doctrines (which need only be stated to carry their refutation upon their face) are received as fundamental truths in physiology and psychology, it will be vain to expect that these sciences can make any progress in the field of utility and practical operations. While such errors prevail, the phenomena, attributed to mesmerism, table-moving and spirit-rapping, will continue to confound the wisdom of the learned and to lead the ignorant and credulous into every species of ridiculous extravagance. Such is the natural tendency of the popular mind when men of science are driven to the subterfuge of denying phenomena clearly demonstrable —not for the want of evidence of their existence, but for the want of something in their philosophy to explain them. Back to Moses, then, let young America, not too old or full of prejudice to learn new truths, go to take a fresh start in physiology and psychology. Physiologists and psychologists will there learn, what the experiments on the crocodile prove, that the blood is the *subjective or the me*, and that all other parts of the body are the *objective or the not me;* or, in the language of Moses, the blood is the life of the flesh and the air is the life of the blood. Life, in the proper Hebrew sense of the term—life, consisting of motion, sensation, will, consciousness and intelligence; these are all implied by the Hebrew word translated life. Neither physicians nor theologians have fully believed in the physiological doctrines taught by Moses. Some of the former and all the latter profess to believe in the prophet, but not in the prophet's doctrines when applied to physiology. It is not as a prophet I quote him, but as a man and a learned physiologist. My experiments on the crocodile, as well as those of Dr. Dowler, show most clearly and positively, that, as far as regards the fundamental principles of the science of physiology, Moses is a great way a-head of either Carpenter or Dunglison. Dowler proves that the blood is the life of the flesh when he irritates a nerve, dissevered from the brain and spine, and produces the phenomena of life and motion in the part to which it is distributed. When the blood was previously poisoned by carbonic acid gas, as in the experiment with the battle-ground crocodile, recorded in this Journal (page 79, vol. 47), not a single symptom of life followed the irritation of the nerves or any other part. Muscular irritability had been destroyed by the carbonic acid destroying the life of the blood. Whereas in other experiments, where the blood had not thus been previously poisoned, or if poisoned, its vitality had been restored by insufflation, then the irritation of any nerve, after it had been divided or after the spine and brain had been destroyed, produced the phenomena of life in the parts to which it was distributed. The brain and nerves, therefore, instead of being the primary seat and type of life, are subordinate agents, or mere conductors of vitality from the fountain of life, the blood, to the flesh and solid structures of the body.

My experiments prove that the life of the blood is derived from the atmospheric air; and that air alone, without any aid from the heart at all, is its main and principal motive power. In other words, the oxidation of the blood in the lungs is the chief motive power ; or, in the language of Mrs. Willard, " the chief motive power of the blood is derived from respiration." Whether caloric, as Mrs. Willard contends, or caloric and electricity combined, be the *Phætonitis equi* of those cars of life, called blood corpuscles, is another question, lying in hypothetical regions I have no desire to explore. It is not the occult cause of things, but the existence of the things themselves, I seek to prove. That there is such a thing as a *hæmatokinetic* or blood-moving power, derived from respiration, is abundantly proved by artificial respiration restoring motion to the blood and bringing to life dead crocodiles. That this hæmatokinetic or blood-moving power can act beyond the periphery of the animal body, is sufficiently proved by those beautiful habitations which the mollusks build, paint and polish for themselves, without the aid of head or hands. Shells are nothing more than the thing called mesmerism in the solid form. Their frame work consists of fibrin thrown off from the body of the animal, chinked or filled in with solid matter thrown out like the fibrin. The stumbling-block, to those educated in the doctrines of solidism and mechanical agencies, is that their philosophy will not admit them to attach ideas of life, motion, sensibility and intelligence, to any substances not provided with an apparatus to move by mechanical means, with nerves, brain, and organs especially designed for hearing, seeing, tasting, smelling and feeling. Yet the beaver and the snail have an additional sense, which has been called the *hygrometic*, enabling them to foretell changes in the weather. No organ has ever been discovered through which such knowledge is communicated. There are millions and myriads of living creatures in the ocean possessing one or more of the above-mentioned senses, and some of them sufficient intelligence to be expert navigators ; yet they are liquid masses having less consistency than the blood, being mere bubbles of jelly inflated with atmospheric air, and without any solid organization whatever. Even the membrane enclosing the radiaries is as foreign to their gelatinous bodies as the shell is to the crustacea. The light, seen in the ocean near the arctic circle and the equator, is emitted by myriads of animals, not only possessing life, sensation and intelligence, but motions as *rapid as meteors.* They are of less consistence than the blood ; the slightest touch resolves them into thin air and an unctuous liquid. They prove that life, with all its essential attributes, does and can exist in the liquid and even in the aeriform state.

The difficulty of believing the Mosaic physiology, that the blood is the life, and air the fountain of life to the blood, is not for the want of facts proving that substances less dense possess life, but is owing to the prejudices of education founded on too narrow a platform. The platform of Harvey, that the chief motive power of the blood is derived from a muscular organ, excludes the larger half of the animal creation. Fishes have no aortic heart to circulate the blood. They have a small, weak muscular organ to assist in propelling the blood into the gills, but they have no heart to propel it through the systemic circulation. The oxygenation of the blood in the gills is a sufficient motive power. In the sturgeon the arteries are cartilaginous tubes, and can give the hæmatokinetic power, derived from the oxygenation of the blood in the gills, no assistance. The heart of the fœtus in utero does not beat time with that of the mother, nor are the blood corpuscles of the same size in the mother and her unborn child; proving that it is not the same blood, and is not circulated by the same forces, as the theory of Harvey supposes. The law, which gives the motive power to the blood of fishes—the oxidation of the blood in the gills—gives the motive power to the fœtal blood; the placenta performing for the fœtus the same office that the gills do for fishes. The fœtus in utero is, physiologically speaking, *a tadpole*, the placenta being its branchiæ or gills. When comparative anatomy is more studied, the radical error of the received doctrines of the circulation will become more apparent.

Dowler and the mesmerizers (I fear he will never pardon me for the association) have done much to expose the errors of the schools on the nervous system. The former has demonstrated repeatedly that the phenomena of sensation, voluntary motions, the will, the passions, and some degree of intelligence, can be re-produced in animals deprived of the brain and spinal marrow. Both have proved that the mind is not a prisoner in the bone called the cranium, as the learned world believe. My experiments prove that the blood, instead of being a lifeless mass, moved only as it is moved by physical forces, is highly vital, and derives from the oxygen of the air, not only its life, but a hæmatokinetic or motive power more active than that which the needle derives from the load-stone; that the motive power thus generated, is not dependent on vascular organization or any organization at all for its manifestations, as is proved by the Articulata and Radiata, and that it can carry the vital blood beyond the immediate periphery of the vascular system, as is proved by the fibrous frame-work in the shells of the Mollusca.

Canal street, New Orleans, June 11th, 1853.

SOURCE OF VITALITY IN THE TEETH.

" RHIZODONTRYPO-NEURHÆMAXIS," AND THE REMOVAL OF THE DENTAL PULP, NOT BASED ON PHYSIOLOGICAL PRINCIPLES, AND THEREFORE IMPRACTICABLE.

[Concluded from page 417.]

In the early development of the dental pulp, the sac (which when calcified is the cementum) plays an important part, being highly vascular; but when the pulp receives its proper dental vessels, it degenerates into a non-vascular, protective membrane; and its present importance and utility with its former, may well be compared to the umbilical vessels of the fœtus, which in its primitive life are the *only* media of vitality; but in after years degenerate into simple, fibrous, impervious ligaments.

The cemental membrane has been found by Dr. Carpenter " to be a substance very *closely* resembling that which *intervenes* in the *growing* bone, *between* its surface and the investing periosteum."* Another evidence of the vitality of the teeth existing alone in their central gan-

* The Italics are mine.

glia, is drawn from the case given by Dr. Miller, as reported in this Journal, Vol. xlvii., No. 12, where a lady with nine teeth *superficially* decayed, in which the sensibility was so much exalted as not to admit of their being filled until it was in some way reduced, was submitted to the pain-destroying influence of chloroform, and six of the nerves cut, "after which the teeth were filled without pain." If the cementum furnishes vitality to any part of the tooth, we should naturally suppose that it would be to its external surface. If it is a source of vitality, it must furnish vessels and nerves, and this being the case an amputation of the central ganglion would not destroy the sensibility in superficial carious cavities, as stated in the above case.

In regard to removing the crowns of teeth that from decay have become useless, and inserting mineral ones ; it is well understood by most scientific surgeon-dentists, that it is not the best of practice, and should, as a general rule, be avoided, though there are cases where it seems the only thing that can be done under the circumstances. Every physician and dentist knows that teeth which have lost their crowns, either by the hand of the dentist or by disease, whether covered by an artificial crown or not, are usually great sources of discomfort from their gradual decomposition, and not unfrequently produce serious diseases of the stomach, jaw, and especially of the nervous system. No unprejudiced mind can fail to be convinced, on removing the fang of a tooth that has for any length of time, or for any reason, been deprived of its central vessels, that it is *dead*—that it leaves its alveolus readily, because absorption has already commenced. It is a fundamental law of the animal economy, that any portion of its structure, losing its vitality, shall early or late be removed ; the length of time occupied being always in proportion to the power in the substance to resist decomposition and the amount and activity of the absorbents by which it is surrounded. On this principle, I attribute the long standing of the fangs referred to in No. 18 of the present volume of this Journal.

In regard to the subject of "amputation" and "*puncture*" of the nerve or its accompanying vessels, I would inquire the size of the instrument with which Dr Miller punctures the desired vessel, in an inferior incisor, when the dental canal (as is often the case) one line from the border of the alveolus is one hundreth of an inch in diameter, and that canal traversed by three vessels—vein, nerve and artery ? And how does the doctor distinguish between the other vessels and the nerve ? How does Dr. Miller account for a puncture of the nerve destroying its sensibility ? In cases of facial neuralgia and sciatica, would they be relieved if the facial and sciatic nerves were thoroughly punctured with a lancet or a fine trocar ? In cases of an irritated ulnar nerve occurring in an amputated fore-arm, would it be relieved of its sensibility if the brachial nerve was well *punctured* ? On taking away one quart of blood or less from the brachial artery, would it diminish the sensibility in its exposed extremity, so that by irritating it with a sharp excavator the patient would experience no pain ? I am strongly inclined to the belief that these cases of puncture are in fact cases of excision, or at least the vessels are so much injured that they are unable to do duty. If depletion is the object, it can be done through the carious cavity, and the patient spared some pain, which is quite an object, especially with the patient. I have no doubt, as Dr. Miller affirms, "that the dental nerves of elderly people become absorbed, and their canals filled with a bony deposit"; but "that the nerve sometimes becomes ossified," is a matter of doubt; yet exostosis frequently occurs in the lining membrane of the alveoli, often involving the fang and causing the destruction of the tooth and its extraction.

From the foregoing I think we may come to the conclusion :—

1st. That the human teeth receive all their vitality from the vessels that enter the pulp cavity.

2d. That the *cementum petrosa* is a non-vascular membrane in the fully-developed tooth ; consequently can have no part in supplying the tooth with vitality, and can serve only as a connecting medium " belonging equally to the alveoli and the tooth."

3d. That the destruction of the central ganglion destroys the vitality of the organ ; therefore any operation contemplating it, with a view to its preservation, is not based on physiological and therapeutical principles, and therefore is " impracticable."

But because this or that operation does not bring the success hoped for, " shall nothing be done " to prolong usefulness and extend existence ? Certainly, the physician and surgeon should call to his aid all the resources of science and art, and with discrimination and judgment such as becomes physicians, apply the means to a perfect cure ; but if this is impossible, let him do all that a humane and sympathizing man can do, to allay the physical and mental disquiet which disease brings, that when it takes its leave (wholly or in part), he may possess the pleasing assurance that in all honesty it has been treated upon pure scientific and practical principles.

It is not to be supposed that the department of dentistry, though in skilful hands, has as yet arrived at a point, either in theory or practice, beyond which there is nothing better. That the profession during the past few years have made great progress and many improvements, is a matter of rejoicing to many that suffer ; and it would be unprofessional and unchristian to call them a " stupid set of fellows," for not knowing twenty, ten or even five years ago, the same, and all other physiological and pathological facts which they now possess, or even for not being acquainted with the operation called " rhizodontrypo-neurhæmaxis."

Rockville, Ct., June 11th, 1853.   M. M. Frisselle, M.D.

SURGICAL OPERATIONS IN CANCEROUS DISEASES.

[At the last meeting of the American Medical Association, Dr. Yandell, of Kentucky, presented a report from Dr. S. D. Gross, of the same State, on the results of surgical operations for the relief of malignant diseases. The following is the concluding portion of it.]

From the facts and statements which have now been presented, embracing the opinions of many of the most intelligent, experienced and distinguished practitioners in different ages, and in different parts of the world, the following conclusions may be legitimately deduced:

First.—That cancerous affections, particularly those of the mammary gland, have always, with a few rare exceptions, been regarded by practitioners as incurable by the knife and escharotics. This opinion, commencing with Hippocrates, the father of medicine, has prevailed from the earliest records of the profession, to the present moment. Nature never cures a disease of the kind ; nor can this be effected by any medicine, or internal remedies, known to the profession.

Secondly.—That excision, however early and thoroughly executed, is nearly always, in genuine cancer, followed by relapse, at a period varying from a few weeks to several months, from the time of the operation.

Thirdly.—That nearly all practitioners, from the time of Hippocrates to the present day, have been, and are still averse to any operation for the removal of cancerous tumors, after the establishment of ulceration, rapid growth, firm adhesion, organic change in the skin, lymphatic invasion, the cancerous dyscracy, or serious constitutional derangements ; on the ground that, if had recourse to, under these circumstances, the malady almost inevitably recurs in a very short time, and frequently destroys the patient more rapidly than when it is permitted to pursue its own course.

Fourthly.—That in all cases of *acute* carcinoma, or, in other words, in all cases of this disease, attended with very rapid development and great bulk of the tumor, extirpation is improper and unjustifiable, inasmuch as it will only tend to expedite the fatal result, which, under such circumstances, always takes place in a very short time.

Fifthly.—That all operations performed for the removal of encephaloid cancer and its different varieties, are more certainly followed by rapid relapse than operations performed upon scirrhus or hard cancer.

Sixthly.—That in nearly all the operations for cancerous diseases, hitherto reported, the history has been imperfectly presented, being deficient in the details which are necessary to a complete and thorough understanding of the subject in each case. This remark is particularly true in reference to the diagnosis of the malady, the minute examination of the morbid structure, and the history of the case after the operation, as to the period of relapse, the time and nature of the patient's death, and the result of the post-mortem examination.

Seventhly.—That cancerous affections of the lip and skin, now usually described under the name of cancroid diseases, are less liable to relapse after extirpation than genuine cancerous maladies, or those which are characterized by the existence of the true cancer-cell and cancer-juice.

Eighthly.—That, although practitioners have always been aware, from the earliest professional records, of the great liability of cancer to relapse after extirpation, a great majority of them have always been, and still are, in favor of operation in the early stage of the disease, especially in scirrhus, before the tumor has made much progress, or before there is any disease of the lymphatic ganglions, or evidence of the cancerous cachexy.

Ninthly.—That many cases of tumors, especially tumors of the breast and testicle, supposed to be cancerous, are in reality not cancerous, but of a benign character, and consequently, readily curable by ablation, whether effected by the knife or by escharotics. It is to this circumstance that we must ascribe the astonishing success which is said to have attended the practice of Hill of Scotland, Nooth of England, and Flajani of Italy.

Tenthly.—That all operators insist upon the most thorough excision possible ; removing not merely the diseased mass, but also a portion of the surrounding and apparently healthy tissues, as well as all enlarged and indurated ganglions.

Eleventhly.—That the practice has always prevailed and still obtains, to save, if possible, a sufficient amount of healthy integument to cover the wound, and to unite, if possible, the wound by the first intention ; on the ground that these precautions will tend much to retard, if not to prevent, a recurrence of the disease.

Twelfthly.—That much stress is laid by writers upon a properly regulated diet, and attention to the bowels and secretions after operation, as means of retarding and preventing relapse.

Thirteenthly.—That there is no remedy, medicine or method of treatment which has the power, so far as we are enabled to judge of its virtues, of preventing the reproduction of the morbid action after operation, no matter how early or how thoroughly it may be performed.

Fourteenthly.—That life has occasionally been prolonged and even saved by operation after relapse, as in some of the remarkable cases mentioned in a previous part of this report ; but that, as a general rule, such a procedure is as incompetent to effect a permanent cure as a first extirpation.

THE BOSTON MEDICAL AND SURGICAL JOURNAL.

BOSTON, JUNE 29, 1853.

Medical Vases.—Among other evidences of the labors accomplished by that indefatigable physician, Dr. Simpson, of Edinburgh, we have received within a few days a pamphlet by him upon the discovery of certain little vases, about an inch high and two-thirds of an inch in diameter, labelled in Greek, *lykion.* They are found in Greece, and occasionally in Italy, particularly in those places where there were Greek settlements in early times. The *lykion* was held by the ancients in the greatest estimation, and from the slight history of its use by practitioners of a remote age, it must have been very costly. Dr. Simpson's notes are full of interest. With praiseworthy enterprise, he has ascertained where the article was procured, and shows that it is still in repute in India, where it has always been prepared. For diseases of the eyes this *lykion* has been celebrated from the times of Dioscorides, Galen, and others equally well known for their attainments in medicine, and was considered far superior to all other remedies for certain affections of the optic apparatus. *Lykion* is in reality known as *ruswut* in Hindostan, and may be purchased at shops in most of the great towns over all India ; and we therefore suggest to medical gentlemen living in ports in the United States from whence vessels are frequently sailing to Calcutta, to send an order for a few ounces. At all events, the oculists might find it to their special advantage to prescribe it. The *ruswut* is an inspissated extract from the wood and roots of several species of *berberis*, growing on the mountains principally of Upper India, and especially near Lahore. Dr. Simpson has a faculty of imparting a peculiar interest to any and every subject upon which he finds leisure to write.

Consumption.—Progress of improvement in the treatment of this sweeping, uncontrolled malady, including pulmonary and laryngeal diseases, is the substance of the title to a pamphlet just received from England, by James Turnbull, M.D., &c., to whom we are indebted for a copy. At this era in medicine, when the idea of specifics is so generally discarded, physicians will be slow to believe that pulmonary consumption is curable when the lungs have become ulcerated, notwithstanding the encouragement held out in this treatise. There are distinct dissertations in the book, on the use of some of the pyrogenic remedies; the use of the alcoholic extract and the tincture of the seeds of the Œnanthe phellandrium; the topical application of the solution of the nitrate of silver in laryngeal diseases; on the employment of inhalations; on hygienic means of treatment, and the application of the sugar of milk as an article of diet. The author is a methodical writer, and quite conversant with the writings and practice of those who have preceded him. Rather than epitomise any of the pages of his short treatise, we shall endeavor to extract such brief paragraphs as will give the reader an idea of Dr. Turnbull's efforts in this ample field of labor.

Purchased Fame.—In an appendix to a treatise on the structure, diseases and injuries of the blood vessels, by Edward Crisp, M.D., which won the Jacksonian prize at the Royal College of Surgeons in 1844, the learned author says, "In this country (England), a man must generally be attached, by purchase, to an hospital, before his works can obtain celebrity." "How is it in this country?"—inquires a gentleman who has never had either a patron or a fortune. "Is true merit noticed without the accompaniment of a strong family influence or its equivalent in real estate and stocks?" The question is open for discussion—although he insists upon it that when merit in a medical aspirant is encouraged, those who bestow the encouragement first ascertain that the individual will neither be in their way or disposed to outgrow his dependence.

Ladies' Physiological Institute.—An act of incorporation for this institution, located in Boston, was obtained in March, 1850. All the members are females, and they have conducted the affairs of the Institute admirably. Usually, a lecture is given once a week. Besides skeletons, models of individual organs, and one of the finest manikins in the city, they have a choice collection of books. A catalogue of them covers ten pages of the last annual report, which speaks well for their course of preparation. With limited pecuniary means, the members have made themselves known and respected for their intelligence, and their praiseworthy determination to study the art of promoting the health of themselves and others. Without claiming to be originators of new doctrines or contemplating innovations upon the usages of society, they simply endeavor to improve their physical well-being, through the teachings of the best lecturers and writers on the laws of physiology.

Dental Toilet Articles.—Such a vast variety of powders, liquids, saponaceous and other preparations, for keeping the teeth in health, are now in the market, that it becomes a matter of serious importance to determine what may be serviceable and what injurious. When these articles emanate from honorable, well-known dentists, who give their names and address with their remedies, we naturally conclude the latter to be good, and that it is perfectly safe to follow the directions given. Each and all of them have too much reputation at stake to hazard it all upon a shilling's worth of any thing that will not stand the test of examination. Trusting to their integrity, therefore, we are disposed to make trial of whatever comes from them, professing to better the condition of the teeth. Dr. Angell's and Mr. Davis's dental soaps have had an extensive sale, and de servedly so, for they are excellent, accomplishing all that the inventors promise. J. A. Cummings, M.D., a medically-educated dentist of Boston, has brought out a dentifrice and a tooth-wash, very elegantly put up, which meets with an extensive patronage. It has the appearance of meriting, and we have no doubt does really merit, the praise implied by its extensive sales.

Manikins.—Inquiries are frequently made, both by letter and through messengers, respecting the cost of manikins, which are now considered quite indispensable in popular lectures on anatomy and physiology. An agency was opened at Albany, some years ago, where M. Azoux had his articles for sale. Why he should have sent the preparations away interior, instead of having them on sale at Boston or New York, cannot be understood. The sales have been fewer in consequence of the agency being out of the way. The following information, which is worth laying aside for reference, is taken from the Water Cure Journal.

"For the benefit of prospective lecturers on Physiology, who may be desirous of obtaining suitable apparatus, with which to illustrate the subject, we have obtained the following particulars with regard to the cost of a suitable cabinet.

"Manikins of the best quality can only be obtained from France. They are no where else manufactured with any thing like the same degree of perfection. The different sizes and prices are as follows. The smallest size, about eighteen inches high, may be had at $90. The second size, four feet high, with seventeen hundred objects, at $350. Same size, with twelve hundred objects, for $200.

"The third size, six feet high, with twelve hundred objects, $400.

"Same size, with seventeen hundred objects, $950.

"French skeletons, wired, ready for use, may be had at prices ranging from $26 to $50.

"The time usually required to import these articles by steamer from Paris, is from six to eight weeks. Payment is always required at the time of purchase.

"Besides the manikin, and skeleton, a set of anatomical drawings, the size of life, representing every part of the human body, colored and mounted, may be had in New York at $25. A complete set is composed of eleven figures, and, in the absence of other specimens, will serve well, in the lecture room, to illustrate physiology and anatomy." '

Imperforate Rectum.—From Dr. Kirby's Journal, the following account of an operation is extracted. It was communicated by J. K. Payne, M.D., of Bangor, Me.—"I attended a female infant, born Dec. 10, 1852, with an imperforate rectum, where the obstruction was situated three inches from the anus. The intestine was entirely closed about an inch, by a tough muscular substance, as if the sides of the rectum had grown together. The anus was natural, but the rectum, from the anus to the obstructed part, was contracted to one half its usual size. As I could not direct a bistoury by the finger to the stricture, I first placed a large-sized *trocar* in the direction of the rectum, through the obstruction, till it came in communication with the intestine beyond. After withdrawing the trocar, I inserted a bistoury to the upper part of the obstruction (using a grooved sound for a director), and made an incision towards the sacrum and down nearly to the anus. Then, distending the rectum with a pair of probe forceps, a copious discharge from the bowels immediately followed. The operation was not performed till the fourth day (the parents would not consent before), when all the symptoms of incarcerated hernia had set in. Those symptoms soon subsided, and the child is now perfectly well. The ring and middle fingers, and all the small toes, were grown together nearly to the ends."

Treatment of Spermatorrhœa.—With the difficulties connected with the treatment of obstinate cases of this malady, most practitioners are familiar. Books without number have been written on the subject; and almost every system of medicine proposes remedies, many of which on trial are found of no value whatever. It is hopeless to undertake to interrupt by medication the repetitions of the misfortune. There are but two methods, we believe, decidedly reliable; one of them is mechanical, the other is left to the ingenuity of the reader to ascertain. For several years past some of the very worst forms in which the disease presents itself, have been terminated in a short time, and the sufferer restored to permanent health, by a mechanical contrivance, which originated, it is believed, in Boston. The way to proceed is this: Take a piece of firm harness leather one inch wide, and make a ring or ferrule, which shall be one eighth of an inch greater in diameter than the penis. Thrust the points of four pins, equi-distant from each other, through the walls of the ring, so that they will project through a little way on the inside, and then cut off the projecting part of the pins on the outside. On retiring for the night, slip the ring on the organ, midway, and insert cotton wool between the two, to keep the pins from pricking the flesh. An emission seldom occurs without a full distension of the penis. The theory of a cure, as well as the facts, are simply these. When an erection takes place, and even before, the uniform enlargement presses the cotton, which yields, causing the points of the pins to enter the flesh. and thus the patient is instantly awakened. This occurs as frequently as distension comes on, and the semen is therefore retained. This, we repeat, is superior to any and all other prescriptions made use of. Last week an instrument was left on sale at Dr. Cheever's, under the Tremont Temple, in this city, that acts precisely like the leather ring. It is made of steel, however, clasping like a dog's collar, according to the size required, and having on its inner edge a row of sharp points. Within this steel ring is another, extremely delicate, which opens to receive the penis, and retains it exactly in the middle. When it begins to distend, the small ring allows the member to enlarge till it strikes the sharp points, and then the individual is awake and safe. After interrupting the emission a few times in this way, the morbid tendency in many cases is removed, and the sickly, feeble youth rallies and regains his health. Other cases may require a more constant use of the remedy, until maturer age and different circumstance render it no longer necessary.

Memoir of Dr. Nichols.—Samuel A. Lord, M.D., has prepared an interesting sketch of the life of the late Andrew Nichols, M.D., of Danvers, reprinted from the communications of the Massachusetts Medical Society. It is concise, but embraces the principal events in the life of a good and trustworthy physician. The subject of Dr. Lord's memoir was neither a blusterer nor a man of iron heart. His sympathies were strong, his efforts untiring in the routine of professional duties ; and as a man, a gentleman and a citizen, he was courteous without being obsequious ; firm, but never obstinate, and in all the relations of life a pattern for those who would rise to distinction by the practice of the social virtues. Our recollections of Dr. Nichols are of a pleasant kind. Hospitality and a consideration for others were prominent traits, which endeared to him a great circle of friends, who sympathize with a bereaved family in their affliction. Dr. N. held a commanding position in the medical councils of the fraternity, that was based on many years of experience and a cultivated understanding.

Public Health.—Notwithstanding the extreme heat of the weather the past week, the health of this metropolis is excellent. No epidemic prevails. Cases of bowel complaint are always liable to appear at the approach of the fruit season ; but that should by no means prevent people from indulging reasonably in all the fully ripe fruits with which the country is blessed. Some few deaths have occurred from imprudence in drinking cold water ; and reports of the sudden extinction of life from excessive heat have appeared in the papers. But a very satisfactory state of the public health appears at present to exist throughout New England.

Medical Electricity.—There has recently been an active competition in the employment of this agent in the treatment of diseases. Several well-informed physicians are giving exclusive attention to it, and with happy effects. Dr. Rogers, Tremont Row, Boston, has a curious and ingenious apparatus for the application of it to the various regions of the body ; and by a judicious administration of the power which in so many ways is made subservient to the purposes of science, has achieved very important results.

Physicians Abroad.—Perhaps a larger number of American physicians were never before in Europe, than at the present time. Nearly every school and city in the Union is represented, and there is also a flood of American students distributed through the schools of London, Edinburgh,

Dublin, Paris, Berlin, Vienna, and other celebrated cities. There is something at each place worth seeing.

Medical Miscellany.—Samuel Martin died at Orwell, on the 11th inst., at the advanced age of 107 years.—All kinds of sickness prevailed at Venezuela, at the last accounts.—Sixty deaths by black vomit were recently reported at Vera Cruz.—Yellow fever and dysentery are raging at Rio Janeiro.—A large number of cases of cholera are said to have appeared at Norfolk, Virg., some of which terminated fatally.—A serious riot occurred in New York, last week, by a mob, who riddled the house of Dr. Geo. A. Wheeler, because some human bones were found on the premises. —Mrs. Elizabeth Dunlap died at Winsboro', S. C., on Friday of last week, at the advanced age of 109 years.—Owen Duffy, of Monaghan County, Ireland, is 122 years old. When 116 he lost his second wife, and subsequently married a third, by whom he had a son and daughter. His youngest son is two years old, his eldest 90. He still retains in much vigor his mental and corporeal faculties, and frequently walks to the county town, a distance of eight miles.—A jury has returned a verdict of $800 against Dr. Crosby, in New Hampshire, for mal-practice in the management of a broken bone.—Dr. John Westcott is the surveyor general of Florida. —Dr. Loring, late surgeon of the Chelsea Marine Hospital, has been appointed post-master of Salem, Mass.—Dr. William Hildebrand, a native of Germany, residing at Mineral Point, Wisconsin, has been appointed U. S. Consul at Bremen.—The New York Medical Gazette states that 29 suicides, 5 murders and 209 cases of insanity are directly traceable to spiritual manifestations as the cause.—Such has been the infectious character of the land speculation fever at Chicago, that even the physicians have caught the disease. Dr. Egan, of that place, represented as a good and worthy man, was recently called to prescribe for a lady. The potions were duly prepared, and when he was about withdrawing she very naturally inquired —" doctor, when are they to be taken?" Quarter down, balance in one, two, and three years!" was the prompt reply. "Good morning, madam," and the doctor bowed himself out with his usual suavity.—A rich bachelor quaker has given $300,000 for building and endowing an asylum for the insane at Baltimore.—Dr. Elisha R. Kane has sailed, as commander of the Arctic Exploring Expedition.—The Female Medical College of Pennsylvania is to have a female faculty; Miss Mory, M.D., of Providence, is one of them. It is located at Perkioomen Bridge, Montgomery Co.— Small-pox is quite common in remote parts of Pennsylvania.

DIED,—In London, by suicide, Dr. Bailey, a medical man of distinction.

MARRIED,—Dr. S. Heath, of Kingsville, Ohio, to Miss A. Hayes.—Dr. John G. Sewell, of New York, to Miss J. W. Gannett.

Deaths in Boston for the week ending Saturday noon, June 25th, 64. Males, 34—females, 30. Inflammation of the bowels, 4—bronchitis, 1—inflammation of the brain, 2—congestion of the brain, 1—consumption, 8—convulsions, 5—cholera morbus, 1—croup, 1—cancer, 1—dysentery, 1— dropsy of the head, 2—drowned, 1—infantile diseases, 5—puerperal, 1—typhus fever, 1—typhoid fever, 2—scarlet fever, 6—hooping cough, 1—disease of the heart, 1—hemorrhage, 1—intemperance, 1—disease of the kidney, 1—inflammation of the lungs, 2—marasmus, 3—measles, 2—mortification, 1—palsy, 2—pleurisy, 1—sun-stroke, 2—teething, 2—thrush, 1.

Under 5 years, 36—between 5 and 20 years, 6—between 20 and 40 years, 10—between 40 and 60 years, 7—over 60 years, 5. Born in the United States, 48—Ireland, 14—England, 1—British American Provinces, 1. The above includes 9 deaths in the city institutions.

. *Bristol (Mass.) District Medical Society.*—At the regular meeting of the Bristol District Medical Society, held at Attleboro', June 8th, 1853, were passed the following preamble and resolutions :—

We, the members of the Bristol District Medical Society, being assured as we are by the Constitution and By-laws of the Massachusetts Medical Society, that its great and leading object was in the beginning, and should continue to be, the promotion of medical science,

And further, believing that the great object for which the Society was formed can never be accomplished until it has disenthralled itself from empiricism of every name and nature,

And again, believing that the parent Society is, at the present time, encumbered by the most dishonest class of empirics that have ever disgraced the medical profession.

And finally, believing that the time has come when she must disenthrall herself of these insidious parasites, or abandon the objects for the promotion of which she was so wisely founded and has been so long and worthily sustained, therefore

Resolved,—That we heartily approve of the course adopted by our sister Society of Essex North, at the annual meeting of the parent Society.

Resolved,—That in our opinion the parent Society ought immediately, and in the most positive manner, to purify itself from all empirical connections.

Resolved,—That in the opinion of this Society it is doing injustice to censure " Thomsonians," " homœopathists," " empirical oculists," &c., or those who consult with outside empirics, while the parent Society *retains,* in full and honorable communion, a class of Jesuitical deceivers, in comparison with whom all other empirics and mountebanks are entitled to the most profound respect.

Resolved,—That in the event the parent Society refuses to grant this just request, we ask of her that boon, which she has recently so liberally extended to a certain class of her communionists, viz., that we may be permitted to withdraw ourselves from all connection with the parent Society.

Resolved,—That this preamble and these resolutions be signed by the President and Secretary, and that the Secretary be instructed to transmit a copy to the Corresponding Secretary of the parent Society, and also to the Secretaries of each of the District Societies.   M. R. RANDALL, *President.*

WM. DICKINSON, *Secretary.*

At the last meeting of the Bristol District Medical Society, held at Attleboro', on the 8th of June, the following preamble and resolutions were adopted.

Whereas,—By the dispensation of an inscrutable Providence, Dr. Phineas Savery has been by death removed from our Society,

Resolved,—That in the death of Dr. Savery the Bristol District Medical Society is deprived of one of its most esteemed and valuable members; *esteemed* for his gentle bearing and many amiable qualities, and *valuable* for his zealous efforts in the promotion of medical science.

Resolved,—That our warmest sympathies, elicited by kindred emotions, are tendered to the family of the deceased.

Resolved,—That these proceedings be published in the Boston Medical and Surgical Journal.

Resolved.—That a copy of the above proceedings be transmitted to the widow of the deceased.   Per order of B. D. M. Society,

WILLIAM DICKINSON, M.D., *Secretary.*

Application to close St. George's Churchyard.—A memorial is now in course of signature from the parishioners of St. Giles's-in-the-Fields, London, to the Home Secretary, praying for an order to close the churchyard in High street, some part of which has been used for interments ever since the year 1117, and another part since the year 1667. So long back as the year 1803, it was stated, in an act of Parliament, that the ground had become extremely offensive and dangerous to the health of the inhabitants of the neighborhood.—*London Lancet.*

THE

BOSTON MEDICAL AND SURGICAL JOURNAL.

Vol. XLVIII.   WEDNESDAY, JULY 6, 1853.   No. 23.

HOOPING COUGH AND ASTHMA.

BY J. C. PERRY, M.D., OF MATAGORDA, TEXAS.

THE recent epidemic of hooping cough was unusually severe, and along the Colorado very fatal. During the acute stage I did not find nitric acid beneficial ; after that had passed, any alterative or nervous sedative seemed to exercise a beneficial effect.

In young children (under 3 years) the disease was attended with high fever, bilious vomitings, inflammation of the bowels, and spinnage-colored stools, which, if neglected or treated with mercurials, generally proved fatal in four or five days.

In such cases I found a solution of nitrate of silver, of from four to five grains to the ounce, administered in teaspoonful doses every three or four hours, to act admirably, relieving the cough, and soon changing the nature of the discharges. Whether it acted as a caustic in passing over the epiglottis and so relieved the irritation there, as the cauterizations used by others, or whether the benefit arose from the powerful alterative and sedative influence it unquestionably exerts upon the gastro-intestinal mucous membrane and nerves, is for experience to determine.

I administered chloroform internally in every stage without benefit. Perhaps I was too cautious. Externally over the throat, on the spine and abdomen, it sometimes seemed to act well.

During paroxysms of asthma I have seen no relief from nitric acid. During the interval, when there has been torpor of the liver, as is apt to follow repeated attacks of the disease, doubtless attributable to the remora of the blood in the organ and destruction of its vessels during the paroxysms, I have thought it very useful, but not otherwise. In the internal use of chloroform, however, we have almost a specific. Administered when the paroxysm is forming it will generally prevent its full development, and given during its height will moderate all the urgent and distressing symptoms. I have used it ever since the discovery of the article, and have been generally successful, if not in curing, at least in palliating. I will give two cases only of many I have treated.

In 1849, saw Miss W., æt. 42, cachectic ; has had cough for years, probably tubercles. Has for fifteen years suffered from asthma after every exposure to cold, and always during the prevalence of the east wind. The paroxysms have become so frequent for the last year that she never breathes freely at night. Has gone through the whole materia medica. Gave chloroform, ten drops every three hours for four doses. Relief in 15 minutes, followed by sound sleep. Continued to take it whenever threatened with a paroxysm, which was less and less frequently for six months, after which time, for two years that I know her history, there was no return of the disease.

In 1852, saw Mrs. H., very fat, æt. 50 ; has been subject to asthma for thirty years. The paroxysms had become more and more frequent, and of longer duration with increase of age. Has one, of late years, every month in summer ; every week in winter. Has tried every remedy, including frequent changes of climate, without relief. She has enlargement of the heart and liver. The paroxysms were the most violent I ever witnessed, attended with intense pain in the head, delirium, small, feeble, very quick pulse, cold sweat, lasting two or three days and going off on supervention of copious expectoration of pure blood ; sometimes over half a pint would be expectorated in a night. During the paroxysm always gave relief and cut it short by giving chloroform, ten to fifteen drops every three hours, for four doses in the twenty-four hours, and a full dose of calomel.

By taking the chloroform on the accession of the first symptom she had succeeded in warding them off for months ; and now, after using nitric acid for two months, has been free from any attack for eight months, and enjoys as good health as the state of her liver and heart will admit.

The latter is not a case of pure asthma ; doubtless there was great congestion of the liver and lungs. But I could give you several cases of pure nervous asthma, in which the relief was even better marked than in these.

It has proved equally efficacious in relieving bronchitis or catarrhus senilis. Since 1849 I have been in the habit of treating neuralgia and the pains of inflamed eyes, by stuffing a thimble with cotton wet in chloroform, and holding it on the lids or on the skin along the course of the nerves. The thimble retains the vapor. I generally keep it applied for three minutes to one spot and change. If the nerve is superficial, it will ease entirely in a few seconds. You can cure some sore throats by applying it at the sides of the larynx. Rheumatic pains can be relieved in the same manner.

I do not know how much originality there is in the foregoing, but I have not read or heard of similar use of this remedy. Try it.—*New Orleans Monthly Medical Register.*

USE OF ANÆSTHETICS IN RIGIDITY OF PERINÆUM IN FIRST LABOR.

BY J. H. BEECH, M.D., OF COLDWATER, MICH.

HAVING a desire to exercise great caution in the employment of new remedies, I began the use of anæsthetics in obstetric practice, only in cases of unusual severity, where pain seemed rather a dangerous than a warning symptom.

At first I was extremely reluctant in admitting them in first labors, desiring to give dame nature a fair chance with new apparatus. A case like the following, not the first which had come under my observation, and I believe not unheard of in the practice of most physicians, suggested the use of anæsthetics for a definite object, under certain circumstances. A young woman in first labor, had proceeded in about the usual manner (except that there was excessive firmness of the os externum) until the head distended the perinæum to its utmost capacity. Venesection and tartarized antimony, &c., had lent their aid ; and the perinæum had been many minutes carefully supported by the hand covered by a napkin, the reluctant *os* was slowly yielding, and time seemed the only additional remedy necessary. The pain, however, was most intolerable, and my patient, although perfectly confiding, and obedient as possible to every word of caution, hitherto, suddenly threw all her energy into one effort, which tossed her from her position, and almost from the hands of her attendants. The result was, a rupture, extending from the *fourchette* backward about two inches ; the posterior commissure being about eight lines from the *raphe*. Reflection brought resolution in regard to future trials of this kind. The course of human events brought cases unlike, and at last a similar one, in nearly all respects. The extreme pain appeared to be the only bar to my prospect of success.

Ether was accordingly administered by inhalation, and to my infinite gratification, the rigid parts yielded like warmed India rubber, and the head passed almost as soon as the subtle fluid had banished the cognizance of pain. The etherization had nearly subsided before the hips escaped.

Again, a similar patient came to my charge, but the whole process of dilatation, both internal and external, had been tardy and unusually painful, although nausea and vomiting were almost constant. The usual methods had been resorted to with that success which patience bestows, until the head bore hard upon the centre of the perinæum.

Several strong uterine and abdominal contractions had exhibited a force sufficient to have made an independent passage, but for the support of the hand. With each effort the perinæum seemed to yield a little, and then contract with all its power, and carry all nearly back to the starting point of last pain. The patient had nearly exhausted self-control, and although there was evidently an enlargement of the *vulva* steadily progressing, delay was dangerous, as there was a strong disposition of the parts to become dry and tender, requiring frequent artificial lubrication.

I knew the patient to be very susceptible to the influence of chloroform, and it was accordingly administered. Its effect was as soon discovered at the seat of difficulty, as by the attendant who gave it, and three or four natural contractions, in quick succession, completed the labor, with slight perception of pain.

I have exhibited both chloroform and ether, to females not primiparous, and have often thought that the external organs relaxed more readily ; whereas, formerly, I had feared injury from the withdrawal of consciousness in the last stage of labor in cases like the above. But agony as effectually destroys self-command as Morpheus himself, and I argue thus: the sentient nerves being quieted, dame nature has the more perfect control.

If the experience of others agrees with my own thus far, anæsthetics are useful adjuvants in labor with rigidity of the soft parts, especially where it possesses the character of clonic spasm.—*Buffalo Med. Jour.*

FAULTS OF MEDICAL WRITERS.

[IN the discourse by Dr. Samuel Jackson before the Philadelphia County Medical Society at its last annual meeting, we find the following remarks on a subject which deserves the attention of the profession generally— especially those who are in the habit, as all should be, of writing occasionally for the press.—ED.]

Let the young doctor do his very utmost in acquiring a habit of writing with *perspicuity, propriety, and precision.* Let him seek no other ornament, for medical language is, like Thomson's loveliness, when "unadorned, adorned the most." No merit will make amends for the want of perspicuity. I can show whole paragraphs in our American books which have no meaning whatever, being similar in this respect to those verbose letters that Queen Elizabeth used to write when she had pre-determined to say nothing. Medical diction ought to use as few words as possible, thus going the shortest way to the end of a thought. An English writer on morbid poisons, wishing to describe the daily progress of the variolous pustule, uses the following verbosity :—" You receive, from a long distance, from Dublin or from Edinburgh, a lancet, on the point of which there is a little dry animal matter. This lancet has pricked the pustule of a patient suffering with smallpox, and the contents of the pustule have been suffered to dry on the lancet. Now with this lancet you make a single puncture in the arm of a healthy person, not previously defended by vaccination or otherwise, and what results ? "

Now suppose this author, Dr. Simon, had wished to describe, also, the effect of a rattlesnake's bite, he might have begun thus :—You receive from a long distance, from Utah or California, a rattlesnake, which Linnæus calls *crotalus,* it may be the species *horridus* or *durissus ;* this dreadful animal has a sacculus of poison at the root of each fang, and when he bites, these sacculi pour forth their deadly contents along a groove in each fang. Now you permit this animal to bite a horse, for an experiment, or perhaps it bites one of you, and what results ? In this multiplication of useless verbiage, a great amount of time is wasted without any compensation.

In a celebrated medical journal, we have this circuitous way of saying that a certain medicine was probably useful in rheumatism : the disease was cured in eleven days ; "and lemon juice, if it was not the principal remedy, certainly exerted an important influence toward the production of that end." What think you, gentlemen, of *producing.* or *leading forward* an end or a cure ? One might suppose that the writer was a cobbler, and that he was talking about the *producing* or the *pulling forward* of his waxed-end.   And then be·bas lemon-juice *making an exertion, and exerting an influence.*

Why should a writer say, " I had recourse to a medicine," if he had not previously used it in the same disease ?   This word means a running backward.   The simple English word *to give,* is often supplanted by the Latin word *to exhibit ;* that is, to make a show of the medicine. A shopkeeper *exhibits* his goods, a physician *gives* or *orders* his medicine.   Celsus took nearly all his ideas from the Greeks, but he did not copy their words.   I believe he never uses the word *exhibere,* but *dare et uti.*   Sometimes he says *adhibere,* but this does not mean *to make a show ;* moreover, it is pure Latin.   His own language was sufficient for him, except in the mere ñaming of diseases ; and hence one reason that his style and manner are universally approved.

It is of no little importance that our young author should not practise the coining of words.   A new idea may require a new‚word, but old ideas will always be most intelligibly introduced by known terms ; hence the great English lexicographer, whose head might well be fancied as swarming with words, introduced only four in all his writings.·   His rule was, " to admit only such as may supply real deficiencies, such as are readily adopted by the genius of our tongue, and incorporate easily with our native idiom."   If a little license be granted, how will you define· its limits ?   How will you definitely measure the old vulgar phrase *too much* ?   A little liberty will prove like moderate drinking, and lead to intemperance.   If every writer of the present times should coin words at his pleasure, and the next generation should adopt them and add to them, what odious gibberish would then fill the air !   It is told of Sir John Mandeville that, when far in northern Asia, with his retinue, their words were all frozen before they could be heard, and that, on coming south, they were suddenly thawed, and filled the air with their liberated voices.   I can hardly credit this fact, as the amiable author does not relate it himself, and yet something similar may happen to the jargon of the present generation ; while confined to books it may pass without much notice, but our successors may find the accumulated vocabulary to become a clattering of unmeaning voices, the mere echoes of our vanity, and as unintelligible as Sir John's thawed vocables.

In the Transactions of the American Medical Association you may find some animating specimens of these important additions to our deficient language.   *Numerism, socialism, sensationalism, subjectivity, progressionist, therapeutication, truths eliminated, annexes of the heart.*   A writer in vol. iv., p. 59, calls impressions *" intuitively-felt relations,"* and then inquires, " Are not all the felt relations based on immediacy and intuition, not on representational and transmitted impressions."   Truly, if men in high places · continue· to pour forth such floods of impurity, men in low places may well complain ; hence I have ventured to notice the subject ; it pertains to *self-education,* which is our present topic.

ACTION OF COD-LIVER OIL.

BY JAMES TURNBULL, M.D., LIVERPOOL.

THE mode in which cod-liver oil acts upon the system is a most interesting subject for inquiry. It has attracted some attention, but has not received all the investigation which its practical importance demands. It is not a matter of mere speculative interest; for, if the mode of action were certainly known, such knowledge would form a sure basis for further improvements in the treatment of consumption and other diseases. Some advance towards a solution of the problem has been gained by the discovery of the fact that other animal oils, as well as cod-liver oil, have a similar, though none of them an equal, efficacy. Dr. T. Thompson found that neats'-foot oil has in some instances no inconsiderable power of arresting phthisis ; and he has recorded cases in which it was of very decided service. I made a trial of it in a case under my care in the Infirmary, but found it more difficult of digestion, and less efficacious than cod-liver oil, after substituting which there was a rapid improvement in the condition of the patient. Train and spermaceti oils have likewise been tried at the Consumption Hospital, and the fact that all of them possess some efficacy has been placed beyond dispute : but the oils obtained from the livers of fish, especially the cod fish, still stand unrivalled in respect to the facility with which they are assimilated by the digestive organs, as well as their power of arresting the progress of tubercular disease.

The germ of many discoveries no doubt lies hidden in the researches of former ages, which were certainly more fruitful in experimental therapeutics than the present, which has, however, by turning its inquiries into the fields of physiology and pathology, laid a better foundation for such researches. It is not unworthy of notice that, nearly a century ago, cod-liver oil was recognized as a remedy of no mean value, though its efficacy in consumption continued unknown ; also that suet dissolved in milk was known as a remedial article of diet in consumption in the time of Dr. Young. Yet it is strange that two such facts should not have been placed together, especially as other kinds of oil and fat had been known to have proved serviceable in consumption, and that thns the discovery should not have been sooner made of the applicability of cod-liver oil to the treatment of tubercular disease.

Organic chemistry is a rapidly advancing science which must soon throw more light upon the *modus operandi* of this remedy, and Liebeg has justly observed, that without a profound knowledge of chemistry and natural philosophy, physiology and medicine will obtain no light to guide them in the solution of their most important problems—that is, in the investigation of the laws of life, the vital processes and the removal of abnormal states of the organism. Now the fact that other oils as well as cod-liver oil have the power of controlling phthisis, proves that the efficacy of this oil does not depend upon the accidental ingredients— the iodine, the bromine, the phosphorus, or the biliary matter, to each of which its peculiar action had been attributed, but upon the essential oily principles. This leads us to ask what is the composition of oils generally, and of cod-liver oil particularly. Oils and fat are generally combinations of fatty acids with oxide of lipyl, which may be separated in the form of glycerine. Lehmann regards them as haloid salts, formed by the combination of a haloid base with an organic acid, and he places together the oxides of ethyl, methyl, and lipyl, as belonging to the same series of compounds. They are also analogous in composition to what Gmelin calls ethers of the third class, and acetate of the oxide of methyl, one of these, bears a certain degree of analogy in its chemical constitution to fats and oils. Again, spermaceti is the cetylate of the oxide of cetyl, and the hydrated oxide of cetyl is considered by chemists to be closely allied to the alcohols, in fact a species of alcohol.

Dr. Winkler states that he has lately found that cod-liver oil differs in composition from all other oils hitherto used in medicine, in this respect, that when saponified with potash it does not yield glycerine, but oxide of propyle, a new body which exists in combination with the oleic and margaric acids, taking the place of the oxide of lipyl in other oils and fats. By means of oxide of lead this body may be separated in a higher state of oxidation as propylic acid. By means of ammonia it may likewise be converted into an alkaloid propylamine, which has also been obtained from ergot of rye, from herring brine, and from the destructive distillation of substances containing nitrogen. It thus appears that there is a sufficient difference in the chemical composition of cod-liver oil to account for its superior efficacy, without attributing it to the accidental ingredients it contains. It has been thought not improbable that, in the ultimate decomposition of fat and oils in the animal economy, the fatty acids are first separated from the base, oxide of lipyl or oxide of propyle; and from margaric acid it is known that there is a descending series of fatty acids, each of which contains two atoms less of carbo-hydrogen than the one above it. As some of these acids are found in the animal economy, it is not improbable that the fatty acids are thus oxigenated by successive subtractions of a certain number of atoms of carbo-hydrogen, until finally reduced to carbonic acid and water; and that after having served various purposes in the nutrition and metamorphosis of the tissues, this portion of oils and fat is thus finally consumed, furnishing fuel for the support of the important function of respiration, and the maintenance of animal heat. With respect to the glycerine separated from the fatty acid, it has been thought by Dr. Lehmann, that it may be converted into lactic acid, which performs an important part in digestion and other processes, and is finally consumed in the process of respiration, for which purpose the alkaline lactates, by their affinity for oxygen, are peculiarly adapted. It would appear, too, that the oxide of propyle is readily oxidated so as to form propylic acid. Oils and fat unquestionably serve other important intermediate purposes in nutrition, as yet very imperfectly understood; and they are essential to the growth of cells as they form the nuclei; that they are however ultimately oxidated and consumed in the process of respiration, scarcely admits of doubt.

Lehmann asserts that there are no acute and but few chronic diseases in which there is not deficient oxidation, and if we consider how much

of our treatment, in most diseases, consists in removing unhealthy secretions, most of which would not exist at all if the function of respiration were vigorously performed, we have much reason to believe that
there is a great amount of truth in this view. This can be clearly shown
to be true of gout, where deficient oxidation prevents the conversion of
uric acid into urea, as well as of some other diseases. I am strongly
disposed to think that deficient oxidation, that completing part of the process of digestion which takes place in the lungs, and consists of excretion as well as absorption, is one of the great causes of tubercular forma-
tions, which are more frequently deposited in these organs than in any
other part of the body. Among the best known causes of tubercular
phthisis, we find many of the conditions which lessen the activity of the
respiratory function, such as—depressing passions, grief and anxiety of
mind, sedentary employments, and above all confinement in prisons;
whilst, on the other hand, active out-door exercise, a cheerful state of
mind, and all those hygienic conditions which promote the free action
of the atmosphere on the blood, tend to avert this disease. Let it not,
however, be supposed that I consider deficient oxidation the sole cause,
as there are facts in relation to other diseases which seem to show that
it is not so. There is much reason, however, to believe that imperfect
digestion, combined with deficient oxidation, or a want of uniformity in
the action of oxygen on the blood, and through this fluid on the whole
system, is the main cause. We should likewise observe, that in proportion as the breathing power of the lungs is impaired by tubercular disease,
the tendency to further deposit is increased, so that the difficulty the physician has in combating the disease is continually increasing with its advance. Hence, too, the fact, that tubercular disease affecting the lungs
is not only more common, but less curable, than when it occurs in any
other organ.

Cod-liver oil appears to improve the quality of the blood by increasing the red corpuscles which are supposed to convey the oxygen from the
lungs to the tissues of the body : by its attraction for oxygen it would
appear to increase the energy of the respiratory function, furnishing
hydro-carbonaceous fuel well suited for this purpose, and thus, as well as
by suppressing the purulent secretions, it would seem to promote a more
uniform action of the oxygen on the blood and system. If this view of
its action be correct, it should lead us to try the effect of other hydro-
carbonaceous bodies, in the hope of discovering some that may be even
more efficacious ; and it should lead us to regulate the diet of consumptive patients with special reference to the function of respiration.—*Report on the Treatment of Consumption.*

LECTURES OF M. VALLEIX ON DISPLACEMENTS OF THE UTERUS.

TRANSLATED FROM THE FRENCH BY L. PARKS, JR., M.D.

NUMBER VII.

I do not dwell, gentlemen, upon the diagnosis in this case. In concert
with M. Danyau, who was good enough to watch the treatment, and of
whose competency and ability I need not remind you, I was able easily

to establish the existence of a complete anteversion. That which interests us now, is to. know to what cause that anteversion may be attributed. The supposition would be evidently improbable that it was caused by the parturition, which was followed by more than ten years of perfect health. No less difficult would it be to refer it to the first miscarriage, succeeding to which the patient experienced only a slight anemia caused by the attacks of hæmorrhage which followed. Besides, after the first abortion, there elapsed two years without the occurrence of the slightest symptom of displacement. But, after the second miscarriage, there was a different state of things. We now see the patient keeping the bed six months, and when she rises she experiences pains in the loins, dragging sensations in the groins, feelings of weight in the pelvis, &c., all these symptoms augmenting during walking. The frequent desire of micturition did not occur, but that symptom has been found absent several times, and is quite possible in a case of anteversion where the uterus is not very heavy and has retained sufficient mobility.

It may be questioned whether the displacement was produced at the time of the abortion, or not till six months after, when the patient attempted to walk. As it was not till the latter period that the pains and dragging sensations made themselves felt, it is supposable that in consequence of the vertical posture, the displacement which probably existed before, manifested itself then, for the first time, by its appropriate symptoms.

I would call your attention, in passing, to the treatment. The presence of the instrument for twenty-four hours was sufficient for the replacement of the body of the uterus. Later, I applied it anew to replace the cervix, although I should now question if this new application was indispensable. The observation of subsequent cases has led me to believe that it might, perhaps, have been omitted, and that we might, after a certain length of. time, and after the complete disappearance of the engorgement, have seen the cervix return spontaneously to its normal situation.

It has been thought that anteversion often produced miscarriage—a question to which I shall revert, at a future time, in speaking of displacements in general. In the case under consideration, you have seen, from the order of succession of the symptoms, that it was the miscarriage which produced the anteversion.

The cases which I have analyzed do not prove that *parturition in very young women*, produces anteversion more easily than at a more advanced age. Two only of our patients have borne children while very young. In one, it is true, the displacement took place a short time after labor, but in the other (Case II.) whose first labor occurred at the age of 17, it was only after two subsequent abortions and, at the expiration of eleven years, that the displacement manifested itself.

In our 18 cases, the first symptoms due to the anteversion followed, 13 times, so closely upon the labor, or the miscarriage, that we cannot attribute them to any other cause. Twice it was impossible for us to ascertain exactly at what epoch these first symptoms appeared. Three times they showed themselves at an epoch too distant from that of child-bearing to enable us to attribute them to that.

Violent Efforts—Falls.—In one of the three last-mentioned cases the real cause of the disease escapes us. But in the two other cases there had been an evident cause, since violent exertion or falls, followed rapidly by the manifestation of the disease, fully account for its occurrence. In no case of this kind has the cause been followed by the effect more rapidly than in a woman treated by me at the " Hôpital Beaujon." The record of her case I here give you.

CASE III.—M. E., æt. 37—cook—entered the Hospital April 16th, 1851. She is of a robust constitution, of high stature, has considerable " embonpoint," a florid complexion, and good muscular development. She never has had any severe disease.

Menstruation commenced at the age of 13 years—scanty, and attended with variations due to hygienic circumstances. At 22 years she met with a fall, after which leucorrhœa set in, and continued till her 34th year. At 32 she bore a child, the labor being severe, and lasting 15 hours, but being followed by no bad symptoms. A year after this childbirth, making an effort to raise a bed (four years having intervened between this event and the time the record of her case commences), she immediately felt in the left hypochondrium a species of crackling, together with pains in the groin. These symptoms redoubled during walking, or defecation, and continued on the increase till 1850—the epoch at which I received this woman under my care at the " Hôpital Sainte-Marguerite." I then ascertained the existence of an anteversion, and not yet being acquainted with the treatment of Prof. Simpson, I had recourse to an instrument devised by M. Meyer, of Berlin. It consisted of a sponge supported by a whalebone stem. The sponge introduced into the vagina behind the cervix pushed it forward so as to raise the uterus, whilst the whalebone handle, forming a spring, was bent over on the abdomen where it was maintained by a girdle. This instrument, though very defective, brought about a slight amelioration, and the leucorrhœa disappeared.

But in 1851, after having had two falls upon the nates in one week, the patient sought me, at the " Hôpital Beaujon," the 16th of April. The menses were fifteen days behind their time. The leucorrhœa, the pains and the constipation had returned. By the " toucher," the speculum, and the sound, I ascertained the existence of anteversion. The uterus was easily brought into place after three days of preparation by means of the sound. The pessary with the immovable stem was applied without difficulty the 21st of April. It was allowed to remain only four days, on account of an abundant menstrual discharge. Replaced the 3d of May, it was thrown out of place at the end of nine days, in consequence of a movement of the patient, when a notable amelioration was at this early period ascertained in the position of the uterus, which, however, had not yet been completely brought into its normal direction. The 16th, re-placed anew, it was removed the 20th, the patient complaining of griping pains in the uterus. These pains preceded by three days the appearance of an abundant menstrual flow, which lasted five days, whilst ordinarily their duration was from one t two days. From this time forward the uterus remained in place, and th symptoms after having persisted for a time soon ceased completely. Th

5th of June the patient was able to leave the Hospital. I saw her again the 6th of July, the 8th of September, and the 7th of October, and, although she was engaged in a laborious occupation, the displacement never returned. The 7th of October, I found, however, the uterus inclined forward, some pains and feeling of weight having been felt since a fall the day before. But one of the former pupils of the Hospital, M. Leclerc, visited the patient, and told me in the month of February last, that all had disappeared, under the influence chiefly of some laxative pills.

You will permit me, gentlemen, not to •discuss the diagnosis in this case, since I cite it to you only to show the influence of the violent effort, and the succeeding falls, as causes of the malady. You must have remarked, in fact, that immediately afterwards the patient experienced the first symptoms, and that from that time to the commencement of our treatment, they were only temporarily amended, and this after the employment of a process of re-placement from which I obtained for her but a transient amelioration. You see, on the contrary, how much more substantial was the cure obtained by means of the uterine pessary, since a very violent fall was not sufficient to re-produce entirely the anteversion, and the slight inclination which was discovered spontaneously disappeared.

Summary.—In summing up what has been taught us by a careful analysis of our cases, we see, gentlemen, that among the principal causes of anteversion are labor at the full term, and miscarriage ; since in the great majority of the cases, one or the other preceded by a very short time the appearance of the first symptoms. It has not been demonstrated to us that a painful and severe labor has had more influence than ordinary parturition. We may add that to this cause is joined the existence of a lymphatic temperament, the predominant elements of which we have found, either alone or united to those of the nervous temperament, in two thirds of the cases (12—18). Does this temperament act as a predisposing cause, by opposing the prompt return of the uterus to its original size after labor, and, by consequence, facilitating its displacement under the influence of the slightest cause? This is a question which it is fair to ask, but which for the moment cannot be completely elucidated.

Not any of our 21 patients had attained the *critical age.* We have met with some other displacements after this age, but not a single anteversion.

Neither have I found a case in which the affection was produced by tumors, or adhesions existing in the neighborhood of the uterus. In all the cases, the organ had preserved sufficient mobility.

When M. Ameline ranges *constipation* among the causes of anteversion, he seems to have taken the effect for the cause. For, even in the cases cited by him, that symptom had not shown itself till after the commencement of the uterine affection.

Can the liver and spleen in a state of hypertrophy press down the intestines in such a manner, and to such a degree upon the uterus, as to cause it to deviate from its position ? M. Ameline thinks so from a case cited by Morgagni (Let. 46, § 16). But, in relation to this isolated fact in science, we have no other information than that furnished by the autopsy. There was found in the vagina a wooden ring covered with incrustations—a clumsy species of pessary which had been employed to support the uterus, and I ask myself if it was not by the unskilful introduction of this ring itself that the displacement was produced.

M. Rayer met with a case of anteversion (cited by M. Ameline) after a peritonitis. What was the influence of this peritonitis? Did it produce adhesions? Details are wanting.—Can the engorgement of the anterior walls occasion an anteversion of the uterus? It is not impossible that it might, since it would render the uterus heavier in front. But, in the case cited by Levat, was the engorgement anterior or posterior?

Murat and M. Patissiér (Diction. des Sciences Méd.) report a case of anteversion, which they believe to have been caused by a *cancer* of the uterus. But, here again, did the cancer precede or follow the anteversion? This is a point on which we have not sufficient information, and you see how difficult it is to arrive at a solution of these questions, with the facts cited by authors who have not undertaken carefully to note everything.

Among the causes given by authors we see parturition still predominate. In 5 cases out of the 18 contained in the thesis of M. Ameline, it is said that the women have had previous labors. With regard to the remainder no mention is made, either on the positive or negative side. Examining the other cases collected by M. Ameline, we find, in one case, that a sudden effort was immediately followed by the first symptoms ; in a second case, borrowed from Mme. Legrand, the displacement was referable to a fall twenty-four hours after delivery ; and, in a third case, for which the above-mentioned writer was indebted also to Mme. Legrand, it was assignable to adhesions of the cervix to the posterior wall of the vagina—adhesions which were seen and felt, so that their existence is incontestable. But, as much cannot be said in relation to a case borrowed from Mme. Boivin, in which the anteversion was believed to have been occasioned by adhesions of the anterior wall of the body to the neighboring organs, from the fact that in the attempt to re-place the uterus, pain was developed in the right groin. We know, in fact, that this manœuvre may produce pain, without the existence of adhesions, and I could cite to you a case of retroversion, in which, though the uterus was very mobile, there was pain in the left groin when it was returned to its place. If this pain had been produced by traction upon adhesions, it ought to have manifested itself, in this case, in the direction of the sacrum.

We see, then, that the assertions of authors confirm the results at which we have arrived by the examination of our cases, and that even after considering the cases cited by them, we may fairly entertain doubts as to the real influence of certain causes, the existence of which we have never recognized in our patients. To sum up, if we unite the cases capable of serving us, in the study of the causes of the affection

Galvanism in Accidents from Lightning.* 461

under consideration, to those collected by myself, we have 31 cases; among which we find,

    18 times, the unquestionable influence of parturition.
    2 "   " doubtful   "   "
    In 4 the cause was a jar—fall—effort—once occurring after delivery.
    1 it was the bulk of the liver and spleen (doubtful).
    1 "   engorgement of the anterior wall, "
    1 "   cancer   "
    1 "   peritonitis   "
    1 "   presumed adhesion of the body of the uterus.
    1 "   adhesion of the cervix to the posterior wall (real cause
            fully established).
    1 "   completely unknown (Case I.).

GALVANISM IN ACCIDENTS FROM LIGHTNING.

To the Editor of the Boston Medical and Surgical Journal.

Sir,—If you think the following sketch of sufficient value for publication in the Journal, you will please insert it.

I was called June 21st, to see a girl about 8 years of age, who had been struck by lightning. She was standing near a window during a thunder shower in the vicinity. The electric fluid came down on the outside of the window case, demolishing it entirely, passed through the side of the house, and then divided into two parts. One portion passed through a cupboard, demolishing its contents; the other passed to the neck and through the body of the child. She was prostrated, and to all appearance dead. Cold water was thrown on her, and a kind of gasping respiration produced; but at the time of my arrival, some forty minutes after the shock had been received, the intervals between the efforts at respiration had become so long that each one appeared to be the last. The body was cold; no pulse; præcordial region still, and only the slightest cardiac impulse to be heard. In this state of things, I applied a powerful galvanic current along the dorsal vertebræ, also warmth and friction to all parts of the body. As soon as the galvanic current passed along her back, respiration and the heart's action improved at once. After the application had lasted for ten minutes, and respiration was in a good degree established, I discontinued the galvanism, when I found the respiration returning to its gasping stage, again attended with rattling in the throat, and complete relaxation. I again applied the galvanic current, and continued it with slight intermissions for an hour or more, when she became able to swallow, though it could hardly be called voluntary. A stimulant was given, which provoked vomiting. After this there was some trouble in removing the congestion which had taken place, and in establishing proper nervous action in the lungs, also in the kidneys and bowels; but emetics, blisters, nitre and turpentine, with stimulating liniments, completed the treatment. In fact, after re-action was established, the case was amenable to ordinary measures, although it was necessary to keep in mind the exciting cause.

The thought naturally suggested is, whether lightning produces death by asphyxia, or by overpowering the nervous system and rendering it insensible to its own proper stimulus. This case would seem to prove the latter to be the fact. I should apply galvanism in all cases of apparent death by lightning, unless more than an hour had elapsed after respiration had ceased, and especially if circulation is dependent on respiration. 　　　　　　　　　　　　　　　T. G. SIMPSON.
Hampstead, N. H., June 30, 1853.

THE BOSTON MEDICAL AND SURGICAL JOURNAL.

BOSTON, JULY 6, 1853.

Medical Education.—Dr. Samuel Jackson's discourse before the Philadelphia County Medical Society, in Dec. 1852, is one of the best medico-literary productions we have read for many a day. It is terse, full of sparkling thoughts, wise suggestions, and historical memoranda; and written very much in the style of Dr. Rush. If medical orators would oftener leave out the physic from their addresses, audiences would be better pleased with their performances. Anecdotal relations, illustrative of character, and the processes by which the lowly and humble rose to distinction and usefulness, never fail to be both interesting and instructive. We have given on a previous page of to-day's Journal, an extract from this address, which appeared suitable for a separate article; but we cannot forbear, in connection with these remarks, from drawing still further upon so rich a treasury of sound wisdom and experience. "The great business of the young doctor's life," says Dr. J., "is to study the interminable book of nature in health, sickness and death; hence his first object ought to be a frequent visiting of the sick. Let him not run away to Europe, but rather let him apply his learning to the more simple diseases of his own country, to those which he hopes to treat all the days of his life. Though he may thus see a less variety, he will certainly see more than he can faithfully study. After he has practised some years, and acquired some fixed and definite knowledge, he may visit foreign countries with some advantage. As the fortune of getting into a hospital can happen to few, he must seek for patients among the poor, laboring day and night among them. Their diseases are generally more simple than those of the luxurious and idle, hence they are better adapted to his inexperinced mind. Their doors will be open to him night and day, so that he can visit them more frequently than he can the rich; they will give him a hearty welcome at any hour, from sunrise to sunrise again. Let him be careful to conduct himself with the same punctilious respect that he would show to his equals. This is required not only by morality, and by all the obligations of a gentleman, but by mere selfishness also; for if he indulge here in a careless bearing, this will become habitual, and he will carry it with him among his superiors; unless, indeed, he be a great actor, or what is etymologically and essentially the same thing, a hypocrite. But the poor are entitled to our respect, for it is only God who knows whether they are not better than their doctor. They are entitled to our gratitude, also, for they are the humble steps to higher ranks and to a lucrative practice. If we find them sometimes troublesome and presumptuous, let us take this as a trial of our patience and of our power of resisting temptation, as pre-paratory to the same trials in the higher walks of life. Remember that the poor have many grievous burdens to bear, of which the rich can form no just estimation. A lady of high rank, walking with Napoleon in St. Helena, reproved her porter sharply for crossing her path ; the great man said to her, in the kindest manner, " Madam, have regard to the burden." Let our young doctor have regard to *the burdens of the poor*, and consider whether, if he were in their place, he would conduct himself better than they. I have descanted a little on this subject, because it pertains to self-education, and because he that neglects it will find, to his sorrow, that he has indeed had a fool for his master."

Disuse of Pork among the Shakers.—For many years past, the Shakers of Massachusetts, and perhaps those of other States, have wholly aban-doned swine-raising, although an acknowledged source of profit to farmers like themselves. Some very wise men may be found among those excel-lent agricultural broad-brims, who on many subjects, supposed to require the exercise of very elevated intellectual endowments, exhibit powers and acquirements which would command respect in any society. They make no display of their knowledge beyond turning it to a practical account on their own industrial territories. In medicine, there are individuals among them who are vigilant students, and prescribe, when occasion requires, with a clear understanding of the symptoms, and the value of the medi-cines they may give. Their village health is proverbial. They seem scarcely liable to the prevailing maladies in their vicinity; and in re-spect to this general immunity from disease, and the consequent length of days, clearly exhibit the advantages of habitual cleanliness, temperance, simplicity of diet, pure air, and an approving conscience. The Shakers have, from the organization of their Societies, been remarkable for their sanatory measures. Pork is not eaten by them, because they find satis-factory evidence that the flesh of domesticated swine is more or less dis-eased ; and they naturally suppose that injury must follow the use of it as an article of human food. A statement was recently made to us by a pro-minent Shaker, connected with this subject, which may be deserving of further consideration. He says that the children in his community never had measles, and, stranger still, they could not take the disorder. A few weeks since, an experiment was instituted which confirmed the truth of this alleged immunity. In order that the disease might be contracted by their children while young, upon the supposition that they were destined, of course, to undergo that specific suffering, as others did, they were sent to see some children " among the world's folks " who were then sick with measles. But the little Shakers did not imbibe the sickness, having remain-ed perfectly well ever since. The reason given by the Shakers them-selves, why their children did not contract rubeola in this case, and why they are not liable to its invasion, is that they have never eaten pork. Whether this be the only cause, or whether it be the effect of the general hygienic regulations of their community, we will not undertake to decide, but leave the subject for the consideration of others.

American Physicians in Europe.—An exclamation of surprise is not unfrequently expressed, that so many medical gentlemen should leave their business the present season, to study in the hospitals of the Old World. It is true that an immense representation from the States is distributed all over Europe. Some of them may devote themselves exclusively to the study of cases in the hospitals of London and Paris; but we think the number of such is small. We have invariably maintained that as many anomalous and instructive cases in medicine and operative surgery occur in our own large cities, in proportion to the population, as may be found in the old hospitals of Great Britain, France or Germany. Yet this going abroad has a wonderfully good influence upon most men, enlarging their powers of contemplation and thought. A tour of a single month, in surveying the magnificent scenery of Switzerland, or the architectural ruins of Italy, convinces Americans that we are not quite so far advanced in all the accompaniments of civilization, as is sometimes imagined. The fact cannot be concealed, that Europe is an extensive field for exploration, where the arts, ages upon ages before the continent of America was discovered, had reached a high degree of perfection. To see men and things, also, under different political aspects, is worth all the discomforts of a voyage, because it furnishes such an abundance of material for after-life reflection. Further, it strengthens in an American the love of his own country. Despotism is felt there, and political liberty is enjoyed here. Physicians can better comprehend the value of their own social, literary, scientific and political privileges, by a jaunt through the misgoverned kingdoms of continental Europe. While it liberalizes and enlarges the sphere of thought, such a trip likewise furnishes each visiter with something to bring back, that must, as a natural consequence, radiating from the domicile of each returned traveller, have a beneficial influence upon the society in which he moves. Physicians, we repeat, need not offer as an apology, that they wish to pursue their professional studies with the superior advantages which may be found abroad. They are variously improved in other respects by a tour, and therefore we are a firm advocate for seasons of relaxation from the routine of professional drudgery. Going to Europe is worth more than it costs, especially to the laborious practitioner of medicine.

Beards.—It would be quite ridiculous to write upon the physiology of the beard. Whether it is best to shave it off or permit it to grow, are questions that have been discussed till few would trouble themselves to read twenty lines upon the subject, with an expectation of being enlightened. There is no getting away from one point, viz., that nature has not taken a hint from civilized man, who crops it close to the skin, but she still persists in starting a crop on the faces of a majority of men of all countries and climates. One permits his beard to twist, mat and curl, to the discomfort of his neighbor, who estimates neatness and refinement according to the skill of the barber. Throughout continental Europe, and over Asia and Africa, the beard is rarely mutilated, and those who wear it are strangers to the throat diseases familiar to us in this part of the world. A disposition to ape the appearance and manners of beard-wearers abroad, leads certain fashionable aspirants in society among us to cultivate a growth quite disproportioned to their age and physical development, while a few, from a freak of oddity, and others through a fanatical whim, permit their's to grow till it resembles the antique Dutch drawings of the patriarchs. We beg to commend to the attention of physicians, in their circuits of practice, the inquiry whether any thing is gained for health by not shaving.

Each town and village will furnish abundant materials for ascertaining whether there is any thing saved or lost to the health of individuals, by permitting their beard to thrive undisturbed.

Copper, a preventive of Cholera.—The writer of a long article in the *Journal de la Société Gallicane*, M. Escallier, labors to prove that in many, if not all, of the large manufacturing establishments of the metals in France, but more particularly in the copper foundries, the operatives suffered but slightly from invasions of cholera. It is a singular historical fact, that in 1849, in a body of one thousand steel workers, only four at most died of cholera. An active inquiry into the condition of mechanics in all the various trades, brought to light very curious facts in regard to the progress of the epidemic among them. But the copper-smiths suffered less than any. Notwithstanding their dissolute habits, in Paris, out of thirteen hundred in one foundry, there were only eight deaths during the prevalence of the cholera in that season. Observations made on this class of men at Impy, Romilly, Villedieu, Falen, and in the copper regions of Siberia, seem to establish the fact that copper, in some manner at present unknown, protects from attacks of spasmodic cholera. Detailed reports might be cited, abounding in statistical minutiæ, collected by responsible medical inquirers, to substantiate these statements. It devolves upon physicians to ascertain in what manner this immunity is secured by that metal. In the vicinity of Lake Superior, should that active copper mining region ever be invaded by the Asiatic scourge, which extended itself to Upper Mississippi a few years ago, an opportunity would present for testing the effects of a cuperous cordon on a scale far surpassing in magnitude any that has been presented in Europe.

Surgeons Protected by Contract.—A significant piece of intelligence is circulating, viz., that Dr. Josiah Crosby, an eminent surgeon of Manchester, N. H., refused to dress a fractured limb, the other day, unless the patient would place himself under bonds not to prosecute in the event the limb should not be perfect. This is the only safe course for surgeons. The rage for obtaining money from surgeons in unsuccessful cases, is only paralleled by the suits against railroad companies. Juries invariably assess heavy damages against both, whenever an opportunity occurs. A professor of surgery in one of the oldest and most respectable Schools of medicine in New England, has recently, as we have before mentioned, been assessed eight hundred dollars by a jury, for alleged mal-practice. Similar cases are of late becoming so common, that blank forms of bonds should be kept on sale, ready to be executed before a Justice of the Peace, whenever an individual sends for a surgeon.

Transactions of the American Medical Association.—Dr. Condie, the Treasurer, has issued a circular, giving the following prices of the forthcoming volume; viz., $5 for a single copy, and two copies for $9. Six copies to institutions and associations, $25; and twenty-five copies for $75. Volumes 5 and 6 may be had, by addressing the Treasurer at Philadelphia, for $8. Intimations are given that the next volume, now in preparation, will be of a high order. Colored illustrations will add much to its value. Delegates to the late meeting in New York, throughout the States, are expected, according to a resolve, to assist in procuring subscribers to the Transactions. To defray the cost of publication, $1,500 will be wanted more than has yet been received.

Practice without Medicine.—B. F. Bowers, M.D., the physician of what is called, in the city of New York, a Half-Protestant Asylum, has publish- ed a report of his doings for ten years, which is principally curious on ac- count of the fact that medicine appears to have been wholly eschewed in the institution. By his own showing, he has done next to nothing, and consequently should have been paid accordingly, if at all. The following is a detached paragraph from his account of the medical administration of the charity.—"There has been no blood-letting in any form, venesection, bleeding, nor cupping ; no emetic, nor cathartic nor blister ; not a grain of calomel nor opium ; not a drop of laudanum nor paregoric has been used, and not more than half a pint of castor oil. The eight gallon jug that used to be filled with castor oil, is now used for lamp oil, and the old me- dicine closet is converted into a wardrobe." Perhaps Dr. Bowers belongs. to the expectant school. If so, his organ of hope in the resources of na- ture, to meet all contingencies in the various phases of disease, must have been large and actively exerted. At any rate, his honesty is commendable in not attributing his success to sugar pills and other useless infinitesimals.

Homœopathy in England.—Besides three Homœopathic Societies, em- bracing a large number of members. there is an annual Congress held by the new School of practitioners in England, which this year is to meet in the city of Manchester. In London there is a Hahnemann Hospital with forty beds ; the London Homœopathic Hospital with thirty ; and the Man- chester Homœopathic Hospital with twenty beds. There are also many dispensaries under their exclusive charge. As instrumentalities for pro- pagating their doctrines, there are seven Homœopathic Journals, spiritedly conducted.

Butter a Substitute for Cod-Liver Oil.—Cod-liver oil is an aliment. which restores and reconstitutes the tissues ; in a word, it is an analeptic medicine, by the aid of which the disorganizing action of tubercle is com- bated. The only inconvenience attending its use is that it is sometimes difficult of digestion.. In this case, M. Trousseau substitutes, with advan- tage for it, the following compound : " Fresh butter, $\mathrecal{3}$iv. ; iodide of potas- sium, gr. $\frac{3}{4}$; bromide of potassium, gr. iij. ; common salt, $\mathrecal{3}$ss. This but- ter is eaten during the day on very thin slices of bread.—*Dublin Med. Press.*

A New Remedy for Warts.—A French writer states, in the " Bulletin de Thérapeutique," that he has observed that the use of a teaspoonful of carbonate of magnesia, morning and night, for a few weeks, was generally attended with the disappearance of the warts on the fingers. Whether this is to be regarded as an effect rather than a coincidence, seems to be ques- tionable. Warts will often fall off after having existed a certain length of time ; hence the success of the incantations and other witcheries resorted to by certain " wart curers." One of the most prompt applications we have tried is the tincture of iodine. By putting a drop of this upon the wart once a day, it will generally fall off in a week. Lunar caustic, nitric acid, potash, &c. will often succeed very well, but are apt, if incautiously applied, to occasion some inflammation and pain.—*Southern Med. and Surg. Journal.*

Medical Miscellany.—Havana is unusually sickly the present season; many seamen from the United States have died there.—Sulphuric acid is represented, on authority, to be a speedy remedy for dysentery, but neither the doses or manner of administration are given.—A committee of the Homœopathic Medical Society of the State of New York, have reported in favor of founding a Homœopathic College. Their language runs thus: " We have the funds for its substantial foundation, and the men for the supply of its respective chairs."—Samuel Rice of Langdon, N. H., recently died at the age of 104 years.—Mrs. Jane Pushee died at Antigonish, N. S., May 5th, aged 105 years, leaving 157 descendants.—A man known as Dr. Watts, was mulcted in a sum of $1,100 damages in New York, for injury inflicted on a patient by giving *Watt's Nervous Antidote.*—A Cincinnati druggist recently, while asleep, swallowed a gold plate, upon which false teeth had been inserted. The plate lodged a short distance below his palate, and will neither go up or down. It causes him great pain, and it is feared that lockjaw will ensue.—Dr. Wieser, of Pennsylvania, has been arrested for attempting to bribe somebody, in a railroad matter.—Watering places are rapidly filling up.—Dr. Burnett's translation of a great work from the German, on Pathological Anatomy, is in press by Gould & Lincoln, of Boston. Dr. Noyes's translation of a volume on the same subject, is nearly completed.—Dr. William H. Van Buren, Professor of Anatomy in the University Medical College, has been chosen Surgeon to the New York Hospital, in the place of Dr. A. C. Post.—Dr. Alexander F. Vaché has been nominated as Physician of the Marine Hospital at Staten Island, N. Y., an office abolished two or three years since, and recently restored by the legislature of the State.—Dr. Arthur P. Hayne has received the appointment of Special Examiner of drugs, medicines, chemicals, &c. at the port of Charleston, S. C. The office had been for some time past filled by Dr. F. M. Robertson.—"Kindness," says Dr. Tschallener, " is the basis of the proper management of the insane. It is my right hand, as earnestness and severity are my left."

To CORRESPONDENTS.—Dr Cartwright's account of a "Decisive Experiment," and Dr. Miner's remarks on Concentrated Medical Agents, have been received.

MARRIED,—At Brockett's Bridge, N. Y., Edw. S. Walker, M D., to Miss Mary Grant.— Z Snow, M.D, of Randolph, to Miss M. A. Crane.—Samuel D. Moses, M.D , of Sumner Co., Tenn., to Miss S. A. Arnold.

DIED,—At Philadelphia, Nathaniel Chapman, M.D., long known as an eminent professor in the University of Pennsylvania, and one of the most distinguished of the medical profession in the United States. He died on Friday of last week. A biographical memoir will doubtless soon be given of him.

Deaths in Boston for the week ending Saturday noon, July 2d, 54. Males, 33—females, 21. Accidental, 2—apoplexy, 1—inflammation of the brain, 1—congestion of the brain, 1—burns and scalds, 1—consumption, 9—cholera infantum, 1—croup, 1—dropsy, 2—dropsy in the head, 2— drowned, 2—infantile diseases, 3—puerperal, 2—epilepsy, 1—erysipelas, 1—fever, 1—typhoid fever, 2—scarlet fever, 3—hooping cough, 1—hemorrhage, 1—disease of the heart, 1—inflammation of the lungs, 3—marasmus, 4—measles, 1—disease of the stomach, 1—suicide, 1—teething, 1— unknown, 3—worms, 1.
Under 5 years, 25—between 5 and 20 years, 7—between 20 and 40 years, 18—between 40 and 60 years, 3—over 60 years, 1. Born in the United States, 45—Ireland, 9.
The above includes 5 deaths at the City Institutions.

Singular Case of Foreign Substances in the Intestinal Canal. By D. HAYES AGNEW, M.D., Philadelphia.—The following case I am induced to report from its very singular character : On examining the body of an individual who, I believe, labored under some mental alienation during life, my attention was attracted to an adhesion between the parietal and visceral layer of peritoneum over the cœcum, upon the separation of which a small opening was perceived through the walls of the intestine, disclosing a dark-looking substance, which, upon examination, proved to be a large mass of straw, little less than an ordinary-sized fist, and firmly impacted in all the space below the ileo-cœcal valve. Noticing the transverse colon very much distended, an incision was made into its cavity, where were found a pair of suspenders, three rollers, and a quantity of thread, interwoven with one another. The webbing, which evidently was his suspenders, exceeded one and a quarter inches in breadth, and must be several feet in length, inasmuch as it extended through the ascending, transverse, and a portion of the descending colon, and doubled in several places upon itself. The rollers were of ordinary muslin, over one inch in width and the same in diameter, but which must have been of much greater size when swallowed, as they had in their progress along the intestines, become unrolled, leaving long ends which were encased within layers of fæculent matter. The peritonitis, which no doubt had been the principal cause of death, was not, however, produced by the escape of any intestinal matter into the serous cavity, no such discharge having occurred. The opening into the cœcum only presented itself after the reflected layer of the peritoneum was separated therefrom. Had life been prolonged, it is highly probable that the ulceration would have extended through the walls of the abdomen, and the cœcal contents passed out by this artificial route.—*Philad. Med. Examiner.*

Health of London during the Week ending May 21.—In the week that ended last Saturday, the deaths registered in London numbered 1098, being nearly the same amount as in the previous week. In the ten corresponding weeks of the years 1843-52 the average number was 900, which, if raised in proportion to increase of population during that period and up to the present time, will give a mortality for last week of 990. Hence it appears that the actual number of deaths last week exceeds the estimated amount by 108. Fatal cases arising from diseases of the respiratory organs continue to decline, but they still exhibit an excess above those of corresponding weeks, for last week they were 174, while the corrected average is only 131. Phthisis destroyed 152 lives, hooping cough 65. The weekly temperature rose 10 deg., and an increase in diarrhœa is the immediate result; this complaint was fatal in 18 and 28 cases in the last two weeks. Typhus in the same time declined from 71 to 58.—*London Lancet, May* 28.

Pounded Ice mixed with Linseed Meal as a Topical Application in Cases of Febrile Tympanitis.—M. Sandras, of Paris, has of late been using the above-mentioned application in cases of fever connected with much abdominal heat and tympanitis. These symptoms were in some cases so intense that the ice melted in fifteen minutes. But as improvement was obtained, it was more than two hours in melting. M. Sandras also used the same cataplasms with much success in the case of a boy affected with severe glossitis and considerable œdema of the sublingual and submaxillary textures. Great discrimination is necessary in the use of these remedies.

THE

BOSTON MEDICAL AND SURGICAL JOURNAL.

| VOL. XLVIII. | WEDNESDAY, JULY 13, 1853. | No. 24. |

ON THE EMPLOYMENT OF INHALATIONS IN CONSUMPTION AND OTHER PULMONARY DISEASES.

BY JAMES TURNBULL, M.D., LIVERPOOL.

THE facts which have been brought forward with reference to the beneficial effects gained by combining local with constitutional means in the treatment of laryngeal diseases, would lead us to expect similar advantages from the direct application by inhalation of volatile remedies to the seat of the disease in pulmonary affections. It can scarcely, however, be said that we have as yet derived an equal advantage from the use of inhalations ; and it may be asked how it is that a mode of treatment, which has been used more or less from the earliest periods, has not furnished more definite and useful results ; and that, notwithstanding the discovery of a new class of remedies—the anæsthetic, such as ether and chloroform—this mode of treatment may still be said to be in its infancy. One reason may perhaps be that the investigation is a difficult matter, and would require to be made thoroughly on a large scale in order to furnish definite results. It is an easier matter for a medical man to prescribe a medicine than to superintend the inhalation of remedies. I believe, too, that our knowledge of the subject has not advanced as much as it might have done, because many who use inhalations prescribe them without any well-defined object beyond the soothing effect, which may often be attributed rather to the watery vapor than to the medicinal agent ; and Dr. Snow has shown that some used for this purpose, such as extract of hyoscyamus, are incapable of being volatilized, and cannot therefore have any effect at all. There are, however, a great variety of volatile agents capable of being used for inhalation, which have never been tried at all ; and, as organic chemistry is constantly adding to their number, there can be little doubt that this is a mode of treatment from which we may yet expect to derive a considerable amount of assistance in the treatment of pulmonary diseases.

My own researches on the use of inhalations being at present incomplete, I should not now have touched upon the subject were it not to direct attention to a mode of treatment which seems to me to be somewhat neglected. I shall examine it, therefore, rather with the view of ascertaining what is the actual state of our knowledge of this mode of treatment, and how far we may reasonably expect to derive benefit from

24

the use of inhalations, than for the purposes of stating the results of my own observations.

When volatile remedies are inhaled, they must produce, besides the general effect resulting from absorption, as occurs with chloroform, a local action on the mucous membrane and its secretions, and hence we should expect them to exert an influence in bronchitis, especially the chronic forms. They must also produce a direct action upon the nerves which supply the mucous membrane, and through them upon the muscular fibres of the bronchial tubes. This would lead us to expect that inhalation of antispasmodic remedies would prove beneficial in spasmodic asthma, a deduction which is confirmed by the results of experience. Some remedies, such as iodine, must, when inhaled, act more directly upon the tissue of the lung itself, than when taken internally, and hence it was thought that they might promote absorption of tubercles of the lungs. But experience has not confirmed this view ; and, when we consider that tubercle is the result of a constitutional disease, there does not appear to be any good ground to expect advantage, until at least the constitutional tendency to deposition has been arrested or removed. There is still another very common morbid condition of the lungs, upon which the inhalation of volatile agents must act directly, viz., ulcerated cavities resulting from tubercular disease. In these cases it would be a vain hope to expect any lasting good from mere local treatment ; but, in conjunction with such treatment as suspends or removes the constitutional disease, it is reasonable to expect benefit from such means. I have never, therefore, used inhalations in those cases where cavities were present in the lungs, except in conjunction with other means, to arrest the disease, and seldom until some decided progress had been made. I conceive, however, that in many cases where the health has been restored by the use of the means which recent improvements have placed in our hands, when the patient has become stout and often apparently well, but has still an open cavity in the lung, it is quite possible that local means may be used with advantage. In such a condition we know that, even after the cavity has contracted, and the process of healing is advancing, the ulcerated surface is liable to become inflamed from exposure to the weather and various other exciting causes ; that the unprotected vessels often allow blood to escape, causing hæmoptysis ; and that there is always more or less purulent secretion, which weakens the system and re-acts upon the constitutional tendency to tubercular disease. There can be no doubt that the want of power to complete the healing of cavities, even after considerable progress has been made, is one reason that patients so often relapse after they have regained an appearance of health. Without overlooking the fact that tubercles generally exist in other parts of the lungs, I consider that the discovery of means which would promote the cicatrization of cavities in these cases of arrested phthisis is a desideratum and a legitimate object of inquiry. Any means which would promote this object would certainly tend to advance still further the treatment of consumption.

Dr. Snow has shown, in a paper on the inhalation of various medicinal substances, that some must be inhaled with the aid of heat, such as opium, morphia, extract of stramonium, and the gum resins ; others with the vapor of water, such as iodine, camphor and creosote ; and a third class of substances, such as hydrocyanic acid, ammonia and chlorine, at the ordinary temperature.   Mead, in his day, recommended fumigations with the balsams in phthisical cases ; and Dr. A. T. Thomson (Cyclopædia of Medicine, Art. Expectorants) has stated that he has seen much benefit from them when inhaled in spasmodic asthma, in shortening the paroxysm and promoting expectoration.   Dr. Snow found that ammoniacum gives off a fragrant, rather pungent odor, which can be inhaled very well by most persons.   He also found inhalation of the watery extract of opium serviceable in relieving the cough, but that morphia was the most pleasant and suitable preparation of opium for inhalation.   Extract of stramonium afforded more or less relief in five or six cases of asthma.   He tried iodine in eighteen cases of consumption at the Brompton Hospital ; in ten of them it was continued for more than a month ; and the conclusion to which he came was, that no benefit could be observed to follow its use.   Oil of turpentine appeared to relieve the cough in a few cases, and likewise camphor.   He used the volatile alkaloid conia in the quantity of one minim diluted with nine of spirit ; the cough was usually relieved, and in two or three cases the breathing also.   It would therefore seem from its volatility, at the ordinary temperature, to be a remedy peculiarly suitable for inhalation, if it could be obtained more easily.   Dr. Snow also found great relief produced in a few cases of bronchitis with difficult expectoration, from inhaling ammonia, twenty drops of the strong solution being mixed with two ounces of water in a Woulfe's bottle.   Chlorine has been much used for inhalation.   It was introduced for this purpose in France, and there seems to be good reason to believe that it has proved of material service in cases of chronic bronchitis, and even in some of phthisis.   With reference to its use in the latter disease, Sir James Clark has observed, "We have tried it in many instances, and it has in several apparently suspended the progress of the disease."   He also states, that it relieved dyspnœa and cough in some cases, though in the majority it produced no amelioration.   Dr. A. T. Thomson has likewise stated, that in cases of asthma the relief it produced was very striking, and that in phthisis he had observed the hectic symptoms abate.

Of the various remedies now mentioned, it is probable that the gum resins and balsams, camphor, conia and chlorine, are the most suitable and useful for inhalation ; but it does not appear that, by inhalation of opium or morphia, any very decided advantage has been gained over the more ordinary mode of exhibiting them.

The vapor of tar was formerly recommended for inhalation, and few medicines have been more used for this purpose than creosote.   Sir Alexander Crichton, in 1823, strongly recommended tar vapor in consumption ; but Dr. Forbes, in a report of cases in which he had tried it, published in the Medical and Physical Journal, stated that he had found it injurious in this disease, though of service in some cases of chronic bronchitis.   He appears, however, to have used it in cases so far advanced, that no benefit could reasonably have been expected from its employment. Creosote has now superseded the use of tar vapor, which does not, from its irritating properties, seem well suited for inhalation, though there can be very little doubt, when we consider the healing power which it has as an external application, that it must exert a similar effect upon the lungs, if it could be used in such a form as to obtain its beneficial influence apart from its irritating properties. Creosote is, perhaps, more generally used by the profession for the purpose of inhalation than any other remedy ; and I believe that when sufficiently diluted with the vapor of water it is one of the most useful. I have found that it has a sedative influence, relieving cough and promoting expectoration, whilst it at the same time not unfrequently lessens the quantity of this secretion both in consumption and bronchitis.

I have already observed that the pyrogenic bodies act upon the mucous and cutaneous surfaces ; and my attention has been directed to other bodies of this class by the fact that many of them have remarkable healing properties when applied to ulcers and chronic cutaneous eruptions, a fact which leads me to expect that this class of bodies may, when fully investigated, furnish a suitable remedy for promoting the healing of pulmonary ulcers, and thus supply the desideratum to which I have. previously alluded. Many of the pyrogenic bodies possess such healing properties in cutaneous diseases in a greater or less degree. From my own experience, I know that ointments made with tar, creosote, spirit of tar, juniper tar oil, and naphthaline, each have such properties, and are valuable remedies in the treatment of skin diseases.

The inference drawn from these facts, has led me to use for inhalation, some other pyrogenic bodies, viz., spirit of tar, juniper tar oil, Persian naphtha, and eupion. The spirit of tar possesses the healing virtues of tar, without its irritating effects ; so much so, that I think it might advantageously supersede the crude substance, as an external remedy. It is more readily volatilized than creosote ; and, when inhaled, it produces generally a mild, stimulating, and often rather a soothing effect upon the lungs. In some instances, however, it has appeared to increase the cough and expectoration, and it is not, therefore, suited for cases of bronchitis until inflammatory action has been. subdued completely, or for cases of consumption until progress has been made in arresting the disease. Without wishing to speak confidently of the remedy, I may state that it has appeared useful in some cases of the latter disease, in conjunction with other treatment. Juniper tar oil (oleum cadinum), which is a valuable remedy in skin diseases, and much used on the Continent, is less volatile than spirit of tar, and it is more irritating when inhaled. Persian naphtha and eupion possess decided anæsthetic properties: the former, when inhaled along with the vapor of water, has in some instances relieved difficulty of breathing in a very remarkable and decided way ; and this fact renders it worthy of trial in spasmodic asthma. Eupion has decided sedative properties, it has relieved cough and difficult breathing, and patients have slept after using it ; but it is not a pleasant remedy to inhale, and it has not unfrequently produced sickness afterwards, so that I should not recommend it to be used for this purpose.

I have used several of the essential oils for the purpose of inhalation. Many of them possess decided antispasmodic properties; and I have found that they have a remarkable power of relieving difficulty of breathing, a property which renders them peculiarly suitable for the treatment of spasmodic asthma. The oil should be dissolved in spirit, and inhaled with the vapor of water, so as to dilute its stimulating properties. The oils of cubebs, turpentine and copaiva, which are pure hydro-carbons, are mild in their action, and produce very little stimulating effect. The oxygenated oils which I have used appeared to be more stimulating in their action on the air-tubes; and some of them have stronger antispasmodic and expectorant properties. The oils of anise seeds and of peppermint are very stimulating, and in general cause too much irritation. Oil of spearmint is milder and anti-spasmodic, relieving difficulty of breathing in asthma, and even in phthisis. Oil of fennel is also mild. The oil of origanum is moderately stimulating and expectorant. I have also used the oils of rosemary and pimenta, which have similar properties. The hydruret of benzoyle, which is the bitter almond oil deprived of its prussic acid (and closely connected with gum benzoin, becoming benzoic acid in a higher state of oxidation), is very irritating and much too stimulating for inhalation.

Chloroform is a remedy which has been much used by some medical men for the purpose of inhalation, not only in asthma, but in a small quantity in consumption, in order to relieve irritable cough. In some cases, I have dissolved the essential oils in chloroform, and given them in this way for inhalation, their volatility being so much increased that they may thus be given on a handkerchief, as chloroform is usually administered.—*Report on the Treatment of Consumption.*

CONCENTRATED MEDICAL AGENTS.

To the Editor of the Boston Medical and Surgical Journal.

Sir,—In a recent number of the Journal, is an article upon the establishment of the American Chemical Institute, by Messrs. Keith & Hendrickson, New York. I hail the universal knowledge and use of concentrated medical agents by the profession, as one of the distinguishing marks between the infinitesimal homœopath, infinitesimally diluted and attenuated—the patent pill-monger and nostrum-vender—or the quack with his secret remedies, together with Major Standstill—and the learned medical profession with their safe and proper medicinal agents, scientifically-prepared and administered. Well may Dr. Jalap retire from the cares and troubles of professional life, since Dr. Jalapine will undoubtedly prove to be the dutiful son who more than makes good his father's place.

I have long since laid aside all those bulky articles of the materia medica, for which I could substitute the concentrated preparations. I am also using several articles which would have offered, by their bulk, insurmountable objections to their general use, had they not been presented in a concentrated form. My patients have already remarked the difference, and are well pleased with the small fine powders, in place of the coarse bulky ones which the crude material offered.

Who, in general practice, would lay aside quinine for Peruvian bark ; strychnine for nux vomica ; morphine for crude opium or the unripe capsules of the Papaver somniferum ; jalap for jalapine ? If no one then will object to the above articles which our fathers prepared and used with so much advantage to themselves and their patients, why should Dr. King's class of practitioners, " whose every obligation begins and ends with themselves " (see page 239, of the present volume of the Boston Medical and Surgical Journal), find fault because their sons have added to the list of concentrated remedies, Podophylline from the Podophyllum peltatum ; Leptandrine from the Leptandria Virginica ; Macrotin from the Macrotrys racemosa or cimicifuga ; or the Hydristine from the Hydrastas Canadensis ; and so on for the whole list of drugs and medicines? So far from any objections being urged against the concentrated remedies by those who have used them, I believe all speak with decided approbation of the improvement which science, in the hands of our indefatigable chemists and pharmaceutists, has made in this particular direction. Some who are afraid of anything that is new may object, as it will require some little time and attention to become well acquainted with the concise description of each medicine, and its precise dose. And I make no doubt but some of our remedial agents will be found to have acquired new powers, instead of losing ; or at least will have a decided advantage in power and certainty of action over the dead chips and barks with which some of our practitioners have been accustomed to load the stomachs of their patients.

Some may object to their use for fear of additional expense, as their patients are poor and they cannot collect their bills, and their time is as much as they can afford to lose, without being subjected to the additional cost of good and certain remedies. In answer to such, I would say, let the overseers of the poor take charge of these patients, if you are not able ; for my part, the convenience and certainty of the concentrated preparations are enough to satisfy me as to cheapness.

In relation to the Macrotin, let me observe that it possesses in full the properties of the root, except its narcotic effects, acting in a peculiar manner upon the uterus, in all uterine diseases, in doses of one to four grains from three to six times a-day ; being as near a specific for uterine diseases as quinine is for intermittent fever.

Newport, Pa., July 1st, 1853.   C. E. Miner.

DECISIVE EXPERIMENT—PROVING THAT THE CHIEF MOTIVE POWER OF THE BLOOD IS DERIVED FROM RESPIRATION, AND THAT THE LIFE OF THE FLESH IS IN THE BLOOD THEREOF.

BY SAMUEL A. CARTWRIGHT, M.D., NEW ORLEANS, LATE OF NATCHEZ.

[Communicated for the Boston Medical and Surgical Journal.]

While writing this article, June 17th, 1853, there is a living witness, in the court-yard of my office, proving the truth of the doctrine taught by Moses—that the life of the flesh is derived from the blood, and the physiological principle, announced some years ago by Mrs. Emma. Willard, that its chief motive power is derived directly and immediately from respiration.   The witness is a live crocodile, upwards of six feet in length, and about two feet in circumference.   Gen. Felix Houston and Dr. Backee saw it yesterday crawling about the yard.   Dr. B. Dowler and some other physicians and individuals have seen it to-day.   It has been visited by a number of scientific men ever since the 13th instant. On that day, at ten minutes of 10 o'clock, A.M., its trachea was tied in presence of Drs. Dowler, Backee, Copes, Wharton, and several others. The temperature of the room was 87°, that of the reptile's body 78°. In twenty minutes after the ligation it fell into a state of asphyxia.   But soon the liver began to act spontaneously, and it had some four or five copious dejections from the bowels.   As the purging progressed it began to recover from the asphyxia, and at length sprang from the table and snapped at the by-standers.   It was supposed that these unlooked-for phenomena might be owing to the trachea not being sufficiently secured to prevent the admission of air into the lungs.   Two additional ligatures were placed upon it.   Yet the heavings of the chest and a sound resembling respiration continued to be observed.   This proceeded, no doubt, from the consumption of the atmospheric air stored away in the large air-sacs, which are known to exist in the lungs of the saurian tribe of animals, and some others that can remain under water a long time without breathing.   The air-sacs answer the purpose of diving bells. After the carbonic acid, retained in the blood by the compression of the trachea, was thrown off by the spontaneous action of the liver, the air contained in the sacs, or natural diving bells, was sufficient to support a low degree of vitality.   With a view of compressing the sides of the air-sacs together, to prevent the air therein from being used by the lungs, and the carbonic acid from escaping, the abdomen, chest and cloaca were compressed by a bandage.   The bandage was applied at 11 o'clk., and in a few minutes the reptile again fell into a state of asphyxia.   At half after 11 o'clock fire was applied to the most sensitive parts of the body.   Some slight twitching of the muscles followed the application, proving that sensation and muscular irritability were not wholly destroyed.   At this stage of the experiment the company left to visit Prof. Riddell's chemical laboratory to witness an experiment the Professor's brother was making.   At fifteen minutes after 12 o'clock the company re-assembled ; having been absent three quarters of an hour, and found the crocodile dead.   Muscular irritability seemed to be entirely destroyed. Fire was repeatedly applied to the most sensitive parts of the body, and not a single movement, twitch or symptom of vitality could be elicited thereby.   After ten minutes had been spent to enable the gentlemen present to try experiments to extort a symptom of vitality, and after they had all convinced themselves that the animal was certainly dead, I proceeded, at twenty-five minutes after 12 o'clock, to make a dissection, and to expose the abdominal and thoracic viscera to view.   The whole extent of the abdomen and thorax was laid open.   A cross incision was also made, and the anterior and lateral walls of the thorax and abdomen were fastened back by hooks, so as to bring the lungs, liver, bowels, and the sac containing the heart, under the direct action of the senses of sight and touch. No twitch or the smallest indication of life was elicited by the dissection. The animal had been previously unbound, and lay on the table—a dead subject undergoing dissection. At length the pericardium was slit open by an incision five inches in length —exposing the heart and its auricle to view. On exposing the heart to the external air, and taking it in the hand, slight twitches or muscular contractions, eight times in a minute, were felt.

At half after 12 o'clock, more than two and a half hours after the ligation, insufflation was commenced by inserting the nozzle of a common-sized fire bellows into the trachea. At this stage of the proceeding the company got tired and began to drop off, being fully convinced that insufflation nor nothing else could restore life. The process of insufflation, in about ten minutes, appeared to begin to change the tissues of the reticular network of the lungs to a brighter color. This was supposed, however, to be owing to the direct action of the external air on the membranes. At length small bloodvessels, barely visible, began to be seen on the exposed surfaces, where none could be seen before—proving that the blood was in motion through the pulmonary tissues. The heart was now felt, and its pulsations had become evidently much stronger and had increased from eight to eighteen beats in a minute. The insufflation was steadily persevered in until 1 o'clock, when the motions of the heart had increased to 34 pulsations. Fire was now applied, and some faint evidences of returning muscular irritability were elicited. An ice-water enema was thrown into the bowels, and the whole surface of the body, including the exposed viscera, was frequently wetted with ice-water. As the weather was very hot, this measure was resorted to, to prevent the blood from undergoing chemical decomposition. At ten minutes after 1, the animal seemed to revive, and made ineffectual efforts to breathe. The intercostal muscles and the diaphragm having been cut, the efforts were fruitless. Soon after this, fire was applied, and it writhed its body and moved its tail. As yet the head appeared to be perfectly dead, the eyes glazed and motionless. At half after 1, it would move and writhe its body on being rubbed with ice. At thirty-five minutes after 1, the bellows was removed, and a metallic tube, with a calibre large enough to admit the little finger, was inserted into the trachea. Dr. Copes sewed up the rent in the pericardium, and also stitched together the muscles of the throat and abdomen, which had been divided by the crucial incisions. The dense skin was pierced by an awl, brought together and secured by sutures. At 3 o'clock the other extremity of the divided trachea was put into the tube, and the divided ends brought together and fastened over the tube. The crocodile was then removed from the table and placed under the hydrant. It breathed freely, opened its eyes, and life and intelligence were restored. Dr. Dowler, being unwell, had left before the resuscitation. Indeed all had left, except Drs. Copes, Wharton and Nutt. I sent for Dowler, and when he returned and saw the crocodile alive, he raised his hands and said, " *glorious experiment.*"

Two days ago, the poor reptile appearing to suffer from the tube in the trachea, I removed it. Dr. Dowler calls every day to see the subject. But I entertain no hopes of its ultimate recovery, as the wounds inflicted on it, in order to expose the viscera to view and to watch the changes which occurred during the passage from death unto life, are of too serious a nature to be cured.

Practical Remarks.—In exposing the viscera, care was taken to avoid cutting any large bloodvessel or piercing the lungs. If much blood be lost, resuscitation cannot be effected from the want of the material to operate on. It is thought, however, that the loss of a little blood is rather beneficial than otherwise, as it enables the remaining mass to move more readily through the lungs, by removing the congestion in the pulmonary capillaries. In measles, when the eruption has been repelled and the skin gets blue and cold, the loss of a little blood from the arm will facilitate the circulation through the lungs, clear the complexion, warm the skin and raise the pulse. In concussions or severe shocks, interrupting the respiratory movements and impairing the action of the heart, the modern practice is to give stimulants and to avoid bleeding until re-action occurs. But too often re-action never does occur, from the blood stagnating in the pulmonary vessels. In such cases, the loss of a little blood will facilitate the transmission of the balance through the lungs by removing the congestion. Dr. Dowler was the first to prove, by practising venesection on the dead subject, that the blood, in certain cases, will not only run out, but will flow in a jet and remove post-mortem congestions. The erroneous theory, that the nervous system is the fountain of life, has caused the old practice of bleeding, vomiting and purging for concussions of the brain and severe shocks of the body, to be abandoned, and the stimulating of the nervous system, to produce re-action, to be substituted for it. The nervous system, deriving its life from the circulating blood, and the blood its life and motion from respiration, cannot be stimulated while the blood is stagnant and the respiratory actions suspended. To restore the respiratory process and to put the blood in motion, is the true indication in such cases.

It also appears, by the facts elicited in the experiment just related, that the application of ice water had a good effect in aiding the insufflation to restore animation. The ice-water injection may also have brought the portal system to aid in decarbonizing the blood.

The experiment shows, that it is not so much the absence of oxygen, as the retention of carbonic acid in the blood, which kills so quickly when respiration is suspended; because, when the liver acted, the animal partly recovered from the asphyxia—but until that great decarbonizer of the blood, second only to the lungs, began to act, the oxygen in the air-sacs was not sufficient to prevent the accumulated carbonic acid in the blood from producing asphyxia. In the cold abstraction of death produced by depravation of oxygen and accumulation of carbonic acid in the blood, and also in some congestive diseases, the application of ice water internally and externally would seem to be much better than hot applications and stimulants. For frozen limbs, snow is known

to be more effectual than any form of heat.   In resuscitating the drowned, stimulants and hot applications are injurious.

The wonderful power of hepatic or bilious purging was well illustrated in the early part of the experiment.   Bilious vomiting or bilious
purging, when the lungs are crippled in their function, often restores
the body to life and energy in cases apparently the most hopeless.   The
frequency of cold congestive diseases in the South, with pulmonary oppression, and the manifest good effects of calomel and such medicines as
excite the liver into action, led, some years ago, to the employment of
mercurial cathartics in almost every ailment, without due discrimination.
In Europe the cases calling for their employment are much less numerous than in southern latitudes.   That method of aiding the lungs, in decarbonizing the blood, is not duly appreciated by European practitioners.
Nor can they see why a patient, who would sink under the action of
the mildest laxative, should rise and walk before a strong mercurial cathartic has ceased to operate.   In typhus, when the lungs began to flag
in their action, a twenty-grain dose of calomel was a favorite remedy
with Dr. Chapman.   The experiment on the crocodile throws some
light on the *modus operandi* of that remedy, and also explains the reason why mercurial purgatives are particularly useful in severe wounds
of the head, concussions of the brain, and other lesions interrupting the
excretion of carbonic acid by the lungs.

, Experiments of this kind are full of practical instruction, and ought
not to be considered as suiting the visionary more than the practical
man.   They tend to prevent the practical man from being led into error
by visionary theories.   .Visionary practitioners do not trouble their heads
about facts.   In contemplating the anatomy of the dead subject, theory
conjectured that the heart was the chief agent in circulating the blood.
But in seeing the dead subject brought to life, with the viscera exposed to
the sight and touch, it plainly appeared that the received theory of the
power which produces the circulation of the blood, is not correct—that
the *primum mobile* of the circulation is in the reticulated pulmonary
tissue and not in the heart.   The reddening of that tissue and the injection of its vessels with blood, was preliminary to the restoration of
the heart's activity.   The nerves, which had been insensible to fire,
hooks and forceps, had their sensibility restored in proportion as the redness, motion and vitality of. the blood were restored—proving that the
life of the nerves and the flesh is in the blood, and that the blood derives its life and motion from respiration.

Dr. Dowler's experiments are forcing physiologists to adopt the doctrine of a diffused sensorium.   He has only published a few scraps of
the evidence proving that doctrine.   He has fully ten volumes of un-
published facts containing evidence in its support, which will be perfectly
irresistible.   1 am not the interpreter of his opinions, but his facts are
common property, speaking for themselves.   Instead of the brain and
nerves being the sensorium, as the Greek and modern philosophers taught
him to believe, his own experiments, Riddell's and mine, will demonstrate positively that the blood is the sensorium, as Moses said it was ; if

by sensorium be meant the life, the sensibility, the will, the passions, and that species of intelligence called instinct.

In a former experiment, reported in vol. xlvii., page 79, of this Journal, in less than an hour after the trachea had been tied, a very fierce and vigorous animal, called the battle-ground crocodile, was handed over to Dr. Dowler and some eight or ten other physicians, to extort a single symptom of life if they could. The heart was still beating, but muscular irritability had been destroyed in all other parts of the body, by the carbonic acid retained in the blood by ligating the trachea. Fire, knives and forceps, on the bare nerves, failed to extort a single symptom of vitality. In that experiment, insufflation of the lungs was not attempted until after the failure to extort any evidences of life or sensibility. When it was attempted, the lungs were found to be too much torn to hold air, and the process was abandoned. But in the present experiment, it was not until an hour and a half after the compression of the abdomen and thorax by a bandage, and more than two hours and a half after the ligation of the trachea, that insufflation was commenced. It not only restored muscular irritability, but it brought the animal to life, and it is living yet, the fifth day after the resuscitation.

The doctrine of Moses that life, with all its attributes of sensation, volition, mobility and intelligence, exists in the blood (the term life, in Hebrew, meaning life with its attributes), is no more difficult to understand than the doctrine of the Greeks and modern physiologists, which presupposes that life, with all its attributes, is located in the pulpy substance called the brain and its appendages. That the Greeks were wrong and Moses right, can be proved not only by the crocodile, but by every turtle and tarapin on the wide earth. When the heads of these animals are cut off, they will continue to make intelligential motions for some time afterwards, and some of them, as my friend Dr. Cornelius S. Baker, of Bucks Co., Penn., has kindly reminded me, will dart out their headless necks at their persecutors (as the snapping turtle, for instance), proving that they are not only alive, but retain the passion of anger without a head, about as well as with it. Such phenomena are perfectly irreconcileable with the received doctrines of modern physiologists and psychologists, or with the philosophy of the Greeks and Romans, but are in beautiful accordance with those doctrines which have come down to us from the Hebrews.

Canal street, New Orleans, June 17, 1853.

SPINAL CURVATURE.

BY E. C. ROGERS, M.D., OF BOSTON.

[Communicated for the Boston Medical and Surgical Journal.]

FEW are aware, even in the medical profession, of the numerous cases of spinal distortion to be met with in society. Indeed, we have heard members of the profession, of no mean repute, and of extensive practice, deny that this derangement was often to be found. It is only where one's attention is specially directed to any particular department of nature, that her testimony in that department will be realized. In no respect is this truth more apropos than in the above.

Let any physician, who attends much to chronic diseases, make it a point to examine the spine carefully. Let him make use of the plumb and line in every case, and we will venture to say that one eighth of his cases will present a very marked palpable deviation from the spinal line. If one is in the habit of merely looking at the tongue, feeling of the pulse, and listening to a few answers to questions concerning feeling pains and aches, he will be most certain to know of but few cases of spinal curvature, perhaps of not one out of five hundred or a thousand of his patients ; and then it will be so extremely marked and glaring, as to require no examination to detect it. Such cases will be those so far advanced as to render them hopeless. Hence physicians of such experience will generally affirm that spinal distortions are not only very rare, but quite, if not wholly incurable ; certainly that, in the great majority of instances, they are irremediable. Whereas the real fact in the case is exactly the reverse of this ; that is, when the whole number of cases of actual curvature is taken into the account, a great majority of them are susceptible of perfect restoration, if proper means be applied. This we shall endeavor to show in the sequel.

Again, it should be considered, that not a very small number of persons, who have curvature of the spine, seldom become known to the physician as chronic patients. It is only in acute attacks that the physician will be called upon ; and then his attention will be drawn wholly to the acute symptoms. And in such cases even a very marked distortion will scarcely be noticed, as the attention is drawn another way ; or if the eye should detect it, the impression upon the mind would be so slight that it would soon lose sight of it.

To show that we are not alone in the opinion, as to the frequency of this affection, we might refer to the authority of a great number of learned surgeons in Europe, who have devoted much talent to its investigation. Bell, Bamfield, Shaw, Duffin, Beale, Copland, Wilson, Lawrence, and numerous others refer to this fact, and name many apparently very slight causes, which operate to effect the evil under consideration ; such causes as are constantly acting in our midst, and are inevitable in their results, unless in some way counteracted. This will be seen more readily when we come to touch upon the object of the spine, its peculiar conformation, its braces and pulleys, so to speak, and the numerous causes which contribute to their deviation from a normal condition.

The human spine is a pillar of support, sustaining the weight (when in the erect position) of the thorax, upper extremities and head—to say nothing of the weight of internal viscera, especially of parts above the diaphragm. Indeed the spine, at its base, sustains nearly the whole weight of the trunk, as well as that of the whole of the head and the superior extremities. For nature does not allow the softer parts of the organism to sustain superincumbent bodies without detriment. Hence all those parts in the trunk are in some way attached to, and dependent from, the spine, namely, by projecting bones, as the ribs, by integuments, tendons, &c.

Now it should be considered, in this connection, that the spine, sustaining so -much weight, is not placed mechanically in the *centre* of the weight to be supported, but only *on one side* of it—on the posterior side ; so that the weight sustained is mostly anterior, or anterio-lateral to the spinal column. It hence follows that the mechanical tendency of the spinal curvatures is anteriorally and anterio-laterally. This is seen in infants before the effort at balancing developes itself. Thus, if the infant, at this early period, be set upright on one of the parent's hands, and the other sustains the trunk, it is seen that the bead falls forward, and leans upon the chest, or forward and sideways, leaning upon the chest and shoulder. If now the hand be removed from the trunk, the whole trunk will fall forward.

From this it is evident that the agent called into action, in acquiring the power of balancing, is one which is directly opposed to the mechanical arrangement of the spine, and the tendency of its superincumbent weight ; that is, for instance—in order for the cervical vertebræ to sustain the head against the tendency of its weight, namely, anteriorly—a power must be exerted within the parts to throw the head posteriorly, and so of the whole form.

This force must represent itself in the muscles, after being originated in the nerve centres, and is one of the first developments of human automatic action. As it acts in opposition to the gravity of the parts, whose tendency is anteriorly, its over-action would be to throw the trunk out of balance posteriorly. Hence after the infant has got over falling forward, it commences falling backward. This naturally excites cautiousness, which, in nervous constitutions, becomes very greatly developed with the balancing power.

From the foregoing it is evident that the erect position is one that is, in the first place, assumed by the power of nerves, muscles and tendons, against the tendency of the weight to follow the law of gravity. The spine alone, then, is not a pillar of support. It is so only when nerves, muscles and tendons act with it. Without it, however, the nerves, muscles, &c., could sustain nothing. With them, it is a flexible, supporting column.

Its flexibility depends upon its being composed of numerous bony parts united to each other by means of an elastic substance interposed between each member. Thus the spine is a connected chain or series of alternate bone and cartilage, or elastic and inelastic substance. This chain is strengthened in its connections by means of ligaments attached to the exterior surfaces, and also by means of muscles and tendons connected with its processes. These being attached to different points of the vertebræ, not only render the spine capable of being sustained upright, but of being curved in any required direction. Hence is it that the spine is not only a flexible, supporting column, but, at any point of it, a fulcrum, upon which muscles are made to act as a counteracting force to gravity.

If the erect posture be assumed as the first position of the spinal column, it must be granted that this posture cannot be maintained without the fulfilment of important conditions, namely,

First, the integrity of those muscles and ligaments, constantly employed as natural stays to the spine, while in the above position.

Second, the integrity of those muscles employed as pulleys to lift the superincumbent weight attached to the spine, when the latter is thrown out of its first position.

Third, equality in the thickness of each separate vertebra and intervertebral substance.

The first and second of the above conditions are evident from the preceding observations. Let us for a moment consider the third.

The elasticity of the intervertebral substance renders the spine capable of being curved slightly in every direction—less posteriorly than in any other, from the arrangement of the processes; more laterally; most in the anterior direction.

On bending the spine in any direction, the vertebræ involved in the curve must approach nearer to each other on the concave side; consequently the intervertebral substance also involved in the curve must become thinner by pressure on the concave side. This being only temporary in the normal curvatures, the intervertebral substance recovers its equal thickness when the spine is brought into its normal line,—that is, nearly perpendicular.

Should the intervertebral substance, however, become thinner anteriorly or laterally, the weight of the superincumbent parts would carry the spine in that direction. This would involve a permanent curvature.

Now it is a well-known fact in physiology, that protracted topical pressure excites local absorption. If in any instance, therefore, protracted topical pressure shall take place on any particular side of the intervertebral substance, its absorption must follow as a natural consequence. The absorption on that side would make it permanently thinner than the opposite side, thus inducing permanent spinal curvature. The vertebræ and intervertebral substance, in the curve of the spine, must become cuniform, aptly illustrated by Bamfield by reference to the stones of an arch.

Again. It must appear, according to principles involved in the foregoing, that the progress of spinal curvature from the first degree, takes place by a *mechanical,* as well as by a physiological law. This will appear from the following. "If a column be perfectly upright, it will bear a considerable weight, as long as it preserves its perpendicularity. But if a weight be affixed to the upper extremity of an *elastic* column, curved to the degree of one, and the same weight be placed upon the upper extremity of another, curved to the degree of three or four—in the latter case the superincumbent weight will tend to increase the bending of the column with a greater force and effect than in the former. Hence the more extensive the curvature, the greater will be the compressing power of the superincumbent weight, and the more rapid the absorption that is established."

From the above facts it must follow, first, that whatever causes operate upon the vertebræ, or the intervertebral substance, to alter their equal thickness, tend to produce spinal deformity. In the second place, that whatever causes operate to weaken or destroy the functional integrity of the muscles and ligaments, which brace the spine, tend to produce permanent spinal curvature.

In the first class of these causes, may be included caries of the vertebræ; ulceration, and the like; also the unequal length of the lower extremities; also the habit of sitting the infant upright before the vertebræ and cartilages are sufficiently consolidated; the habit many acquire of leaning in a particular direction, either to favor an affected point, as that of the side, or pit of the stomach, &c. &c., or from the nature of a particular employment, as that of shoemakers, seamstresses, &c.

In the second class of causes may be included the incautious endeavors of parents to make their infants " sit alone," when the ligaments and muscles attached to the spine are yet too weak to act as sufficient braces, especially in cases of infants of scrofulous diathesis, the retardation of muscular development from dentition, scrofula, &c. Also, certain forms of derangement of the digestive and reproductive system, which reflect their influence by sympathy upon the muscles of the spine, through the visceral ganglia. Also affections of the sexual system, and the last named, which reflect their influence upon the motor centres of the spinal system. Also certain affections of the brain, which reflect upon the spinal muscles.

Many of these, after acting as the first causes of curvature, may cease, but the curvature itself remain, and become in turn, in many instances, an exciting cause of other diseases; such as affections of the heart, lungs, spleen, liver, stomach, intestines, kidneys, bladder, uterus, spinal centres, &c., occasioning palpitations of the heart, dyspnœa, pain in the region of the liver, spleen, stomach, causing constipation, spasms, urinal suppression, derangements of the catamenia, and a hundred other symptoms.

Now it must be a very important question to every person laboring under spinal curvature, in whose cases especially any of the above consequences arise, what possibility is there of relief, if not of cure.—A few physicians have contended that there is no cure for spinal distortions. Others oppose this denial with an array of numerous cases where it has been removed; not only in cases of lateral curvature, but in those of incurvation and excurvation. Indeed we could name not a few English writers, of no mean repute, who have detailed unquestionable cases of complete restoration. It is certain, however, that in all cases of true anchylosis, a cure could not be effected. Nor would it be advisable to think of attempting the usual methods, in those cases where the curvature is very extreme, and has been of very long standing,—where for instance the thorax and all the internal organs have become shaped to the deformity,—even should it be possible to bring the spine into its perfect figure. So far, however, as a partial relief of consequent ills is concerned, that is another question, which most physicians are not disposed to hesitate in attempting. Most of us are ready to exhibit a " dose of something," if it be but a " pill " or a " globule." We have all the humanity to " *try that.*" Indeed, in what instance, simple or complex, would a physician refuse to " try what simple means he *had at hand* " to afford relief? True, he might weary of " trying " in such cases, especially when nearly every thing

" *at hand* " failed.   But even then, would it be wise to turn the wretch adrift, rather, I may say, to sink under the impression there was no spar, not even a straw on life's tide that could help to buoy him up a little longer ?

There are cases of curvature, however, where it would be extremely unwise not to attempt a positive cure, if safe and appropriate means could be made use of.   But here the question arises, what means are safe and appropriate ?

The general answer is—such as would act—1.   With reference to the physiological law of the muscles, tendons and ligaments connected with the spinal column.   2.   The anatomical structure of the bones and cartilages of the spine.   3.   The law of local absorption from topical pressure.   4.   With specific reference to the pathological condition of the vertebræ, and the intervertebral substance.   5.   With reference to the specific *mechanical* tendency of the curvature and the superincumbent weight, which are to be overcome.

Every well-educated physician will admit that if these points can all be made to harmonize in any set of means, and the first causes of the curvature are not kept still in play, and no true anchylosis, nor destruction of substance, as in caries and the like, exists, it would be quite unpardonable not to make a trial of them.   There are very few, who would stand in the way of such a trial, and all good souls, whose judgments became convinced, would heartily commend such means.

If the editor permits, we may endeavor, in a future number, to exhibit some of the means indicated.

THE BOSTON MEDICAL AND SURGICAL JOURNAL.

BOSTON, JULY 13, 1853.

Homœopathy—Its Tenets and Tendencies.—Not long ago, we had occasion to speak of the indomitable energy as well as literary industry of Dr. Simpson, of Edinburgh.   He is greatly distinguished, and it has been brought about by an untiring exercise of every talent with which Providence entrusted him.   This is the legitimate way of rising above the circumstances which would keep a man in ignorance and idleness.   Be incessant, be importunate, and fortune will smile kindly on your efforts.   Dr. Simpson is always busy.   He never waits for leisure, but takes time by the forelock.   Labor with him is the first element of enjoyment.   In the midst of a vast practice, and besides his duties as a public lecturer, Dr. Simpson is scarcely ever without some kind of a book or pamphlet in the process of construction.   Before us is a beautifully printed octavo, of 292 pages, entitled *Homœopathy ; its Tenets and Tendencies—Theoretical, Theological and Therapeutical.*   Of course, from such a source, it must possess merit, and in Edinburgh it has passed through a third edition, which implies that somebody reads it.   There are twenty chapters, in which the keen-sighted author has sifted the pretensions of the new school of practitioners so finely, that their infinitesmal doses could hardly pass his scrutiny.

It is really a logical argument, accompanied by the most potent of instrumentalities, facts, to prove that homœopathic medicines, and no medicines, are essentially the same thing. His knife is so sharp that he slices off the heads of medical pretenders before they begin to feel the edge. Should the work be republished here, it would have a run ; but if not, those of our neighbors who may wish to read what Dr. Simpson has said on this exciting topic, are welcome to the use of our copy.

Memphis, Tenn.—Its Health and Mortality.—By a resolve of the Medical Society of Memphis, 1500 copies of a report by Charles T. Quintard, M.D., were published at the expense of the society. Memphis is in lat. 35deg. 8m. north, and long. 90deg. 6m. west, and is situated on a high bluff. After a close analysis of former and later tabular records, it appears, according to this gentleman, that "nearly one third of the diseases that have proved fatal in Memphis, are attributed to the digestive apparatus." Dr. Quintard charges this upon the atmosphere. We are led to suppose there is excessive filthiness in the streets. Water cannot run off, and scavenger carts belong to the reminiscences of a past epoch. Dr. Quintard appeals to the brotherhood respecting the present "creamy mud, through which all pedestrians have waded laboriously." According to this report, Memphis is shamefully neglected by the municipal officers. The business of the city is on the increase, but health and longevity will not be found within its borders, if something is not speedily accomplished by its board of health. With a fine climate, and an elevated locality, where thorough drainage might be economically established, villainous smells rise up to meet the senses, while other nuisances abound and multiply, to the disgust, if not to the positive detriment of the people. Dr. Quintard exhibits a clear and familiar acquaintance with his subject, besides having the moral courage to expose the negligence of the magistrates.

Spirit-Rapping Mania.—Grave men and women, who converse sensibly upon ordinary subjects, are still found to be excessively disturbed by any remark that carries with it a shadow of doubt in regard to the truth or importance of the spiritual revelations of the so-called mediums. The employment of a spirit-rapper is a profitable one. Individuals who would higgle with a hard-working mechanic, and beat him down two cents in the price of a day's wages, pay cheerfully for rapping nonsense, whatever may be the price demanded. People moving in circles supposed to be particularly intelligent, as often as otherwise, are the greatest dupes. Consequently there are the upper ten thousand dollar rappers, who receive a large fee, and the vulgarians, who cheat each other for amusement, without any fee. One of the curious circumstances in connection with this singular furor, is the fact that however placid, kind, courtly and obliging the believers in this "mystery" may naturally be, the moment they discover a disposition to cavil at the silly statements of what *they know, and what they have heard with their own ears,* their ire is up, they fly in a passion, and bedlam shows itself in exhibitions of temper, over which many of them will mourn hereafter, when reminded of this insane devotion to a humbug. A paper is now regularly published in this city, exclusively devoted to heralding the intercourse between the inhabitants of this and the unseen world. In New York, the brotherhood of rappers are a little in advance of us in Boston, as is shown by the following advertisement

from a recent newspaper of that city. "This evening, Henry Clay and
J. C. Calhoun will deliver a lecture through the mediumship of Rev. R.
P. Wilson, Spiritually Magnetized, at Hope Chapel. Subject—The true
principles of Government. One part of the lecture will be dictated by H.
Clay, and the other by J. C. Calhoun. Commence at 8 o'clock.—Admission 25 cents."

Travelling Quacks.—Quite a new system of quackery is beginning to
be extensively practised. The operator gives notice that such enormous
demands are made upon him for assistance, that the only way of meeting
them is to make announcements, that on Monday, for example, he may be
found in Philadelphia, Tuesday in New York, and Wednesday in Boston.
All who are desirous of availing themselves of the transcendant skill of
the very celebrated and most eminently distinguished Dr. Bolus are notified that they must be punctual in their attendance at his apartments. A
few editorial notices on the day previous to his arrival, intimating the immense benefit to be derived from consulting this remarkable physician,
prepare the minds of that great multitude who are always trying the
latest new thing, and they are accordingly promptly on the ground. Some
of these individuals increase the demand for their services by lecturing on
the all-important specifics they have at their benevolent disposal.

Berkshire Medical College.—A circular from the thriving and well-conducted medical institution, located in western Massachusetts, reminds us
to refer the profession to it as a thorough school of medicine, one that is
economical for students, and under the administration of a learned faculty.
In all the various changes which have characterized the country schools
of medicine, the Berkshire has been distinguished for continued energy,
talent, and a high-toned conservative spirit. Dr. Timothy Childs, a son
of the founder, now in the chair of Anatomy and Physiology, has just returned from Europe, bringing a knowledge of the latest improvements and
discoveries; and, better still, a disciplined mind—thus giving him, with
his eminent qualifications, the ability to infuse a vigor into the daily course
of instruction, that will redound to the increasing reputation of the College.

Mineral Springs.—No country abounds with such a variety of medicinal waters as ours. Besides the sulphur, graduated down to the flavor of
the broth of Weisbaden, we have warm and hot, sweet and sour, astringent and laxative, clear and clouded, and, in short, every variety of medicated waters are, in various parts of the country, copiously gushing out
of the earth. Among them all, here at the north, the Saratoga Springs
have always been in the ascendant. Since the discovery of the Iodine,
and the increasing consumption of the excellent water of the Empire
Spring, Saratoga presents new attractions for invalids. As all who might
derive benefit from them, cannot leave home, physicians are reminded that
the water may be had in Boston, fresh from the fountains, bottled daily
at Saratoga, and delivered in this city the same evening. Mr. Green, one
of the proprietors, is extremely particular in regard to securing each bottle
so that atmospheric air is completely excluded, while the escape of any
property belonging to the water is guarded against, and the patient actually has all the medicinal advantages from it in his own house, that he
would were he drinking at the aperture in the rock through which it is
perpetually boiling.

Deformities of the Human Frame.—A treatise on the nature and treat‑ment of the deformities of the human frame, by W. J. Little, M.D., of London, is a great work. It is great, because it is a practical treatise on every possible form and variety of distortion and malformation to which the body is liable, with minute instructions as to the remedy for such as can be benefited by art, accompanied by a vast number of illustrations. We have not seen a volume, for a long while, that is more needed for the medical libraries of the United States, and it is desirable that it should be re-published immediately. Conditions of the body, as described in this thoroughly-prepared book, are recognized in every town and city in this country. Great advances have been made in orthopedic surgery among us, within the last few years; but there is abundant room for more; and the series of lectures which Dr. Little has recently carried through the press, would, if studied, essentially contribute to uniformity of practice, and to further success. Fourteen years ago, the author gave the medical public instruction on the nature and treatment of club-foot, and analogous distortions, with and without surgical operations. He now presents him‑self, laden with experience, and fortified at every point by a careful series of observations, the value of which is apparent to the reader in passing from one page to another. Under the following heads, the different va‑rieties of deformities are considered, viz.:—deformities from wounds and diseases of the joints, accidents, rheumatism, &c.; from spasm, paralysis, burns, habitual retention in one position; from rickets, weakness and cur‑vatures of bones; from congenital distortions, club-foot and club-hand; from congenital malformations and monstrosities; from distortions of the spine. One hundred and sixty engravings and diagrams enhance the practical value of Dr. Little's labors.

In walking the streets, one is struck with the numbers passing him who are suffering from distorted limbs, club-feet, projecting sternums, wry necks, depressed shoulders, crooked spines, stiff joints, &c., which might, to a very considerable extent, be relieved. A lack of confidence in the re‑sources of surgery, or an ignorance of the improvements and discoveries which are constantly taking place, explains in some measure the existence of these physical embarrassments. A distinct department in the medical colleges, for particular instruction in orthopedic surgery, would be hailed with satisfaction, and add to the reputation of the institution that first creates such a chair.

ERRATUM.—The Female Medical College, referred to in the Journal of June 29th, is located in Philadelphia, and not in the place there stated.

To CORRESPONDENTS.—The following papers have been received:—A Lecture on Medical Delusions, by Dr. J H. Nutting; a second paper by Dr. Cartwright on the Hygienics of Tempe‑rance; Meeting of the Rhode Island Medical Society; and several documents relating to the late mal-practice trial in New Hampshire.

Deaths in Boston for the week ending Saturday noon, July 9th, 77. Males, 41—females, 36. Accidental, 2—apoplexy, 1—inflammation of the bowels, 3—inflammation of the brain, 1—con‑gestion of the brain, 1—burns and scalds, 2—consumption, 16—convulsions, 3—croup, 1—dysen‑tery, 1—dropsy, 1—dropsy in the head, 3—drowned, 1—infantile diseases, 4—puerperal, 1—erysipelas, 1—typhus fever, 2—scarlet fever, 1—hooping cough, 2—disease of the heart, 1—in‑flammation of the lungs, 5—congestion of the lungs, 1—marasmus, 5—measles, 2—old age, 5.—palsy, 3—pleurisy, 1—teething, 4—tumor, 1—unknown, 2.
Under 5 years, 32—between 5 and 20 years, 9—between 20 and 40 years, 7—between 40 and 60 years, 16—over 60 years, 13. Born in the United States, 47—Ireland, 26—British American Provinces, 1—Germany, 1—Denmark, 1—France, 1.

Bite of a Rattle-Snake—Cure.—By J. C. BLACKBURN, M.D., Flat Shoals, Geo.—I was called a few days since to visit a negress, some 8 miles from my office, who had been bit by a large rattle-snake. I saw her eight hours after the wound had been inflicted, which was on her ankle. I found the patient deathly sick; cold rigors running over her; pulse 120, small, quick, and thread-like; the entire left leg was swollen to twice its normal size; in a word, I thought she was moribund. She complained of no pain in the affected limb, and even insisted that she had not been bitten. I commenced giving her corn whiskey by the gill, and pushed the remedy until she had taken *two quarts* within twelve hours, when discovering some symptoms of inebriation, it was discontinued. In the mean time I applied warm emollient poultices to the wound, after having applied a cupping glass for one hour. In three days this negress was well and at her usual labor. —She took no medicine save the whiskey, and on the second day a dose of Epsom Salts.

The question here presents itself, would the usual remedies have been attended with success in this case? Had I not considered her in a moribund condition, she doubtless would have been treated, not *empirically*, but *scientifically*. I will remark, however, that this is the *fourth* case, that I have treated successfully with corn-whiskey, occurring from the poison of venomous reptiles. I had oftentimes seen ardent spirits recommended in snake bites, prior to my having prescribed it. My confidence in the remedy never was fully established until witnessing a rash act of a man while in a beastly state of inebriation. He caught a large rattle-snake and held it notwithstanding he was bit several times, until the snake becoming so greatly incensed bit himself, which soon relieved it from its confinement. The reptile speedily died. The man never complained of the least pain or uneasiness.—*Nelson's American Lancet.*

Bill to restrain the Practice of Inoculation in Canada.—At the close of the recent session of Parliament, on the 14th of June, the Governor General was pleased to give his sanction to the following Bill:—intituled, "An act to restrain the injurious practice of inoculating with the smallpox."— The preamble and enacting clause of the Bill read thus:—"Whereas it is highly expedient to restrain the injurious practice of inoculating with the natural smallpox (variola); Be it enacted, &c., That any person who shall produce or attempt to produce, by inoculation with variolous matter, or by wilful exposure to variolous matter, or to any matter, article or thing impregnated with variolous matter, or wilfully by any means whatsoever the disease of smallpox in any person in this Province, shall be liable to be proceeded against and convicted summarily before any two Justices, and for every such offence shall, upon conviction, be imprisoned for any term not exceeding one month."—*Montreal Medical Chronicle.*

Turpentine in Hæmoptysis.—Long experience has taught Dr. Lange, (of Kœnigsberg), that the spirit of turpentine acts more promptly in hæmoptysis than the different methods usually employed in that affection, such as tannin, common salt, acetate of lead, alum, nitrate of potash, cold applications and leeching. The efficacy of turpentine in the treatment of hæmoptysis, has been already recognized by Copland, Wiltshire and others, but this corroboration of it deserves to be recorded. —*Gazette des Hopitaux.*

THE

BOSTON MEDICAL AND SURGICAL JOURNAL.

| VOL. XLVIII. | WEDNESDAY, JULY 20, 1853. | No. 25. |

THE PHILOSOPHY OF MEDICAL DELUSIONS.

BY J. H. NUTTING, M.D., STAFFORD SPRINGS, CT.

[Communicated for the Boston Medical and Surgical Journal.]

NOTHING, except Religion, has had so many delusions connected with it as Medicine. Alike remedial in their nature, no sooner had man "brought death into the world and all our woe," than they began their mission of good to man. Religion aimed at healing the moral maladies of man. Nor could he, though in rebellion against his Maker, throw off all religion. Its elements were implanted in his nature ; and driven by a sense of guilt and impending danger, he has devised a thousand schemes for the redemption of his soul. Nothing has been too costly, nothing too cruel, nothing too revolting, nothing too senseless and absurd, for men to rush into. Witness the costly structures of Hindooism ; the horrid orgies of the Mexican priests ; the senseless mummeries of Buddhism ; the penances of the Romish church, and the wild ravings of fanatical sects! Ignorance, wilful blindness, and the corruption of the heart, have all lent their power to delude. "And as they did not like to retain God in their knowledge, He gave them over to believe a lie." Nor can one survey the religious history of the race, without doubting whether man is possessed of reason, or whether he is not "more foolish than the brutes that perish." But the infinite value of the soul has not been jeopardized by being left to the vain imagination of man. Infinite Benevolence has not only left some sparks of celestial wisdom glittering amid the rubbish of the human soul, but has even condescended to concentrate the full radiance of that wisdom on man's path ; and if he be now deluded, it will be through wilful perverseness and guilt. There is an unerring standard to which all religious theories may be brought, and delusion stamped on each that differs from that. Nor with that stamp upon them, can their advocates challenge for them either the respect or consideration of any.

Nor has the same Benevolence left the maladies of the body uncared for. "The tree whose leaf is for the healing of the nations," abounds in various forms throughout the globe. "There is balm in Gilead, and a physician there." But the balm must be sought with diligence, and the teachings of the physician studied with the greatest care. There

25

are the elements of the true medical system, implanted in the physical nature, as are those of the moral in the soul. But the former, unlike the latter, have no concentration of divine light thrown upon them. It is left for human reason to follow up the hints of Nature ; to take the oracular responses of the Physician, scattered like those of the Sybil, and combine them into one harmonious whole.

The possibility of doing this, coupled with the strong desire to ward off physical suffering, has made physicians. in every age. But there has been no standard of medical truth, except the ambiguous teachings of Nature, and few have been able, even to a limited extent, to read these aright. Hence the best physicians have been constantly deluding themselves and their patients. While they elucidated much of truth, they mingled with it much of error. Hence the firmly-established medical theories of one age, have in the next been neglected, or shown to be false. The physician for whom his contemporaries have decreed an apotheosis, has been hurled from his preëminence by his successors.

Medicine must ever be limited in its powers. It cannot raise the dead, nor prevent entirely the accession of disease, nor confer the boon of earthly immortality. But these are what men most desire. " Skin for skin, yea, all that a man hath, will he give for his life," was declared in regard to the man of Uz ; and acting under this passionate desire for life, the multitude have ever despised the modest pretensions of true medical science, while they have been loud in their applause of the arrogant assumptions of quackery. " The elixir of life " was the great desideratum, and quackery was ever ready to assert its possession of the invaluable boon. Hippocrates, and Galen, and Avicenna, no mean names, labored hard, by patient research and observation, to lay firmly the foundations of medical science. Nor without success, for many of their principles still stand as monuments of their labor, and the correctness of their judgment. But Paracelsus, the prince of quacks, could burn their works in the market place, and the multitude applauded the act. He, too, had the secret of immortality ; yet he died miserably at an early age, with a bottle of his elixir in his pocket.

The history of medicine, I had almost said, was a history of delusion. The wrecks of systems lie scattered all along its course, and often these systems formed a part of what was then regarded as true medical science. But while system after system has been wrecked, the truths which formed their nucleus have been increasing in number and importance, from age to age. False systems and theories have enveloped them in their mists ; but when increasing light has scattered these mists, the truths have remained. Unlike the thousand systems of quackery, which, when destroyed, leave no trace behind, this increasing centre of truth has come down from age to age, conferring blessings on all within its influence. And now this stream of truth has become a mighty river. Anatomy has shown the minute structure of nearly every tissue ; and physiology, aided by the microscope, has unveiled the functions of almost every organ ; while hygiene has pointed out the laws of health, and pathology the laws of disease, with the unnumbered changes effected in the living body by its invisible but potent foes ; and a rational system of therapeutics has taken the place of the absurdities formerly practised. Those old-time men were men of no mean powers, but they lacked all the appliances of modern art. Nor is it any disparagement to medical science that there has been so much of error mingled with it. With what science has this not been the case? Yet with all its errors, there has been truth enough mingled to preserve it through a long series of ages. System after system of quackery, on the other hand, has arisen, and even while boastingly predicting the destruction of the old system, have themselves been forgotten; and though system after system now make the same boast, they are yet but of a day, and, like their predecessors, will be remembered only with contempt.

It is true, Medicine is yet imperfect, nor are all its professors perfect even in the knowledge which it affords. But if we compare the medical science and practice of the present day, with that of the time of our Saviour, or even with that of a century ago, we shall see that it has made wonderful advances. And its progress will be still more wonderful; but it will be limited in its powers, and will still be, as it has been, an object of contempt to the unthinking. The man writhing on the bed of pain will give it no credit unless it cause that pain at once to cease. The friends of the deceased will upbraid it, because it kept him not back from the grave, never reflecting that man has "a time to die." Quackery, with its brazen tongue, will still proclaim its boasted powers, and the multitude will fall down and adore, while the modest voice of true science will be unheard. They would indulge each appetite and passion, and yet escape the penalty. Science reiterates, "The soul that sinneth it shall die." Quackery asserts, "Ye shall not surely die; indulge your appetites and passions, here is a balm for every evil that indulgence brings. Have your practices brought sickness on you? I can restore to health. Is youth fading? I have a panacea for your ills. Is death claiming you as his victim? I can unlock his grasp, and send you back to life. Ye shall not surely die." The unthinking multitude will receive these arrogant assumptions as the oracles of truth.

In surveying the medical history of the past, we hardly know which to wonder at most, the effrontery and boldness of quackery, or the credulity and perseverance of patients. It matters not that, like the woman in scripture, they have expended all their living and suffered many things of the physicians, nor been healed of any; they are just as ready to swallow each new pill, and drink each new potion, which the boldness of quackery may invent; till, however against their wills, they find out the truth of the old Greek epigram —"Death is the physician that cures," and sink into his embrace.

The sources of medical delusions are similar, however these may differ in form. To write the history of all medical delusions, would be a task too great for one man, and even if it were done, one might say, with the evangelist, "I suppose the world could not contain the books that would be written." It will therefore be more to the purpose to trace out the sources of medical delusions, giving the history of such as best illustrate the mode in which they arise. This will be my object, nor will it grieve me to expose quackery, whether under the garb of ignorance, or covering its shame with the fair parchments of medical colleges.

It is somewhat difficult to define clearly a medical delusion. So easily are truth and error mingled on this subject, and so difficult is it for even the best physician to determine what is due to his treatment, and what is due to the recuperative powers of nature, that many things have been admitted as legitimate medical knowledge, which the researches of after times have shown to be false. The discovery of the circulation of the blood, overturned a multitude of theories and conclusions which had before stood as truths ; and so with each succeeding discovery. Nor is it certain that many things in our present medical system, will not one day give place to more correct views. Not but that many principles are established beyond a doubt. Thus the principles of inflammation had been established by the experience and observation of many physicians ; and of late the microscope has shown, to the eye, the truth of the conclusions at which they had arrived. So with many other principles. These being strictly conformable to the operations of Nature, may be considered as established. But there are many others, resting only on probable evidence, which future investigation may show to be false.

The sources of medical delusions are many, and each delusion usually springs from several of them. The first source I shall notice, is in the *Nature of Medical Reasoning.*

This must, of course, rest on observation, or, as it is commonly termed, experience. But it cannot be properly termed experience, since this applies rather to what affects the subject of it, than to what one person observes in another. One person may observe the effects of grief in another, while he experiences nothing of the kind. Nor will he by any means have as clear an apprehension of its nature and effects, as though he had himself felt it. The same difference exists between what is usually termed medical experience, and true experience. Medical experience is, then, but an observation of the visible effects of the disease or remedy which the patient experiences. The uncultivated mind can form little idea of the grief it may behold in the person of cultivation and refinement. A cultivated mind alone can properly observe these effects. The value, then, of medical experience will depend entirely on the capacity of the observer. It can have no value above that of ordinary observation ; nor is it worthy of the credence given to the observation of physical phenomena, since the physician is obliged, in a great measure, to depend on the sensations of the patient, as described by him ; and any one at all conversant with disease, knows how often the sensations are perverted, and how often effects are considered as having taken place, which a further examination shows had no existence but in the imagination of the patient. A very extensive experience may therefore afford no correct basis for medical reasoning. On the contrary, the more extensive an incorrect experience or observation in medicine may be, the more incorrect will be the reasoning and practice founded upon it.

In addition to this, the connection between cause and effect is for the most part concealed. In ordinary phenomena, although we cannot explain how or why one act stands in the relation of cause to another, yet we know, from the obvious results, that they are thus related. Why the impulse of one body on another should cause the latter to move, is beyond our power to explain. We know that the impulse is the physical cause of the motion, since it is the uniform consequence of an impulse, and no other known cause can possibly come in to produce this effect. But in medical experience, or observation, it is not so. We administer a drug, and a certain result follows ; yet we can only say " *vel post hoc, vel propter hoc.*" Either it took place after it, or ' on account of it. We can effect no changes by merely therapeutic means, which Nature may not under favorable circumstances effect alone. And we know that the same changes are often effected independently of medical interference. Hence we cannot, in any given case, say with certainty that a given change is the result of our interference. Nor does it render it *certain*, even if we have often administered the same medicine with the same result. Nature, in one case, may have effected the change, and in another it may have been the result of our interference. Other causes, even, may have come in to effect the change, of which we know nothing. Still, if the same results follow upon a repetition of the medicine under similar circumstances, we are at liberty to consider the change as probably the effect of the administration of the medicine. In some cases it may even amount to a certainty ; as when, in an acute inflammation, a copious depletion reduces it at once. But this class of cases is comparatively small. For the most part, the results of medical treatment are spread over a considerable period of time. Nature, in these cases, has time to effect great changes. The medicine is given, and may, it is true, stand as the cause of the changes, or it may, with the Peruvian proverb, but have amused the patient, while Nature has performed the cure. The delusions arising from this source will be considered more at length hereafter.

Another fruitful source of medical delusions, is found in the *Difficulty of determining the Exact Nature of the Disease.* This is rather a branch of the difficulty arising from the nature of Medical Reasoning, than a distinct source.

There are, besides death, many diseases which no art can cure. When these have taken hold on man, his days are numbered. Science and art may indeed assuage the pang, and smooth the descent to the grave, but the deadly arrow has been fixed too deeply to be withdrawn. When once Hercules had put on the poisoned robe of the faithless Dejanira, the poison went through the very bones, nor could his celestial origin avert the fatal result. Nor is it for the disgrace of the medical art, that these are beyond her skill. Death hath universal power over mortals ; and, though science hath disarmed many of his ministers of their potency, he will doubtless possess some over which art will have no control, till Death shall have yielded up his power to Him that is mightier than he.

The difficulty of determining these diseases, has been a fruitful source of delusion. In their external character, they for the most part resemble affections readily amenable to medical art. The skilful physician perceives the difference ; and while he loses his patient, feels that he has done what he could, but had met his superior in power. Not so the mass. Undisciplined in mind, they perceive only the resemblance ; and hence, when another case occurs *resembling* this, but differing in its essential character, and which recovers, they are loud in their condemnation of the first physician, and vociferous in their praises of him who has cured a patient " just like that."

Cancer is a disease of this kind. It is what physicians call a heterologous growth ; that is, a series of cells, unlike those of the healthy tissue, is produced among the healthy tissues, and these multiply till the frightful results of this terrible disease take place ; and these cells are always the same. In its early stages, especially, it resembles, in its external characters, a simple non-malignant tumor. The microscope, however, shows the cancer cells ; and the experience of the world has thus far shown, that when once these peculiar cells are produced in a part, nothing but the entire abscision of the part will check them ; and that, even then, in a majority of cases, the germs of these cells will be found so widely disseminated in the blood, that they will speedily spring up, and form new growths like the first. The skilful physician perceives this character in a tumor, and pronounces it hopeless without an operation, and doubtful with it. In another, resembling this in external appearance, he fails to find these cells, and it recovers. No noise is made about it, for no great cure has been performed, nor is true science either noisy or brazen tongued. But the *cancer doctor* comes, with loud boasts of skill, and finding a simple non-malignant tumor, he will not, or cannot, see it to be such, and if the tumor disappears while he is giving his syrups, he has done what the regular physicians could not—cured a cancer ! And the multitude applaud him for his skill. There was no cancer in the case, but his own insufferable ignorance and arrogance, surpassing in malignancy the fatal disease he pretends to have cured.

[To be continued.]

HYGIENICS OF TEMPERANCE, OR WATER AND ALCOHOL CONTRASTED ON LAWYERS.

BY SAMUEL A. CARTWRIGHT, M.D., NEW ORLEANS, LATE OF NATCHEZ.

[Communicated for the Boston Medical and Surgical Journal.]

SOME weeks ago the writer had the honor to receive a lengthy communication from a theologian of high standing and great influence—the Rev. Dr. C. K. Marshall, of Vicksburg, Mississippi—earnestly calling on him for the results of the observation and experience of the medical profession in regard to the physical effects of alcoholic beverages on the different classes of people. It appeared from the communication, and the documents accompanying it, that an organized opposition was being made in Mississippi against the only king who has any sway there—that being hard pressed by the reverend gentlemen and others, the advocates of alcohol had sought refuge in the strong and inaccessible fortress of medical science. They claimed protection from medicine, and demanded allegiance to alcohol by virtue of the theory (or rather the assumption) that the use of distilled liquors, in moderation, by persons in health, is useful in preventing disease, bracing the system against sudden changes in the weather, and in giving the body strength, vigor and endurance under fatigue and exposure;—that its general use, in some form or other, is almost indispensable in those parts of the South where the fogs are heavy, the musquitoes troublesome, and nature has furnished nothing but rain and river water to drink. The reverend gentleman wished much to know, whether the medical faculty would sustain the advocates of alcohol in these positions and pretensions? and whether the span of life was lengthened or shortened by the daily use of alcohol in any form? On such grounds, the question, in regard to the claims of alcohol to medical protection, is strictly one, which none but physicians have a right to decide or sit in judgment upon.

Having no authority to speak for the medical profession, the writer simply proposes to contrast the effects of water as a beverage with those of alcoholic drinks, from facts derived from his own experience and observation, and to answer the reverend gentleman by giving the result of the contrast through the appropriate organs of the profession—the Medical Journals.

In a former article on the Hygienics of Temperance, the writer gave a summary of his observations on one class of citizens, the physicians themselves, residing in the locality where he formerly practised. That article was intended as a part of his reply to the reverend gentleman's interrogatories, and was written with a hope that it might draw the attention of abler men to the important subject. It was also thought that it might be useful to the junior members of the profession.

Before going further, it may be necessary to premise, for the benefit of juniors, who have not got through their studies, and for seniors, who have not kept up with the progress of the sciences, that alcohol belongs to the Ethyl group of Lowig (the latest and most voluminous chemical authority of Germany). Ether or letheon is also a compound of the radical, ethyl. The former is an oxyhydrate, and the latter an oxide of ethyl. Chloroform is a compound of formyl. The compounds of ethyl and formyl are kindred in properties. None of them are found in nature, but are creatures of the chemist's alembic, as much so as the steam engine is of the mechanician. An important question has arisen, whether they ought not all to be kept exclusively under the control and direction of those who know where, when and how to use them? The oxide of ethyl, like chloroform, is the realization of the fabled waters of Lethe; while alcohol, which is an oxyhydrate of ethyl, is even more than the realization of the fabled potion, used by Circe, in transforming the companions of Ulysses into swine. The vapor of the oxide of ethyl, when breathed, destroys the will and renders the body insensible to impressions: but it should be remembered that all spirituous liquors contain a greater or less quantity of ethyl in the form of an oxyhydrate; the vapor of which affects the will and the senses, rendering those, who come within the sphere of such exhalations, less competent to govern their passions and inclinations. In other words, the atmosphere, within and around those places where spirituous liquors are retailed, contains ethyl—a substance palsying the will and depriving man of his free agency. The contaminating influences of an atmosphere containing ethyl cannot be avoided without avoiding the places charged with it. A few have such strong wills as not to be sensibly influenced by it, but in the great majority of mankind the will is so weak as to be affected by the smallest quantity in the air. Moral persuasion is lost upon such. Indulgence in drinking creates a greater susceptibility to such influences, until those, who see their error and wish to reform, are unable to do so. The smallest taint of ethyl in the air, from some neighboring distillery, or retail liquor shop, will cause them to break the most solemn vows ; and often with tears in their eyes to be led, against their better judgment, to seek the cup, which they know is causing their ruin. Some would rush to it at the cannon's mouth if they knew the match was being applied, so completely are they deprived of a will of their own. It is a penal offence to poison springs and wells, but there is no penalty attached to poisoning the air with ethyl. Whether there should not be, is a question highly important in a political as well as in a medical and moral point of view. Ours is not properly a land of liberty while the oxyhydrate of ethyl, vulgarly called spirituous liquors, is not only permitted to taint the air with its exhalations, but to be infused in the water which thoughtless youth and ignorant, peaceful citizens are tempted to drink ; transforming them into lawless, reckless, dangerous madmen, more numerous and mischievous, a greater restraint upon the liberty of the majority, and a greater nuisance to society, than the marauders of Mexico or the banditti of Italy.

Before giving countenance or encouragement to the general use of such an agent, by the people at large, on the strength of a vague theory, that it is useful to ward off disease and to enable them to endure fatigue and exposure, it is important that every physician should take the necessary means to ascertain whether such a theory be true or not. It should be well considered and tested by experience and observation, the only sure method of arriving at truth. In a former article on the Hygienics of Temperance, it was shown that that theory prevailed in Natchez thirty years ago, and as far as a certain class was concerned—the physicians themselves—the practice of drinking ardent spirits, in what is called moderation, time and experience proved to be highly pernicious— and instead of lengthening, cut short the thread of life.

And now for the voice of time and experience in regard to the lawyers and other professional men. What does it say ? It says, in a tone too clear, loud and plain to be mistaken—that as it was with the doctors of Natchez and vicinity, so has it been with the lawyers. The lawyers of that city and vicinity, thirty years ago, who were in the habit of using alcoholic beverages in the place of plain water between meals, like the doctors who followed the same practice, are all dead long ago. There is not one left. Even to bring down the time to twenty years, there is not one left. While of the temperate lawyers of the same locality, from twenty to thirty years ago, all are living at the present time, June, 1853—minus a number *less* than the natural decrease of mankind, incident to the most healthy countries, as set forth in the Carlisle tables of mortality. The bench and the pulpit have scarcely lost a member except from accident or old age. The temperate lawyers, with the exceptions just mentioned, are not only all living, but they are all rich, although they began life poor. The contrast arrived at by consulting time and experience is so great, that it may be said that death is in alcohol and life is in water, when used as a common beverage. That plain, good, pure water is better than alcohol in any form to enable the human system to endure fatigue and exposure, and to give both body and mind strength and vigor, the history of the above-mentioned classes would plainly prove. The proofs, in regard to one of them, may be read in the history of the Mexican war, requiring nothing more to be added, than that Major General John A. Quitman is the model of a temperate man in all things—except politics, where, if he runs into extremes, it is from the same principle, which, in war, impels him to advance nearest to the foe. Another of the temperate lawyers of Natchez, 28 to 30 years ago, is the Hon. Robert J. Walker, late Secretary of the Treasury, and present Minister to China. Although he never broke through the massive walls of the houses of Monterey with a pickaxe, or stormed Chepultepec, yet he swam Pearl river a cold frosty night without catching cold. The writer is assured, by a creditable person who was with him, that the natural treble tones of his voice, at a political meeting the next day, were not altered or reduced to a bass. His travelling companion of the canteen was too hoarse to speak, although the future holder of the nation's purse, after swimming the river, got a boat and ferried him and the horses across. Capt. John B. Nevitt, for more than thirty years has resided on his estate near Natchez, and been the master spirit at political meetings, yet he never drank as much as half a pint of ardent spirit in all his life—proving that fiery zeal in politics is not incompatible with perfect temperance. He and his other temperate shipmates, under Decatur before Tripoli, proved that water as a beverage is better than opium-eating to give celerity of motion, as the American sword, in their hands, against the Turkish cimetar, was like the lightning's flash. Col. Henry Chotard, a resident of the same vicinity, the same length of time, and of the same temperate habits, three times repelled three fierce assaults of the British regulars on his cannon, and so far won the applause of Gen. Jackson as to be mentioned by name in his despatches as one of the three who " *by their intrepidity saved the artillery.*"—(See Niles's Register, vol. vii., page 357, giving an official account of the important battle of the 23d of December below New Orleans.) His sobriquet, " My Lord Chesterfield of Adams Co.," from his high degree of polish and urbanity of manners, is sufficient to show the folly of some young men who fall into intemperate habits from the fear of being regarded as rustic or clownish.

Space will not permit to speak of all the temperate lawyers, judges, divines and politicians of Natchez thirty years ago, who are now living. Joseph E. Davis, Esq., is one of them ; both he and his younger brother, Col. Jeff. Davis, the hero of Bona Vista, and the present Secretary of

War, are so very temperate that they had rather be shot at than to drink a bumper of ardent spirit; yet no men excel them in energy of mind. The Hon. Powhatan Ellis, for two terms the Nestor of the U. S. Senate, and former Minister to Mexico; ex-senator Gen. John Henderson, who made Spain tremble for Cuba; and Gen. Felix Houston, the John the Baptist who prepared the way for Texian Independence—are all old Natchez lawyers, owing the energy of their character and their good health at the present day to their rejecting alcohol and using water as a beverage. His Excellency Gov. Poindexter, a Natchez lawyer of more than thirty years ago, becoming crippled and bed-ridden under the alcoholic theory, so fashionable in his day, repudiated it—went back to water as a beverage—recovered the use of his limbs, rejuvenated, and again entered the political arena, giving his opponents such sharp thrusts, that the editors of the Globe named him "the devil's darning needle." Their Honors Judges Turner, Perkins, Cage, McGehee, Boyd, Black and Montgomery, are all living at the present day in the possession of their faculties, with nothing but their great wealth to trouble them. They are as temperate as preachers. So are the two renowned brothers, Colonels Claibornes, natives; so are J. A. McMurren, Esq., R. M. Gaines, Esq., A. Buckner, Esq., and M. W. Ewing, Esq., Natchez lawyers of thirty years ago, Kentuckians, with houses full of children. The Rev. J. C. Barruss, the Rev. Messrs. Drake, Curtis, Van-Court, Smilie, Page, Chase, Fox, Fyler, Winans, and the Rev. Dr. Potts, the present pastor of Grace Church, New York, were the principal clergymen in and about Natchez twenty-five to thirty years ago. They are still living. The deaths among the clergy and judges have been less than half the natural mortality indicated by the Carlisle tables. Judge Ogden, of the little town of Vidalia, opposite Natchez, has moved away, but is living yet, nearer a century than three score and ten. Like Judge John Perkins, also of the same side of the river, he is the personification of temperance.

It is unnecessary to go into further particulars in drawing a contrast between water and alcohol as beverages. The temperance casket has been opened, and many jewels of great price have been shown; that of alcohol has also been unlocked, and the more numerous gems lodged there for safe keeping are turned to dust and ashes. Alcohol, that promised to preserve, has been the slow devouring fire to consume them. The human system will often withstand an occasional dose, even a heavy dose, of poison, and recover from its effects; but the stoutest frame will sink under its daily use in portions ever so small. Some of the above-mentioned professional men, classed as temperate, occasionally partook of that slow but potent poison to the blood, alcohol, but let a sufficient time intervene to recover from its effects before taking more; and it appears that they have long since renounced it. It is the daily use of alcohol—particularly between meals—though in quantities regarded as small, which is so highly pernicious.

In the progress of physiology an important fact has been developed, that those, who use water as a beverage, consume more oxygen, than those who partake of spirituous liquors. Although the physical effect of alcohol in diminishing the quantity of oxygen consumed was known to Prout and others, and may be found recorded by Dunglison in his article on respiration, yet its value, as an overwhelming argument against alcoholic beverages in every form, is not clearly seen, but will be, when certain late revelations, made by the crocodile on the dissecting table, become generally known and have time to correct some fundamental errors which have crept into physiology in regard to the motive power of the blood and the primary seat of life. ' They prove, that the oxygen of the air is the chief motive power of the blood, and that that fluid is the primary seat of life as Moses said it was. But until this new doctrine be acknowledged, no short cut can be taken to demonstrate the poisonous properties of alcoholic drinks in small quantities upon the human system, by arguments drawn from the laws governing the organism. The truth will have to be ascertained by the slow and toilsome process of experience and observation. The result, obtained by that sure and safe method, proves that there exists a wide contrast between water and alcohol used as beverages by professional men.

The result of the effects of each on the people at large, of the same locality and at the same period of time, can be told in fewer words, but the labor of arriving at it by the same method is vastly greater ; so much so, that if the large quantity of statistical matter, which has been collected since he made the call upon the writer, as preliminary to the induction to extract truth, hid among so many particulars, could be seen by the Rev. gentleman, he would doubtless find an ample apology for the delay in replying to his interrogatories.

Canal st., New Orleans, June 28, 1853.

CASE OF VENEREAL CHANCRE PRODUCED BY SODOMY.

BY N. R. MOSELEY, M.D., OF PHILADELPHIA.

[Communicated for the Boston Medical and Surgical Journal]

In the month of February last, I was requested by an office pupil to visit John Mc————, aged 35, of good general health and robust constitution. The patient was troubled with a sore just within the verge of the anus, which had been growing worse for several weeks. As no contaminating disease was suspected, he had been treated with mild local remedies without benefit. Upon making an examination I found, one half an inch above the termination of the mucous membrane of the rectum, what appeared to be a large Hunterian chancre. The genital organ was unaffected, and the parts about appeared healthy, with the exception of a little tenderness and swelling in the right groin. My opinion was that the man had syphilis, as his subsequent acknowledgment and facts proved. It seems that about five weeks previous to my visit, the man had been on a drunken frolic, and was one night arrested in the street and committed to one of the city lock-ups for safe keeping until morning. While in this place, another man, put there for the same offence, did some time during the night (mistaking his bed-fellow) commit an outrage upon his person, which he was unable to resist, although conscious of the transaction. This individual, as I have since learned, had at the time small venereal ulcers upon the glans penis.—Under the use of calomel and opium, with the local application of black wash, our patient soon recovered.

July, 1853.

DIFFERENT MODES OF ARRESTING HEMORRHAGE FROM THE EX-TRACTION OF TEETH.

BY BENJAMIN WOOD, M.D., NASHVILLE, TENN.

DR. A. SALTONSTALL, of Columbus, Ohio, Miss., reports a case (Am. Jour. Dental Science, Oct. 1852), of hemorrhage from the extraction of a tooth, which, having resisted the usual means—astringents, escharotics and compression—was arrested by an artificial fixture acting both as compress and actual cautery. He "took a piece of pure silver plate, and cut it in shape to fit between the teeth and cover the lips of the orifice about the eighth of an inch on each side. This was bent to fit the parts, and heated to a white heat, and suddenly applied to the place, where it remained several days. When it was removed the coagulum came away with it. The orifice was examined, and a very delicate covering, resembling tissue paper, had formed over it."

Dr. Levison, of England, in an article published about a year ago, says, that in cases of excessive hemorrhage, where the ordinary styptics cannot be depended upon, "we may arrest the dangerous hemorrhagic flow with certainty by destroying the vessels with the bi-chloride of zinc," and gives cases where this agent, as a last resort, had been successful in his hands. In alveolar hemorrhage, pieces of cotton dipped into the bi-chloride were forced down to the alveolar cavities. It was attended, however, with great pain.

It may be remarked that in some cases where success is ascribed to the last remedy employed, the result may have been owing to a natural stasis of blood from exhaustion of the patient; such hemorrhages sometimes continuing for hours, until after fainting, and then ceasing altogether without any intervention. An interesting case of the kind was related to us a few years ago by a reliable lady who was herself the subject. The bleeding had continued with but occasional and partial intermissions for three days. On the night of the third it ceased, and she retired, but about midnight she was awakened by a renewed flow of blood. Exhausted by the loss of blood and sleep, she merely arranged a wash-bowl upon a chair so as to receive the blood as it flowed from her mouth, and with her head supported by a pillow, she soon fell asleep. In this position she was found early the next morning, in a state of unconsciousness. The bleeding had effectually ceased.

It is fortunate that these cases rarely occur. We have had but few that were troublesome. Besides the use of nitrate of silver (which as a styptic we have found more reliable than anything else that we have used), and the application of pressure, we have in two or three instances resorted to a partial *torsion of the bloodvessels* at the bottom of the alveolar cells. This depends upon the principle that the mouths of the vessels contract more readily when lacerated than when divided with a smooth cut, or broken short off, as may happen in extracting a tooth, and that mechanical irritation has a tendency to induce contraction. The *modus operandi* (as we received it while under pupilage, from our brother, Dr. J. S. Wood) consists in passing a stylet or an ordinary excavator of the proper shape, to the bottom of the socket, until a twinge of pain is felt, and then giving the instrument a sudden turn, so as to twist or lacerate the artery—its situation being indicated by the impression made upon the nerve which it accompanies.

We know of but one instance in this vicinity, of death having occurred in consequence of the kind of hemorrhage under notice. This was in Russellville, Ky., about two years ago. The patient's tooth was broken in extracting, leaving a portion of the fang which could not be gotten out. Pressure, as well as styptics, &c., was tried, but without arresting the hemorrhage, the man dying, according to the recollection of our informant, in about fifteen hours after the operation. We would like very much to be favored with a report of the case in full.

In case a tooth is broken and the bleeding proceeds from the pulp cavity or nerve canal, the obvious means of arresting it would be to plug the orifice with a metallic or wood stopping. A hickory peg or sliver would perhaps be as good as anything. If the orifice be too small to receive a stopping, it should be enlarged by means of a drill.

Pressure applied directly to the bleeding vessels and retained in its place is reliable in such cases of hemorrhage; but there is sometimes considerable difficulty experienced in its application. A ready and effectual means is to roll up pellets of cotton firmly in the fingers, of a size to suit the alveolar cells, and introduce them with considerable force, notwithstanding it be attended with considerable pain, as it always is, we believe, when the hemorrhage has continued for some time. They may be wet with some styptic solution, or coated with powdered lunar caustic. After the first pellet has been introduced, we usually fill the remainder of the cavity with one of a larger size, and if it be a molar tooth with two or three bi-furcations, cover the whole with a third, sufficiently large for the purpose but no larger, crowding the edges under the margins of the gums, which, in ordinary conditions, where the blood possesses its due amount of fibrin, and is of a plastic character, will be found to adhere to the cotton with sufficient tenacity to retain it in its place. It will be safest to let this stopping remain until loosened by the suppurative process. If not thrown off, however, or removed in the course of a few days, the pellets thus introduced are apt to prove the source of great suffering in the sockets, bespeaking the inflammatory action preparatory to suppuration; but when this occurs we think they may be removed at once, regarding it as evidence that active reparation has commenced.

The "waxed cones" recommended by Dr. B. B. Brown, which are made by cutting a piece of linen previously coated with melted beeswax, into tapering strips, and rolling these in a form to suit the sockets to which they are to be applied, may be used to great advantage in many cases.—*Southern Journal of Medical and Physical Sciences.*

CHLOROFORM IN A CASE OF INFANTILE CONVULSIONS.

BY W. C. WILLIAMSON, M.R.C.S.L., ETC., MANCHESTER.

SINCE it is important that all examples of the application of a new remedy should be placed on record, whether the result has been successful or not, the following case, in which a young infant was kept under the influence of chloroform for a period of sixty hours, merits publication.

Mrs. R——— was confined of a fine male child, March 19th. Some little time after her confinement both her breasts became the seats of mammary abscess, hence the infant was compelled to have recourse to artificial food, which, however, did not appear to disagree with it. On Friday morning, April 29, it was seized with a slight convulsion, which recurred on the evening of the same day, and during the three subsequent days it suffered from three or four fits daily, each attack continuing about twenty minutes. The fits gradually became more severe ; some continued three or four hours without remission, though not very violent ; others, which usually woke him up from sleep, when he uttered a sharp scream, were much more severe, though of shorter duration. Of these latter ones the child appeared to have an instinctive dread. Ultimately the fits were unceasingly present whenever the child was awake. During the first two or three days the child's bowels were a little confined, and afterwards the motions became rather slimy and greenish, but no obvious source of irritation could be detected. There was no feverishness or heat of head, except during the more violent fits, and even then the scalp was less hot than might have been anticipated at the commencement. The fontanelle was neither raised nor depressed, but towards the end of the convulsive attacks it became decidedly depressed.

The congestion and lividity produced by the fits gradually increased, and, owing to the difficulty of giving nourishment, the child soon began to lose flesh. The quick succession of the convulsions made it impossible sometimes to give food for twelve hours together.

A leech was applied to the temple, warm baths employed, mild alterative doses of mercury with chalk and ipecacuanha powder, administered internally, along with other remedies calculated to allay irritation and remove any irritant likely to be lodged in the bowels ; but none of these remedies appeared to have the slightest influence either for better or worse. Under these circumstances, since the child was rapidly sinking, Dr. Bardsley and myself determined to have recourse to chloroform. I commenced the use of it at 9 o'clock on the evening of Friday, May 8th. The child was then in a violent convulsion, which had continned for several hours. I folded a thin muslin handkerchief into a hollow funnel-shaped form, and after dropping half a drachm of chloroform into the hollow cavity, I inverted it over the nose of the convulsed infant, holding it about an inch from the face, so as to allow a free current of air to reach the respiratory organs. In about two minutes the convulsion gave way, and the child went to sleep. The effect of the chloroform passed off in a few minutes, when it was again applied, and thus the child was kept quiet for some hours.

I soon found that by slightly releasing the infant from the influence of the chloroform, but without allowing the convulsions to regain their power, it was possible to give a supply of food, which was swallowed eagerly and with great facility. This alone was an important advantage gained from the chloroform, since previous to its administration the child was obviously sinking from inanition.

For some hours I administered the chloroform myself, but afterwards entrusted it to an intelligent nurse, who was instructed to apply it the moment the child exhibited any movements indicating returning consciousness. This treatment was continued without a moment's interruption, until 9 o'clock on the subsequent Monday, when the use of the chloroform was suspended, the infant having then been under its influence sixty hours, sixteen ounces having been used. Its appearance was now decidedly improved ; its flesh was more firm, and the sunken eye and livid countenance were exchanged for a much more healthy aspect. The convulsions exhibited no disposition to return, and up to the present period (May 30) the infant has enjoyed perfect health.

In this case I have not the slightest doubt that the chloroform was instrumental in saving the patient's life ; I can scarcely conceive recovery to have been possible without its aid. No injurious effects, however trivial, appeared to accrue from its use, and I am satisfied that, if necessary, we could have employed it for a much longer period without evil consequences.

It is of course important to ascertain to what class of convulsive attacks this new remedy is applicable. In the present instance, though the condition of the patient was masked at its commencement, in its latter stages the disease assumed the adynamic type. It is obviously in such cases that we should be most likely to obtain benefit from the combination of the stimulating and sedative properties of the anæsthetic agent. It is a curious circumstance that such a modified use of it as allowed of the action of the muscles of deglutition, was nevertheless sufficient to control the convulsions.—*London Lancet.*

THE BOSTON MEDICAL AND SURGICAL JOURNAL.

BOSTON, JULY 20, 1853.

Prosecution for Mal-practice.—We have already alluded to the case of Dr. Dixi Crosby, the Professor of Surgery at Dartmouth College—against whom a verdict has been rendered for damages in a suit for mal-practice. If Dr. Crosby had no more to do with the patient than was represented in the testimony, the verdict appears unrighteous beyond example. A scheme

is imagined to have been devised for breaking down the professor. Somebody is evidently weary of hearing Aristides called "the just;" in other
words, by driving off an old surgeon, there is a chance of dropping into
his place. Some of the papers in Vermont and New Hampshire have
published the particulars of the trial, and we append a synopsis of the
case from one of them, the Vermont Chronicle.

"In April, 1845, Dr. Crosby was called upon to visit one Lorenzo Slack,
of Norwich, Vt., who had been severely injured by the fall of a bank of
earth upon him; but declined going on account of sickness. A physician
residing in Vermont, who was present at the time, volunteered to go and
see the injured man, and did go. Another neighboring physician was also
called, and the two upon examination found the left thigh of Slack badly
broken, high up, in two places. Regarding it as a severe case, they concluded to go to Hanover, and consult Dr. Crosby in regard to dressing the
injury, and also procure splints for the purpose. They did go, and on examination of books there, decided to use a particular kind of splint, and
ordered it to be made. At their earnest solicitation, Dr. C. went to Norwich, and assisted in putting the patient into the splint, which had been
previously prepared. Here ended all connection of Dr. C. professionally
with the case. He only saw him once afterwards—about two weeks after
the injury—and then called at the earnest request of the attending physician, and gave some general advice to the patient on the importance of
remaining as quiet as possible, to facilitate the healing of his limb, expressly stating to him that he assumed and could take no professional
responsibility in his case. Slack remained at the house where he was
carried after receiving his injuries, a month or more, under the care of a
respectable physician of Norwich, during which time the fracture healed
remarkably well, and the leg was not more than a quarter of an inch
shorter than the other at the time, when, against the remonstrance and
protest of his physician, he insisted upon being carried to his home. He
was thus carried—he recovered with a bad limb, and about six years afterwards commenced an action against Dr. C. for mal-practice, which has
resulted in a verdict by the jury in favor of the plaintiff."

Perkins Institution for the Blind.—Whatever is undertaken for the
purpose of promoting the happiness of the unfortunate, should be encouraged. It is no part of selfishness, in the commonly received sense of the
term, to organize a charity school for instructing poor children in a particular district, because they may be a burden to the community and occupants
of prisons, in the course of events, if they are neglected; nor is it selfishness that prompts people to sustain an institution for the deaf and dumb,
or for the still more to be pitied idiots. The same might be said of various other charities, which are diffusing an immense amount of comfort to
the body, while the moral and mental culture received through them makes
known the beauties and consolations of a virtuous life, and its reward
hereafter, to thousands who must otherwise have died, as they began to
live, in wretchedness and ignorance.—A copy of the twenty-first annual
report of the Perkins Asylum for the Blind, at South Boston, brings to
mind its long-known and fully-tested excellences. Quietly, and without
show, the blind are there taught to be useful members of society. All their
powers are developed, and, in the multitude of their blessings, some of
them scarcely feel that, to be without vision, is the greatest of afflictions.

Dr. Howe's success in bringing out the intellectual powers of the pupils, by means of books they can read with the ends of their fingers, is one of the proudest and most important events of the age. We feel as though it was not fully appreciated by the world. Happening to be in England, during the exhibition of all nations, it was a gratification to witness the high estimate in which the invention of type to raise the letters on paper, was held. Being within sight of the edifice in which this vast labor was first undertaken and completed, that has done more for the progress of humanity than can be estimated, the citizens of Boston are too generally strangers to processes and efforts that excite the admiration of Europe. This report chronicles the constant improvements in this important branch of charitable effort. None of us should be so exclusively absorbed in the details of medicine, as to remain insensible to or uninterested in an effort which accomplishes anything for the halt, the maimed, and the blind. We recommend to our professional brethren to acquaint themselves with the system and success of the Perkins Asylum, and also with the course now being pursued in the management of idiotic children, at the same institution.

Meeting of Superintendents of Insane Asylums.—On the 10th of May last, a congress of medical superintendents of the principal institutions for the insane, in the various States, was convened at Baltimore, and some account of it was given in the Journal at the time. This was the eighth annual meeting. The object of these meetings is to interchange civilities, discuss questions considered of importance in advancing the interests of that unhappy class of patients placed under their care; and lastly, to spread abroad, for the benefit of others, the results of their experience and discoveries. The members were all men of decided talents; energetic, philosophical inquirers; and as writers, some of them have an extensive reputation. The Journal of Transactions, just published, indicates an active session, which must have been as satisfactory to the members as it will prove beneficial to the world.

Dr. Clark's Address.—This address bears a critical examination. As president of the Medical Society of the State of New York, a fitting opportunity was offered him, at its last meeting, for making an exhibition of his powers. The discourse, it seems, was delivered before a mixed audience of physicians, legislators, and ladies. Each must have heard much to admire, while the general scholar could not have been otherwise than gratified at the versatility of the orator's talents. If medical meetings were thrown open to the public more frequently, the effect would be decidedly advantageous. The people would soon discriminate between the claims of mere pretenders, and the sterling acquirements of the members of a learned profession. Were our anatomical cabinets also kept open, daily, for the free inspection of citizens and strangers, as they are all over Europe, instead of being blue chambers, to which the vulgar refer in a whisper, as awful places, where dead men's bones are boiled in a cauldron, medical science would be better appreciated, and medical men find their receipts augment. This course will certainly be brought about by the next generation of physicians, in all the cities where there are medical schools and hospitals.

The Hydropathists—their Water-cure Almanac.—No sect or school was ever more persevering than the hydropathists. Nothing disturbs or discourages them. Ridicule, the most potent engine of attack, does not even excite their wrath. Buildings are erected at great cost, with accommodations for administering water scientifically, inside or out; and though the owners have repeatedly failed and the property has passed into other hands, the disciples are never discouraged. The more unfortunate they have been in their outlays for accommodating the unwashed believers, the greater is their activity in selecting new localities for carrying on their curative plans, by means of wet sheets, cold douches, sit baths and aquatic manipulations. Their publications are numerous, and issued in the same determined spirit which characterizes all their efforts. Whether read or not, paid for or given away, it is all the same to the water-cure philanthropists. They commenced in the United States, with a determination to wash the people of their woes, and thus far they have faithfully persevered. Some very accomplished physicians, by some hocus pocus, difficult to comprehend, have given in their adhesion to the party, and are devoting their exclusive attention to boarding and curing patients at their new-founded aquatic establishments. As an instrumentality in this work, humble, but nevertheless powerful upon a large class of minds, is the illustrated "Water-cure Almanac," annually published by Fowler & Wells, New York. It goes, often, where a heavy volume could not be sent. Its facts as well as arguments may be understood by a child, while they are sometimes such as would convert a judge to the water practice, should he happen to cast his eyes over its unpretending leaves. Because this little work is insignificant, its real power is unsuspected ; yet a mightier machine could not be set in motion for enlarging and sustaining the system of hydropathy. Learned gentlemen express their surprise that this tom-foolery of cold-water treatment, as they are pleased to call it, does not die out in New England. The reason is plain enough on looking over the pages of this Almanac and some kindred publications, which are addressed to the masses, among whom its patrons are found, converts multiplied, and stock taken for erecting new establishments.

Liability of Physicians and Surgeons.—Since a few gentlemen, for self-preservation, have decided not to engage in certain kinds of professional services, without a written agreement to protect them against prosecutions for mal-practice, the doctrine has been proclaimed that they cannot legally fortify themselves in this manner. They are not only obliged, it is said, to practise, if called upon, but must stand the racket of a law-suit into the bargain, if a patient wants to raise a sum of money. One of the Massachusetts newspapers assumes that medical men are like common carriers, and can be compelled to act at the bidding of the public. The reasoning is in this wise. When they put out a sign, it is to be presumed they consider themselves competent to prescribe, and perform operations ; and the community, believing such to be the fact, feels a degree of security, in cases of emergency. But if they call upon them, and physicians and surgeons refuse to act, or they act unskilfully, the party employing them has a right to demand damages at a tribunal of justice. Either way, the lawyers pretend that they have us at their mercy. On the other hand, no surgeon or physician, having a particle of self-respect or independence of character, would put himself knowingly at the mercy of an unprincipled knave, whose pleasure would be to ruin him if money could be obtained thereby. If, in these cases of alleged mal-practice, it could be proved, and that beyond question, that a patient died who might have been saved by his physician, but who wilfully and criminally refused to exert himself to do so, then an action might be sustained. Such supposable circumstances, however, are not likely to occur, for who, as a witness, would dare say, absolutely and without qualification, that death might have been prevented ?

Dr. Hamilton's Address.—As usual, in the Buffalo Medical College the graduates are publicly addressed. Dr. Hamilton, the present season, discharged that duty most acceptably. He is a terse writer, original, and always to the point. The young gentlemen cannot readily forget his advice ; neither can they pursue a course more advantageous for themselves and society, than the one pointed out by their distinguished friend and instructer. We are fully expecting that Dr. Hamilton will gratify the medical public with an original work on surgery, for which he is admirably qualified.

Medical Miscellany.—Dr. S. B. Hunt is to be associated hereafter with Dr. Austin Flint in the editorial management of the Buffalo Medical Journal. Dr. Hunt has been a contributor to that Journal, and has shown himself possessed of good literary and scientific attainments.—A splendid accession to the ranks of the spiritual rappers has been made in London, by the professed belief of a great Dr. Somebody whose name is not recollected.—Dr. Darling, known extensively in New England as a popular lecturer on anatomy and physiology, was lecturing in England a while since, on *biology.*—What has become of the hundreds of itinerant professors of animal magnetism, with which the country was flooded a year since ?—Yellow fever is exceedingly prevalent at Kingston, in the Island of Jamaica.—Dr. Charles A. Davis, of Lowell, Mass, has received the appointment of surgeon of the U. S. Marine Hospital, at Chelsea.—A ship carpenter lately bled to death at East Boston. A man also died from the extreme loss of blood in consequence of the extraction of a tooth.—Dr. Alexander Mayer, of Paris, announces a great discovery—heating boilers, cooking, &c., by means of friction, instead of fuel.—Dr. Peasley's case of shoulder-joint operation is to be had in a pamphlet.

To Correspondents —Papers by Dr. Colby, of Stanstead, Canada, Dr. Jones, of Boston, Dr. Moseley, of Philadelphia, and " A Southerner," have been received.

Married,—Dr. John A. Stevens, of Ogdensburgh, N. Y., to Miss F. E. Tower.

Died,—In New York, by suicide, Dr. A. H. Post, a dentist from Connecticut.

Deaths in Boston for the week ending Saturday noon, July 16th, 58. Males, 34—females, 24. Inflammation of the bowels, 2—disease of the bowels, 2—congestion of the brain, 2—consumption, 8—convulsions, 4—cholera infantum, 1—cholera morbus, 1—cancer, 1—dysentery, 1—diarrhœa, 1—dropsy, 1—dropsy in the head, 2—infantile diseases, 8—puerperal, 1—erysipelas, 1—fever, 1—typhus fever, 2—hooping cough, 1—homicide, 1—intemperance, 2—disease of the liver, 1—marasmus, 5—measles, 2—old age, 2—scrofula, 1—suicide, 1—teething, 2—unknown, 1.
Under 5 years, 33—between 5 and 20 years, 2—between 20 and 40 years, 13—between 40 and 60 years, 6—over 60 years, 4. Born in the United States, 42—Ireland, 16.

Rhode Island Medical Society.—The *forty-second* annual meeting was held in Providence, June 29, 1853. Drs. Channing, Adams, Hayden and Homans, of Boston, were present as guests of the Society.

The annual discourse was read by Dr. Ely, of Providence, on the subject of *Fatty Degeneration.* It was listened to with interest, and a copy was requested for publication.

The Trustees of the Fiske Fund announced that no prizes had been awarded for dissertations the past year.

Several honorary members were elected, among whom were D. Humphreys Storer, M.D., and Henry J. Bigelow, M.D., of Boston.

The officers elected for the ensuing year are :—

President—Joseph Mauran, M.D., of Providence.

1st Vice President—Sylvanus Clapp, M.D., of Pawtucket.

2d Vice President—Ariel Ballou, M.D., of Woonsocket.

Recording Secretary—Edwin M. Snow, M.D., of Providence.

Corresponding Secretary—J. W. C. Ely, M.D., of   "

Treasurer—George P. Baker, M.D., of   "

Censors.—S. A. Arnold, M.D., Providence; T. C. Dunn, M.D., Newport; J. J. Smith, M.D., Chepachet; Otis Bullock, M.D., Warren; E. Fowler, M.D., Woonsocket; H. Cleveland, M.D., Pawtucket; J. H. Eldridge, M.D., East Greenwich; R. Brownell, M.D., Providence.

The occasion passed off very pleasantly, though no special business of public interest was transacted.

Parasites in the Profession— Queries.—MR. EDITOR,—In the number of your Journal for June 29th, are a singular series of resolutions, passed by the Bristol District Medical Society. One is at a loss to know *whom,* or *what* class of men, they are so much annoyed with. They say, "It is doing injustice to censure Thomsonians, homœopathists, empirical oculists, &c., while the parent society *retains,* in full and honorable communion, a class of Jesuitical deceivers, in comparison with whom, all other empirics and mountebanks are entitled to the most profound respect." In their preamble, they call them (supposed to be the same class), "insidious parasites," &c. From the manner in which Thomsonians, homœopathists, &c., are named, we should infer that *none of these* belong to this anomalous class which cause so much vexation to the members of the Bristol District. If they are none of these, who are they? What kind of "*parasites*" do they mean? Have they any newly-discovered ones, which are *anonymous?* Can they not give them some *name* that they may be known by?   INQUIRER.

Essex North District Medical Society.— To the Editor, &c.,—At a meeting of the Essex North District Medical Society, held in Bradford, July 7, 1853, the following *resolution* was passed *unanimously,* and it was voted that a copy be sent to your Journal for publication.

M. ROOT, *Sec'ry E. N. D. Med. Soc.*

Byfield, July 13, 1853.

Resolved, That all pretensions to homœopathy, hydropathy, or other exclusive systems of medical practice, when held up in advertisements or otherwise, as means of obtaining business, in preference to other members of the medical profession, are quackish ;—and are sufficient cause, when proved, for exclusion or expulsion from this Society.

THE

BOSTON MEDICAL AND SURGICAL JOURNAL.

Vol. XLVIII.   WEDNESDAY, JULY 27, 1853.   No. 26.

VERATRUM VIRIDE IN FEVERS.

To the Editor of the Boston Medical and Surgical Journal.

Sir,—I have lately seen the attention of physicians called to the anti-febrile power of the American hellebore. I used it thirty years ago, not only in typhus fever, but in acute rheumatism. My experience of its effects in fever was not favorable to its use. I used the saturated tinct. of the root, as prepared by Dr. Norwood. The tinct. alone was used, and also combined with laudanum when I wished to obviate its cathartic effects, and reduce very much the frequency of the pulse. In all cases of typhus fever, in which I used it, or saw it used, the convalescence was very slow. In acute rheumatism, when given in repeated doses to produce the full effect of vomiting, the cure was perfect, but the death-like effect on the patient was always very alarming to himself as well as his friends; and in future attacks I could never prevail on those who had used it, to submit to its effects again. I was uniformly told that they would rather die than take it. It evidently caused a fatal result in one case of rheumatism, in a scrofulous habit, but otherwise a healthy man. He had been treated, by his attending physician, by bleeding, calomel and cathartics. After this he was put under the full effect of veratrum so as to operate as an emetic. At the time he took it, the glutæi and the muscles about the small of the back were much swollen. The prostrating effects of the hellebore were so great that the swollen part became dark during the time of collapse, and never recovered, but terminated in gangrene. It was in this condition that I first saw him. Since that time I have never given the hellebore in acute rheumatism, but have substituted colchicum.

A lover of whiskey clandestinely took a dram of what he supposed bitters, but which proved to be a tincture of hellebore prepared as a wash for a horse, the effects of which were nearly fatal. Dr. F. W. Adams, now of Montpelier, Vt., first introduced the tincture of hellebore in febrile diseases into practice in this place, about the year 1819. Its effects in fever, rheumatism and croup formed the subject of his inaugural dissertation in 1822. It so happened that a child, to whom it was administered by his direction, died with croup at the very time of writing his thesis. Whether Dr. A. continues to use the hellebore in fevers, I can-

26

not say, but I am aware that he had a more favorable opinion of its effects than I had. In order to produce its full effect in acute rheumatism, I think I gave about thirty drops of the saturated tincture, and repeated once in six hours till vomiting was induced. I never knew it effect a cure in acute rheumatism, unless it was given so as to produce its full effects. Since I abandoned the use of hellebore I have given colchicum in tincture or powder, and repeated every four or six hours till it caused vomiting and catharsis. One course will sometimes answer, but it is often necessary to go through a second.

Notwithstanding Dr. Norwood's experience, I certainly could not recommend it as a safe emetic. As Dr. Adams has had more experience in its use than any other man, I presume, by an application to him, any physician would be able to get the results of his experience. I think he has still a favorable opinion of its effects, but I am sure that he does not consider it specific in fever, as there were several deaths from typhus under his practice after he left this place for Boston.

Stanstead, Canada, July 8, 1853.   M. F. COLBY, M.D.

MR. EDITOR,—Having perused the above remarks by Dr. Colby, on the use of the hellebore, I can confirm them so far as they relate to the effects of this medicine in fevers. I studied medicine with Dr. F. W. Adams, and used the hellebore in fevers and other inflammatory complaints at the commencement of my practice ; but finding recovery very slow, and the patients often very much prostrated after its use, I entirely abandoned it in typhus fever. I recollect seeing Dr. C. administer it thirty years ago in a case of acute rheumatism. I, however, differ from him in regard to its effects in that disease, believing it not necessary to give it to the extent of producing emesis, as I have successfully treated acute rheumatism by giving it in doses short of producing its prostrating effects. I administered it successfully under Dr. Adams's direction in one case of croup ; in others, afterwards, it failed. I am now on a visit at the north ; as I reside in Georgia, I may have an opportunity to witness its effects there, of which I will keep you informed.

Very truly yours,   DANIEL DUSTAN.
Stanstead, Can., July 12, 1853.

===

OPERATIONS FOR THE RADICAL CURE OF INGUINAL HERNIA.

To the Editor of the Boston Medical and Surgical Journal.

SIR,—In a communication, published a few weeks since in the Journal, upon medical testimony, allusion was made to an untried operation by which I supposed a radical cure might be effected in cases of inguinal hernia—and which probably might be identical or similar to that practised with success by Dr. Heaton.

I have been asked by physicians if I suppose that I have discovered a new principle of cure ; or, if it is proposed to do a new operation merely, to close the abnormal abdominal aperture, upon principles taught, understood and believed to be correct by surgeons and physicians generally.

I will answer them, and invite instruction by stating my views upon the subject of hernia briefly, so far as may be necessary in consideration of the operations proposed for the radical cure—referring to the structures concerned, as if the general descriptions by the best authors were embodied in or attached to this article in some form ; or supposing each reader to be familiar with the subject, and not desiring a frequent repetition of technical terms, which, according to a distinguished modern surgeon's observation, " are too often applied to parts of the same tissue in such a way as to create confusion, and render these structures, and the changes produced upon them, exceedingly complicated ; while, in reality, they are extremely simple, and easy to be understood." A slight restrospective glance may be pleasant and profitable before examining the modern inventions for radical cure of hernia.

Monsieur Dionis says in his lectures and demonstrations of chirurgical operations in the royal garden at Paris—

" 'Tis a mistake to believe that hernias or descents are modern distempers ; for although we are told that they were not formerly known, and that it is but within the compass of a few past years that we have seen so many persons afflicted with them, 'tis not only because they were little known to the vulgar, but because the ancients took care to hide them—most of those who had them not daring to disclose them to any person. But after the invention of very commodious bandages to repulse the parts to their natural place, and several medicaments to restrain and fortify the relaxed fibres, those who before that time concealed these infirmities, no longer made a scruple of discovering them in hopes of a cure by it."

There were " operations," too, in those days, which Dionis condemns, saying to his pupils, as he was about to describe them, that " he was certain they would condemn them, too," but gave as a reason for his showing the manner of their performance, that " a good chirurgeon should be acquainted with the good and ill of his profession, in order to follow the first and avoid the last."

It is not necessary to describe either the bandages of the hernia doctors, the remedy of the Prior of Cabrieres, or any of the famous plasters, used and " published by the king's goodness ;" or those other kinds, the formulæ of which are kept secret by their inventors; according to Dionis, " they were no more effectual than the others."

Modern surgeons have also discovered, that " hernia is a more frequent disease than has been heretofore supposed " ; and urge as a cause that in " some families it is an hereditary disease."

All that relates to the retention of the bowel by artificial support, and to the operation for the relief of strangulation, is at this day so well taught by books and professors, that pupils do not require an extraordinary exercise of the perceptive faculties to at least understand the principles upon which the modern practice rests, even if their judgment and skill are not quite equal in every emergency to decide upon the necessity of, or to perform the required manipulations. But in the approaches to the radical cure of hernia by operation, it is not certain that modern surgeons are much in advance of Monsieur Dionis, his predecessors and contemporaries.

The cause of hernia, according to Dionis, is a rupture of the peritoneum; " and to cure these sorts of ruptures," he says, " we must endeavor to close the lips of this wound in the peritoneum and to keep them in a posture that they may unite and grow together." He disapproves of the operation of Celsus, and does not advise his pupils to practise it.

With all the light anatomy has thrown upon the structures or tissues concerned in hernia; with all the assistance physiological inquiry has given as to the functions of these tissues, their modes of formation, as primitive developments or as reparatory processes; with all the crusades against the abdominal canal and rings by progressive heroic surgery, no fixed principle has been deduced, either from hypothesis or experiment, by which the abdominal openings referred to may be permanently closed against the descent of a hernial sac and its contents, which has been replaced with or without strangulation.

The names of the inventors of some of the modern operations for radical cures will be omitted; the manifest absurdities of some plans, the complete failure of others, and the hazard of the experiment, condemn them, and are safeguards against frequent repetitions. And if it be admitted that cures are recorded after some operations, and perhaps as a consequence of them, we have no proof that the operators had discovered the principle involved, as future efforts on the same plan overthrew the monuments of success the previous accidental cures had erected.

Modern surgeons seem to agree that the " pins of Bonnet," the " scarifications of Velpeau," the " sutures of Belmas," and the injections of Pancoast and others, are all intended to " *obtain a cure by causing an adhesive inflammation of the walls of the sac* " in cases of hernia.

This declaration as to the walls of the sac, is not sufficiently clear, perhaps—if we suppose that adhesion of the internal surface of the sac is expected to be produced by peritoneal action. Radical cure in all cases, would not follow, if the adhesive action was accomplished with or without inflammation, irrespective of the form of operation.

I do not know what is the understood theory of cure by the application of trusses, which compares favorably with other plans promulgated, as regards results.

There are surgeons who favor the doctrine that inflammation is not necessary to the cure of hernia, or any other disease, nor to repair the injuries inflicted by wounds whether by accident or from operation. These surgeons would consider a proposition, to cause adhesion in the walls of a hernial sac by inflammation, with the intention to prevent thereby the re-appearance of the hernia, as impracticable and unsound. To discuss the question, opens the entire theory of tissue formation and all the doctrines of inflammation received at the present day. It will be passed at this time, to be considered briefly hereafter.

Upon the inflammation theory is based the modern operations for radical cure of hernia. They succeed, and they fail—although inflammation is present, and sometimes, as is stated by the operators, in excess.

Inflammation is present in operations for strangulated hernia occasionally. How often are radical cures recorded after the wounds of the operation are healed. Now suppose adhesion to be formed between the internal surfaces of a hernial sac, with or without inflammation; or suppose lymph to be deposited between the pillars of the ring, with no specific organization or characteristics of a normal structure—are such deposits to be relied on to prevent hernial descents? Adventitious deposits are liable to absorption—and the attendant growths of what is termed acute inflammation usually are absorbed as the process of discussion goes on. Notwithstanding these failures, surgeons rely upon inflammation to produce radical cure of hernia.

It is asked—is there any operation that can be relied on for a cure? In the nature of things, is it possible or not? Do the reparatory principles active in the human organization forbid the attempt? If so, inquiry and experiment in this direction are useless. If success is among the probabilities, let inquiry and experiment go on.

The possibility cannot be disputed, for cures occur under various modes of treatment. The probability is strong, not taking into the account actual cases, and the assertions of the operators and the cured, for physiology favors the theory of reparation, and skilful surgery may direct the action. In addition, we have the statements of a practical surgeon that a cure by operation is a fixed fact, which he does, and will continue to demonstrate, and that at a proper time he will explain the principle of the cure and the mode of operation by which the action is induced.

[To be continued.]

LECTURES OF M. VALLEIX ON DISPLACEMENTS OF THE UTERUS.

TRANSLATED FROM THE FRENCH BY L. PARKS, JR., M.D.

NUMBER VIII.

SYMPTOMS.—It is very important to investigate the symptoms which show themselves before the commencement of treatment, since these strictly appertain to the disease. We proceed, consequently, to examine them with the greatest attention, intending to give, at a future time, a description of the modifications they undergo in consequence of treatment.

Mode of commencement of the Symptoms.—The first appearance of the symptoms was, in one case only, sudden—instantaneous; in another, it was rapid. And it is worthy of remark that, in these two cases, the disease set in as a sequence to violent shocks, efforts or falls. In all the other cases, it was difficult, and, in one patient (Case I.), it was entirely impossible to fix the epoch of the commencement. The symptoms were, in all these cases, produced slowly—gradually. There was, at first, pain in the groins or in the thighs—then, walking became difficult and painful.   Subsequently, there set in leucorrhœa—frequent desire of micturition—various troubles in the digestive organs, inducing loss of strength and emaciation.   From this time, the disease was fully confirmed.

Symptoms of the Disease when confirmed.—If, now, we examine the different symptoms, separately, in order to be able to appreciate their relative degree of importance, we find them in conformity with the following description, viz.:

Pain.—*Spontaneous pain* existed in 19 out of the 20 cases, in which its existence was investigated.   There occurred, however, in the patient, whose case makes the exception (Case I.), that peculiar sensation during micturition of which I have spoken to you.   This pain was situated 17 times in both groins, once in one groin, and once in the hypogastrium.   In this last case there were symptoms of metritis.   This pain was not always of equal intensity on the two sides, a circumstance to be explained, in general, by a lateral inclination of the uterus complicating the anteversion. Ordinarily, the pain was more marked on the side towards which the uterus was inclined, though sometimes the reverse was the case.   The same may be said of the pains in the thighs, which were found in the 19 cases.   We found pains in places at a distance from the uterus, as follows, viz., five times occupying the walls of the chest, it was owing once to muscular rheumatism, and four times to an intercostal neuralgia, corresponding once only with the lateral inclination of the uterus, which was a complication of the anteversion.   Four times there was pain, more or less obstinate, in the loins, there being in my notes no further details on this head, either because the patient could not indicate the precise seat of the pain, or because the point was not noted.   In two cases only, in one of which hæmorrhoids were also present, there was pain in the region of the sacrum.   Once, finally, the pain was intense in the perinæum, while, at the same time, there was difficulty in defecation.

In three cases, where there was *pain arising from some extraneous cause* (douleur provoquée), there was in one, metritis; in the second, muscular rheumatism; in the third, intercostal neuralgia—the painful spots which characterize this last malady not presenting themselves on the walls of the abdomen.

Feeling of Weight in the Pelvis.—There was, five times, a sensation of weight in the region of the perinæum.   In these cases the cervix was very bulky.   Could this sensation of weight be owing to engorgement of the cervix ?   I do not venture to reply in the affirmative, for, while it is true that I have never met with this symptom, when there was no engorgement; on the other hand, I have often seen the cervix engorged without its existence.

Micturition.—In 15 cases out of the 19, in which I was able to obtain an exact account of the symptoms, *micturition was frequent,* and sometimes painful.   In the four other cases the uterus was possessed of great mobility.   It is possible that being in these cases less bulky and less heavy than in the others, it was more easily raised by the bladder, and thus permitted to the latter more distension.   This, however, is but a theoretical explanation, and the fact was not strictly demonstrated, although thus much has been fully established, that it is the pressure of the body of the uterus upon the bladder which produces the frequent desire of passing the urine, as I was able to satisfy myself, in a case where, having introduced the sound for the purpose of reducing a simple retroflexion, I exaggerated the movement, and carried the body of the uterus forward, at the same time that I pushed the cervix backward with the finger in such a manner as to simulate an anteversion. The womb maintained itself in this position for some hours, during which micturition was much more frequent than usual.

Defecation.—Eleven times the bowels were confined, and their evacuation difficult. I have not found that there existed any evident relation between the feeling of weight at the perinæum and this constipation, which seemed to me rather to coincide with the augmentation in the bulk of the cervix and the pains at the top of the sacrum.

All these symptoms are, as is manifest, quite easily explained by the vicious position of the uterus, and by the uterine engorgement. We proceed, now, to the examination of those of another order, which, without being as peculiarly characteristic of the disease, nevertheless have their importance.

Menstruation.—The menses, diminished once, were in two cases more abundant than before the disease. Further, in one of these two last cases, they took place at diminished intervals, and in the other there set in veritable attacks of *hæmorrhage*. This case is sufficiently interesting to be reported with a few details.

CASE IV.—Marie S., æt. 28 years—seamstress—of a bilious and sanguine temperament—of a constitution originally quite strong—menstruated regularly from her 16th year. Her health was always perfect till she reached the age of 17. Her first pregnancy then occurred, which was very painful, and terminated in abortion, at the third month. The abortion, the cause of which escapes us, was followed by griping sensations, and by severe pains in the loins and groins, attended with fever and delirium. At the end of eight days, she was transported to " l'Hôtel Dieu," where the physician, she says, introduced his entire hand into the vagina, after which the pains ceased, the hæmorrhage alone persisting. The patient remained three weeks at the Hospital.

Afterwards she had four new pregnancies, which were carried to the full term, her last confinement having taken place in 1849. Each labor, though not severe, was followed by grave symptoms—by inflammation, which it was necessary to combat with applications of leeches, and which required a course of treatment of from fifteen to eighteen days' duration. In the intervals there was leucorrhœa, and the menses were irregular, painful and often profuse.

Six months before we saw her the metrorrhagia became more frequent and more profuse. At the same time the patient experienced a pain in the right iliac fossa, which extended itself the following month to the hypogastrium. Then followed frequent desire of micturition—obstinate constipation—severe pains during walking, which was very difficult and very painful—inappetency—epigastric pains after eating. The patient lost flesh and strength, and could not stand erect, bending over exceedingly in walking. Twice she was obliged to enter " l'Hotel Dieu ;"

the first time in the department of M. Horteloup, which she left at the end of fifteen days, having been somewhat relieved by cupping ; the second time, in the wards of M. Louis, who recognized the disease, and sent the patient to me without having commenced treatment.

I received her at the " Hôpital-Beaujon," the 16th of October, 1851, and ascertained the existence of an anteversion with slight displacement to the left side. The anterior surface of the body was not extended horizontally, but described a slight curve, with its concavity in front, as if there was a commencing anteflexion. The cervix, which was bulky, presented some granulations. The sound penetrated to the distance of $7\frac{1}{2}$ centimetres. After two applications of the sound, of which one was fatiguing and painful for her (for on that occasion the examination was prolonged for nearly twenty minutes, being made by M. Dubois, Mme. Charrier and other persons, successively, who confirmed my diagnosis), the patient experienced extreme lassitude, and slight chills, the menses appearing three days before their time. The flow was profuse, and continued till the 23d, accompanied by pains in the loins and at the hypogastrium.

The sound, introduced the 24th and 25th, gives rise to an inconsiderable flow of blood. Nevertheless, the stem-pessary is applied the 25th, and after remaining seven days, is removed because quite a profuse hæmorrhage set in. It is re-applied four other times, being left on the second occasion (the 22d of the month) for three days only, in consequence of a new hæmorrhage appearing. On the third application, which is made the 28th, it remains four days, and this time is taken away on account of the appearance of the menses, at their habitual epoch. The flow lasted four days, unattended with pain, and at its cessation leaves the uterus less heavy, but with no change as to its displacement. On being applied, for the fourth time, the stem-pessary remains thirteen days, being withdrawn on the appearance of a little blood, which turns out, this time also, to be the menstrual flow, from five to six days in advance of its time. The uterus slants a little forward, but no longer lies transversely.

The 7th of January the stem-pessary is applied for the fifth time, remaining fifteen days without causing unfavorable symptoms. The patient goes, comes, feels better, recovers her *embonpoint*, and when the apparatus is removed, the uterus is found in its normal direction. I saw the patient again the 29th of March and the 2d of May. The general health was perfect, and the anteversion had not returned.

In this case, upon the diagnosis of which no doubt can be entertained, there was, besides the anteversion, a certain degree of metritis with tendency to hæmorrhage. In this metrorrhagia there is nothing which should astonish you, as certain interesting researches made by Dr. Hérard, upon this subject, show hæmorrhage from the womb to be one of the most constant symptoms of metritis.

As to the anteversion itself, it is very difficult to fix the epoch of its commencement, for though the patient assigns it to a date, six months previously to coming under my care—the time when she began to experience pain—we see, on the other hand, that for a very long time, her menstruation was irregular, painful and harassing, and that the patient was far from enjoying good health.

The readiness with which this hæmorrhage returned, after each introduction of the sound, shows us plainly that the tissue itself of the uterus was not, at the time, in the normal state. This accounts to us for
the manifestation of the febrile symptoms, with sensibility of the uterus,
which was heavier and more bulky after the first application of the
stem-pessary. But, all these symptoms, which were increased by the
pressure of the instrument, were without gravity, and promptly disappeared after it was removed, and a few leeches had been applied to
the hypogastrium.

A circumstance quite worthy of remark, and which assuredly has not
escaped you, is that the further we advanced in the treatment, the better
the stem-pessary was borne, so that, finally, it remained thirteen, and
then fifteen days, without occasioning hæmorrhage. This point is important to notice, because if it had not been understood, either the patient might not have been watched with sufficient attention, after the
early application of the instrument, and the latter have been left in
the uterus long enough to cause serious symptoms ; or else, we might
have allowed ourselves to be too easily discouraged by the re-appearance,
after each application, of symptoms which required its removal, and
might have abandoned the treatment, as liable to danger. If this had
been done, we should not have obtained a cure—now a confirmed one
—of a very grave affection, and one capable by means of the attacks
of hæmorrhage which were the consequence of it, to place the life of
the patient in danger. There was, after the discontinuance of the
treatment, a short period of congestion of the uterus, and a slight tendency to the re-production of the anteversion. But very simple means
were sufficient to dispel the congestion, and maintain the organ in its
normal position, by rendering it lighter. Now, in proportion as the
engorgement shall diminish, as it will, in consequence merely of
the re-placement of the organ, the cure will become more and more
solid.

One remark only, I offer upon this case— that the modes of treatment
previously employed had been of no avail. Cupping alone had been
of some relief, but only by diminishing the phlogosis, since it had no distinct action on the displacement.

DR. NUTTING ON THE PHILOSOPHY OF MEDICAL DELUSIONS.

[Continued from p. 494.]

ANOTHER source of delusion is found in the *Impossibility of determining
accurately on the Results of Treatment.*

We have thus, in addition to the difficulties in the way of correct
medical reasoning, no means by which we can arrive at certain conclusions as to the treatment founded upon it. Nor have we any means of comparing the results of quack treatment, with that of the scientific physician, so that the mass can see the difference. In law, if a pettifogger
venture into court, no sooner does he commence his plea, than the bar
and bench perceive his ignorance. But in medicine, no pleas are made.

There is no public exhibition of talents or learning.   Nor are there any statistics showing the relative mortality under the different treatment, or the relative number of cures : and by these I mean, not *escapes*, nor simple recoveries, for the latter will take place in a majority of all cases of disease if not interfered with ; but cases in which the power of the disease has been broken, and convalescence hastened by the treatment.   Could such statistics be secured, they would place the different systems on their true merits.   But this is impossible in the present state of things.

Not only have we no means of bringing quackery to this test, but, as Dr. Rush has remarked, " there are no greater liars in the world than quacks, except their patients."   They will misrepresent, either from ignorance or on purpose, both the nature and treatment of their cases.   No dependence can be placed on their reports, as every physician can testify. Every tumor or sore is a cancer.   The last and favorable stage of lung fever is consumption, because the patients cough and raise.   If they can fix on no other disease, the *liver* is full of ulcers, or more than half wasted away.*   If in any of these cases, the patient recovers, as often they cannot well help doing, then they have cured these several diseases, and the report of it is trumpeted abroad by the patient and his friends ; for every patient wishes it understood that he was the sickest person that ever survived.

A fourth source of medical delusions is found in the *Influence of the Imagination.*

The power of this faculty over certain persons is well known.   Its perverted influence in highly nervous persons, is especially evident in respect to disease and its treatment.   Reason, judgment, and the will even, are often completely under its control.   The power of motion is lost, the voice gone, the whole system prostrated, and the mind apparently ruined.   The loss of muscular power depends partly on an inability to will, and partly on actual debility induced by the perverted influence of the imagination.   The former of these has, however, the greater power, since if the exercise of the will can be secured, the muscular power is usually instantly regained.   It is in cases of this kind that quacks accomplish their wonderful cures, by which the lame leap and walk, and those who have not spoken aloud for weeks, regain all at once the full power of their voices.   Examples of this kind are, unfortunately, too numerous to need reciting.

Another example of the power of this faculty, is found in the production of various sensations of pain, which are readily dissipated by

---

* The author was called, last year, to see a hypochondriacal woman, affected with prolapsus uteri, and chronic irritation of the liver. She had been attended by two Thomsonians. The following conversation ensued between us at one visit :—" Doctor, don't you think my liver is terribly affected ?" " No, indeed, why do you ask that ?" " Why Dr. P. told me he thought it was more than half wasted away. and Dr. C. said it was full of ulcers the year before." " Humph !" " Could I live if it was rotted away so ?" " Could you live, if your head were half rotted off ?" " Why no, but he said it was a common thing for the liver to rot away, and that if there was a piece left as large as a hen's egg, it would grow again. He said he had as lief his liver would rot away so, as not." " So had I, that *his* would." The woman finally got as well as the hypochondria would let her. The same " Dr. P." used to give cod liver oil in the last stage of lung fever, because, he said, they had the consumption.

affecting the imagination. To the patient, these pains are for the time real, but the manner in which they are dissipated shows they could not depend on any physical lesion. It is in cases of this kind, that the bread-pill treatment becomes effectual; and if I mistake not, its aristocratic offspring, Homœopathy, reaps its fairest laurels among the same.

Again, the imagination, aided by a soothing effect on the nervous system, has the power of removing some real pain. These pains, which are termed *nervous*, are the ones most easily affected, and perhaps the only ones which can be removed by this means. The influence of simply soothing movements upon the head, in case of nervous headache, is well known. The effect is often heightened, if the imagination be affected at the same time. Thus Perkins persuaded his patients that they were cured by electric currents excited by the brass and steel rods with which his manipulations were performed. It was at length discovered, that pine rods could be substituted with equal effect, if the patient did not know it. So popular did this delusion become, that in this State, clergymen, including Pres. Dwight; lawyers, and judges, certified in the most confident manner to its efficacy. In England it was still more popular. The nobility embraced it, an infirmary was established in which it alone was used, and more than five thousand cures were reported within a short time after it was opened. And among these, were the whole list of acute diseases. Its advocates predicted, in the most confident manner, that within twenty years the old drugging and bleeding system of practice would be entirely abandoned. But a fifth of that period had hardly elapsed, before the delusion was exposed, and Perkins, with his tractors and infirmary, ceased to be spoken of but with contempt. Does not the early history of this tractor treatment bear some resemblance to that of the favorite *pathies* of the present day? Nor do I doubt that the latter part of its history will have a still closer resemblance to the latter part of theirs.

Another source of delusion is found in the *Ignorance of the mass as to the proper Power of Medicine and Physicians.*

In the administration of medicine, the object is to assist nature to throw off disease. Nor can it be otherwise than pernicious, when given for any other purpose. A man's recovery, therefore, is not rendered certain in proportion to the amount of drugs taken. Yet this is the sentiment of many; and the physician is often obliged to give something, when he knows nothing is needed, in order to satisfy the patient's wish to take. Well is it for the patient if he gives only the homœopathic globule, or its equivalent, the bread pill. A man gets up in the morning, and feels languid and dull. He may have been living in constant violation of the laws of health, and begins to feel the effects of it. His first question is, what shall I take? not, as it should be, what change in my habits of life will remove the evil? It is TAKE, TAKE. As repentance is most irksome to the moral transgressor; so is physical reformation to him who breaks the laws of health: and as the one would give " the fruit of his loins for the sin of his soul;" so to the other no drug is too nauseous, no application too painful, if by their use he can avoid the necessity of reforming his habits. But as in the former case, all these devices for the redemption of the soul, but add to its guilt, and sink it deeper in perdition ; so this dosing with drugs, but adds to the physical derangement, and sinks the man deeper in physical perdition. And as it matters not with the moral transgressor, that the experience of thousands has proved the utter futility of such devices; so with the physical transgressor, it matters not that thousands have been filled to sur- feiting with nauseous drugs, and without relief. Such is the utter folly of both, that they pursue the same beaten track, rather than reform —closing their eyes and ears to all the evidence against them from with- out—nay, smothering the voice of reason and conscience within.

Their error consists in ascribing to drugs a power they do not possess. They take it for granted that they have not only the power to renovate the system, but to counteract the influence of their pernicious habits. Yet any one may see that nature is fully as much assisted in following the hints she gives, in a change of habits, as by filling the system with drugs,·which at best are but a necessary evil. I say an evil, for all drugs, except iron and a few others, which constitute important parts of the system, must act as poisons, if they act at all. Emetics, whether ipe- cac. or lobelia, act simply from their poisonous qualities. The same is true of the whole list of medicines. But as, in the moral world, one evil is made to counteract the effects of another ; so in medicine, the effects of a poison are made to counteract the effects of a disease. But whether any article is a poison, depends wholly on the relation which it bears to the system. Thus any drug, which in a healthy state disturbs, in any degree, the healthy performance of any function, is so far a poison. But in an altered state of the system, these very substances may contri- bute to the restoration of a healthy action, and thus lose their poisonous qualities. On the other hand, beef-steak, by no means a poison in a healthy state, becomes, in a diseased state, a poison of great power.

In an acute disease, a prompt medical interference may be demanded. But in a majority of cases, more dependence is to be placed on the re- cuperative powers of nature, than on the direct influence of drugs. In such cases, if nature be not too much encumbered by wrong habits, she will in time effect a cure. Nor will drugs alone suffice to accomplish it. A general derangement of the system has taken place, and conside- rable time must elapse before it can become regulated. And we may here see how quackery gains applause in these cases. During the first part of the time, a regular physician is usually employed. He may assist nature, but fails of a cure, as the time for that has not yet arrived. He is therefore dismissed, and some of the irregular practitioners are employed—perhaps several of them, before the cure is complete. The patient gets a full supply of pills, syrups, bitters, and *promises* in abun- dance. The latter establish the superiority of these over the regular physician, for *he* never promised.. Faith is strong, and they wait pa- tiently a great while, and at length are well. It is " *post hoc,*" but · they and their doctor reckon it " *propter hoc* " ; and the superiority of the quack, or quack medicine they took *last,* is fully established.

It is this idea which has emptied box after box of Brandreth's, and Moffat's, and Morrison's, and a thousand others' pills, down the gaping throats of real or imaginary patients. The cases in which the promised cures failed, are never inquired for; but the single cases of recovery after taking these, like the prizes in a lottery, fill every eye.

I have dwelt thus fully on this source of delusion, because it seems an important one. And there is another which gives rise to much delusion in connection with this; and that is, *The Inordinate Desire of Life.*

" Ere hope, sensation fails."

Men dread the passage to another world, and shrink from it with alarm. Nor are they ever ready for it. Hence, if attacked with fatal disease, they snatch at straws. In their extremity they cherish the hope that a medicine may be found, which shall disarm the king of terrors, and give them back to life. It matters not that science knows no such drug; nor that thousands, like themselves, have searched with anxious eye through the whole list, and died without it. Such a drug they know must exist, and they pursue it with the utmost pertinacity, taking box after box, and bottle after bottle, of all the thousands of nostrums which the ingenuity and cupidity of crafty men can invent. This *may* cure, and that *may* cure, and they try all. So, too, doctor after doctor is called, each time taking one more ignorant than the one before. The regular physician, finding no room for hope, gives no promise of recovery, and is discarded for one who will. He, failing to cure, is dismissed for one more ignorant still; for each promises more confidently, in proportion to his ignorance, and they feed delusive hope on these promises, although they know them to be " empty as the wind." At length, having tried the whole round of ignorance, death lays them in their resting place. They have expended their means for that which could do them no good, and have helped feed the whole army of rapacious quacks, ever ready to feed on the extremities of such as these.

Another source of medical delusion is found in the *Utter Ignorance of even educated men, of the Nature and Extent of Medical Knowledge.*

It seems taken for granted, that there are no fixed principles in medicine; that disease, and the action of remedies, are all hap-hazard—the one coming when it may chance to, or, when God, by a miraculous intervention, sends it; and that the action of remedies is equally without law. On such notions as these, they found their idea of medical science. This, also, they consider as a mixture of luck and chance, having in it no fixed principles, and being what one may acquire in a month, as well as in a life time. If you are successful in practice, they will say that you are *lucky* or *fortunate* in not losing your patients. But there is no *luck* nor *fortune* about it. You do not go to your patients and pour down their throats whatever you may happen to, and trust fortune for the result. Having made yourself master of what knowledge is to be attained, you investigate your case, till you find the exact nature of the disease, and then you select that remedial agent which your own observation, or that of others, has shown best adapted to remove the disease. If you are successful, it is because you have done this. But here is no *luck.* The whole matter is as much the result of fixed laws, as any other result of a physical cause. The all-wise

Governor of the Universe has not left disease out from his general plan. Certain causes, acting upon the human system under certain circumstances, will invariably produce disease. Certain remedies, under certain conditions, will invariably assist nature to throw off disease. There is no luck in this. The truly successful physician is he who ascertains these laws, and acts in accordance with them. The really *un*successful physician is he, who proceeds in ignorance, or in disregard of these laws. A truly successful physician is no more lucky than a successful machinist. Nor is an unsuccessful one any more *unlucky*. And by success, I mean not the acquisition of noisy applause, or sudden wealth. These follow the ignorant and knavish quack, more readily than the scientific and honest physician. The physician's knowledge does not consist in knowing that this drug is good for this symptom or disease, and that for that. He has rules for his art, but principles for his science ; and without a fair knowledge of these, he is no physician at all. But to know these, he must first know the structure and functions of the system in health. Then he must know the nature of disease, and what abnormal conditions it will produce in the various organs ; what effect it will have on the vital functions, and what lesions will give rise to the complex and multiform manifestations of disease. Then he must know the nature and effect of his remedial agents, and how to select that one, or that course of medical treatment or regimen, which will best secure the remedial effect required. Without a good degree of this knowledge, no man ought to presume to administer as a physician. Nor can one attain it without time and labor. A *physician* cannot spring up in a night, like Jonah's gourd. A *quack* may ; but the fruit he will bear, will be apples of Sodom and clusters of Gomorrah. No man needs careful study more than the physician, and no man must more carefully employ his judgment and reason than he.

But the class to whom we refer, are wiser than all the physicians o learning—" yea, than seven men that can render a reason." Is a man sick ? they have a remedy for every symptom, and these are generally infallible : but if they are not, then they have enough in number to make up what they lack in power, and the patient must take the whole, because they *may* do him good. at least some of them. But of all forms of quackery, deliver us from this luck-and-chance, hap-hazard form. Thomsonism, and homœopathy, and hydropathy, and the whole class like them, have a " method in their madness." They admit some principles, and their position may be found. But this luck-and-chance quackery has no method in it, no truth at its foundation, and no consistency with itself.

It is these false notions, which make medical grannies of both sexes. It is this which starts the benevolent lady with her pills, or her syrups; or her homœopathic globules, on her round of visits to the sick, often leading her to set aside the prescription of the regular physician and fois hers in its place, to the great detriment of the patient. It is this which makes natural-born doctors, and root doctors, and seventh-son doctors " *et id omne genus.*" It is this which makes the *weaker* of our clerg interfere with the prescriptions of the physicians, that makes them elo quent in praise of the absurdities of homœopathy, or ready, like Behemoth, " to draw up a river into their mouth " in their zeal for hydropathy ; or affixes their names to the thousands of quack medicines, certifying to their efficacy in statements which a school boy in physiology would laugh at for the utter ignorance they displayed, and involving medical theories too absurd for any man to conceive, except him, who having a smattering of theology, therefore concludes himself a master of all the intricacies of medical science.* To the clergyman in his sacred capacity, I look with the most profound respect ; but to the clergyman as a medical quack, with the most unmixed contempt. Such men are ready to prescribe at once, when a skilful physician would hesitate long.

" Fools madly rush, where angels fear to tread."

But it by no means follows, that because they know something of theology, they know anything of medicine ; nor because they have a box of pills, or can make a syrup, that they are competent to treat disease ; nor even if they have heard of a medicine which is reputed to have cured a given disease, that they are under obligation to force it into the throat of every sick man they may see. These seem driven by a sort of necessity to interfere with the treatment of the sick, and not a few patients have lost their lives by this foolish interference.

[To be continued.]

THE BOSTON MEDICAL AND SURGICAL JOURNAL.

BOSTON, JULY 27, 1853.

Williams's Principles of Medicine.—The fourth edition, with additions, of the " Principles of Medicine, comprising General Pathology and Therapeutics, and a brief general view of Etiology, Nosology, Demeiology, Diagnosis, Prognosis and Hygienics," by Charles J. B. Williams, M.D., edited by Meredith Clymer, M.D., has just been published by Messrs. Blanchard & Lea. This new edition is as nearly true to the standard of medicine, as understood in these days of progression, as it could be made. Having, on former occasions, given our views of it, and having also often spoken of the praiseworthy efforts of the publishers in reproducing the most valuable medical works that appear in Europe, it is quite unnecessary to do more on this occasion than to present a brief synopsis of the contents of Dr. Wil-

* The value of certificates to the efficacy of patent medicines, even when honestly given, may be estimated from a circumstance which occurred while the author was in the office of the late Dr. A. G. Welch, of Lee, Mass. A farmer, of general intelligence and acknowledged probity, came to the office, from the town of Tyringham, where Dr. W. had formerly practised, and asked if he could give him some more of the pills, such as he gave him in 1814. Dr. W. had no recollection of giving him any, but remembered being in attendance on his family for the spotted fever. "Well," said the man, " I was sick then, and you gave me some pills which cured me right up, and have kept me well ever since!" This was in 1848. The man would have sworn to that statement of the efficacy of some common cathartic pills !

In 1850, I saw a published certificate, by a young lady, of a complete cure of consumption by a Dr. Fitch, of New York. Four months after it was given, I acted as a pall-bearer to assist in laying her in the grave—a victim to that fell destroyer. She was the last of eight of his patients whom he had cured, or promised to cure, that I had seen laid in the grave within a year !

liams's work, which is a well printed octavo, of 476 pages, in seven elaborate chapters, besides an appendix. A preliminary discourse on the principles of medicine, is followed by a philosophical dissertation on *etiology*, or the causes of disease. Chapter II., pathology; III., proximate elements of disease; IV., structural diseases; V., classification, symptoms and distinction of disease; VI., prognosis—foreknowledge, or results of disease. Nothing has escaped the indefatigable author, in the particular line of his investigations, and the work is therefore a full, perfect treatise, abounding in useful matter, which should be familiar to every medical practitioner.

Diseases of the Liver.—The fact that a single organ may be subject to a catalogue of diseases, the description and treatment of which fills a tome of 468 pages, octavo, impresses the student with the frailty of humanity in its physical organization. Of the functions and importance of the liver, in all animals, no new evidence is needed. If it is impaired in any respect, the whole system must suffer, and life be jeopardized by obscure internal derangements, which it is the appropriate business of the pathologist to investigate. Messrs. Blanchard & Lea, of Philadelphia, have favored us with a specimen copy of the second edition of *Diseases of the Liver*, by George Budd, M.D., from the last improved London edition, with colored plates and wood cuts—the plates on copper beautifully colored. Gall stones, abscesses, encysted tumors, &c., are minutely portrayed. There are five chapters, embracing every shade of disease which has been detected in this viscus. As a whole, it is probably the most complete work extant on the subject. When it first appeared in this country, a hearty commendation was given it by the medical press. With the emendations and additions which have been given to the new edition, it stands without a competitor. The second chapter, on inflammation of the liver, is worth the price asked for the whole work.

Belmont Med. Society Transactions.—This is from an Ohio institution, which from the day of its organization has been distinguished for energy and progress. There are no sleeping members in it. Their labors in 1852 and '53, presented in this report by the society, are creditable to their industry. An essay on ethics, by Dr. R. Hamilton, of Morristown, is a good article. Another, by Dr. John G. Affleck, of Bridgport, abounds with historical memoranda, terse sentiments, sound common sense and profound philosophical deductions. No wonder the medical meetings of the society are well sustained, while such men write and speak. They would give vitality to any kind of association. "Why are medical meetings so intolerably dull?" is a question not unfrequently propounded. One reason may be found in the determination of a combined few, to make the association an instrumentality for promoting selfish ends. In the second place, those the least qualified to open their mouths, generally fancy themselves oracles of wisdom, and therefore engross all the time. Modest men soon discover the direction which things are taking, and stay away. If a society does not die at once, under such leaden pressure, it dies gradually. But when gentlemen are permitted by the hunkers to infuse a little originality, intermingled with vivacity, there is a hope of life and the accomplishment of something for the advancement of science. In respect to the qualities, both social and professional, which insure longevity and honorable mention at home and abroad, the Belmont Medical Society is a model one.

Dr. Sweetser's Valedictory.—These leave-taking discourses are by no means the melancholy sermons a stranger to our medical college system might suppose. Nobody weeps on account of the pathos of the discourse, or swoons when the orator assures a class of graduates that this last public act severs their connection forever with the faculty. But the opportunity is rather embraced as a fitting occasion for impressing the minds of the graduate with a sense of their obligations to God and society. We like the custom, and trust it will be kept up in all coming time. At the Castleton (Vt.) Medical College, William Sweetser, M.D., who sustains the chair of theory and practice, and who is an author of celebrity, recently addressed those who had finished their educational course. His duty was well performed. Without being heavy, and therefore tedious, the discourse was happy in several respects, and is characterized by dignity and truth.

Causes and Prevention of Suits for Mal-practice.—A report to the Mass. Medical Society, on the foregoing subject, has come to us in a separate form, detached from the documents containing the transactions of the society. After reading the ten pages, we defy any one to determine, from the directions therein contained, how to stop a lawsuit. Were a treatise written upon the subject of preventing a house from burning, it would be no more ridiculous. A bucket of water would be worth more than the book. So in reference to preventing lawsuits for mal-practice: refusing to give one's services to people who are disposed to prosecute their professional adviser in order to cheat him out of a bill, or obtain money for miscalled damages, is the shortest way of keeping out of the difficulty.

Harvard Natural History Society.—At the University, Cambridge, Mass., the under graduates sustain a Natural History Society. An annual address is usually given by some person distinguished for attainments in the branches of knowledge cultivated by the members, which in May of the present year, was delivered by the Rev. Thomas Hill, of Waltham. This Journal is not precisely a proper medium for discussing the merits of the the learned gentleman's effort. We shall take the responsibility, however, of departing from the ordinary course, far enough to express our gratification with the performance. Some parts of it are really excellent. The author, who can discourse thus, possesses no ordinary mind. In the Society referred to there are, no doubt, many naturalists in the germ. Age and experience will enable them, at seasonable periods, to render to the world an account of their stewardship.

New Hampshire Asylum for the Insane.—A report of the institution, embracing an account of its condition in 1852 and 53, by John E. Tyler, M.D., the Superintendent, brought down to June last, must be very satisfactory to the people of New Hampshire. There is no flourish of trumpets, but a simple business-like account of what has been done in respect to the inmates, and a statement of the financial condition of the charity.

On the 31st of May there were 70 males and 73 females remaining under treatment. Ill health, domestic troubles, disappointments, excesses and masturbation, are among the prominent causes of their insanity. Of the eleven counties comprising the State, Merrimack, Hillsborough, Rockingham and Grafton furnish the largest number of lunatics. Merrimack takes the lead among them all. What moral causes are operating in that particular section, to lead to madness, is open for investigation. The whole number of patients since 1843, the year when they were first received, has been 1059. Dr. Tyler very properly suggests several improvements in the household—such as a decent cooking apparatus, furnaces that will not smoke, more cheerful halls, gas lights, &c., which the Trustees ought to provide at once. Dr. Tyler appears, by this official document, to be a systematic, prudent, philosophical man, who comprehends the duties of his position.

Dr. Warren's Address.—For some years past, Dr. John C. Warren has been President of the Society of Natural History in Boston. He engages in the labors of the members in a manner most encouraging to the young, advantageous to the interests of science, and honorable to himself. The address to which this paragraph refers, was written for the occasion of the anniversary meeting in May. It gives a condensed history of the Transactions of a body of learned men, who are unobtrusively advancing our acquaintance with all the kingdoms of nature. Dr. Warren has no competitor in industry: early and late, from youth to age, he has never relaxed from one uninterrupted course of elevated study. This is the highway to influence and distinction among men. With so many examples of the personal happiness resulting from a life of literary and scientific diligence, aside from the eminence which invariably pertains to it, how unfortunate for the world that multitudes of minds are wasted on frivolous pursuits, which neither benefit themselves nor contribute to the common store-house of knowledge.

St. Louis University.—From the prospectus of the medical department of this institution, it is certain that a strong faculty has been organized. John B. Johnson, M.D., late of the University of Missouri, has been elected to the chair of clinical medicine and pathological anatomy. He is a New England man, armed with indomitable energy, and eminently qualified to give a brilliant course of lectures. Dr. Pope, the surgeon, whom not to know, argues one's self unknown, has a reputation that must give eclat to any school. Thirty-three students were graduated in medicine in March. The elements of thrift and progress are perceptible in this College.

Dr. Dwight Nims has received the appointment of Postmaster at Homer, N. Y.—Mr. Wilson, of Flushing, L. I., has recently recovered a verdict of $2,500 in the King's County Circuit Court, against a Dr. Snell for malpractice in treating the arm of the plaintiff's son, which was fractured at the elbow by a fall.—The human voice has been heard across the Straits of Gibraltar, a distance of ten miles. This only happens in peculiar states of the weather. The sound of a military band has been heard seventy miles on a clear frosty morning.

Medical School of Harvard University.—The following gentlemen have received the Degree of Doctor of Medicine since the semi-annual examination in March :—

Horace Walter Adams, A.B., Harvard. *Absorption.*

Zabdiel Boylston Adams, A.B., Bowdoin. *Muscæ volitantes.*

Samuel Coleman Blake. *Dyspepsia.*

Algernon Coolidge. *Pulmonary emphysema.*

Edward Brooks Everett, A.B., Harvard. *Sprains.*

John Henry Gilbert. *Pericarditis.*

Joseph Clay Habersham. *Morbid appearances of the Countenance.*

John Alonzo Sidney Hannity.   St. Mary's College, Dublin. *Liver, its diseases and their treatment.*

William Henry Heath. *Opium.*

William Nourse Lane. *Caries of the vertebræ.*

William Hussey Page. *Typhoid Fever.*

Joaquim Antonio Alves Ribeiro. *Hygiene.*

Nathan Payson Rice, A.B., Harvard. *Foreign bodies in the air-passages.*

Horatio Robinson Storer, A.B., Harvard. *Florula Cantabrigiensis medica.*

Jerome Charles Street. *On the Surgical treatment of obstructions that affect mucous canals.*

John Ware, jr., A.B., Harvard. *Some of the principal diseases of the teeth, and the operations for their removal.*

Richard Henry Wheatland, A.B., Harvard. *Diabetes.*

John Samuel Whiting, A.B., Harvard. *Typhus Fever; in what respects it differs from Typhoid Fever.*   J. B. S. JACKSON,
Dean of the Medical Faculty.

To CORRESPONDENTS.—The following communications have been received, and will be published in turn as expeditiously as space will admit :—Water and Alcohol contrasted on the People proper : Disuse of Pork among the Shakers ; Additional Muscle of the Eye ; Hysteria ; Natural and Artificial Induction of Hæmatosis ; Improvements in Medical Practice ; Southern Typhoid Fever ; and the concluding portions of articles already commenced. The verses by N. are inadmissible.

MARRIED,—At Woonsocket, R. I., on the 12th inst., Dr. J. Samuel Bassett, of Paterson, N. J., to Caroline Augusta Bissell.

DIED —At Wallingford, Vt , John Fox, M D , 71, an eminent physician, and one of the oldest practitioners of the State — At Louisville, Kentucky, Charles Caldwell, M.D., said to have been the oldest physician in the United States. He was a pupil of Dr. Rush. For a series of years Dr. Caldwell has been distinguished for his general learning and profound attainments in medical science. A memoir of his life will unquestionably soon appear.—At Chicago, Illinois, Dr Beselin, a German practitioner, accomplished and well esteemed. He presented a bill for attendance on a lady ; but instead of being paid, he was arrested for taking liberties with the patient—which so mortified him, that he shot himself—By suicide at the west, Dr. John G. Bird —At Frankfort, Me , Dr. Edward Abbott, 70 —At Columbia, Dr. H. D Jones, formerly of Conn., 23.—By suicide, in Virginia, Dr. D. W. Petrie, late of Oswego, N. Y —In Buffalo, N Y., Dr. Joseph Peabody, from Norwich, Conn., 59—In Burlington, Vt., July 5th, Ashbel S. Pitkin, M D., aged 44.

Deaths in Boston for the week ending Saturday noon, July 23d, 92. Males, 50—females, 42. Accidental, 2—inflammation of the bowels, 6—inflammation of the brain, 1—disease of the brain, 4—consumption, 19—convulsions, 3—cholera infantum, 8—cholera morbus, 3—croup, 4—dysentery, 3—diarrhœa, 1—dropsy, 1—dropsy in the head, 3—infantile diseases, 8—scarlet fever, 2 —hooping cough, 1—disease of the heart, 3—intemperance, 1—inflammation of the lungs, 4— disease of the liver, 1—marasmus, 3—measles, 2—old age, 1—palsy, 2—smallpox, 1—teething, 5—unknown, 1.

Under 5 years, 53—between 5 and 20 years, 7—between 20 and 40 years, 15—between 40 and 60 years, 9—over 60 years, 8. Born in the United States, 66—Ireland, 18—England, 4—British Provinces, 1—Scotland, 1—Germany, 2. The above includes 5 deaths at the City institutions.

Patients who never pay —The True Flag relates the following story, how a physician got rid of a patient who never paid a bill.—" Hum ! So you don't feel any better after the pill and draught, eh ? That's bad ! We must try a more energetic course of remedies, then. Come in this afternoon, and we'll take fifteen ounces of blood from you, put a blister on the pit of your stomach, a mustard plaster on your back, then electrify you, shave your head, and administer a dose of calomel. That may prove efficacious." The patient kept away.

Sulphate of Quinidin.—Dr. Thomas Humphreys, of Birmingham, writes as follows to the Editor of the London Lancet.

Allow me through the medium of your valuable journal, to inform medical men that an article called sulphate of *quinidin* is being extensively substituted for sulphate of quinine. Trommer's test, as given below, will easily detect this unwarrantable substitution. I would just observe that sulphate of quinidin is worth about 5s. 6d. per ounce, and sulphate of quinine about 10s. per ounce.

" *Trommer's Test.*—The solubility of quinidin in ether, compared with that of quinine, is but slight ; ten grains of pure sulphate of quinine dissolves in sixty drops of ether and twenty drops of spirit of ammonia, while only *one grain* of sulphate of quinidin is soluble in the same quantity of fluid ; and in proportion quinine containing quinidin will always be less soluble than pure sulphate of quinine.

Medical Miscellany.—Cases of cholera occasionally appear in southern ports.—Dr. Alfred Crare, of San Francisco, late Alexandria, Va., was shot in a duel and died soon after. He was the challenger—his age 25. —Yellow fever is destructive at Carthagena.—Dr. Daniel Asbury, of Charlotte, N. C., has written encouragingly on the gold mining prospects of that State. He says that the Gold Hill Mine has yielded $1.500.000 since 1843.—The Female Medical College of Pennsylvania has just conferred the title of M.D. on Miss Charlotte G. Adams, of Boston, and eight other ladies.—A woman who was born at Lyons in 1713, died on the 15th of May, at the age of 140 years. Two years more would have carried her to the age of the Countess of Desmond, who died in Ireland at 142.—Edward Cranson, the Kentish giant, said to be the largest boned man in Europe, measures 7 feet 6 inches, weighs 35 stone, can reach perpendicularly 10 feet 6 inches, and is under 21 years of age.—Smallpox has been destroying the Cheyenne and Snake Indians, near Utah, the Mormon city, to a dreadful extent. On one occasion they piled up the bodies of three hundred victims to the malady, and burned them.—-Dr. Thomas Harris, chief clerk of the Naval Bureau of Medicine and Surgery, has been discharged.—Yellow fever, in its worst form, is raging at St. Thomas. Several cases have also appeared at New Orleans.—-Dr. P. W. Leland, of Fall River, Mass., has been appointed Collector of that port.—Dr. N. G. Trow, of Sunderland, Mass., is president of a musical convention.—Dr. J. B. Bartlett, of Somerville, Mass., has been elected president of the Mystic Corporation.—Andrew M'Farland, M.D., late medical superintendent of the N. H. Asylum for the Insane, is the author of an essay on *draining and subsoil* ploughing, which took a prize of the State Agricultural Society.—M. M. Rogers, M.D., is the author of a work on scientific agriculture.

Lightning Source UK Ltd.
Milton Keynes UK
UKHW021631081118
331957UK00011B/1361/P